Medical Terminology

A Programmed Learning Approach
to the Language of Health Care

Second Edition

Medical Terminology

A Programmed Learning Approach to the Language of Health Care

Second Edition

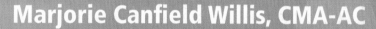

Marjorie Canfield Willis, CMA-AC

Program Director
Medical Assisting/Medical Transcription Programs
Orange Coast College
Costa Mesa, California

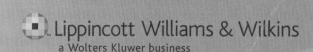

. Lippincott Williams & Wilkins
a Wolters Kluwer business
Philadelphia · Baltimore · New York · London
Buenos Aires · Hong Kong · Sydney · Tokyo

Acquisitions Editor: Julie K. Stegman
Senior Managing Editor: Heather A. Rybacki
Managing Editor: Linda Francis
Marketing Manager: Hilary Henderson
Manufacturing Coordinator: Margie Orzech
Designer: Risa Clow
Compositor: Aptara, Inc.
Printer: RR Donnelley

Lippincott Williams & Wilkins
351 West Camden Street
Baltimore, MD 21201

530 Walnut St.
Philadelphia, PA 19106

DISCLAIMER

Care has been taken to confirm the accuracy of the information presented and to describe generally accepted practices. However, the authors, editors, and publisher are not responsible for errors or omissions or for any consequences from application of the information in this book and make no warranty, expressed or implied, with respect to the currency, completeness, or accuracy of the contents of the publication. Application of this information in a particular situation remains the professional responsibility of the practitioner; the clinical treatments described and recommended may not be considered absolute and universal recommendations.

Printed in China

First Edition, 2002

Library of Congress Cataloging-in-Publication Data

Willis, Marjorie Canfield.
   Medical terminology : a programmed learning approach to the language of health care / Marjorie Canfield Willis. – 2nd ed.
      p. cm.
   Includes index.
   ISBN-13: 978-0-7817-9283-7
   1. Medicine–Terminology. I. Title.
   R123.W4758 2007
   610.1'4–dc22

                          2007004818

The publishers have made every effort to trace the copyright holders for borrowed material. If they have inadvertently overlooked any, they will be pleased to make the necessary arrangements at the first opportunity.

To purchase additional copies of this book, call our customer service department at **(800) 638-3030** or fax orders to **(301) 223-2400**. International customers should call **(301) 223-2300**.

Visit Lippincott Williams & Wilkins on the Internet: http://www.LWW.com. Lippincott Williams & Wilkins customer service representatives are available from 8:30 am to 5:00 pm, EST.

8 9 10 11 12

RRS1306

Dedicated to the memory of

Dell A. Canfield,

my father, my inspiration

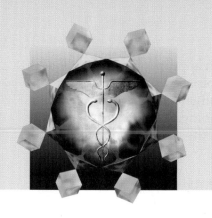

Preface to the Student

SUMMARY OF OBJECTIVES

Upon completion of this text, you will be able to:

⚜ Describe the origin of medical language.

⚜ Analyze the component parts of a medical term and use basic prefixes, suffixes, and combining forms to build medical terms.

⚜ Explain the common rules for proper medical term formation, pronunciation, and spelling of medical terms.

⚜ Define basic terms and abbreviations used in documenting health records.

⚜ Identify common pharmaceutical terms and abbreviations used in documenting medical records.

⚜ Identify the common forms used in documenting the care of a patient.

⚜ Identify common anatomical terms related to the major systems of the body.

⚜ Identify common terms related to symptoms, diagnoses, surgeries, therapies, and diagnostic tests related to the major systems of the body.

⚜ Explain common terms and abbreviations used in documenting medical records related to the major systems of the body.

GETTING STARTED

Goals and Planning

To reach the goal of learning the language of health care, you'll need a reasonable plan for completion. Follow the study path that this text and/or your instructor provides, and work the necessary study time into your personal schedule.

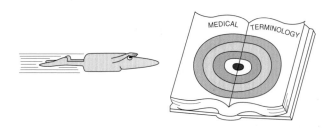

Organizing the Starter Set of Flash Cards

A "starter set" of common prefixes, suffixes, and a selected number of combining forms are provided on flash cards at the back of the text. These cards are a base on which to build, and you should review them often. Each component in the starter set is numbered and colors coded according to division: prefixes are printed on peach cards, **combining forms** appear on **purple cards**, and suffixes are found on green cards. The term component is printed on the front of the card, and its meaning, including a term example, is on the back. Reinforce your learning by drawing lines to separate the components in each of the term examples, and write definitions for each in the margins.

Using a punch, put a hole in the top of each flash card. Loop each card through a key chain or ring holder to make a "rotary file." This method keeps groups of cards together and prevents them from becoming lost or scattered. Within this file, group together associated cards for components related to color, size, position, direction, and so on.

Making Additional Flash Cards

It is highly recommended that you make flash cards for all of the additional term components introduced in each body system chapter. You can even extend the use of the flash cards to include abbreviations, symbols, and terms found throughout the text. The act of writing out your own cards gives you an added memory boost.

To create additional flash cards, you can follow the example of the cards provided in the starter set (using 3 × 5″ cards). If your stack of flash cards becomes large and cumbersome, you may want to try the **frugal flash card** method illustrated below, so named because it consolidates paper and is inexpensive.

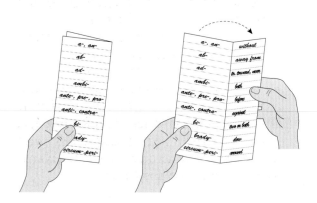

To create frugal flash cards:
1. Fold a piece of 8½ × 11″ lined paper in half lengthwise, creating two columns.
2. Write the word component, symbol, or term on the first line of the first column, and write its definition on the **same** line in the second column.
3. Skip a line and write the next word component, symbol, or term, and write its definition on the **same** line in the second column.
4. Continue listing terms with their corresponding definitions until you reach the bottom of the paper.
5. Fold the paper at the lengthwise crease so that the word component, symbol, or term is listed on one side of the paper and the definition appears on the other side of the paper. This allows you to flip from one side to the other, "flashing" and reinforcing the meanings of the terms. Use the other side of the paper in the same way.

Snatching Moments!

Carry your flash cards with you at all times. During most days, there are times when you can snatch a moment to use your flash cards. You will feel less stress when waiting in a line or for an appointment if you know that you can use that time for studying.

STUDY TIPS

Using Your Senses

An effective memory depends on intricate processes that recall mental images of sights, sounds, feelings, tastes, and smells. For this reason, try to include as many senses as possible in the process of reinforcing learning.

SEE IT	Employ your visual sense (sight) by making and repeatedly reviewing your flash cards.
SAY IT	Pronounce each component out loud three times as you flash each card to reinforce your auditory sense (hearing).
WRITE IT	Write and rewrite responses to programmed review sections before highlighting the correct answers. Make flash cards by hand using pleasant colored paper and ink to satisfy your kinesthetic sense (feeling).

Mnemonics Can Help

Mnemonics, referring to any device for aiding memory, is named for the goddess of memory in Greek mythology. Mnemonic techniques link things to be remembered with clues for their recall using the stimulus of images, sounds, smell, touch, etc. Consider the following applications:

- Make up rhymes or stories that help to differentiate between meanings. For example: *peri-*, the prefix meaning "around," is often confused with *para-*, the prefix meaning "along side of." Use the two components in a sentence to compare their meanings; for example, I sat *para* (**alongside of**) Sarah on the merry-*peri*-go-**around**. Often the most absurd associations can help you to remember. It doesn't matter if they don't make sense to anyone but you!
- Make up songs and rhythms to help remember facts. Take a song you are familiar with like "Row, row, row, your boat . . ." and insert words with definitions that are in tune with the song.
- Draw pictures depicting term components for reinforcement.

Memory Drill

Give yourself a memory drill by listing word components, symbols, or terms on one side of a paper and then filling in the definitions from memory. Write corrections in red ink. Make a list of the incorrectly defined components on a separate paper, and complete the drill again. Repeat this process until you have identified which terms you most frequently get incorrect. Spend additional time studying those troublesome terms.

ADDITIONAL RESOURCES

Take advantage of the many fun and interactive learning activities provided on the **CD-ROM** included with this text. You'll find a variety of exercises to help you remember medical terminology and to reinforce what you've learned in the text, including:

- **Exercises by Chapter** – unscored exercises allow you to choose the types of activities that best suit your learning style, including:
  - *multiple choice, fill-in-the-blank*, and *true/false* questions to support learning
  - *figure-labeling* exercises to reinforce your knowledge of both medical terms and basic anatomy
  - *matching games* in which you match combining forms or terms with definitions
  - *spelling bee* to help you recognize and correctly spell medical terms
  - *case studies* that use actual medical records so you can apply your learning to real-world examples
- **Review or Test Mode** – study a single chapter or multiple chapters in a Review or Test environment to test your knowledge; question types are randomized and include multiple choice, fill-in-the-blank, true/false, and spelling bee

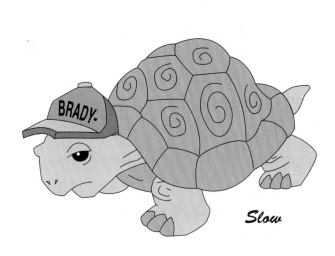

Slow

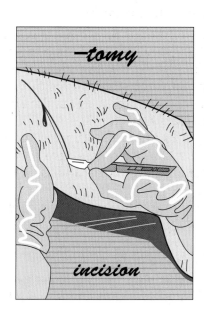

-tomy

incision

- **Pronunciation Drill** – audio pronunciations organized both A-to-Z and by chapter; select individual terms to hear the pronunciation, or "play all" terms from a chapter sequentially
- **Dictionary** – electronic glossary of all key terms from the book organized both A-to-Z and by chapter; definitions provided by *Stedman's*
- **Flash Cards** – interactive flash cards that can be reviewed electronically

- **Answers to Medical Records For Additional Study** questions

READY, SET, GO!

Everything is laid out for you to proceed with your study. The techniques employed here have proven beneficial in learning and are geared toward efficient memorization. Be creative and enjoy the learning process!

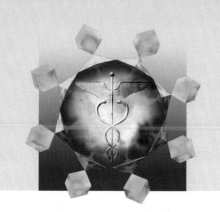

Preface to the Instructor

The second edition of *Medical Terminology: A Programmed Learning Approach to the Language of Health Care* provides a sequential, programmed process for learning medical language that is intended to meet the needs of students working independently or within a classroom. The approach is self-directed. Learning segments are presented in self-study increments followed by programmed review frames for immediate feedback and reinforcement. Diagrams, illustrations, and term tips support learning segments, and practice exercises at the end of each chapter provide additional reinforcement. Learning builds from an understanding of the origin of medical terms and basic term construction, to the comprehension of more difficult terms and concepts encountered in relation to the body systems and medical specialty areas. The process culminates in applying the knowledge to understanding selected medical records.

TEXT OVERVIEW

The first two chapters deliver the basics for understanding the language of health care. Chapter 1 introduces basic term components (prefixes, suffixes, and a selected number of combining forms) and shows how these structures are combined to form medical terms. Rules of pronunciation, spelling, and formation of singular and plural forms are included. Medical word components introduced in this chapter are used repeatedly throughout the text. They are included in the starter set of flash cards for medical term components in the back of the text. Chapter 2 explains how medical terms will be learned and reinforced throughout the text using health records. Common forms, formats, abbreviations, symbols, and methods of documenting patient care are introduced. This helps students understand basic communication between professionals, including physician/provider orders and prescriptions. This chapter prepares students for medical record analyses in succeeding chapters.

Chapters 3 through 15 cover terms related to body systems. Additional combining forms are introduced along with terms related to symptoms, diagnoses, tests, procedures, surgeries, and therapies. After mastering the programmed portions and review exercises, completion of medical record analyses provides further reinforcement of learning through application of knowledge.

The Student CD-ROM included with the text contains additional activities to reinforce learning. The Exercises by Chapter module presents a variety of activities, including multiple choice, true/false, figure-labeling, fill-in-the-blank questions, spelling bees, and matching games, so the student may choose those that that best match his or her learning style. The Review or Test Modes option allows the student to simulate a true testing environment, and allows them to study a single chapter at a time or to study content from multiple chapters. Other activities include a pronunciation drill with 2,000 terms (organized both alphabetically and by chapter), a glossary of terms from *Stedman's Medical Dictionary*, electronic flash cards, and answers to the Medical Record Analyses: For Additional Study included in the text.

NEW TO THIS EDITION

- Chapter Checklists at the beginning of each chapter outline learning tasks related to the text and accompanying CD

- Summary of Chapter Abbreviations and Acronyms at the end of each chapter
- Summary of Chapter Terms with pronunciations and page references at the end of each chapter
- New and revised photographs illustrating pathologies and the latest health care technology
- Addition and clarification of pertinent terms throughout the text
- Expanded programmed review sections
- Addition of up-to-the-minute information regarding medical abbreviations and symbols that are deemed to be error prone and dangerous

SPECIAL FEATURES

- A Student CD-ROM with a variety of learning activities to reinforce understanding
- An online Faculty Resource Center for instructors at **thepoint.lww.com**, with PowerPoint slides, a ready-made testbank, and additional activities and ideas for use in the classroom
- A starter set of common medical term components on flash cards
- Self-study instructional increments followed by programmed reinforcement
- A unique health record orientation in Chapter 2
- Medical Record Analyses at the end of each body system chapter
- Relevant, full-color illustrations
- Practice Exercises for each chapter to meet all learning styles and needs
- Anatomy review with labeling exercises
- Term Tips related to spelling, common pitfalls, and more
- Three valuable appendices, including:
  - a glossary of medical term components (prefixes, suffixes, and combining forms)

listed both from term component to English definition and from English definition to term component
  - a glossary of medical abbreviations and symbols
  - commonly prescribed drugs, including therapeutic classifications

INSTRUCTOR RESOURCE CENTER AT thePOINT

Visit thePoint at **http://thepoint.lww.com/ WillisProgrammed2e** to access resources designed specifically to help instructors teach more effectively and save time. There you'll find:

- *Instructor's test generator* with more than 500 questions, encompassing individual chapter tests and a comprehensive exam
- *PowerPoint slides* for each chapter organized by learning objectives
- *Lesson plans* for each chapter
- *Sample course schedules*
- *Body system overviews*
- *Suggestions for classroom enhancement*
- Our unique *LiveAdvise tutoring service*
- *Image bank*
- Customized course content for use with your *learning management system*, such as **thePoint LMS** (LWW's exclusive learning management system), **WebCT**, or **Blackboard**
- and more!

A solid understanding of medical terminology provides an essential foundation for any career in health care. The *Medical Terminology: A Programmed Learning Approach to the Language of Health Care, 2nd Edition*, product suite makes learning and teaching medical terminology a rewarding and exciting process.

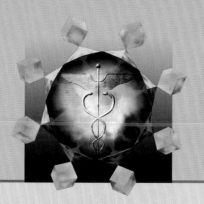

User's Guide

Medical Terminology: A Programmed Learning Approach to the Language of Health Care, Second Edition, is not just a textbook – it is a complete learning resource that will help you understand and master medical terminology. To achieve this, the author and publisher have included tools throughout the text to help you work through the material presented. Please take a few moments to look through this User's Guide to familiarize yourself with the features that will enhance your learning experience.

INTRODUCTORY CHAPTERS

The first two chapters set the stage for learning throughout the text. Chapter 1 provides analysis of **basic term components and rules** for forming, spelling, and pronouncing medical terms.

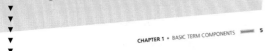

Self-Instruction: Rules for Constructing Terms

Study the following:

COMBINING FORM	MEANING	FLASH CARD ID#
angi/o, vas/o, vascul/o	vessel	CF-5
cardi/o	heart	CF-8
enter/o	small intestine	CF-15
esophag/o	esophagus	CF-17
gastr/o	stomach	CF-20
hem/o, hemat/o	blood	CF-23
hepat/o	liver	CF-24
oste/o	bone	CF-40
ur/o, urin/o	urine	CF-56

SUFFIX	MEANING	FLASH CARD ID#
-al, -eal	pertaining to	S-1
-ectasis	expansion or dilation	S-8
-ectomy	excision (removal)	S-9
-ia	condition of	S-13
-itis	inflammation	S-17
-logy	study of	S-19
-megaly	enlargement	S-22
-stomy	creation of an opening	S-40
-tomy	incision	S-41

PREFIX	MEANING	FLASH CARD ID#
oligo-	few or deficient	P-28
para-	alongside of, abnormal	P-30
peri-	around	P-8

Once you understand the basics of constructing medical terms, the next steps are to memorize common term components and to learn the rules for joining medical term components correctly. Study the following five basic rules, and use them to construct words using the components provided in the *Rules for Constructing Terms* Self Instruction box above.

Programmed Review: Five Basic Rules for Constructing Terms

ANSWERS	REVIEW
	1.13 A combining vowel is used to join root to root as well as root to any suffix beginning with a consonant (any letter except a, e, i, o, or u): *hepat/o* + *-megaly* is spelled hepatomegaly
enlargement of the liver	and is defined as _____

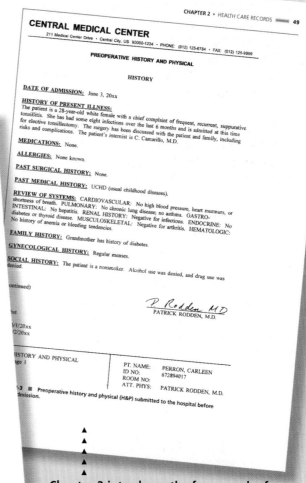

CENTRAL MEDICAL CENTER
211 Medical Center Drive • Central City, US 90000-1234 • PHONE: (012) 125-6784 • FAX: (012) 125-9999

PREOPERATIVE HISTORY AND PHYSICAL

HISTORY

DATE OF ADMISSION: June 3, 20xx

HISTORY OF PRESENT ILLNESS:
The patient is a 28-year-old white female with a chief complaint of frequent, recurrent, suppurative tonsillitis. She has had some eight infections over the last 6 months and is admitted at this time for elective tonsillectomy. The surgery has been discussed with the patient and family, including risks and complications. The patient's internist is C. Camarillo, M.D.

MEDICATIONS: None.

ALLERGIES: None known.

PAST SURGICAL HISTORY: None.

PAST MEDICAL HISTORY: UCHD (usual childhood diseases).

REVIEW OF SYSTEMS: CARDIOVASCULAR: No high blood pressure, heart murmurs, or shortness of breath. PULMONARY: No chronic lung disease; no asthma. GASTRO-INTESTINAL: No hepatitis. RENAL HISTORY: Negative for infections. ENDOCRINE: No diabetes or thyroid disease. MUSCULOSKELETAL: Negative for arthritis. HEMATOLOGIC: No history of anemia or bleeding tendencies.

FAMILY HISTORY: Grandmother has history of diabetes.

GYNECOLOGICAL HISTORY: Regular menses.

SOCIAL HISTORY: The patient is a nonsmoker. Alcohol use was denied, and drug use was denied.

(continued)

P. Rodden, M.D.
PATRICK RODDEN, M.D.

...1/20xx
...2/20xx

HISTORY AND PHYSICAL
...age 1

...-3 ■ Preoperative history and physical (H&P) submitted to the hospital before ...dmission.

PT. NAME:	PERRON, CARLEEN
ID NO:	672894017
ROOM NO:	
ATT. PHYS:	PATRICK RODDEN, M.D.

Chapter 2 introduces the framework of **health care documents** so that real-life medical records can be used to reinforce the understanding of terms presented in the subsequent body system chapters.

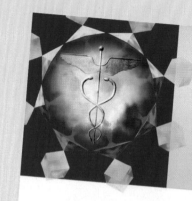

CHAPTER

5

Cardiovascular System

CHAPTER CHECKLIST

Use the chapter checklists at the beginning of each chapter to orient you to the materials and to help you set learning goals.

▶ ▶ ▶ ▶

✓ Chapter 5 Checklist

	LOCATION
☐ Read Chapter 5: Cardiovascular System and complete all programmed review segments.	pages 207-250
☐ Review the starter set of flash cards and term components related to Chapter 5.	back of book
☐ Complete the Chapter 5 Practice Exercises and Medical Record Analysis 5-1.	
☐ Complete Medical Record Analysis 5-2 For Additional Study.	pages 256-262
☐ Complete the Chapter 5 Exercises by Chapter.	pages 263-264
☐ Complete the Chapter 5 Review and Test Modes.	CD-ROM 💿
☐ Review the Pronunciation Drill for the Chapter 5 terms.	CD-ROM 💿
	CD-ROM 💿

BODY SYSTEM OVERVIEW

Chapters 3 through 15 open with a **body system overview**. The overview establishes a basis for each chapter, introducing the body system and laying the foundation for your work.

▶ ▶ ▶ ▶

CARDIOVASCULAR SYSTEM OVERVIEW

The cardiovascular system consists of the heart (Fig. 5-1) and blood vessels, which work together to transport blood throughout the body.

🔴 The heart is a muscular organ that pumps blood throughout the body.

🔴 The heart consists of four chambers: the **right atrium** and **left atrium** (upper chambers), and the **right ventricle** and **left ventricle** (lower chambers).

🔴 The heart is divided into right and left portions by the **interatrial septum** and the **interventricular septum**.

🔴 Heart valves open and close to maintain the one-way flow of blood through the heart.

🔴 The heart has three layers: the **endocardium**, which lines the interior cavities of the heart; the [myocar]dium, which is the thick, muscular layer; and the **epicardium**, which is the outer [ ] [s]ac.

[ ] the heart is a loose, protective sac called the **pericardium**.

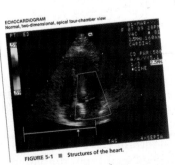

STRUCTURES OF THE HEART (arrows indicate path of blood flow)

◀ ◀ ◀ ◀ ◀ Detailed illustrations present a visual overview of each body system being presented.

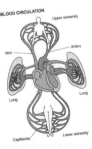

ECHOCARDIOGRAM
Normal, two-dimensional, apical four-chamber view

BLOOD CIRCULATION

FIGURE 5-1 ▬ Structures of the heart.

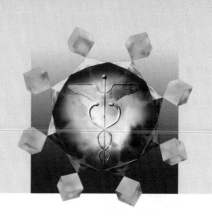

Contents

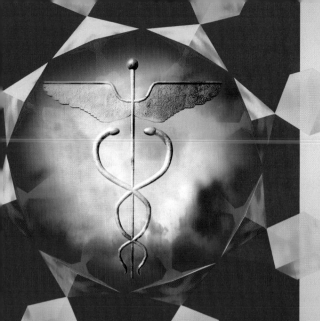

Basic Term Components

✓ Chapter 1 Checklist

	LOCATION
☐ Read Chapter 1: Basic Term Components and complete all programmed review segments.	pages 1-30
☐ Review the starter set of flash cards presenting term components.	back of book
☐ Complete the Chapter 1 Practice Exercises.	pages 31-37
☐ Complete the Chapter 1 Exercises by Chapter.	CD-ROM
☐ Complete the Chapter 1 Review and Test Modes.	CD-ROM
☐ Review the Pronunciation Drill for the Chapter 1 terms.	CD-ROM

INTRODUCTION

Most medical terms have Greek or Latin origins. These terms date back to the founding of modern medicine by the Greeks and the influence of Latin when it was the universal language in the Western world. Other languages, such as German and French, also have influenced medical terms. Many new terms are derived from English, which is considered to be the universal language today. Most of the terms related to diagnosis and surgery have Greek origin, and most anatomic terms come from Latin.

Once you understand the basic medical term structure and know the commonly used prefixes, suffixes, and combining forms, you can learn the meaning of most medical terms by analyzing their component parts. Those mysterious words, which are almost frightening at first glance, will soon seem commonplace. You will learn to analyze each term you encounter with your newfound knowledge and the help of a good medical dictionary.

This chapter includes the most common prefixes and suffixes and a selection of common combining forms. More combining forms and other pertinent prefixes and suffixes are added in following chapters as you learn terms related to specific body systems. This chapter also provides basic rules for proper medical term formation, pronunciation, and spelling.

START NOW

Remove the starter set of flash cards at the back of the text and organize them as recommended in the *Getting Started* section. Make the most of each moment of study time available to you. The key to success in building a medical vocabulary is memorizing the basic structures in this chapter.

How to Use Programmed Learning Segments

Take time to study the material in each self-instruction frame before starting a review segment. Key term components included in the flash card starter set are identified by letter and number. Locate and use them for additional reinforcement.

Remove the Reveal Card from the back cover of the text. Place the card over the left column of the page to hide the responses to the questions in the learning material in the right column. Slide the card down the page to reveal the answer only after you have written your response in the fill-in space on the right. Use a pencil so that you can quickly erase any inappropriate response and replace it with the correct one. Go over all the correct responses with a highlighter for additional reinforcement.

You can move at your own pace given the time allotted. Between study periods, use the Reveal Card as a bookmark.

TERM COMPONENTS

Study the flash cards for the term components listed below in preparation for the programmed review that follows.

 ## Self-Instruction: Term Components

Study the following:

TERM COMPONENT	CATEGORY	MEANING	FLASH CARD ID#
lip	root	fat	
lip/o	combining form	fat	CF-28
~emia	suffix	blood condition	S-10
hyper-	prefix	excessive	P-19
protein	root	protein	

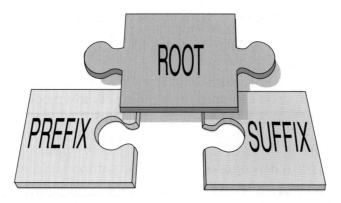

Most medical terms have three basic component parts: the root, the suffix, and the prefix. Each term is formed by combining at least one **root** (the foundation or subject of the word) and a **suffix**

(the word ending that modifies and gives essential meaning to the root). A **prefix** is placed at the beginning of a term only when needed to further modify the root or roots.

Programmed Review: Three Basic Components

ANSWERS	REVIEW
THE ROOT AND SUFFIX	
fat foundation or subject blood condition	**1.1** In the word lipemia, *lip* (meaning _____) is the root and _____ of the term. It is modified and given essential meaning by the suffix -*emia*, meaning _____ _____.
root, fat suffix, blood condition fat blood	**1.2** Breaking down and defining the key components in a term often defines the term or gives clues to its meaning. In the term lipemia, *lip* is the _____ that means _____, and -*emia* is the _____ that means _____ _____. Memorizing key medical term components makes it possible to decipher that the term refers to the condition of _____ in the _____. Note that lipemia is synonymous with lipidemia (formed from *lip, -oid,* and -*emia*).
THE PREFIX	
prefix beginning, modify excessive	**1.3** The prefix is a term component placed at the beginning of a term when needed to further modify the root or roots. For example, in the term hyperlipemia, *hyper-* is a _____ placed at the _____ of the term to further _____ the meaning of the term to denote _____ fat in the blood.
ADDITIONAL ROOTS	
root protein	**1.4** Often, a medical term is formed from two or more roots. For example, in the term hyperlipo**protein**emia, the addition of the _____ *protein* further defines the word to indicate an excessive amount of fat and _____ in the blood.

Combining Forms and Combining Vowels

When a medical term has more than one root, the roots are joined together by a vowel, usually an "o." As shown in hyper/lip/o/protein/emia, the "o" is used to link the two roots, and it provides easier pronunciation. This vowel is known as a **combining vowel.** "O" is the most common combining vowel ("i" is the second most common) and is used so frequently to join root to root or root to suffix that it is routinely attached to the root and presented as a **combining form.**

Programmed Review: Combining Forms and Combining Vowels

ANSWERS	REVIEW
root, combining form, o combining vowel i	**1.5** In *lip/o, lip* is the _____ and *lip/o* is the _____ _____ (a root with a combining vowel attached). The vowel ___ is the most common _____ _____ , and ___ is the second most common.

This text uses combining forms rather than roots for easier term analysis. Each is presented with a slash between the root and the combining vowel. Hyphens are placed after prefixes to indicate their placement at the beginning of a medical term, and hyphens are placed before suffixes to indicate their link at the end of a term.

 ## Programmed Review: Overview of Term Components

ANSWERS	REVIEW
root, suffix, prefix	**1.6** Most medical terms have three basic component parts: the _____, _____, and _____.
foundation or subject	**1.7** The root is the _____ of the term.
suffix	**1.8** The _____ is the word ending that modifies and gives essential meaning to the root.
prefix	**1.9** The _____ is the component at the beginning of a term that is used when needed to further modify the root.
two	**1.10** Often, a medical term is formed by _____ or more roots.
combining vowel, o	**1.11** When a medical term has more than one root, it is joined together by a _____ _____, usually an ___.
root, vowel	**1.12** A combining form is a _____ with a _____ attached.

Note that each component depends upon the other to express the meaning of the term. Few components can stand alone.

CONNECTING TERM COMPONENTS TO CONSTRUCT MEDICAL TERMS

Study the flash cards for the term components listed below in preparation for the instruction and review that follows.

Self-Instruction: Rules for Constructing Terms

Study the following:

COMBINING FORM	MEANING	FLASH CARD ID#
angi/o, vas/o, vascul/o	vessel	CF-5
cardi/o	heart	CF-8
enter/o	small intestine	CF-15
esophag/o	esophagus	CF-17
gastr/o	stomach	CF-20
hem/o, hemat/o	blood	CF-23
hepat/o	liver	CF-24
oste/o	bone	CF-40
ur/o, urin/o	urine	CF-56

SUFFIX	MEANING	FLASH CARD ID#
-al, -eal	pertaining to	S-1
-ectasis	expansion or dilation	S-8
-ectomy	excision (removal)	S-9
-ia	condition of	S-13
-itis	inflammation	S-17
-logy	study of	S-19
-megaly	enlargement	S-22
-stomy	creation of an opening	S-40
-tomy	incision	S-41

PREFIX	MEANING	FLASH CARD ID#
oligo-	few or deficient	P-28
para-	alongside of, abnormal	P-30
peri-	around	P-8

Once you understand the basics of constructing medical terms, the next steps are to memorize common term components and to learn the rules for joining medical term components correctly. Study the following five basic rules, and use them to construct words using the components provided in the *Rules for Constructing Terms* Self Instruction box above.

 ## Programmed Review: Five Basic Rules for Constructing Terms

ANSWERS	REVIEW
	1.13 A combining vowel is used to join root to root as well as root to any suffix beginning with a consonant (any letter *except* a, e, i, o, or u): *hepat/o* + *-megaly* is spelled hepatomegaly
enlargement of the liver	and is defined as _____.

ANSWERS	REVIEW
excision (removal) of a vessel	**1.14** A combining vowel is *not* used before a suffix that begins with a vowel: *vas/o* + *-ectomy* is spelled vasectomy and is defined as ___removal of a vessel___ _____.
inflammation of the heart	**1.15** If the root ends in a vowel and the suffix begins with the same vowel, drop the final vowel from the root and do *not* use a combining vowel: *cardi/o* + *-itis* is spelled carditis and is defined as ___inflammation of the heart___.
pertaining to the heart and esophagus	**1.16** Most often, a combining vowel is inserted between two roots even when the second root begins with a vowel: *cardi/o* + *esophag/o* + *-eal* is spelled cardioesophageal and is defined as ___pertaining to the heart and esophagus___ _____.
pertaining to alongside of the small intestine	**1.17** Occasionally, when a prefix ends in a vowel and the root begins with a vowel, the final vowel is dropped from the prefix: *para-* + *enter/o* + *-al* is spelled parenteral and is defined as ___pertaining to alongside of___ ___the small intestine___.

Note that all these rules have exceptions. Follow the basic guidelines set forth in this text, but be prepared to accept the exceptions as you encounter them. Rely upon your medical dictionary for additional guidance.

In the following review, construct words using the rules previously provided and give the meaning for each term.

Programmed Review: Putting the Rules into Practice

ANSWERS	REVIEW
angiectasis expansion or dilation of a vessel	**1.18** *angi/o* + *-ectasis* is spelled ___angiectasis___ and means ___dilation of a vessel___.
gastrotomy incision in the stomach	**1.19** *gastr/o* + *-tomy* is spelled ___gastrotomy___ and means ___incision in the stomach___.
hematology study of blood	**1.20** *hemat/o* + *-logy* is spelled ___hematology___ and means ___study of blood___.

ANSWERS	REVIEW
gastroenterostomy creation of an opening (between) the stomach and small intestine	**1.21** *gastr/o + enter/o + -stomy* is spelled _gastroenterostomy_ and means _creation of an opening between_ _the stomach and small intestine_ _____.
oliguria condition of deficient urine	**1.22** *oligo- + ur/o + -ia* is spelled _oliguria_ and means _condition of deficient urine_ _____.
ostectomy excision (removal) of bone	**1.23** *oste/o + -ectomy* is spelled _ostectomy_ and means _removal of bone_ _____.
pericarditis inflammation around the heart	**1.24** *peri- + cardi/o + -itis* is spelled _pericarditis_ and means _inflammation around the_ _heart_ _____.

DEFINING MEDICAL TERMS THROUGH WORD STRUCTURE ANALYSIS

You can usually define a term by interpreting the suffix first, then the prefix (if one is present), and then the root or roots.

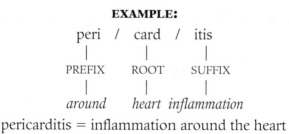

EXAMPLE:

peri / card / itis

PREFIX   ROOT   SUFFIX

around   heart inflammation

pericarditis = inflammation around the heart

You sense the basic meaning of the term pericarditis by understanding its components; however, the dictionary clarifies that the term refers to inflammation of the pericardium, the sac that encloses the heart.

Beginning students often have difficulty differentiating between prefixes and roots (or combining forms) because the root appears first in a medical term when a prefix is not used. It is important to memorize the most common prefixes (those in your starter flash card set) so that you can tell the difference. Also, keep in mind that a prefix is used only as needed to further modify the root or roots.

THE FORMATION OF MEDICAL TERMS

Study the flash cards for the term components listed next to prepare for the review that follows.

Self-Instruction: Patterns of Term Formation

Study the following:

COMBINING FORM	MEANING	FLASH CARD ID#
cardi/o	heart	CF-8
vascul/o	vessel	CF-5

SUFFIX	MEANING	FLASH CARD ID#
-ac, -al, -ar	pertaining to	S-1
-dynia	pain	S-2
-ium	structure or tissue	S-18
-logy	study of	S-19
-rrhaphy	suture	S-34
-rrhexis	rupture	S-36

PREFIX	MEANING	FLASH CARD ID#
endo-	within	P-15
epi-	upon	P-16
sub-	below or under	P-36

All medical terms are built from the root. Prefixes and suffixes are attached to the root to modify its meaning. Two or more roots are often linked together before being modified.

The following examples show the common patterns of medical term formation using the root *cardi* (heart) as a base. Using the term components listed earlier, define the term as you examine each pattern. Also, make a note of the rule used for forming each term.

 ## Programmed Review: Patterns of Term Formation

ANSWERS	REVIEW
pertaining to the heart	**1.25** Root/Suffix *cardi/ac* means ___pertaining to the heart___.
structure or tissue upon the heart	**1.26** Prefix/Root/Suffix *epi/card/ium* means ___structure or tissue upon___ ___the heart___.
pertaining to below or under and within the heart	**1.27** Prefix/Prefix/Root/Suffix *sub/endo/cardi/al* means ___pertaining to below___ ___or under and within the heart___.
pertaining to the heart and vessels	**1.28** Root/Combining Vowel/Root/Suffix *cardi/o/vascul/ar* means ___pertaining to the___ ___heart and vessels___.

ANSWERS	REVIEW
study of the heart	**1.29** Root/Combining Vowel/Suffix *cardi/o/logy* means _study of the heart_.
pain in the heart	**1.30** Root/Combining Vowel/Suffix (Symptomatic) [page 18] *cardi/o/dynia* means _pain in the heart_.
rupture of the heart	**1.31** Root/Combining Vowel/Suffix (Diagnostic) [page 19] *cardi/o/rrhexis* means _rupture of the heart_.
suture of the heart	**1.32** Root/Combining Vowel/Suffix (Operative) [page 19] *cardi/o/rrhaphy* means _suture of the heart_.

Acceptable Term Formations

As you learn medical terms, you can have fun experimenting with creating words, such as *glyco* (sweet) + *cardio* (heart) = sweetheart! However, in the real medical world, a term must be accepted by the medical community for it to be considered a legitimate word. Often, there seems to be no reason why a particular word form became acceptable. If in doubt, always check your medical dictionary for the correct spelling, formation, or precise meaning of a term.

A FEW EXCEPTIONS

Most medical terms are formed by the combination of a root or roots that are modified by suffixes and prefixes, as shown earlier in this section. Occasionally, terms are formed by a root alone or by a combination of roots.

EXAMPLES:

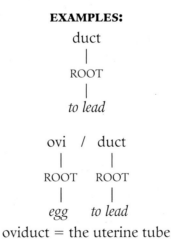

oviduct = the uterine tube

Sometimes, a term is formed by the combination of a prefix and suffix.

EXAMPLE:

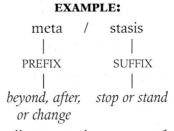

metastasis = the spread of a disease, such as cancer, from one location to another

SPELLING MEDICAL TERMS

Correct spelling of medical terms is crucial for communication among health care professionals. Careless spelling causes misunderstandings that can have serious consequences. The following list shows some of the pitfalls to avoid.

1. Some words sound the same but are spelled differently and have different meanings. Context is the clue to spelling. For example:

   ileum (part of the intestine)   ilium (part of the hip bone)

   sitology (study of food)   cytology (study of cells)

2. Other words sound similar but are spelled differently and have different meanings. For example:

   abduction (to draw away from)   adduction (to draw toward)

   hepatoma (liver tumor)   hematoma (blood tumor)

   aphagia (inability to swallow)   aphasia (inability to speak)

3. When letters are silent in a term, they risk being omitted when spelling the word. For example:

   "pt" has a "t" sound if found at the beginning of a term (e.g., pterygium), but both the "p" and "t" are pronounced when found within a term (e.g., nephroptosis [něf-rop-tō′sis])

   "ph" has an "f" sound (e.g., diaphragm)

   "ps" has an "s" sound (e.g., psychology)

4. Some words have more than one accepted spelling. For example:

   orthopedic   orthopaedic

   leukocyte   leucocyte

5. Some combining forms have the same meaning but different origins that compete for usage. For example, there are three combining forms that mean uterus:

   hyster/o (Greek)

   metr/o (Greek)

   uter/o (Latin)

RULES OF PRONUNCIATION

When you are beginning to learn how to pronounce medical terms, the task can seem insurmountable. Saying a term out loud for the first time can be a tense moment! The best way to make sure you get it right is through preparation: study the basic rules of pronunciation found in this chapter; repeat the words after hearing them pronounced on the CD-ROM accompanying this text or after your instructor has said them; and to try to keep the company of others who use medical language. You'll soon discover that there is nothing quite like the validation you feel when you correctly say something "medical" and no one flinches! Your confidence will build with every word you use.

Use these helpful shortcuts to master the pronunciation of medical terminology:

SHORTCUTS TO PRONUNCIATION

CONSONANT	EXAMPLE
c (before a, o, u) = k	cavity, colon, cure
c (before e, i) = s	cephalic, cirrhosis

CONSONANT	EXAMPLE
ch = k	cholesterol
g (before a, o, u) = g	gallstone, gonad, gurney
g (before e, i) = j	generic, giant
ph = f	phase
pn = n	pneumonia
ps = s	psychology
pt = t	ptosis, pterygium
rh, rrh = r	rhythm, hemorrhoid
x (as first letter in a word) = z	xerosis

Phonetic spelling for the pronunciation of most medical terms in this text is provided in parentheses below the term. The phonetic system used here is basic and has only a few standard rules. The macron and breve are the two diacritical marks used. The macron (¯) is placed over vowels that have a long sound:

ā in day

ē in bee

ī in pie

ō in no

ū in unit

The breve (˘) is placed over vowels that have a short sound:

ă in alone

ĕ in ever

ĭ in pit

ŏ in ton

ŭ in sun

Vowels that are not accented have a flat sound:

a in mat

e in bed

i in hip

o in got

u in put

The primary accent (′) is placed after the syllable that is stressed when saying the word. Monosyllables do not have a stress mark. Other syllables are separated by hyphens.

SINGULAR AND PLURAL FORMS

Plurals are usually formed by adding "s" or "es" to the end of a singular form. The following are common exceptions for forming plurals of Latin and Greek derivatives. Study the exceptions to prepare for the review that follows.

Self-Instruction: Singular and Plural Forms

SINGULAR ENDING	EXAMPLE	PLURAL ENDING	EXAMPLE
-a	vertebra *vĕr'tĕ-bră*	-ae	vertebrae *vĕr'tĕ-brā*
-is	diagnosis *dī-ag-nō'sis*	-es	diagnoses *dī-ag-nō'sēz*
-ma	condyloma *kon-di-lō'mă*	-mata	condylomata *kon'di-lō-mah'tă*
-on	phenomenon *fĕ-nom'ĕ-non*	-a	phenomena *fĕ-nom'ĕ-nă*
-um	bacterium *bak-tēr'ē-yŭm*	-a	bacteria *bak-tēr'ē-ă*
-us*	fungus *fŭng'gŭs*	-i	fungi *fŭn'jī*
-ax	thorax *thō'raks*	-aces	thoraces *thō-rā'sēz*
-ex	apex *ā'peks*	-ices	apices *ap'i-sēs*
-ix	appendix *ă-pen'diks*	-ices	appendices *ă-pen'di-sēz*
-y	myopathy *mī-op'ă-thē*	-ies	myopathies *mī-op'ă-thēz*

*The words *virus* and *sinus* follow the usual rule of adding "s" or "es" to form the plural (viruses and sinuses) instead of using the Latin plural ending *-i*.

Programmed Review: Singular and Plural Forms

ANSWERS	REVIEW
t	**1.33** The *pt* in *pterygium* has a/an ____ sound.
ovaries, ova	**1.34** An ovum is an egg produced by an ovary. There are two _____ in the female that produce eggs or _____.
k	**1.35** The *ch* in *chronic* has a/an ____ sound.
metastases	**1.36** The spread of cancer to a distant organ is called metastasis. The spread of cancer to more than one organ is _____.
s	**1.37** The *c* in *cirrhosis* has a/an __s__ sound.
verrucae	**1.38** A verruca is a wart. The term for several warts is _____.

ANSWERS	REVIEW
z	**1.39** The *x* in *xerosis* has a/an _____ sound.
condyloma	**1.40** Condylomata are genital warts. One genital wart is a ____condyloma____.
j	**1.41** The *g* in *genital* has a/an ___ sound.
index	**1.42** Indices is a plural form of ____index____.
thrombi	**1.43** A thrombus is a clot. Several clots are termed ____thrombi____.
n	**1.44** The *pn* in *pneumatic* has a/an __n__ sound.

BUILDING A VOCABULARY

The key to building a medical vocabulary is to know and understand the basic term components. To start you on your way, study and memorize the following lists of common prefixes, suffixes, and combining forms used in medical language. Each of these term components is included on a flash card in the starter set. Organize the flash cards as suggested in each section. Draw lines to separate the components in each of the example terms found on the cards, and write definitions in the margins to prepare for review exercises.

Refer to Appendix A for a summary list of prefixes, suffixes, and combining forms.

Common Prefixes

Prefixes are term components found at the beginning of a term when needed to further modify the root or roots. A list of commonly used prefixes organized into categories follows. Each is included on a flash card in the starter set. Organize the cards into the categories listed here. Draw lines to separate the components in each of the example terms shown on the cards, and write definitions in the margins in preparation for the review exercises.

 ## Self-Instruction: Common Prefixes

Study the following:

PREFIX	MEANING	FLASH CARD ID#
NEGATION		
a-, an-	without	P-1
anti-, contra-	against or opposed to	P-5
de-	from, down, or not	P-10
POSITION/DIRECTION		
ab-	away from	P-2
ad-	to, toward, or near	P-3

PREFIX	MEANING	FLASH CARD ID#
circum-, peri-	around	P-8
dia-, trans-	across or through	P-11
e-, ec-, ex-	out or away	P-13
ecto-, exo-, extra-	outside	P-14
en-, endo-, intra-	within	P-15
epi-	upon	P-16
inter-	between	P-21
meso-	middle	P-23
meta-	beyond, after, or change	P-24
para-	alongside of or abnormal	P-30
retro-	backward or behind	P-35
sub-, infra-	below or under	P-36

QUANTITY OF MEASUREMENT

bi-	two or both	P-6
hemi-, semi-	half	P-18
hyper-	above or excessive	P-19
hypo-	below or deficient	P-20
macro-	large or long	P-22
micro-	small	P-25
mono-, uni-	one	P-26
oligo-	few or deficient	P-28
pan-	all	P-29
poly-, multi-	many	P-31
quadri-	four	P-33
super-, supra-	above or excessive	P-37
tri-	three	P-39
ultra-	beyond or excessive	P-40

TIME

ante-, pre-, pro-	before	P-4
brady-	slow	P-7
tachy-	fast	P-38
post-	after or behind	P-32
re-	again or back	P-34

PREFIX	MEANING	FLASH CARD ID#
GENERAL PREFIXES		
con-, syn-, sym-	together or with	P-9
dys-	painful, difficult, or faulty	P-12
eu-	good or normal	P-17
neo-	new	P-27

Study the flash cards for the prefixes listed above in preparation for the following review.

Programmed Review: Common Prefixes

ANSWERS	REVIEW
away to, toward, or near around across or through out or away one, bi	**1.45** Several prefixes modify position or direction when used in a term. **Ab**duction is used to describe movement __away__ from the body, and **ad**duction describes movement __toward__ the body. **Circum**duction is movement that is __around__. A **dia**gonal is an angle that moves _____. **In**version refers to turning in, and **e**version means to turn _____. **Uni**lateral refers to __one__ side, whereas __bi__ lateral means both sides.
below or under upon across or through within, intra outside between inter, out away, below or under infra	**1.46** **Sub**cutaneous pertains to __below__ the skin. **Epi**dermal refers to something __upon__ the skin, whereas **trans**dermal pertains to __across__ the skin. **Intra**dermal pertains to __within__ the skin. That which is within a cell is __intra__ cellular. **Extra**cellular pertains to __outside__ a cell. *Inter-*, a prefix meaning __between__, is used in the term describing that which is between cells: __inter__ cellular. **Ec**centric is situated __out__ or __away__ from center. *Infra-*, a prefix meaning __below__, is used to indicate a position below the part to which it is joined. For example, __infra__ umbilical refers to a position below or under the umbilicus (navel).
within endo, middle meso outside, ecto	**1.47** Layers of embryonic tissue are named for their position. *Endo-*, meaning __middle__, is used to describe the innermost layer, or __endo__ derm. *Meso-*, meaning __middle__, is used to name the middle layer, or __meso__ derm. *Ecto-*, meaning __outside__, is used to identify the outer layer, or __ecto__ derm.

ANSWERS	REVIEW
exo endo within	**1.48** Glands that secrete within the body are the endocrine glands, and those that secrete outside are the ___exo___crine glands. An instrument to examine within the body is an __endo__scope. When something is encapsulated, it is held ___within___.
deficient excessive hypo hyper below above above, excessive above excessive beyond ultra	**1.49** *Hypo-* means below or ___deficient___, and *hyper-* means above or ___excessive___. A patient with a deficient level of blood glucose (sugar) has a condition of __hypo__glycemia. A condition of excessive blood glucose is ___hyper___glycemia. **Hypo**thermia is a condition in which the body temperature is ___below___ normal, whereas **hyper**thermia is a condition of body temperature well ___above___ normal. Like *hyper-*, *super-* and *supra-* are prefixes meaning ___above___ or ___excessive___. **Supra**renal pertains to a location ___above___ the kidney. **Super**numerary pertains to numbers that are above or ___excessive___ (too many to count). *Ultra-* is a prefix meaning ___beyond___ or excessive. The term describing high-frequency sound beyond that which can be heard by humans is known as ___ultra___sound.
large small macro, micro	**1.50** *Macro-* refers to something ___large___ or long, and *micro-* refers to something ___small___. A large cell is called a ___macro___cyte. A small cell is called a ___micro___cyte.
mono-, one bi-, tri- quadri-, many one many three four	**1.51** *Uni-* and ___mono-___ are prefixes meaning ___one___. The prefix for two is ___bi-___, three is ___tri-___, and four is ___quadri-___. *Multi-* and *poly-* mean ___many___. **Mono**neuropathy describes the disease of ___one___ nerve, whereas polyneuropathy involves ___many___ nerves. A triangle has ___three___ sides. **Quadri**plegia is a condition of paralysis of all ___four___ limbs.
all Pan	**1.52** *Pan-* is a prefix meaning ___all___. A panacea is a cure-all. ___Pan___sinusitis refers to an inflammation of all of the sinuses.
semi- one-half	**1.53** The two prefixes meaning one-half are *hemi-* and ___semi-___. **Semi**lunar pertains to a half-moon shape. **Hemi**cephalic pertains to ___one___-___half___ of the head.

ANSWERS	REVIEW
without an a, painful, difficult, or faulty dys a	**1.54** *A-* and *an-* are prefixes meaning _____without_____. *An-* is used before a vowel. For example, aerobic pertains to air, and ____aerobic pertains to without air. A patient without the ability to speak has a condition called ___phasia. *Dys-* is a prefix meaning _____. **Dys**phasia is a condition of difficult speech. A condition of difficulty swallowing is termed __dys_phagia. The patient without the ability to swallow has _____phagia.
contra-, against or opposed to anti	**1.55** Two prefixes meaning against or opposed to are *anti-* and _____. A **contra**ceptive is _____ conception. An _____inflammatory drug acts against or opposed to inflammation by reducing it.
from, down, or not again before backward or behind	**1.56** **De**activated refers to something that is _____ active. When something is **re**activated, it is made active _____. **Pro**active refers to an action made _____. **Retro**position refers to a structure that is _____.
fast slow, tachy brady slow fast	**1.57** *Tachy-* is a prefix meaning _____, and *brady-* means _____. A condition of fast heart is _____cardia. A condition of slow heart is _____cardia. **Brady**pnea refers to _____ breathing, whereas **tachy**pnea refers to _____ breathing.
before pre around, after Neo	**1.58** Natal pertains to birth. **Ante**natal is the time _____ birth, also known as the _____natal period. **Peri**natal is the time _____ birth, and **post**natal is the time _____ birth. _____natal pertains to newborn.
good or normal painful, difficult, or faulty	**1.59** *Toc/o* is a combining form meaning labor. **Eu**tocia is a condition of _____ labor, and **dys**tocia is a condition of _____ labor.

ANSWERS	REVIEW
together	**1.60** *Con-*, *syn-*, and *sym-* are prefixes meaning _together_ or
with	_with_. A **con**genital disorder is one that an infant is born
with	_with_. *Dactyl/o* is a combining form meaning finger or toe.
	Syndactylism is a condition of fingers or toes that are fused
together	_together_. *Syn-* appears as *sym-* before b, p, ph, or m.
	For example, the term describing the condition in which different
sym	species are able to live together is _sym_biosis.

Common Suffixes

Suffixes are endings that modify the root. These endings give the root essential meaning by forming a noun, verb, or adjective. The two basic types of suffixes are simple and compound. Simple suffixes form basic terms. For example, the simple suffix *-ic* (pertaining to) combined with the root *gastr* (stomach) forms the term gastric (pertaining to the stomach). Compound suffixes are formed by a combination of basic term components. For example, the root *tom* (to cut) combined with the simple suffix *-y* (a process of) forms the compound suffix *-tomy* (incision); the compound suffix *-ectomy* (excision or removal) is formed by a combination of the prefix *ec-* (out) with the root *tom* (to cut) and the simple suffix *-y* (a process of).

Compound suffixes are added to roots to provide a specific meaning. For example, combining the root *hyster* (uterus) with *-ectomy* forms hysterectomy (excision of the uterus). Noting the differences between simple and compound suffixes will help you to analyze medical terms.

Suffixes in this text are divided into four categories:

1. Symptomatic suffixes, which describe the evidence of illness
2. Diagnostic suffixes, which provide the name of a medical condition
3. Surgical (operative) suffixes, which describe a surgical treatment
4. General suffixes, which have general application

A listing of commonly used suffixes follows. Each suffix is included on a flash card in the starter set. Organize the cards into the four categories of suffixes. Draw lines to separate the components in each of the example terms found on the cards, and write definitions in the margins to prepare for the review exercises.

Self-Instruction: Common Suffixes

Study the following:

SUFFIX	MEANING	FLASH CARD ID#
SYMPTOMATIC SUFFIXES **(Word Endings That Describe Evidence of Illness)**		
-algia, -dynia	pain	S-2
-genesis	origin or production	S-11
-lysis	breaking down or dissolution	S-20

SUFFIX	MEANING	FLASH CARD ID#
-megaly	enlargement	S-22
-oid	resembling	S-24
-penia	abnormal reduction	S-27
-rrhea	discharge	S-35
-spasm	involuntary contraction	S-38

DIAGNOSTIC SUFFIXES
(Word Endings That Describe a Condition or Disease)

-cele	pouching or hernia	S-4
-ectasis	expansion or dilation	S-8
-emia	blood condition	S-10
-iasis	formation or presence of	S-15
-itis	inflammation	S-17
-malacia	softening	S-21
-oma	tumor	S-25
-osis	condition or increase	S-26
-phil, -philia	attraction for	S-29
-ptosis	falling or downward displacement	S-32
-rrhage, -rrhagia	to burst forth (usually blood)	S-33
-rrhexis	rupture	S-36

SURGICAL (OPERATIVE) SUFFIXES
(Word Endings That Describe a Surgical [Operative] Treatment)

-centesis	puncture for aspiration	S-5
-desis	binding	S-6
-ectomy	excision (removal)	S-9
-pexy	suspension or fixation	S-28
-plasty	surgical repair or reconstruction	S-30
-rrhaphy	suture	S-34
-tomy	incision	S-41
-stomy	creation of an opening	S-40

GENERAL SUFFIXES
(Simple or Compound Suffixes That Have General Application)
Noun Endings (suffixes that form a noun when combined with a root)

-ation	process	S-3
-e	general indicator that a word is a person, place, or thing	S-7

SUFFIX	MEANING	FLASH CARD ID#
-ia, -ism	condition of	S-13
-y	condition or process of	S-42
-ium	structure or tissue	S-18

Adjective Endings (suffixes that form an adjective when combined with a root)

-ac, -al, -ar, -ary, -eal, -ic, -ous, -tic	pertaining to	S-1

Diminutive Endings (suffixes meaning small)

-icle, -ole, -ula, -ule	small	S-16

Other General Suffixes

-gram	record	S-12
-graph	instrument for recording	S-12
-graphy	process of recording	S-12
-iatrics, -iatry	treatment	S-14
-logy	study	S-19
-logist	one who specializes in the study or treatment of	S-19
-ist	one who specializes in	S-19
-meter	instrument for measuring	S-23
-metry	process of measuring	S-23
-poiesis	formation	S-31
-scope	instrument for examination	S-37
-scopy	process of examination	S-37
-stasis	stop or stand	S-39

Don't be rolled over by the

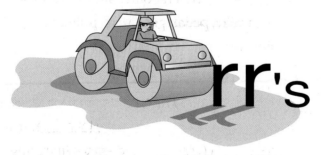

rr's

We have the Greeks to thank for the suffixes with **double rr's**. Take a careful look at each so that you will spell them correctly in a term!

Suffix	Meaning	Example
-rrhea	discharge	pyorrhea (a discharge of pus)
-rrhage or -rrhagia	to burst forth (usually blood)	hemorrhage (a burst forth of blood)
		menorrhagia (a burst forth of blood during menstruation)
-rrhexis	rupture	angiorrhexis (a rupture of a vessel)
-rrhaphy	suture	nephrorrhaphy (a suture of the kidney)

Each component also has an *h*, and *-rrhaphy* has two!

Study the flash cards for the suffixes listed on the previous pages in preparation for the following review.

Programmed Review: Common Suffixes

ANSWERS	REVIEW
stomach prefix, upon -ium, suffix structure, tissue condition of process of process, noun	**1.61** *Gastr/o* is a combining form meaning _____. In epigastrium, *epi-* is the _____ meaning _____, and _____ is the _____, a noun ending meaning _____ or _____. The noun endings *-ia* and *-ism*, as seen in the terms pneumon**ia** and hypothyroid**ism,** refer to a _____ ___. The *-y* ending in atrophy indicates a condition or _____ ___. The suffix in extravas**ation** denotes a _____. The *-e* in erythrocy**te** is a _____ marker.
-ic pertaining to upon, epigastrium -eal pertaining to esophagus pertaining to	**1.62** In epigastric, use of the suffix _____ forms an adjective that means _____ ___ the stomach—specifically referring to the tissue region _____ the stomach known as the _____. In gastroesophageal, _____ is the adjective ending that modifies the term to mean _____ ___ the stomach and _____. Several other suffixes form adjectives, as noted in the terms cardi**ac**, ped**al**, glandul**ar**, pulmon**ary**, esophag**eal**, hypno**tic**, and fibr**ous**, and also mean _____.
ending pain enlargement discharge, involuntary contraction symptomatic, illness	**1.63** A symptomatic suffix is a term _____ used to describe evidence of illness. The suffixes *-algia* or *-dynia* (meaning _____), *-megaly* (meaning _____), *-rrhea* (meaning _____), and *-spasm* (meaning _____) are examples of suffixes used to form _____ terms that describe evidence of _____.

ANSWERS	REVIEW
gastralgia or gastrodynia epigastralgia gastrospasm rrhea gastromegaly	**1.64** The symptomatic term that describes stomach pain is _____. Pain located in the tissue upon the stomach is termed _____. Involuntary contraction of the stomach is called _____, and the discharge of gastric juice from the stomach is termed gastro_____. Enlargement of the stomach is termed _____.
pain examination stomach within gastroscope	**1.65** Physical examination and test procedures are key to identifying the cause of symptoms in order to make a diagnosis. A diagnosis is the name of a condition or disease. In evaluating the cause of a symptom such as gastrodynia, or ____pain____ in the stomach, a gastroscopy or _____ of the ____stomach____ may be performed. The specific endoscope (instrument to examine ____within____) used in gastroscopy is called a _____.
endings diagnosis gastritis iasis gastromalacia pouching, hernia gastrocele blood, burst forth gastrorrhagia stasis	**1.66** Diagnostic suffixes are word ____endings____ used to describe a condition or name of a disease, called a ____diagnosis____. If, on gastroscopic examination, the physician notes an inflammation of the stomach, a diagnosis of ____gastritis____ is made. The presence of a stone in the stomach is termed gastrolith____iasis____. A finding of softening of the stomach wall is referred to as ____gastromalacia____. The suffix *-cele,* meaning ____pouching____ or ____hernia____, is used in the term describing a pouching or hernia of the stomach: _____. Hemorrhage, a term referring to bleeding, was formed by the link of *hem/o,* a combining form meaning ____blood____, with *-rrhage,* a suffix meaning to ____burst____ ____forth____, usually in reference to blood. Using the suffix *-rrhagia,* the condition of bursting forth of blood from the stomach is called _____. The suffix meaning stop or stand is used in the term describing efforts to stop hemorrhaging blood: hemo____stasis____.
stomach suffix, study of	**1.67** Gastroenterology, a term formed by a link of *gastr/o* (meaning ____stomach____), *enter/o* (meaning small intestine), and *-logy* (a ____suffix____ meaning ____study of____), is the name of the medical specialty involved with the study of gastrointestinal conditions. Using the suffix referring to one who specializes in the

ANSWERS	REVIEW
gastroenterologist	study or treatment of, the physician who specializes in the treatment of the stomach and intestines is called a _gastroenterologist_.
condition, increase stenosis gastrostenosis	**1.68** Many symptomatic and diagnostic terms use the suffix *-osis* to indicate a _condition_ or _increase_. For example, when combined with *sten/o*, a combining form meaning narrow, the term for a condition or increase of narrowing is _stenosis_. A narrowed condition of the stomach is therefore called _gastrostenosis_.
endings operative -tomy, gastrotomy gastrectomy downward displacement, stomach pexy gastroplasty gastrostomy gastrorrhaphy -centesis -desis	**1.69** Once a diagnosis is made, treatment follows. Some treatments require surgery. Operative suffixes are term _endings_ that describe a surgical or _operative_ treatment. The first step in a surgical procedure is to make an incision, the suffix for which is _-tomy_. An incision in the stomach is called a _gastrotomy_. Given a diagnosis of stomach tumor, a surgical remedy might involve a partial or complete removal of the stomach, called a _gastrectomy_. Gastroptosis, defined as a falling or _downward_ _displacement_ of the _stomach_, may necessitate a surgical suspension or fixation, called a gastro_pexy_. The operative term describing a surgical repair of the stomach is _gastroplasty_. In some cases, the creation of an opening is required, such as to bypass a diseased part. The creation of a new opening in the stomach is called _gastrostomy_. Perforation of the stomach requires suturing, the operative term for which is _gastrorrhaphy_. When fluid builds up within the abdominal cavity as a result of illness or injury, a puncture for aspiration is required. The suffix meaning puncture for aspiration is _-centesis_. The surgical suffix specifically referring to binding of tissue is _-desis_.
-icle -iole, -ula, -ule	**1.70** Other general suffixes are commonly seen in health records. Those referring to diminutives (something small) are _-icle_, _-iole_, _-ula_, and _-ule_, as seen in the terms vent**ricle**, bronch**iole**, mac**ula**, and ven**ule**.

ANSWERS	REVIEW
record	**1.71** You'll find several general suffixes describing diagnostic testing. For example, *-gram* is a suffix meaning _record_. An electrocardiogram (ECG) is a record of the electrical conduction of the heart. The instrument for recording an ECG is called an
graph	electrocardio_____ machine. This process of recording is
electrocardiography	referred to as _____. The suffix *-metry* is a suffix
measuring	referring to the process of _____. A thermometer is
instrument	an _____ for measuring temperature.

Common Combining Forms

The following table shows selected combining forms (roots with vowels attached) to give you a start toward building medical terms. Each is included on a flash card in the starter set. Organize the cards into categories such as the ones in the following list. Review the cards by drawing lines to separate the components in each example term, and write definitions in the margins in preparation for the review exercises. Additional combining forms are introduced at the beginning of Chapters 3 through 15 on the body systems, and Appendix A contains a summary list of combining forms. Study the entire starter set of flash cards in preparation for the next review.

 ## Self-Instruction: Common Combining Forms

Study the following:

COMBINING FORM	MEANING	FLASH CARD ID#
COLORS		
cyan/o	blue	CF-12
erythr/o	red	CF-16
leuk/o	white	CF-27
melan/o	black	CF-30
SUBSTANCES		
aer/o	air, gas	CF-4
hem/o, hemat/o	blood	CF-23
hydr/o	water	CF-26
lip/o	fat	CF-28
py/o	pus	CF-49
ur/o, urin/o	urine	CF-56

COMBINING FORM	MEANING	FLASH CARD ID#
ORGANS/STRUCTURES		
abdomin/o, lapar/o	abdomen	CF-1
acr/o	extremity or topmost	CF-2
aden/o	gland	CF-3
angi/o, vas/o, vascul/o	vessel	CF-5
arthr/o	joint	CF-6
cardi/o	heart	CF-8
cephal/o	head	CF-9
col/o, colon/o	colon	CF-10
cyt/o	cell	CF-13
derm/o, dermat/o, cutane/o	skin	CF-14
enter/o	small intestine	CF-15
esophag/o	esophagus	CF-17
gastr/o	stomach	CF-20
hepat/o	liver	CF-24
hist/o	tissue	CF-25
my/o, muscul/o	muscle	CF-32
nas/o, rhin/o	nose	CF-33
nephr/o, ren/o	kidney	CF-35
neur/o	nerve	CF-36
or/o	mouth	CF-38
oste/o	bone	CF-40
pneum/o, pneumon/o	air or lung	CF-47
GENERAL COMBINING FORMS		
carcin/o	cancer	CF-7
crin/o	to secrete	CF-11
esthesi/o	sensation	CF-18
fibr/o	fiber	CF-19
gen/o	origin or production	CF-21
gynec/o	woman	CF-22
lith/o	stone	CF-29
morph/o	form	CF-31
necr/o	death	CF-34

COMBINING FORM	MEANING	FLASH CARD ID#
onc/o	tumor or mass	CF-37
orth/o	straight, normal, or correct	CF-39
path/o	disease	CF-41
ped/o	child or foot	CF-42
phag/o	eat or swallow	CF-43
phas/o	speech	CF-44
phob/o	exaggerated fear or sensitivity	CF-45
plas/o	formation	CF-46
psych/o	mind	CF-48
scler/o	hard	CF-50
son/o	sound	CF-51
sten/o	narrow	CF-52
therm/o	heat	CF-53
tox/o, toxic/o	poison	CF-54
troph/o	nourishment or development	CF-55

◈ Programmed Review: Common Combining Forms

ANSWERS	REVIEW
kidney combining, form suffix study, kidney	**1.72** *Nephr* is a Greek root meaning ___kidney___. Combined with an "*o*", it becomes *nephr/o*, a ___combining___ ___form___. *Nephr/o* cannot stand alone as a term. At the least, it needs a ___suffix___ to give it essential meaning. In the term nephrology, the addition of the suffix -*logy* forms a term with a specific meaning: ___study___ of the ___kidney___.
stone, -iasis presence or formation of kidney stones, o suffix ren/o	**1.73** In nephrolithiasis, the link of *nephr/o* to *lith*, a root meaning ___stone___, and the suffix ___-iasis___ forms the term referring to the ___presence or formation of kidney stones___. The combining vowel for *lith* is ___o___. Notice that the vowel was not used when linked to -*iasis*, because the ___suffix___ began with a vowel. Nephrolithiasis is a renal disease. Renal is a term formed using ___ren/o___, the Latin combining form meaning kidney.

ANSWERS	REVIEW
combining form abdomen lapar/o abdomen	**1.74** *Abdomin/o* is a _____ _____ meaning _____, the central part of the body trunk. Note that the spelling of *abdomin/o* is different from the anatomic part it represents. Another combining form meaning abdomen is _____. A laparoscope is an instrument used to examine the _____.
water head	**1.75** *Hydr/o* is a combining form meaning _____. A person with hydrocephaly has a condition of water (fluid) within the _____.
acro topmost, acro	**1.76** An enlarged extremity is called _____megaly. *Acr/o* also means _____. A person with _____phobia has a fear of high places.
gen/o origin or production cancer	**1.77** The suffix meaning origin or production is *-genesis*. The combining form meaning origin or production is _____. The suffix *-genic* pertains to _____. Carcinogenic pertains to the origin or production of _____.
melan/o, leuk/o erythr/o, cyan/o black skin, white red cyan	**1.78** Several combining forms are listed in the starter set related to color: black is _____, white is _____, red is _____, and blue is _____. Melanoma, referring to a _____ tumor, is a common cutaneous cancer, or _____ cancer. A leukocyte is a _____ cell. Erythroderma refers to _____ skin. When the skin turns blue from lack of oxygen, it is termed _____osis.

LEVELS OF ORGANIZATION IN THE BODY (Fig. 1-1)

Study the entire starter set of flash cards to prepare for the review that follows.

🔷 Programmed Review: Cells/Tissues/Organs/Systems

ANSWERS	REVIEW
    small	**1.79** The term cell, meaning small room, was used to describe the structures first observed in 1665 by Robert Hooke as he examined cork using a microscope, an instrument to examine something _____. He noted that the small cells were part of a larger web of

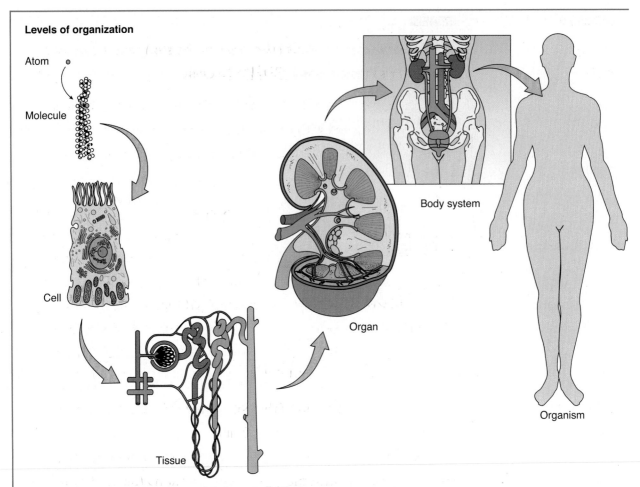

Levels of organization

Atom

Molecule

Cell

Tissue

Organ

Body system

Organism

FIGURE 1-1 ■ **Levels of organization in the body.**

ANSWERS	REVIEW
cell	woven tissue. Using *cyt/o*, a combining form meaning _____, the study of cells that comprise the human body became known as
cyto, histology form morphology	_____logy and the study of tissue as _____. *Morph/o*, a combining form meaning _____, is used to name the study of the form and shape of cells and tissue: _____.
larger organs urine pertaining to	**1.80** Body cells combine to form tissues, and combinations of tissues compose the organs necessary for body functions. Organs act together as part of the _____ body systems. For example, the kidneys are _____ that function to filter blood as part of the urinary system (*urin/o* means _____ and *-ary* means _____).
ren/o urology	**1.81** The Greek combining form for kidney is *nephr/o*, and the Latin is _____. The medical specialty concerned with the study and treatment of the urinary tract is called _____. The

ANSWERS	REVIEW
nephro	physician who particularly specializes in the study and treatment of the kidneys is known as a _____logist.
patho pathologist	**1.82** Examination of body cells and tissues is part of the medical specialty concerned with the study of disease, known as _____logy. The physician who is a specialist in the study of disease is called a _____.
formation faulty new -oma carcinoma oncology	**1.83** *Plas/o* is a combining form meaning _____, and *dys-* is a prefix meaning bad, difficult, or _____. Dysplasia is the term used to describe abnormal cell and tissue development, and neoplasia, referring to a condition of _____ formation, is the term used to describe the formation of cells and tissue into tumor. The suffix for tumor is _____. A cancerous tumor is called a _____. The specialty concerned with the study of tumors and cancers is _____.
dermat/o skin study dermatologist	**1.84** The largest organ of the body is the skin. *Cutane/o* is the Latin combining form, and *derm/o* and _____ are the Greek combining forms, that mean _____. Dermatology is the specialty involved with the _____ and treatment of skin diseases. The specialist is called a _____.
Oste/o joint muscle correct foot	**1.85** The musculoskeletal system provides support and gives shape to the body. Bones, which form the skeleton, are covered with muscle to supply the forces that make movement possible. _____ is the combining form for bone, and *arthr/o* is the combining form meaning _____, the hinge between bones. *My/o* and *muscul/o* are the combining forms for _____. *Orth/o*, meaning straight, normal, or _____, and *ped/o*, meaning child or _____, were combined to form the term orthopedic (pertaining to the specialty related to the musculoskeletal system).
heart, vessels blood hematology cell	**1.86** The cardiovascular system consists of the _____ and _____ that transport blood throughout the body. Blood provides transport for oxygen, nutrients, wastes, etc. *Hem/o* and *hemat/o* are combining forms meaning _____. The study of blood is called _____. It includes analysis of blood and its cellular components. *Cyt/o* means _____. Cells of the

ANSWERS	REVIEW
red leukocytes blood, suffix poison py/o, formation pus	blood include erythrocytes, or __red__ cells, and __leukocytes__, or white cells. Hemopoiesis is a term referring to the formation of __blood__, and *-emia* is the __suffix__ that means blood. Toxemia is a condition of blood __poison__. Leukocytes are blood cells that fight infection. They are present in pus, the fluid produced by inflammation of tissue. The combining form for pus is __py/o__. Pyopoiesis describes the __formation__ of __pus__.
air or lung nose nas/o	**1.87** *Pneum/o*, meaning __air or lung__, is the key combining form of the respiratory system, the body system responsible for the exchange of gases (oxygen and carbon dioxide) within the body. The nose is the first structure to receive oxygen. *Rhin/o* is the Greek combining form meaning __nose__. The Latin combining form with the same meaning is __nas/o__.
Neur/o	**1.88** The nervous system is a complicated network of nerves and fibers that control all functions of the body. __Neur/o__ is the combining form for nerve.
within, to secrete	**1.89** The ductless glands of the endocrine system affect the function of organs by the secreting hormones. *Endo* means __within__, and *crin/o* means __to secrete__.
mouth esophagus, stomach small, large liver	**1.90** The gastrointestinal system provides for digestion and elimination. Combining forms related to key structures of the tubular digestive tract are *or/o* (meaning __mouth__), *esophag/o* (meaning __esophagus__), *gastr/o* (meaning __stomach__), *enter/o* (meaning __small__ intestine), and *col/o* or *colon/o* (meaning __large__ intestine). *Hepat/o* is the combining form for __liver__, the organ that produces bile necessary for digestion.
logist gynecology	**1.91** The male and female reproductive systems produce the sex cells and maintain the organs necessary for production of human offspring. The physician who specializes in the treatment of the male and female urinary system, as well as the male reproductive system, is called a uro__logist__. Treatment of the female reproductive system involves two medical specialties: obstetrics and __gynecology__ (study of woman).

PRACTICE EXERCISES

Circle the correct meaning for the following term components:

1. inter-
   a. difficult   b. between   c. within   d. out, away   e. behind

2. ultra-
   a. across   b. excessive   c. against   d. around   e. without

3. anti-
   a. beside   b. outside   c. against   d. around   e. away from

4. a-
   a. double   b. both   c. two   d. without   e. against

5. bi-
   a. without   b. upon   c. excessive   d. two   e. back, again

6. pre-
   a. against   b. out   c. toward   d. before   e. after

7. poly-
   a. many   b. few   c. above   d. before   e. after

8. neo-
   a. birth   b. death   c. origin   d. new   e. disease

9. peri-
   a. many   b. all   c. alongside of   d. attraction for   e. around

10. hyper-
    a. below   b. after   c. beyond   d. excessive   e. deficient

11. -plasty
    a. surgical repair   b. cancer   c. tumor   d. excision   e. incision

12. -megaly
    a. development   b. tumor   c. fixation   d. enlargement   e. softening

13. -itis
    a. excision   b. condition   c. abnormal reduction   d. formation   e. inflammation

14. -rrhagia
    a. discharge   b. suture   c. rupture   d. burst forth   e. repair

15. -penia
    a. discharge   b. fixation   c. rupture   d. reduction   e. suspension

16. necr/o
    a. fear   b. death   c. black   d. tumor   e. large

17. toxic/o
    a. development   b. poison   c. pus   d. swallow   e. black

18. acr/o

    a. gland   b. blue   c. air   d. extremity ✓   e. red

19. angi/o

    (a. artery) ✗   b. heart   (c. vessel)   d. red   e. gland

20. cyt/o

    a. color   b. sac   c. blue   d. colon   (e.) cell ✓

21. melan/o

    a. death   b. disease   (c. black) ✓   d. dissolution   e. large

*After verifying that you have circled the correct answers, go back over questions 1-21 and write the correct term component for each of the meanings listed.

Circle the correct term component for the following meanings:

22. kidney

    a. enter/o   b. gastr/o   (c. ren/o) ✓   d. hepat/o   e. necr/o

23. large

    a. poly-   b. -malacia   c. -oma   d. hyper-   (e. macro-) ✓

24. record

    a. -meter   b. -metry   (c. -gram) ✓   d. -graph   e. -graphy

25. surgical fixation

    a. -ptosis   b. -plasia   c. -penia   (d. -pexy)   (e. -plasty)

26. condition or increase

    (a. -itis)   b. -iasis   (c. -osis)   d. -ium   e. -ous

27. excision

    a. -tomy   b. -stomy   (c. -ectomy) ✓   d. -centesis   e. -cele

*After verifying that you have circled the correct answers, go back over questions 22-27 and write the meaning for each term component listed.

Circle the correct plural for the following words:

28. vertebra

    a. vertebray   b. vertebras   (c. vertebrae) ✓ d. vertebrus   e. vertebraes

29. bulla

    (a. bulli) ✗   b. bullia   (c. bullae)   d. bullas   e. bullata

30. speculum

    a. speculata   b. speculumes (c. specula) ✓   d. speculae   e. speculuma

31. fungus

    (a. fungi) ✓   b. fungae   c. funges   d. funguses   e. fungea

32. stoma

    (a. stomata)   (b. stomatae) ✗ c. stomes   d. stomatus   e. stomatum

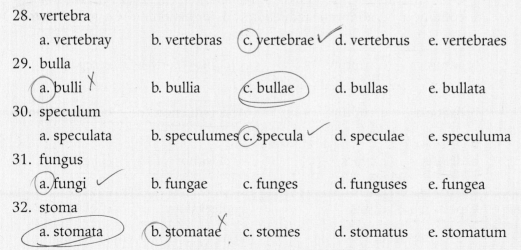

33. macula
    a. maculus   b. maculas   c. maculi   d. maculae   e. maculies

34. radius
    a. radii ✓   b. radiusos   c. radiuses   d. radia   e. radiis

35. diagnosis
    a. diagnosa   b. diagnoses   c. diagnosses   d. diagnosi   e. diagnosae

Circle the operative term in each of the following:

36. a. nephroptosis   b. hemolysis   c. angiectasis   d. colostomy ✓   e. necrosis

37. a. vasorrhaphy   b. hematoma   c. gastrocele   d. endoscope ✗   e. cardiorrhexis

38. a. morphologic   b. adenolysis   c. abdominocentesis ✓   d. osteomalacia   e. polyrrhea

→ incision of the colon

*After verifying that you have circled the correct answers, go back over questions 36-38 and define each of the terms.

Circle the correct spelling:

39. a. nephroraphy ✗   b. nephrorrapy   c. nephrorrhaphy   d. nephrorrhapy

40. a. abdominoscopy ✓   b. abdemenoscopi   c. abdomenscopy   d. abdominoschope

41. a. perrycardium   b. pericardium ✓   c. periocardium   d. paracardium

For each of the following words, identify the term components (prefixes [P], combining forms [CF], roots [R], and suffixes [S]) by writing them on the lines below the word. Then, define the word according to the meaning of its components.

EXAMPLE:

hyperlipemia

$$\underline{\quad hyper \quad} / \underline{\quad lip \quad} / \underline{\quad emia \quad}$$
$$\qquad\quad P \qquad\qquad R \qquad\qquad S$$

DEFINITION: above or excessive/fat/blood condition

42. microlithiasis

$$\underline{\quad micro \quad} / \underline{\quad lith \quad} / \underline{\quad iasis \quad}$$
$$\qquad P \qquad\qquad R \qquad\qquad S$$

DEFINITION: ___presence of formation of a small stone___ ✓

43. sympathy

$$\underline{\quad sym \quad} / \underline{\quad path \quad} / \underline{\quad y \quad}$$
$$\qquad P \qquad\qquad R \qquad\qquad S$$

DEFINITION: ___together with the condition or process of disease___ ✓

44. toxoid

$$\underline{\quad tox \quad} / \underline{\quad oid \quad}$$
$$\qquad R \qquad\qquad S$$

DEFINITION: ___resembling poison___ ✓

45. mesomorphic

$$\underline{\quad meso \quad} / \underline{\quad morph \quad} / \underline{\quad ic \quad}$$
$$\qquad P \qquad\qquad R \qquad\qquad S$$

DEFINITION: ___pertaining to the middle form___ ✓

46. pancytopenia

_____pan_____ / ___cyto___ / ___penia___
P   CF   S

DEFINITION: ___abnormal reduction of all cells___

47. metastasis

___meta___ / ___stasis___
P   S

DEFINITION: ___beyond / stop___

48. acrodynia

___acro___ / ___dynia___
CF   S

DEFINITION: ___pain in the extremities___

49. tachycardia

___tachy___ / ___card___ / ___ia___
P   R   S

DEFINITION: ___condition of a fast heart___

50. pyogenesis

___pyo___ / ___genesis___
CF   S

DEFINITION: ___production of pus___

51. adenitis

___aden___ / ___itis___
R   S

DEFINITION: ___inflammation of the gland___

52. macrocephalous

___macro___ / ___cephal___ / ___ous___
P   R   S

DEFINITION: ___pertaining to the large head___

53. paracentesis

___para___ / ___centesis___
P   S

DEFINITION: ___along puncture for aspiration___

54. ultrasonography

___ultra___ / ___sono___ / ___graphy___
P   CF   S

DEFINITION: ___process of recording beyond sound___

55. orthopedic

___ortho___ / ___ped___ / ___ic___
CF   R   S

DEFINITION: ___pertaining to normal foot___

56. angiomegaly

___angio___ / ___megaly___
CF   S

DEFINITION: ___vessel enlargement___

69. cyano/tic
    ‾CF‾ ‾S‾
    blue/pertaining to
70. extra/vas/ation
    ‾P‾ ‾R‾ ‾S‾
    outside/vessel/process
71. hyper/ troph/ y
    ‾P‾ ‾R‾ ‾S‾
    above or excessive/
    nourishment or
    development/
    condition or process
    of
72. c. supra-

73. d. re-
74. c. pre-
75. c. post-
76. b. de-
77. c. mono-
78. e. trans-
79. c. super-
80. b. infra-
81. a. exo-
82. c. ante-
83. b. dys-
84. b. ab-
85. b. pro-
86. b. poly-

87. c. brady-
88. d. circum-
89. a. an-
90. b. bi-
91. c. hemi-
92. f. melan/o
93. a. tri-
94. h. erythr/o
95. g. quadri-
96. b. leuk/o
97. e. uni-
98. c. cyan/o
99. d. bi-
100. i. oligo-

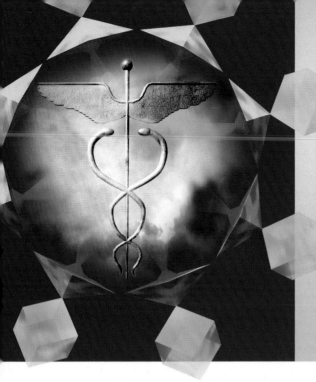

Health Care Records

COMMON RECORDS USED IN DOCUMENTING THE CARE OF A PATIENT

To put your knowledge of medical terminology into use, you need to see how this language is used in everyday communication about patients. Learning the common abbreviations, symbols, forms, and formats used in recording patient care will help you to comprehend medical record documentation.

The History and Physical

The record that serves as a cornerstone for patient care is the **history and physical (H&P)** (Fig. 2-1). The H&P documents the patient's medical history and findings from the physical examination. It is usually the first document to be generated when a patient **presents** for care, and is most often recorded at a new patient visit or as part of a consultation.

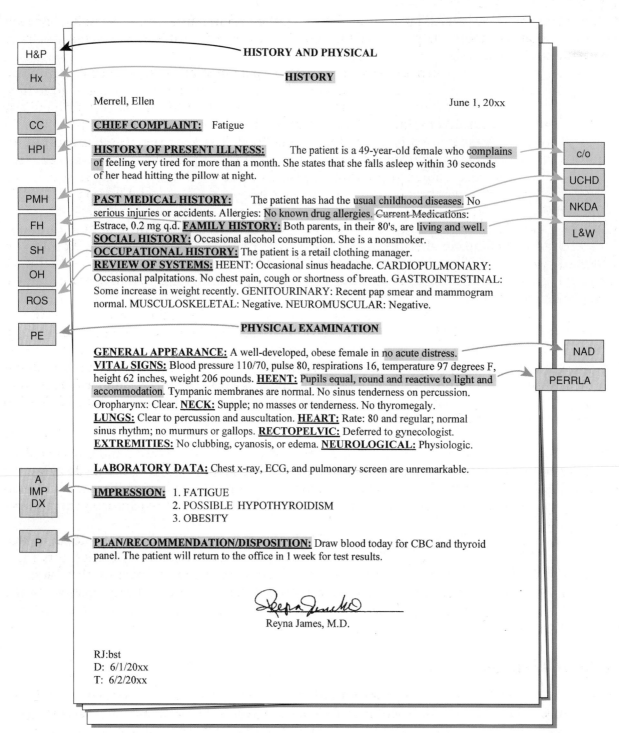

FIGURE 2-1 ■ History and physical (H&P).

The first portion of the H&P, the **history (Hx)**, documents **subjective information** from the patient's personal statement about his or her medical history and includes information regarding past injuries, illnesses, operations, defects, and habits. It begins with the **chief complaint (CC)**, the patient's reason for seeking medical care. The chief complaint is usually brief, and is often recorded in the patient's own words, which are indicated by quotation marks (e.g., CC: "flu"). Often, especially in handwritten notes, the abbreviation **c/o (complains of)** is used. Details of the complaint are documented in the **present illness (PI)**, or **history of present illness (HPI)**, noting the duration and severity of the complaint (i.e., how long the patient has had the complaint, and how bad it is). Notations about the patient's **symptoms (Sx)**, which are subjective evidence of illness, indicate what the patient is experiencing.

Information about the patient's **past history (PH)**, or **past medical history (PMH)**, is recorded next. This includes a record of information about the patient's past illnesses, starting with childhood, and it includes surgical operations, injuries, physical defects, medications, and allergies. The abbreviation **UCHD (usual childhood diseases)** is used here to record that the patient had all the "usual" or commonly contracted illnesses during childhood. The abbreviation **NKA (no known allergies)**, or **NKDA (no known drug allergies)**, indicates that the patient has had no known allergic reaction to a previously administered drug. The **family history (FH)** includes the state of health of the immediate family members (mother, father, and siblings), and the **social history (SH)** notes the patient's recreational interests, hobbies, and use of tobacco and drugs, including alcohol. A record of work habits that may involve health risks is included in the **occupational history (OH)**.

The history is complete after documenting the patient's answers to questions related to the **review of systems (ROS)**, or a **systems review (SR)**, a head-to-toe review of the functions of all body systems. This review makes it possible to evaluate other symptoms that may not have been previously mentioned.

After the subjective data are recorded, the provider begins a **physical examination (PE)**, or a **physical (Px)**, to obtain **objective information**, facts that can be seen or detected by testing. **Signs,** or objective evidence of disease, are documented, and selected diagnostic tests are performed or ordered when further evaluation is necessary. Several abbreviations are used to document the findings of the physical examination, such as **HEENT (head, eyes, ears, nose, and throat)**, **PERRLA (pupils equal, round, and reactive to light and accommodation)**, **NAD (no acute distress)**, and **WNL (within normal limits)**.

The identification of a disease or condition is recorded in the **impression (IMP)**, **diagnosis (Dx)**, or **assessment (A)**, which is made after the evaluation of all subjective and objective data. Often, when one or more diagnoses are in question, a **differential diagnosis** is made using the abbreviation **R/O (rule out)**. The possible conditions are identified, and further investigation, often involving diagnostic tests and procedures, is done to **rule out** or eliminate each suspect and to verify the final diagnosis.

Final notations include the health care provider's **plan (P)**, also called the **recommendation** or **disposition.** Here, the provider outlines strategies designed to remedy the patient's condition, including instructions to the patient and orders for medications, diagnostic tests, or therapies.

Often, physicians are required to dictate a current H&P before admitting a patient to the hospital (e.g., for elective surgery). When the patient is to have surgery, this report is often called a **preoperative H&P.**

Progress Notes

After the initial H&P is recorded, **progress notes** are used to document the patient's continued care. The **SOAP** method of documenting a patient's progress is most common. The letters represent the order in which progress is noted as each complaint or problem is addressed (Fig. 2-2):

S:	**Subjective**	that which the patient describes
O:	**Objective**	observable information (e.g., test results and blood pressure readings)
A:	**Assessment**	patient's progress and evaluation of the plan's effectiveness; any newfound problem or diagnosis is also noted here
P:	**Plan**	decision to proceed or to alter the plan strategy

Make flash cards and memorize the following abbreviations used in documenting a history and physical examination and progress notes so that you will recognize them in the health records found throughout this text.

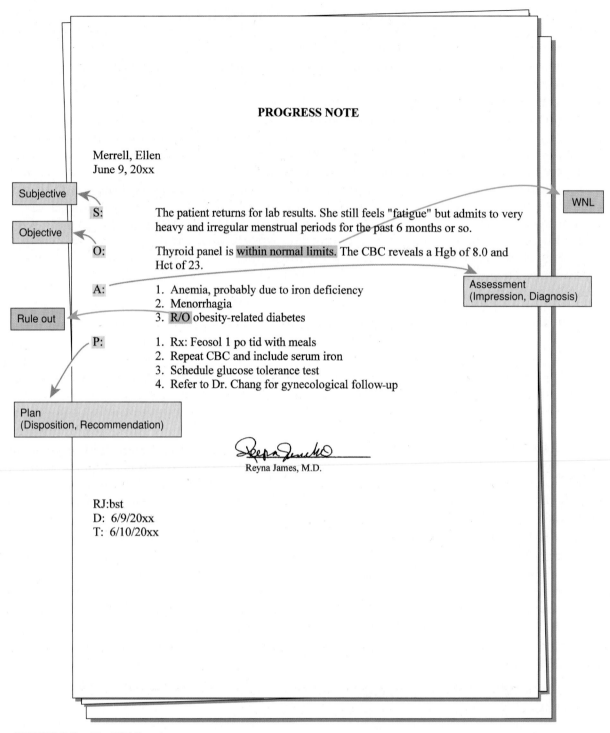

FIGURE 2-2 ■ SOAP note.

 ## Self-Instruction: Common Abbreviations Used in the History and Physical and Progress Notes

Study the following:

ABBREVIATION	EXPANSION
A	assessment
A&W	alive and well

ABBREVIATION	EXPANSION
CC	chief complaint
c/o	complains of
Dx	diagnosis
FH	family history
HEENT	head, eyes, ears, nose, and throat
H&P	history and physical
HPI, PI	history of present illness, present illness
Hx	history
IMP	impression
L&W	living and well
NAD	no acute distress
NKA, NKDA	no known allergies, no known drug allergies
O	objective information
OH	occupational history
P	plan (recommendation, disposition)
PE, Px	physical examination
PERRLA	pupils equal, round, and reactive to light and accommodation
PH, PMH	past history, past medical history
R/O	rule out
ROS, SR	review of systems, systems review
S	subjective information
SH	social history
Sx	symptom
UCHD	usual childhood diseases
WNL	within normal limits

 ## Programmed Review: Common Abbreviations Used in the History and Physical and Progress Notes

ANSWERS	REVIEW
history and physical	**2.1** The H&P, or _____ _____ _____, is the first document generated in the care of a patient. It is divided into
history	two categories: the Hx, or _____, which provides all
subjective	_____ information obtained from the patient, including his
physical	or her own perceptions; and the Px, or _____, or PE,
physical examination	or _____ _____, which records all
objective	_____ information that can be seen or verified by the examiner.

ANSWERS	REVIEW
chief complaint complains of present illness history, present illness symptoms	**2.2** The first thing that is noted in the history is the CC, or _____ _____, or what the patient c/o, or _____ _____. It is a brief explanation of why the patient is seeking medical care. Further details about the complaint are noted in the PI, or _____ _____, or HPI, or _____ of _____ _____, to report how long the patient has had the complaint and how bad it is. All subjective evidence of disease that the patient reports is noted as Sx, or _____.
past history, past medical history usual childhood diseases no known allergies, no known drug allergies	**2.3** The history continues by gathering information regarding past injuries, illnesses, operations, physical defects, medications, and allergies in the PH, or _____ _____, or PMH, or _____ _____ _____. UCHD notes that the patient had the _____ _____ _____, or commonly contracted illnesses during childhood. NKA, or _____ _____ _____, and NKDA, or _____ _____ _____ _____, indicate that the patient has had no known allergic reaction to a previously administered drug.
family history social history occupational history review of systems systems review	**2.4** "Father, age 58, mother, age 54, brother, age 32, all L&W" is an example of an FH, or _____ _____. Notes about recreational interests, hobbies, and use of tobacco and drugs, such as alcohol, are noted in the SH, or _____ _____. Work habits that may involve health risks are included in the OH, or _____ _____. The history is complete after the patient answers questions related to a review of the functions of the body systems in the ROS, or _____ _____ _____, or SR, _____ _____.
physical physical examination signs head, eyes, ears nose, throat, pupils	**2.5** The second portion of the H&P is the Px, or _____, or PE, or _____ _____. Objective evidence of disease, called _____, are documented, and selected tests are ordered and the findings recorded. Common abbreviations include HEENT, which means _____, _____, _____, _____, and _____; PERRLA, which means _____

ANSWERS	REVIEW
equal, round, reactive, light accommodation, within normal limits no acute distress	_____, _____, and _____ to _____ and _____; WNL, which means _____ _____ _____; and NAD, which indicates _____ _____ _____.
impression, diagnosis assessment rule out	**2.6** The identification of a disease or condition is recorded in the IMP, or _____; the Dx, or _____; or the A, or _____. This is made after all subjective and objective data are evaluated. When one or more diagnoses are in question, a differential diagnosis is made using the abbreviation R/O, or _____ _____.
plan recommendation, disposition	**2.7** An outline of strategies designed to remedy the patient's condition is noted in the provider's P, or _____, which is also called a _____ or _____. This section includes the provider's instructions to the patient and orders for medications, diagnostic tests, or therapies.
progress	**2.8** After the initial history and physical is recorded, _____ notes are used for further documentation of the patient's care. The letters "SOAP" represent the order in which progress is noted:
subjective	S: _____; that which the patient describes
objective	O: _____; observable information (e.g., test results or blood pressure readings)
assessment	A: _____; patient's progress and evaluation of the effectiveness of the plan
plan	P: _____; decision to proceed or alter the plan strategy

Hospital Records

The **history and physical** (Fig. 2-3) is often the first document entered into the patient's hospital record and is commonly required before elective admission for surgery. **Physician's orders** (Fig. 2-4) list the directives for care prescribed by the doctor who is attending to the patient. The **nurse's notes** (Fig. 2-5) and **physician's progress notes** (Fig. 2-6) chronicle the care throughout the patient's stay. In a difficult case, a specialist may be called in by the attending physician, and a **consultation report** is filed. If a surgical remedy is indicated, a narrative **operative report** (Fig. 2-7) is required of the primary surgeon. In this report, a detailed account of the operation is given, including the method of incision, technique, instruments used, types of suture, method of closure, and the patient's responses during the procedure and at the time of transfer to recovery. The anesthesiologist, who is in charge of life support during surgery, must file an **anesthesiologist's report**, which covers the anesthesia details, including the drugs used, the dose and time given, and the patient's vital status throughout the procedure. When a surgery or procedure involves a reasonable risk to the patient, an **informed consent** form must be signed by the patient to show that he or she has been advised of the risks and benefits of the proposed treatment as well as any alternatives. **Ancillary reports** note any additional procedures and therapies, including **diagnostic tests** and **pathology reports** (Fig. 2-8).

The final hospital document, which is recorded at the time of discharge, is the **discharge summary** (also termed the **clinical resume**, **clinical summary**, or **discharge abstract**). It is a summary of the patient's hospital care, including the date of admission, diagnosis, course of treatment, final diagnosis, and date of discharge (Fig. 2-9).

The sample medical records in Figures 2-3 through 2-9 chronicle the medical care of Carleen Perron, a 28-year-old woman who was seen in consultation by Dr. Patrick Rodden, an ear, nose, and throat (ENT) specialist who recommended a surgical remedy for the repeated infections she has had over the past 6 months.

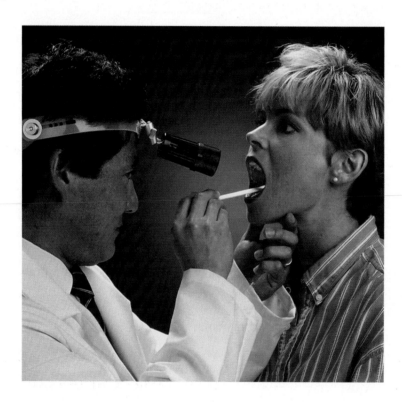

CENTRAL MEDICAL CENTER

211 Medical Center Drive • Central City, US 90000-1234 • PHONE: (012) 125-6784 • FAX: (012) 125-9999

PREOPERATIVE HISTORY AND PHYSICAL

HISTORY

DATE OF ADMISSION: June 3, 20xx

HISTORY OF PRESENT ILLNESS:
The patient is a 28-year-old white female with a chief complaint of frequent, recurrent, suppurative tonsillitis. She has had some eight infections over the last 6 months and is admitted at this time for elective tonsillectomy. The surgery has been discussed with the patient and family, including risks and complications. The patient's internist is C. Camarillo, M.D.

MEDICATIONS: None.

ALLERGIES: None known.

PAST SURGICAL HISTORY: None.

PAST MEDICAL HISTORY: UCHD (usual childhood diseases).

REVIEW OF SYSTEMS: CARDIOVASCULAR: No high blood pressure, heart murmurs, or shortness of breath. PULMONARY: No chronic lung disease; no asthma. GASTRO-INTESTINAL: No hepatitis. RENAL HISTORY: Negative for infections. ENDOCRINE: No diabetes or thyroid disease. MUSCULOSKELETAL: Negative for arthritis. HEMATOLOGIC: No history of anemia or bleeding tendencies.

FAMILY HISTORY: Grandmother has history of diabetes.

GYNECOLOGICAL HISTORY: Regular menses.

SOCIAL HISTORY: The patient is a nonsmoker. Alcohol use was denied, and drug use was denied.

(continued)

P. Rodden MD
PATRICK RODDEN, M.D.

JR:bst

D: 6/1/20xx
T: 6/2/20xx

HISTORY AND PHYSICAL Page 1	PT. NAME: PERRON, CARLEEN ID NO: 672894017 ROOM NO: ATT. PHYS: PATRICK RODDEN, M.D.

FIGURE 2-3 ■ Preoperative history and physical (H&P) submitted to the hospital before surgical admission.

CENTRAL MEDICAL CENTER

211 Medical Center Drive • Central City, US 90000-1234 • PHONE: (012) 125-6784 • FAX: (012) 125-9999

PREOPERATIVE HISTORY AND PHYSICAL

PHYSICAL EXAMINATION

VITAL SIGNS: Afebrile, alert, oriented, normotensive. Blood Pressure: 124/80. Pulse: 84. Respirations: 18.

HEENT: PERRLA (pupils equal, round, and reactive to light and accommodation). Tympanic membranes are clear. Light reflex is present. No sinus tenderness on percussion. Oropharynx: Clear. Hypertrophic tonsils. No exudates. Nasopharynx: No masses. Larynx: Clear.

NECK: Supple; no masses or tenderness. No cervical adenopathy.

LUNGS: Clear to percussion and auscultation.

HEART: Rate: 84 and regular; normal sinus rhythm; no murmurs or gallops.

RECTOPELVIC: Deferred.

EXTREMITIES: No peripheral edema. No ecchymoses.

NEUROLOGICAL: Physiologically intact.

IMPRESSION: Chronic, recurrent tonsillitis. The patient is admitted for an elective tonsillectomy.

P. Rodden MD
PATRICK RODDEN, M.D.

JR:bst
D: 6/1/20xx
T: 6/2/20xx

HISTORY AND PHYSICAL PAGE 2	PT. NAME: PERRON, CARLEEN
	ID NO: 672894017
	ROOM NO:
	ATT. PHYS: PATRICK RODDEN, M.D.

FIGURE 2-3 ■ *Continued.*

CENTRAL MEDICAL CENTER

211 Medical Center Drive • Central City, US 90000-1234 • PHONE: (012) 125-6784 • FAX: (012) 125-9999

DOCTOR: PLEASE STATE PERTINENT CLINICAL INFORMATION WHEN ORDERING RADIOLOGY PROCEDURES

WRITE WITH BALLPOINT INK PEN; PRESS HARD

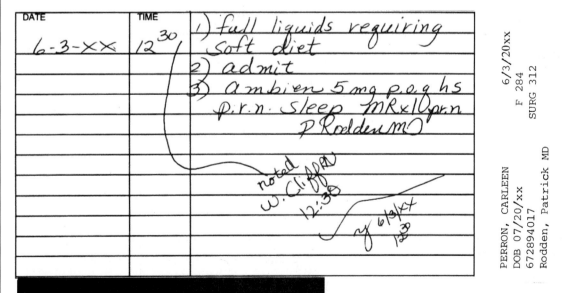

WRITE WITH BALLPOINT INK PEN; PRESS HARD

PHYSICIAN'S ORDERS

FIGURE 2-4 ▬ Physician's orders: orders written by the anesthesiologist and surgeon and noted by the nursing staff during the patient's surgical care.

CENTRAL MEDICAL CENTER

211 Medical Center Drive • Central City, US 90000-1234 • PHONE: (012) 125-6784 • FAX: (012) 125-9999

DOCTOR: PLEASE STATE PERTINENT CLINICAL INFORMATION WHEN ORDERING RADIOLOGY PROCEDURES

WRITE WITH BALLPOINT INK PEN; PRESS HARD

DATE	TIME	
6/3/xx	0800	T.O. Dr Rodden / G. Glen RN
		Consent for tonsillectomy
		P Rodden, MD
		RB noted
		P Carson RN
		6/3/xx
		0800 Q Good RN 6-3-xx 0830

6/3/20xx
F 284
SURG 312

PERRON, CARLEEN
DOB 07/20/xx
672894017
Rodden, Patrick MD

WRITE WITH BALLPOINT INK PEN; PRESS HARD

DATE	TIME	
6/3/xx	10:00	ANESTHESIA POST-OP CARE
		1.) MASK O₂ 8L/MIN
		2.) VS PER PACU ROUTINE
		3.) DILAUDID (HYDROMORPHONE)
		1mg IV q 15 min (max of 4mg/hr)
		4.) ZOFRAN 4mg IV q 4h p.r.n.
		nausea
		5.) MAY BE DISCONTINUED WHEN
		AWAKE & VS STABLE X 1h
		Robert Jung, MD
		noted 6-3-xx
		P Carson RN
		10¹⁰

6/3/20xx
F 284
SURG 312

PERRON, CARLEEN
DOB 07/20/xx
672894017
Rodden, Patrick MD

PHYSICIAN'S ORDERS

FIGURE 2-4 ■ *Continued.*

DATE	TIME	REMARKS
6/3/xx	0615	admitted & oriented to room 312. In no acute distress. VS stable. Afebrile NPO maintained. Condition stable K. Brown RN
6/3/xx	0800	To OR via gurney - awake & oriented accompanied by her mother - condition stable K. Brown RN
6/3/xx	1110	Returned from PAR drowsy but arouses easily. Skin warm & dry. Color pink - VS stable. Throat dry unable to take sips of water very well - no nausea - c/o severe sore throat medicated x̄ with IM pain medication with desired effect - mother very supportive & remains @ bedside. Using a bedpan but unable to urinate - IV infusing well K. Brown RN

**CENTRAL MEDICAL CENTER
PATIENT'S PROGRESS NOTES
GENERAL CARE & TREATMENT**

PT. NAME: PERRON, CARLEEN
ID NO: 672894017
ROOM NO: 312
ATT. PHYS: PATRICK RODDEN, M.D.

FIGURE 2-5 ■ Nurse's notes: a recording by the nursing staff of the patient's progress made during general care and treatment.

DATE	TIME	REMARKS
6/3/xx	10^05^	op note
		Chronic recurrent tonsillitis
		Procedure: tonsillectomy
		Surgeon: P. Rodden MD
		Anesthesiologist: Robert Jung MD
		Procedure tolerated well
		P Rodden MD
6/3/xx	12^20^	post op check
		VS stable
		C/o pain & poor p o fluid intake
		Will keep pt overnight for observation
		Plan to DC in am
		P Rodden MD
6/4/xx	08^00^	Doing much better – no bleeding
		taking liquids freely
		DC'd on fluids
		Given Rx for tylenol.
		RTO in 48h
		P. Rodden MD

CENTRAL MEDICAL CENTER **PHYSICIAN'S PROGRESS NOTES**	PT. NAME: PERRON, CARLEEN ID NO: 672894017 ROOM NO: 312 ATT. PHYS: PATRICK RODDEN, M.D.

FIGURE 2-6 ■ Physician's progress notes: physician's notations of the patient's progress throughout care.

CENTRAL MEDICAL CENTER

211 Medical Center Drive • Central City, US 90000-1234 • PHONE: (012) 125-6784 • FAX: (012) 125-9999

OPERATIVE REPORT

DATE OF OPERATION: June 3, 20xx.

PREOPERATIVE DIAGNOSIS: Chronic tonsillitis.

POSTOPERATIVE DIAGNOSIS: Frequent, recurrent tonsillitis.

SURGEON: Patrick Rodden, M.D.

ASSISTANT SURGEON: None

ANESTHESIOLOGIST: Robert Jung, M.D.

ANESTHESIA: General.

SURGERY PERFORMED: Tonsillectomy.

DESCRIPTION OF OPERATION: After general anesthesia induction, with intubation, the McGivor mouth gag and tongue retractor were utilized for exposure of the oropharynx. Local anesthetic consisting of 6 mL of 0.5% Xylocaine with 1:100,000 epinephrine was utilized. Tonsillectomy was carried out using dissection and air technique. The right tonsillectomy electrocoagulation Bovie suction was utilized for hemostasis. Examination of the nasopharynx was normal.

The patient tolerated the procedure well and went to the recovery room in good condition.

P. Rodden MD
PATRICK RODDEN, M.D.

JR:as
D: 6/3/20xx
T: 6/4/20xx

OPERATIVE REPORT	PT. NAME:	PERRON, CARLEEN
	ID NO:	672894017
	ROOM NO:	312
	ATT. PHYS:	PATRICK RODDEN, M.D.

FIGURE 2-7 ■ Operative report: surgeon's account of surgical procedure.

CENTRAL MEDICAL CENTER

211 Medical Center Drive • Central City, US 90000-1234 • PHONE: (012) 125-6784 • FAX: (012) 125-9999

PATHOLOGY REPORT

PATIENT: PERRON, CARLEEN
            28 Y (FEMALE)

DATE RECEIVED: June 3, 20xx.   DATE REPORTED: June 4, 20xx

GROSS:

Received are two tonsils each 2.5 cm in greatest diameter.

MICROSCOPIC:

The sections show deep tonsilar crypts associated with follicular lymphoid hyperplasia. No bacterial granules are seen.

DIAGNOSIS:

CHRONIC LYMPHOID HYPERPLASIA OF RIGHT AND LEFT TONSILS.

Mary Needham MD
MARY NEEDHAM, M.D.

MN:gds

D: 6/4/20xx
T: 6/5/20xx

FIGURE 2-8 ■ Pathology report.

COMMON DIAGNOSTIC TESTS AND PROCEDURES

Diagnostic tests and procedures are an integral part of patient care. Analyses of urine, stool, and blood specimens are found among the earliest recorded efforts to understand conditions of disease. The advance of technology has led to the development of many highly sophisticated laboratory tests, examples of which will be introduced in this text as they pertain to a specific body system. The two most common laboratory tests that are performed as part of a general health inquiry or to rule out a particular condition are the complete blood count, or CBC (*see* Fig. 6-7), and urinalysis, or UA (*see* Fig. 13-8).

It is valuable for health care professionals to recognize common diagnostic tests and procedures as well as the types of technology used to produce them.

	MEDICAL RECORDS USE
THAT CONDITION WHICH AFTER STUDY IS DETERMINED TO BE THE REASON FOR ADMISSION TO THE HOSPITAL PRINCIPAL DIAGNOSIS - *Chronic tonsillitis*	
	474.00
FINAL DIAGNOSIS - NO ABBREVIATIONS	*474.00*
Same	
SECONDARY DIAGNOSIS:	
—	
COMPLICATIONS AND/OR COMORBIDITY:	
—	
PRINCIPAL OPERATION/PROCEDURES(S)/TREATMENT RENDERED:	
Tonsillectomy	
SECONDARY OPERATIONS/PROCEDURES:	

CONDITION ON DISCHARGE *Stable*

☐ DISCHARGE INSTRUCTIONS   ☐ PRE-PRINTED INSTRUCTIONS GIVEN

MEDICATIONS *Tylenol*

PHYSICAL ACTIVITY *Bed rest*

DIET *full liquid*

FOLLOW-UP *office in 48 h*

DATE OF SUMMARY IF DICTATED:

DATE ADMITTED: *6/3/XX*		DATE DISCHARGED: *6/4/XX*		ATTENDING PHYSICIAN *P. Rodden*		M.D.

FOR MED. RECORDS USE ONLY	ASSEMBLY *SL*	ANALYSIS *Mc/37*	CODED *NZ*	KEYED *L4*	FINAL CHECK *S*		*06/03/20XX*
CONSULTANTS:				AA	/		
				DP	R48		
				SC	1212		

CENTRAL MEDICAL CENTER

**DIAGNOSIS RECORD/
DISCHARGE SUMMARY**

FIGURE 2-9 ■ Discharge summary (abstract): final report documented at time of discharge. This abstract is more commonly seen in outpatient surgery. See Medical Record 13-2 (page 662) for an example of a typical inpatient summary.

Diagnostic Imaging Modalities

Methods of diagnostic imaging have rapidly expanded since Wilhelm Roentgen discovered x-rays in 1885. By using x-rays, physicians and scientists could see through the body to produce images of the skeleton and other body structures. However, the radiation used to produce x-rays was found to be **ionizing**, a process that changes the electrical charge of atoms and has a possible effect on body cells. Overexposure to ionizing radiation can have harmful side effects (e.g., cancer), but over the years, researchers and scientists have found new ways to produce images that require significantly lower doses of radiation and minimize the risk to the patient.

Further advancement has led to the discovery and use of other imaging modalities (or techniques) that fall under the umbrella of the medical specialty known as **radiology**. Common ionizing modalities include radiography (x-ray), computed tomography (CT), and nuclear medicine. Common nonionizing modalities that present no apparent risk include magnetic resonance imaging (MRI) and sonography (US).

IONIZING IMAGING

Radiography (X-ray)

Radiography is an imaging modality that uses x-rays (ionizing radiation) to produce images of the body's anatomy for the diagnosis of a condition or impairment. An image is created when a small amount of radiation is passed through the body to expose a sensitive film. The image is called a **radiograph** (Fig. 2-10).

> **TERM TIP**
>
> In radiology, *-graph* is the preferred suffix used to refer to an x-ray record. It is taken by a **radiologic technologist**, also known as **radiographer,** and is interpreted or read by a **radiologist,** a physician specializing in the study of radiology.

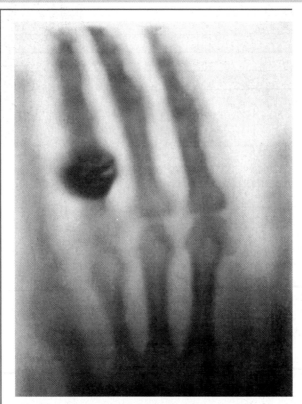

FIGURE 2-10 ■ First published radiograph, showing the hand and signet ring of Professor Roentgen's wife, produced on December 22, 1895.

ANSWERS	REVIEW
study of radiograph radiologic technologist radiologist cancer	meaning radiation, and the suffix *-logy,* meaning _____ ____. The x-ray image is called a _____. It is taken by a radiographer or _____ _____ and then interpreted by a physician who specializes in the study of radiology, called a _____. Ionizing radiation has an effect on body tissue, and overexposure can have harmful side effects, such as _____.
CT process of recording tomo computer	**2.10** The application of computer technology to medical imaging was first applied with the development of computed tomography, which is abbreviated as _____. *Tom/o,* a combining form meaning to cut, and the suffix *-graphy,* meaning _____ ____ _____, give clues to how the CT scanner operates. The scanner is used to take a series of cross-sectional or _____graphic x-ray films that are converted by a _____ into a three-dimensional picture on a screen.
radionuclide organ ionizing isotope gamma function	**2.11** Nuclear medicine imaging, or _____ _____ imaging, is another modality using _____ radiation. The technique involves the injection or ingestion of a radioactive _____ that emits gamma rays. An image is produced using a _____ camera to detect the distribution of the gamma rays. Radionuclide organ images are useful in determining the size, shape, location, and _____ of body organs.
risk, magnetic resonance imaging sonography, magnet radio soft sound recording	**2.12** Two major nonionizing imaging modalities have shown no apparent _____ to patients: MRI, or _____ _____ _____, and ultrasound, or _____. MRI uses a large _____ and _____waves to visualize anatomic structures within the body, especially _____ tissues. Sonography, from the combining form *son/o,* meaning _____, and the suffix *-graphy,* meaning a process of _____, uses high-frequency sound waves to produce body images.

COMMON MEDICAL RECORD TERMS RELATED TO DISEASE

The following terms related to disease are common in medical records. Learn them as a foundation on which you will build as your vocabulary expands.

 ## Self-Instruction: Disease Terms

Study the following:

TERM	MEANING
acute *ă-kyūt'*	sharp; having intense, often severe symptoms and a short course
chronic *kron'ik*	a condition that develops slowly and persists over a period of time
benign *bē-nīn'*	mild or noncancerous
malignant *mă-lig'nănt*	harmful or cancerous
degeneration *dē-jen-ĕr-ā'shŭn*	gradual deterioration of normal cells and body functions
degenerative disease *dē-jen'ĕr-ă-tiv di-zēz'*	any disease in which deterioration of the structure or function of tissue occurs
diagnosis *dī-ag-nō'sis*	determination of the presence of a disease based on an evaluation of symptoms, signs, and test findings (results) (*dia* = through; *gnosis* = knowing)
etiology *ē-tē-ol'ŏ-jē*	study of the cause of a disease (*etio* = cause)
exacerbation *ek-zas-ĕr-bā'shŭn*	increase in the severity of a disease, with aggravation of symptoms (*ex* = out; *acerbo* = harsh)
remission *rē-mish'ŭn*	a period in which symptoms and signs stop or abate
febrile *feb'ril*	relating to a fever (elevated temperature)
idiopathic *id'ē-ō-path'ik*	a condition occurring without a clearly identified cause (*idio* = one's own)
localized *lō'kăl-īzd*	limited to a definite area or part
systemic *sis-tem'ik*	relating to the whole body rather than to only a part
malaise *mă-lāz'*	a feeling of uneasiness or discomfort; often the first indication of illness
marked *markt'*	significant

TERM	MEANING
morbidity *mōr-bid'i-tē*	sick; a diseased state
mortality *mōr-tal'i-tē*	the state of being subject to death
prognosis *prog-nō'sis*	foreknowledge; prediction of the likely outcome of a disease based on the general health status of the patient along with knowledge of the usual course of the disease; often noted in one word (e.g., "Prognosis: good")
progressive *prō-gres'iv*	pertaining to the advance of a condition as the signs and symptoms increase in severity
prophylaxis *prō-fi-lak'sis*	a process or measure that prevents disease (*pro* = before; *phylassein* = guard)
recurrent *rē-kŭr'ĕnt*	to occur again; describes a return of symptoms and signs after a period of quiescence (rest or inactivity)
sequela *sē-kwel'ă*	a disorder or condition usually resulting from a previous disease or injury
sign *sīn*	a mark; objective evidence of disease that can be seen or verified by an examiner
symptom *simp'tŏm*	subjective evidence of disease that is perceived by the patient and often noted in his or her own words
syndrome *sin'drōm*	a running together; combination of symptoms and signs that give a distinct clinical picture indicating a particular condition or disease (e.g., menopausal syndrome)
noncontributory *non-kŏn-trĭ'byū-tōr-ē*	not involved in bringing on the condition or result
unremarkable *ŭn-rē-mark'ă-bel*	common; not out of the ordinary or significant

Programmed Review: Disease Terms

ANSWERS	REVIEW
sign	**2.13** Originating from the Latin word for a mark, the term _____ is used to describe objective evidence of disease that can be seen or verified by an examiner. The subjective evidence of disease that is
symptom	perceived by the patient is a _____. Many different signs
malaise	and symptoms manifest disease in the body. The term _____ is used to describe a patient who feels unwell. A patient is considered to
febrile	be _____ if he or she has an increase in body temperature, and
a	to be ___febrile if he or she is without a fever. Conditions limited to a
localized	definite area or part are considered to be _____, whereas those
systemic	that are _____ affect the whole body.

ANSWERS	REVIEW
acute chronic progressive exacerbation remission recurrent	**2.14** Some conditions have intense, often severe or _____ onset, whereas others that are _____ develop slowly and persist over time. A condition is considered to be _____ when the symptoms and signs advance with increased severity. A flare-up, or _____, occurs when there is an increase in the severity of symptoms. A condition is said to be in _____ during the period in which signs and symptoms have stopped. The term _____ describes a return of symptoms and signs after a period of inactivity.
not degeneration	**2.15** Degenerative disease occurs as a result of gradual deterioration of tissue with loss of function. The prefix *de-*, meaning from, down, or _____, is used in the term describing this process: _____.
etiology idiopathic malignant, benign marked	**2.16** The cause or _____ of a disease is often unknown. A condition is considered to be _____ when there is no clear identifying cause. If a condition is cancerous, it is termed _____, and if it is noncancerous, it is _____. A patient with significant weakness can be said to have _____ weakness.
diagnosis prognosis	**2.17** The doctor makes a _____ when naming a disease and gives a _____ when predicting its likely outcome.
prophylaxis	**2.18** A _____ is a process or measure that prevents disease.
syndrome	**2.19** The term describing a combination of symptoms and signs that give a distinct clinical picture is called a syndrome. For example, hot flashes, weight gain, mood swings, and irregular menstruation are signs and symptoms that indicate a woman is going through menopause, a condition known as menopausal _____.
sequela sequelae	**2.20** A sequel is something that follows something else. The medical term that refers to a disorder or condition that results from a previous disease or injury is called _____. The plural of sequela is _____.
noncontributory unremarkable	**2.21** When patient care data are not related to bringing on or causing a condition, they are said to be _____. Similarly, information that is not significant or out of the ordinary is said to be _____.

MEDICAL RECORD ABBREVIATIONS

The following table lists common medical abbreviations used in patient care documentation. They represent "acceptable" terms that are used extensively throughout this text. Remember that individual medical facilities provide their own list of acceptable terms and abbreviations that may not be used elsewhere. Memorize the terms and abbreviations from this list, and plan to adapt them to the variations you encounter.

ERROR PRONE ABBREVIATIONS AND SYMBOLS

Medical errors caused by illegible writing and misinterpretations of medical abbreviations and symbols have led health care agencies, such as the Joint Commission on Accreditation of Healthcare Organizations (JCAHO), to require that medical facilities publish lists of authorized abbreviations for use by all personnel, including a list of abbreviations and symbols that are unacceptable.

In this text, the abbreviations and symbols that have been identified as error prone are in **red** and the preferred use noted in brackets ([ ]). Depending on the medical facility, the use of these abbreviations and symbols may or may not be deemed to be acceptable; therefore, it is very important to study them so that you can properly interpret their meaning if they are used in a medical record. Those included on the official JCAHO "Do Not Use" list are marked by an asterisk (*).

 ## Self-Instruction: Medical Facilities and Patient Care Abbreviations

Study the following:

ABBREVIATION	MEANING
MEDICAL CARE FACILITIES	
CCU	coronary (cardiac) care unit
ECU	emergency care unit
ER	emergency room
ICU	intensive care unit
IP	inpatient (a registered bed patient)
OP	outpatient
OR	operating room
PACU	postanesthetic care unit
PAR	postanesthetic recovery
post-op or **postop**	postoperative (after surgery)
pre-op or **preop**	preoperative (before surgery)
RTC	return to clinic
RTO	return to office
PATIENT CARE	
Ⓑ	bilateral
BRP	bathroom privileges

ABBREVIATION	MEANING
CP	chest pain
DC or D/C	discharge, discontinue [spell out *discharge* or *discontinue*]
ETOH	ethyl alcohol
Ⓛ	left
Ⓡ	right
ⓜ	murmur
pt	patient
RRR	regular rate and rhythm
SOB	shortness of breath
Tr	treatment
Tx	treatment or traction
VS	vital signs
T	temperature
P	pulse
R	respiration
BP	blood pressure
Ht	height
Wt	weight
WDWN	well-developed and well-nourished
y/o or y.o.	year old
#	number or pound; if used before a numeral, it means number (e.g., #2 = number 2); if used after a numeral, it means pound (e.g., 150# = 150 pounds)
C	Celsius, centigrade
F	Fahrenheit
♀	female
♂	male
°	degree, or hour
↑	increased
↓	decreased
∅	none or negative
♀	standing
♀	sitting
○−	lying

Programmed Review: Medical Facilities and Patient Care Abbreviations

ANSWERS	REVIEW
emergency care unit ER outpatient inpatient intensive care unit operating room postanesthetic care unit	**2.22** The patient seeking emergency care is often seen in the ECU, or _____ _____ _____, most commonly known as the hospital _____. Depending on the circumstances of the accident or illness, the patient is treated as an OP, or _____, or is admitted as an IP, or _____. Sometimes, in a critical case, the patient is transferred directly to the ICU, or _____ _____ _____. If surgery is necessary, it is performed in the OR, or _____ _____, after which a period of recovery is made in the PACU, or _____ _____ _____.
patient treatment vital signs, temperature pulse, respiration, blood pressure bathroom privileges chest pain, shortness of breath return to office discharge	**2.23** While hospitalized, the pt, or _____, is seen by the attending physician and is cared for by the nursing staff. The doctor writes orders for all Tx, or _____, including how often the VS, or _____ _____ (T, or _____; P, or _____; R, or _____; and BP, or _____ _____), are to be taken and whether the patient is to have BRP, or _____ _____. The nurses must document the care and report any abnormal findings, such as CP, or _____ _____, and SOB, or _____ _____ _____. The doctor usually asks the patient to RTO, or _____ ____ _____ within a few days of DC, or _____, from the hospital.

PHARMACEUTICAL ABBREVIATIONS AND SYMBOLS

Pharmaceutical abbreviations and symbols are frequently used in documenting patient care. They are found throughout the medical record. Efficient medical record keeping and effective communication among health care workers depends on knowledge of commonly used pharmaceutical abbreviations and symbols.

Units of Measure

Both the metric and apothecary systems are used to express pharmaceutical units of measure. Consult your medical dictionary for a complete listing of units of measurement and conversion formulas.

THE METRIC SYSTEM

Metric is the most commonly used system of measurement in health care. It is a decimal system based on the following units:

meter (m)	length (39.37 inches)
liter (L)	volume (1.0567 U.S. quarts)
gram (g or gm)	weight (15.432 grains)

THE APOTHECARY SYSTEM

The apothecary system is a method of liquid and weight measures that was used by the earliest chemists and pharmacists. The liquid measure was based on one drop. The weight measure was based on one grain of wheat. Although the small apothecary measures are rarely used, the larger ones (e.g., fluid ounces) are still common.

 # Self-Instruction: Units of Measure

Study the following:

ABBREVIATION	MEANING
METRIC	
cc	cubic centimeter; 1 cc = 1 mL [use the metric equivalent *mL*]
cm	centimeter; 2.5 cm = 1 inch
g or **gm**	gram
kg	kilogram; equal to 1,000 grams or 2.2 pounds
L	liter
mg	milligram; equal to one-thousandth (0.001) of a gram
mL or **ml**	milliliter; equal to one-thousandth (0.001) of a liter
mm	millimeter; equal to one-thousandth (0.001) of a meter
cu mm or **mm³**	cubic millimeter
APOTHECARY	
fl oz	fluid ounce
gr	grain
gt	drop (*gutta* = drop)
gtt	drops
dr	dram; equal to 1/8 ounce
oz	ounce
lb or **#**	pound; equal to 16 ounces
qt	quart; equal to 32 ounces

ABBREVIATION	MEANING	LATIN†
a.m.	before noon	ante meridiem
b.i.d.	twice a day	bis in die
d	day	
h	hour	hora
h.s.	at the hour of sleep (bedtime) [spell out *bedtime*]	hora somni
noc.	night	noctis
p̄	after	post
p.c.	after meals	post cibum
p.m.	after noon	post meridiem
p.r.n.	as needed	pro re nata
q	every	quaque
q.d. (*)	every day [NEVER USE: spell out *every day* or *daily*]	quaque die
qh	every hour	quaque hora
q2h	every 2 hours	
q.i.d.	four times a day	quarter in die
q.o.d. (*)	every other day [NEVER USE: spell out *every other day*]	quaque altera die
STAT	immediately	statium
t.i.d.	three times a day	ter in die
wk	week	
yr	year	

MISCELLANEOUS

ABBREVIATION	MEANING	LATIN†
AD	right ear [spell out *right ear*]	auris dextra
ad lib.	as desired	ad libitum
amt	amount	
aq	water	aqua
AS	left ear [spell out *left ear*]	auris sinistra
AU	both ears [spell out *both ears*]	auris unitas
c̄	with	cum
NPO	nothing by mouth	non per os
OD	right eye [spell out *right eye*]	oculus dexter
OS	left eye [spell out *left eye*]	oculus sinister
OU	both eyes [spell out *both eyes*]	oculi unitas

ABBREVIATION	MEANING	LATIN†
per	by or through	
p.o.	by mouth	per os
PR	through rectum	per rectum
PV	through vagina	per vagina
Rx	recipe; prescription	
s̄	without	sine
Sig	label; instruction to the patient	signa
s̄s̄	one-half [spell out *one-half* or use *1/2*]	semis
wa	while awake	
x	times or for; *x6* means *six times* while *x2d* means *for two days*	
>	greater than [spell out *greater than*]	
<	less than [spell out *less than*]	
i̇	one (modified lowercase Roman numeral i)	
i̇i̇	two (modified lowercase Roman numeral ii)	
i̇i̇i̇	three (modified lowercase Roman numeral iii)	
i̇v	four (modified lowercase Roman numeral iv)	
I, II, III, IV, V, VI, VII, VIII, IX, X	uppercase Roman numerals from 1 to 10	

†The original Latin is supplied when applicable.

◆ Programmed Review: Common Prescription Abbreviations and Symbols

ANSWERS	REVIEW
before, ā	**2.32** Ante, meaning _____, is abbreviated as ____. Before
a.m., before meals	noon is abbreviated _____, and a.c. stands for _____ _____.
after, p̄	Post, meaning _____, is abbreviated ____. After noon is
p.m., after meals	abbreviated _____, and p.c. stands for _____ _____.
d, noc, h.s.	Day is abbreviated _____, night as _____, and bedtime as _____.
STAT	Some medications must be taken immediately or _____. If a

ANSWERS	REVIEW
as needed lib. NPO b.i.d., t.i.d. four, wk yr, q qh q2h, for x7d x10, every day every other day Do Not Use NEVER spelled	medication is taken p.r.n., it is taken _____ _____. If the patient can have as much as desired, the abbreviation is ad _____. Sometimes, such as before surgery, the doctor wants the patient to take nothing by mouth, or _____. Some drugs are taken twice a day, or _____; three times a day, or _____; or q.i.d., or _____ times a day. Week is abbreviated _____, and year is abbreviated _____. The abbreviation for every is ____. Every hour is abbreviated _____. Every 2 hours is abbreviated _____. The symbol x, meaning times or _____, is used to abbreviate the words "for seven days" as _____ and "ten times" as _____. Use of **q.d.**, meaning _____ _____, and of **q.o.d.**, meaning _____ _____ _____, are error-prone abbreviations on the official "____ _____ _____" list provided by JCAHO and should _____ be used. They should be _____ out instead.
I, II, III IV, V, VI, VII,VIII, IX, X ī, īī īīī, īv, s̄s̄ c̄, s̄	**2.33** Roman numerals 1 through 10 are written as ____, ____,____, ____, ____, ____, ____, ____, ____, and ____, respectively. The modified lowercase Roman numeral that means one is ____. Two is ____, three is _____, and four is _____. The symbol for one-half is _____, for with is ____, and for without is ____.
   OD OS OU AD, AS, AU spelled >, < spelled	**2.34** Sinister, meaning left, and dexter, meaning right, are referenced in abbreviations for the eyes and ears. The right eye, or oculus dexter, is abbreviated as _____. The left eye, or oculus sinister, is abbreviated _____. Oculi unitas, referring to both eyes, is abbreviated _____. Auris refers to ear. The right ear is abbreviated as _____, the left ear as _____, and both ears as _____. Because abbreviations related to the eyes and ears have been misinterpreted, it is recommended that they be _____ out instead. The symbols for greater than (__) and less than (__) have also been confused with each other, and it is recommended that they also be _____ out instead.

⬥CAUTION⬥ **Examples of Error-Prone Abbreviations and Symbols**

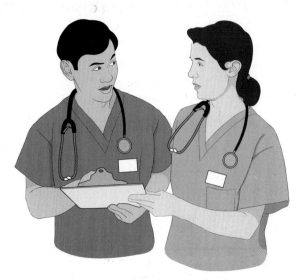

Listed below is a sampling of abbreviations and symbols deemed to be error-prone, including the risk for misinterpretation and the preferred use. Those included on the official "Do Not Use" List published by the Joint Commission of Accreditation on Healthcare Organizations (JCAHO) are marked by an asterisk (*).

A comprehensive list of error-prone abbreviations, symbols, and dose designations is available through the Institute for Safe Medication Practices (http://www.ismp.org/). JCAHO provides the official "Do Not Use" List on their website (http://www.jointcommission.org/).

ERROR PRONE ABBREVIATION	MEANING	RISK	PREFERRED USE
AD, AS, AU	right ear, left ear, both ears	mistaken as OD, OS, OU (right eye, left eye, both eyes)	spell out *right ear, left ear*, or *both ears*
OD, OS, OU	right eye, left eye, both eyes	mistaken as AD, AS, AU (right ear, left ear, both ears)	spell out *right eye, left eye*, or *both eyes*
cc	cubic centimeter	mistaken as units	use the metric equivalent *mL*
DC, D/C	discharge, discontinue	mistaken for "discontinue" when followed by medications prescribed at the time of discharge	spell out *discontinue* or *discharge*
h.s.	bedtime	mistaken as "half-strength"	spell out bedtime
q.d. (*)	every day	mistaken for q.i.d. when the period after the "q" is sloppily written to look like an "i"	**NEVER USE** – spell out *every day* or *daily*

ERROR PRONE ABBREVIATION	MEANING	RISK	PREFERRED USE
q.o.d. (*)	every other day	mistaken for q.d when the "o" is mistaken for a period	NEVER USE – spell out *every other day*
SC, SQ, sub-Q	subcutaneous	mistaken for SL (sublingual) or 5Q ("5 every")	spell out *subcut* or *subcutaneously*
s̄s̄	one half	mistaken as "55"	use *one-half* or ½
>, <	greater than, less than	mistaken for each other	spell out *greater than* or *less than*

RECORDING DATE AND TIME

The date and time are usually required in entries in a medical record. Always include the month, day of the month, and the year (e.g., 12/25/xx); sometimes eight digits are required (e.g., 01/08/20xx). Military time is often used to indicate the exact time of day (Fig. 2-16).

STANDARD	MILITARY	STANDARD	MILITARY
1:00 a.m.	0100 (zero one hundred hours)	1:00 p.m.	1300 (thirteen hundred hours)
2:00 a.m.	0200 (zero two hundred hours)	2:00 p.m.	1400 (fourteen hundred hours)
2:15 a.m.	0215 (zero two fifteen hours)	2:15 p.m.	1515 (fifteen hundred fifteen hours)
3:00 a.m.	0300 (zero three hundred hours)	3:00 p.m.	1500 (fifteen hundred hours)
4:00 a.m.	0400 (zero four hundred hours)	4:00 p.m.	1600 (sixteen hundred hours)
4:30 a.m.	0430 (zero four thirty hours)	4:30 p.m.	1630 (sixteen hundred thirty hours)
5:00 a.m.	0500 (zero five hundred hours)	5:00 p.m.	1700 (seventeen hundred hours)
6:00 a.m.	0600 (zero six hundred hours)	6:00 p.m.	1800 (eighteen hundred hours)
7:00 a.m.	0700 (zero seven hundred hours)	7:00 p.m.	1900 (nineteen hundred hours)
8:00 a.m.	0800 (zero eight hundred hours)	8:00 p.m.	2000 (twenty hundred hours)
9.00 a.m.	0900 (zero nine hundred hours)	9:00 p.m.	2100 (twenty-one hundred hours)
10:00 a.m.	1000 (ten hundred hours)	10:00 p.m.	2200 (twenty-two hundred hours)
11:00 a.m.	1100 (eleven hundred hours)	11:00 p.m.	2300 (twenty-three hundred hours)
12:00 p.m. (noon)	1200 (twelve hundred hours)	12:00 a.m. (midnight)	2400 (twenty-four hundred hours)

REGULATIONS AND LEGAL CONSIDERATIONS

Medical record documentation is created by physicians caring for the patient and by other authorized health care professionals involved with patient care. State, federal, and private accrediting agencies (e.g., JCAHO) provide specific guidelines that regulate how medical records are kept, including proper format for all forms, use of appropriate terminology and accepted abbreviations, protocol for personnel having access to records, and responsibilities for documentation.

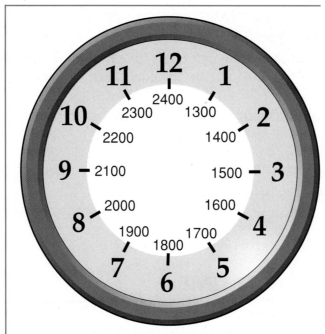

FIGURE 2-16 ■ Military and standard time.

CORRECTIONS

Sometimes mistakes are made when making an entry in a medical record. Careful clarification of the error is essential. The format may vary according to specific facility or organizational guidelines. Generally, if a mistake is made in a handwritten entry, it should be identified by drawing a single line through it, then writing the correction in the margin above or immediately after the mistake. Include the date and the initials of the person making the correction. The use of correction fluid is forbidden!

The medical record often becomes evidence in medical malpractice cases. Obliterations and signs of possible tampering can be construed as trying to withhold information or covering up negligent wrongdoing. Complete and accurate record keeping is your best defense against any possible legal action (Fig. 2-17).

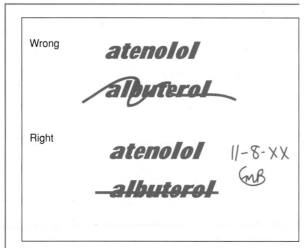

FIGURE 2-17 ■ Proper correction of a handwritten chart entry.

CHAPTER 2 ACRONYMS AND ABBREVIATIONS

ABBREVIATION	EXPANSION
A	assessment
ā	before
a.c.	before meals
AD	right ear
ad lib.	as desired
a.m.	before noon
amt	amount
aq	water
AS	left ear
AU	both ears
A&W	alive and well
Ⓑ	bilateral
b.i.d.	twice a day
BP	blood pressure
BRP	bathroom privileges
C	Celsius, centigrade
c̄	with
cap	capsule
CAT	computed axial tomography
CBC	complete blood count
CC	chief complaint
cc	cubic centimeter
CCU	coronary (cardiac) care unit
cm	centimeter
c/o	complains of
CP	chest pain
CT	computed tomography
cu mm or mm³	cubic millimeter
d	day
DC or D/C	discharge; discontinue
dr	dram
Dx	diagnosis
ECU	emergency care unit
ER	emergency room
ETOH	ethyl alcohol

ABBREVIATION	EXPANSION
F	Fahrenheit
FH	family history
fl oz	fluid ounce
g or gm	gram
gr	grain
gt	drop
gtt	drops
h	hour
HEENT	head, eyes, ears, nose, and throat
H&P	history and physical
HPI	history of present illness
h.s.	hour of sleep (bedtime)
Ht	height
Hx	history
ICU	intensive care unit
ID	intradermal
IM	intramuscular
IMP	impression
IP	inpatient
IV	intravenous
JCAHO	Joint Commission on Accreditation of Healthcare Organizations
kg	kilogram
L	liter
Ⓛ	left
lb	pound
L&W	living and well
ⓜ	murmur
mg	milligram
mL or ml	milliliter
mm	millimeter
MRA	magnetic resonance angiography
MRI	magnetic resonance imaging
NAD	no acute distress
NKA	no known allergies
NKDA	no known drug allergies
noc.	night

ABBREVIATION	EXPANSION
NPO	nothing by mouth
O	objective information
OD	right eye
OH	occupational history
OP	outpatient
OR	operating room
OS	left eye
OU	both eyes
oz	ounce
P	plan; pulse
p̄	after
PACU	postanesthetic care unit
p.c.	after meals
PE	physical examination
per	by or through
PERRLA	pupils equal, round, and reactive to light and accommodation
PH	past history
PI	present illness
p.m.	after noon
PMH	past medical history
p.o.	by mouth
post-op or postop	postoperative (after surgery)
PR	through rectum
pre-op or preop	preoperative (before surgery)
p.r.n.	as needed
pt	patient
PV	through vagina
Px	physical
q	every
q.d.	every day
qh	every hour
q2h	every two hours
q.i.d.	four times a day
q.o.d.	every other day
qt	quart
R	respiration

ABBREVIATION	EXPANSION
Ⓡ	right
R/O	rule out
ROS	review of systems
RRR	regular rate and rhythm
RTC	return to clinic
RTO	return to office
Rx	recipe; prescription
S	subjective information
$\bar{s}$	without
SC, SQ, or sub-Q	subcutaneous
SH	social history
Sig	label; instruction to the patient
SOB	shortness of breath
SR	systems review
$\bar{\bar{s}}s$	one-half
STAT	immediately
suppos	suppository
Sx	symptom
T	temperature
tab	tablet
t.i.d.	three times a day
Tr	treatment
Tx	treatment; traction
UA	urinalysis
UCHD	usual childhood diseases
US or U/S	ultrasound (sonography)
VS	vital signs
wa	while awake
WDWN	well-developed and well-nourished
wk	week
WNL	within normal limits
Wt	weight
x	times or for
x-ray	radiology
y/o or y.o.	year old
yr	year

Write out the expanded term or meaning for each abbreviation:

25. CC _____

26. OH _____

27. PR _____

28. BRP _____

29. PACU _____

30. PH _____

31. D/C _____

32. Sig: _____

33. ER _____

34. ICU _____

35. R/O _____

36. NPO _____

37. L&W _____

38. BP _____

39. AU _____

40. Sx _____

41. VS _____

42. ROS _____

43. pt _____

44. OD _____

45. H&P _____

46. Tx _____

47. Dx _____

48. HPI _____

Match the following terms with their meanings:

49. febrile	D	a.	period in which symptoms stop
50. syndrome	E	b.	probable outcome of a disease
51. chronic	G	c.	name of a disease based on history, examination, and testing
52. remission	A	d.	elevated temperature
53. etiology	J	e.	set of symptoms characteristic of a particular disease or condition
54. malignant	I	f.	increase in severity with aggravation of symptoms
55. prognosis	B	g.	developing slowly over time
56. diagnosis	C	h.	limited to a definite area or part
57. exacerbation	F	i.	cancerous
58. localized	H	j.	the study of the cause of a disease

Match each definition with its corresponding abbreviation or term:

59. the route of oral medications _____ D

60. place for surgery _____ H

61. as desired _____ F

62. progress note _____ I

63. after surgery _____ G

64. pound _____ J

65. as needed _____ B

66. by injection _____ C

67. before surgery _____ A

68. immediately _____ E

a. preop

b. p.r.n.

c. parenteral

d. p.o.

e. STAT

f. ad lib.

g. postop

h. OR

i. SOAP

j. #

Write the meaning for the following pharmaceutical phrases:

69. VS q h ×4h, then q2h _____

70. ī p.o. q.i.d. p.c. h.s. _____

71. aspirin (ASA) gr īī s̄s̄ _____

72. 650 mg p.o. q4h p.r.n. temp >101° _____

73. ī suppos PR q noc. p.r.n. _____

74. gt ī OU t.i.d. ×7d _____

75. cap īī p.o. STAT, then ī p.o. q6h _____

76. 15 mL p.o. q 6 h p.r.n. pain _____

Write the standard pharmaceutical abbreviations for the following:

77. one suppository in the vagina at bedtime

_____

78. two drops in left ear every 3 hours

_____

79. one capsule by mouth two times a day, morning and evening

_____

80. two by mouth immediately, then one by mouth every 6 hours

_____

81. five hundred milligrams by mouth four times a day for 10 days

_____

Give the meaning for the following error-prone abbreviations, identify why each abbreviation is commonly misinterpreted, and list the preferred term for each:

	Abbreviation	Meaning	Mistaken for	Preferred Term
82.	q.d.	_____	_____	_____
83.	q.o.d.	_____	_____	_____
84.	OS	_____	_____	_____

85. AD _____ _____ _____
86. AU _____ _____ _____
87. > _____ _____ _____
88. D/C _____ _____ _____
89. cc _____ _____ _____

Give the military times for the following standard times:

90. 1:00 a.m. _____0100_____
91. 2:30 p.m. _____1530_____
92. midnight _____2400_____
93. 1:00 p.m. _____1300_____
94. 7:00 p.m. _____1900_____
95. 4:50 p.m. _____1650_____

Match the following chart entries with the corresponding health record abbreviation :

96. works as a security officer ____E____ a. UCHD
97. advised to lower salt intake ____H____ b. HPI
98. father, age 88, L&W; mother, age 78, died, stroke ____G____ c. PE
99. quit smoking 2 years ago, drinks alcohol socially ____F____ d. CC
100. Diagnosis: tonsillitis ____I____ e. OH
101. c/o lower back pain ____B____ f. SH
102. pain in lower back for 2 weeks, worse at night ____D____ g. FH
103. no reaction to any previously administered drug ____J____ h. P
104. had all commonly contracted childhood diseases ____A____ i. A
105. Lungs: clear. Heart: regular rate and rhythm ____E____ j. NKA

From the following list of diagnostic imaging modalities, identify which use ionizing radiation and which use nonionizing radiation by circling the correct choice:

106. **computed tomography** ionizing radiation nonionizing radiation
107. **magnetic resonance imaging** ionizing radiation (nonionizing radiation)
108. **radiography** (ionizing radiation) nonionizing radiation
109. **radionuclide organ imaging** ionizing radiation nonionizing radiation
110. **sonography** ionizing radiation nonionizing radiation

Match the following imaging modalities with their descriptions:

111. computed tomography ____E____ a. standard x-rays
112. magnetic resonance imaging ____D____ b. gamma rays
113. radiography ____A____ c. ultrasound waves
114. radionuclide organ imaging ____B____ d. radio waves
115. sonography ____C____ e. three-dimensional x-rays

MEDICAL RECORD ANALYSIS

Medical Record 2-1

PROGRESS NOTE

CC: 37 y.o. ♂ c̄ diabetes c/o swelling of the Ⓡ foot and calf ×3d

S: There is no Hx of trauma, pain, SOB, or cardiac Sx, smoker ×12 yr, s̄s̄ pkg q.d., denies ETOH consumption
Meds: parenteral insulin q.d. NKDA

O: Pt is afebrile, BP 140/84, P 72, R 16, lungs are clear; abdomen is benign s̄ organomegaly; muscle tone and strength are WNL; there is swelling of the Ⓡ calf but s̄ erythema or tenderness

A: Edema of Ⓡ calf of unknown etiology

P: Schedule STAT vascular sonogram of lower extremities; pt is to keep the leg elevated × ii d, then RTC for follow-up and test results on Thursday (or sooner if ↑ edema, SOB, or CP)

QUESTIONS ABOUT MEDICAL RECORD 2-1

1. What is the sex of the patient?
   a. male
   b. female

2. Where was the patient seen?
   a. emergency room
   b. outpatient office or clinic
   c. inpatient hospital
   d. not stated

3. What is the condition of the patient's abdomen?
   a. shows signs of cancer
   b. internal organs are enlarged
   c. internal organs are not enlarged
   d. muscle tone and strength are weak

4. How much does the patient smoke per day?
   a. one package
   b. two packages
   c. half a package
   d. none; patient quit smoking 12 years ago

5. How is the patient's insulin administered?
   a. orally
   b. transdermally
   c. infusion through implant
   d. by injection

6. What is the cause of the patient's complaint?
   a. unknown
   b. fever
   c. shortness of breath
   d. trauma

7. When should the sonogram be performed?
   a. immediately
   b. within 2 days
   c. at the time of follow-up
   d. only if symptoms persist

8. How long should the patient's leg be kept elevated?
   a. 1 week
   b. 2 weeks
   c. 1 day
   d. 2 days

Medical Record 2-2

POSTOP MEDS FOR LAPAROTOMY

1. Vicodin (hydrocodone and acetaminophen), ī tab p.o. q3h p.r.n. mild pain, or īī tab p.o. q3h p.r.n. moderate pain
2. Demerol (meperidine), 100 mg IM q3h p.r.n. severe pain
3. Tylenol (acetaminophen), 650 mg p.o. q4h p.r.n. oral temp ↑ 100.4°F
4. Ambien (zolpidem), 10 mg p.o. h.s. p.r.n. sleep
5. Mylicon (simethicone), 80 mg, ī tab, chewed and swallowed q.i.d.
6. Dulcolax (bisacodyl) suppos, ī PR in a.m.

QUESTIONS ABOUT MEDICAL RECORD 2-2

1. How is the Demerol to be administered?
   a. by mouth
   b. within the vein
   c. under the skin
   d. within the muscle

2. What is the Sig: on the Mylicon?
   a. one every other day
   b. one twice a day
   c. one three times a day
   d. one four times a day

3. What is the Sig: on the Dulcolax?
   a. one suppository in the rectum in the morning
   b. one suppository taken orally before noon
   c. two suppositories before breakfast
   d. one suppository as needed in the morning

4. When should the Ambien be administered?
   a. each night
   b. at bedtime
   c. as needed
   d. every hour

5. What are the instructions for administering Vicodin in the case of moderate pain?
   a. one tablet every three hours
   b. three tablets every hour
   c. two tablets every three hours
   d. three tablets every three hours

6. How should Tylenol be administered?
   a. one dose every four hours as needed
   b. one dose every four hours only if patient has a temperature of 100.4°F or higher
   c. one dose every four hours as long as the patient's temperature does not go over 100.4°F
   d. one dose every hour up to four per day

7. Laparotomy refers to which of the following?
   a. a puncture in the abdomen
   b. excision of the stomach
   c. a puncture of the stomach
   d. an incision in the abdomen

Medical Record 2-3

FOR ADDITIONAL STUDY

Michael Marsi has had chronic health problems in the last 2 years and has been seeing Dr. Spaulding, his personal physician, regularly during recent months. Dr. Spaulding uses problem-orientated medical records and writes a new SOAP progress note at each patient visit. Mr. Marsi has come to see Dr. Spaulding today because he feels worse than usual. Medical Record 2-3 is the progress note from today's appointment. Dr. Spaulding handwrote it herself during the patient's visit.

Read Medical Record 2-3 (page 96) for Michael Marsi, then write your answers to the following questions in the spaces provided.

QUESTIONS ABOUT MEDICAL RECORD 2-3

1. How old is Mr. Marsi? _____

2. Where was the treatment rendered? _____

3. List the three elements of the patient's complaint.

   a. _____

   b. _____

   c. _____

4. In your own words, not using medical terminology, briefly summarize Mr. Marsi's history:

   _____

   _____

   _____

5. Which of the following is not mentioned at all in this history?

   a. the prescription medication Mr. Marsi takes

   b. Mr. Marsi's smoking habit

   c. Mr. Marsi's activity level at work

   d. Mr. Marsi's consumption of alcohol

6. Dr. Spaulding and Mr. Marsi talked at length about Mr. Marsi's symptoms and how they have changed recently, and then Dr. Spaulding examined Mr. Marsi. List three objective findings that she noted in this examination.

   a. _____

   b. _____

   c. _____

7. Dr. Spaulding's assessment is that Mr. Marsi has _____

   _____.

   However, she also wants to make sure Mr. Marsi does not have _____

   _____.

8. Dr. Spaulding's treatment plan involves four areas. List the specific plan(s) for each of these.

   a. Diagnostic tests ordered: _____

   _____

   b. Instruct the patient to change his personal habits (and how): _____

   _____

   _____

   _____

   c. Drug prescribed (including how much and when): _____

   _____

   d. Future diagnostic check and/or action to take: _____

   _____

9. When is Dr. Spaulding expecting to see Mr. Marsi again? _____

   _____

Medical Record 2-3

FOR ADDITIONAL STUDY

PROGRESS NOTES

Patient Name: _Marsi, Michael_

DATE	FINDINGS
2-3-xx	CC 51 y.o. ♂ c/o dizziness x3wk and headaches 5-6 xTwk. Today he woke c̄ numbness in (L) leg and hand
	S Hx of ↑BP x 4yrs Smoker x 20 yrs – 1 pkg/day ⊖ CP ⊖ SOB. occipital headaches in a.m. moderate fat diet – 3 beers q̄ noc. MEDS: Dyazide ī daily NKDA
	O BP 150/100 (R) arm L̄ Ht 68" Wt 198# T 98.7° P 76 R 15 Heart RRR s̄ (m) Lungs clear HEENT – WNL
	A Hypertension (HTN) R/O congestive heart failure (CHF)
	P Chest x-ray (CXR) and electrocardiogram (ECG) today ↓ ETOH to ī beer q̄ noc. DC smoking Rx: Vasotec (enalapril) 5 mg tab ī p.o. daily ↑ exercise to 3x wk for 20-30 minutes Stop if CP, SOB, or dizzy ↓ fat and cholesterol in diet recheck BP in ī wk RTO sooner if CP, SOB or dizzy
	JR Spaulding MD

ANSWERS TO PRACTICE EXERCISES

1. H&P
2. Hx
3. CC
4. HPI
5. PMH
6. FH
7. SH
8. OH
9. ROS
10. PE
11. A, IMP, or Dx
12. P
13. c/o
14. UCHD
15. NKDA
16. L&W
17. NAD
18. PERRLA
19. subjective
20. objective
21. WNL
22. assessment (impression, diagnosis)
23. rule out
24. plan (disposition, recommendation)
25. chief complaint
26. occupational history
27. per rectum
28. bathroom privileges
29. postanesthetic care unit
30. past history
31. discontinue or discharge
32. instructions to patient
33. emergency room
34. intensive care unit
35. rule out
36. nothing by mouth
37. living and well
38. blood pressure
39. both ears
40. symptom
41. vital signs
42. review of systems
43. patient
44. right eye
45. history and physical
46. treatment or traction
47. diagnosis

48. history of present illness
49. d
50. e
51. g
52. a
53. j
54. i
55. b
56. c
57. f
58. h
59. d
60. h
61. f
62. i
63. g
64. j
65. b
66. c
67. a
68. e
69. vital signs every hour for 4 hours, then every 2 hours
70. one by mouth, four times a day, after meals and at bedtime
71. two and one-half grains of aspirin
72. 650 milligrams by mouth every 4 hours as needed for temperature greater than 101°F
73. one suppository through the rectum every night as needed
74. one drop in both eyes three times a day for 7 days
75. two capsules by mouth immediately, then one by mouth every 6 hours
76. fifteen milliliters by mouth every six hours as needed for pain
77. suppos i PV h.s. or i suppos PV h.s.
78. gtt ii AS q3h or ii gtt AS q3h

79. cap i p.o. b.i.d. a.m. and p.m. or i cap p.o. b.i.d. a.m. and p.m.
80. ii p.o. STAT, then i p.o. q6h
81. 500 mg p.o. q.i.d. x10d
82. every day, mistaken for q.i.d. (four times a day); spell out "every day" or "daily"
83. every other day, mistaken for q.d. (daily) or q.i.d. (four times a day); spell out "every other day"
84. left eye, mistaken for opposite eye or ears; spell out "left eye"
85. right ear, mistaken for opposite ear or eyes; spell out "right ear"
86. both ears, mistaken for both eyes or right or left ear/eye; spell out "both ears"
87. greater than, mistaken as less than; spell out "greater than"
88. discharge or discontinue, mistaken for each other; spell out either "discharge" or "discontinue"
89. cubic centimeter, mistaken as "units"; use metric equivalent "ml" or "mL"
90. 0100 hours
91. 1430 hours
92. 2400 hours
93. 1300 hours
94. 1900 hours
95. 1650 hours
96. e
97. h
98. g
99. f
100. i
101. d

102. b
103. j
104. a
105. c
106. ionizing radiation

107. nonionizing radiation
108. ionizing radiation
109. ionizing radiation
110. nonionizing radiation
111. e

112. d
113. a
114. b
115. c

ANSWERS TO MEDICAL RECORD ANALYSIS

Medical Record 2-1: Progress Note

1. a   2. b   3. c   4. c   5. d   6. a   7. a   8. d

Medical Record 2-2: Postop Meds for Laparotomy

1. d   2. d   3. a   4. b   5. c   6. b   7. d

Medical Record 2-3: For Additional Study

See CD-ROM for answers.

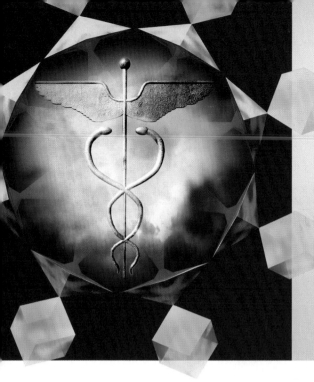

Integumentary System

INTEGUMENTARY SYSTEM OVERVIEW

The integumentary system (Fig. 3-1) consists of the following tissues:

- Skin (also called the **integument**)
- Hair
- Nails
- Sweat glands
- Sebaceous glands

There are four functions of the integumentary system:

- Protects the body from injury
- Protects the body from intrusion of microorganisms
- Helps to regulate body temperature
- Houses receptors for the sense of touch, including pain and sensation

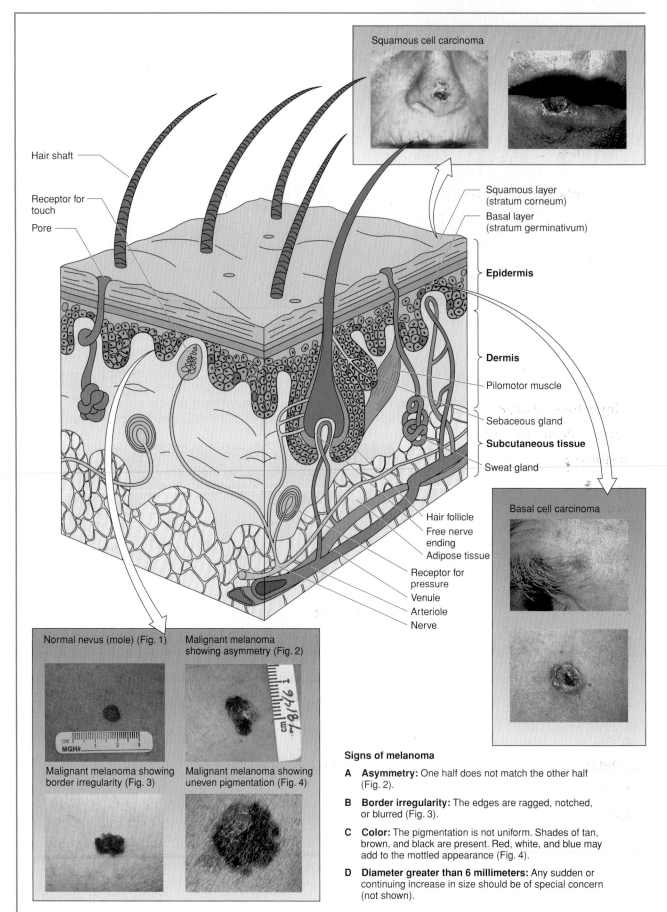

Squamous cell carcinoma

Hair shaft

Receptor for touch

Pore

Squamous layer (stratum corneum)

Basal layer (stratum germinativum)

Epidermis

Dermis

Pilomotor muscle

Sebaceous gland

Subcutaneous tissue

Sweat gland

Hair follicle
Free nerve ending
Adipose tissue
Receptor for pressure
Venule
Arteriole
Nerve

Basal cell carcinoma

Normal nevus (mole) (Fig. 1)

Malignant melanoma showing asymmetry (Fig. 2)

Malignant melanoma showing border irregularity (Fig. 3)

Malignant melanoma showing uneven pigmentation (Fig. 4)

Signs of melanoma

A **Asymmetry:** One half does not match the other half (Fig. 2).

B **Border irregularity:** The edges are ragged, notched, or blurred (Fig. 3).

C **Color:** The pigmentation is not uniform. Shades of tan, brown, and black are present. Red, white, and blue may add to the mottled appearance (Fig. 4).

D **Diameter greater than 6 millimeters:** Any sudden or continuing increase in size should be of special concern (not shown).

FIGURE 3-1 ■ The skin.

The skin has three layers:

❋ The **epidermis** consists of several layers of stratified squamous (scale-like) epithelium.

    1. Cells are produced in the innermost (basal) layer, moving the older cells up toward the surface.

    2. Cells that are pushed up flatten, fill with a hard protein substance called **keratin**, and die.

    3. Layers of packed dead cells accumulate in the outermost (squamous) layer, where they are sloughed off.

❋ The **dermis,** which is the connective tissue layer, contains blood vessels, nerves, and other structures (*see* Fig. 3-1). Collagen fibers make the skin tough and elastic.

❋ The **subcutaneous layer** below the dermis is composed of loose connective tissue and adipose (fatty) tissue.

Self-Instruction: Combining Forms

Study the following:

COMBINING FORM	MEANING
adip/o, lip/o, steat/o	fat
derm/o, dermat/o, cutane/o	skin
erythr/o	red
hidr/o	sweat
hist/o, histi/o	tissue
kerat/o	hard
leuk/o	white
melan/o	black
myc/o	fungus
onych/o	nail
plas/o	formation
purpur/o	purple
scler/o	hard
seb/o	sebum (oil)
squam/o	scale
trich/o	hair
xanth/o	yellow
xer/o	dry

Programmed Review: Combining Forms

ANSWERS	REVIEW
skin dermatology dermatologist skin under	**3.1** *Derm/o* and *dermat/o* are Greek combining forms meaning _____. The medical field specializing in the study of the skin is _____. The physician who specializes in the study and treatment of the skin is called a _____. *Cutane/o* is a Latin combining form meaning _____. Subcutaneous therefore pertains to _____ the skin.
cell tissue, histology production tissue	**3.2** Recall that *cyt/o* means _____. Cells with specialized functions combine to form varying types of tissue. *Hist/o* is a combining form meaning _____. The study of tissues is called _____. Histiogenic pertains to the origin or _____ of _____.
plas/o faulty condition of dysplasia	**3.3** The combining form meaning formation is _____. *Dys-* is a prefix meaning painful, difficult, or _____, and *-ia* refers to a _____ _____. Therefore, the term used to describe a condition of (faulty) abnormal development of tissue is _____.
upon epi scale, pertaining to squamous	**3.4** The prefix *epi-*, meaning _____, is used in naming the outer tissue layer of the skin, called the _____dermis. The combining form *squam/o* means _____. The suffix *-ous* means _____ _____. The flat, scale-like cells of the epidermis are aptly called _____ cells.
black darker cells	**3.5** The pigment called melanin is found in the basal layer of the epidermis. The combining form *melan/o* means _____, and people with more melanin have _____ skin. Melanocytes are the _____ in the basal layer that produce melanin.
Kerat/o skin keratin	**3.6** _____ is the combining form that means hard. Keratin is the hard protein substance found in the basal layer of the _____. Keratosis is a condition characterized by an overgrowth of cells having a large amount of _____.
trich/o hair	**3.7** Hair follicles are found in the dermis layer of the skin. The combining form for hair is _____. Combined with the suffix meaning rupture, trichorrhexis is the term describing _____ that is broken or split.

ANSWERS	REVIEW
sebum, seb/o sebum	**3.8** Sebaceous glands, which open to the hair follicles in the skin, produce _____ (oil). The combining form is _____. Seborrhea refers to an overproduction of _____ by these glands.
water sweat hidro	**3.9** *Hydr/o*, a combining form meaning _____, stems from the Greek word hydros. A similar component, *hidr/o*, stemming from the Greek word hidros, means _____. The formation of sweat is termed _____poiesis.
fungus myc/o	**3.10** Mycosis refers to any condition caused by a _____. The term was coined using the combining form _____.
nail, softening onycho fungus or fungal	**3.11** The combining form *onych/o* refers to the fingernail or toe_____. Recall that *-malacia* is a suffix meaning _____. An abnormal softening of the nails is therefore called _____malacia. Onychomycosis refers to a _____ infection (condition) of the nails.
lip/o fat adip/o sub fat, inflammation, fat	**3.12** Several combining forms refer to body fat. The term lipid is from the combining form _____. Liposuction therefore refers to the procedure for suctioning _____ from body tissues. The adjective adipose, meaning fatty, is from the combining form _____. Adipose tissue is found below the dermis in the _____cutaneous layer of the skin. A third combining form, *steat/o*, also refers to _____. Steatitis refers to an _____ of _____.
white leuko	**3.13** The combining form *leuk/o* means _____. It is used to form the term for a partial or total absence of pigment in the skin, known as _____derma.
erythr/o red red skin	**3.14** The combining form _____ means red. Erythema therefore refers to skin that is _____. Erythroderma is another term referring to _____ _____.
purple purple blood	**3.15** The meaning of the combining form *purpur/o* is easy to remember, because it sounds like the color _____. Purpuric lesions are _____ because they result from hemorrhages, or the bursting forth of _____ into the skin.
xanth/o yellow	**3.16** The combining form _____ refers to the color yellow. A xanthoma is a _____ skin tumor.
skin xer/o, dry	**3.17** Xeroderma is a term meaning dry _____. The combining form for dry is _____. Xerosis is a condition of pathologically _____ skin.

Self-Instruction: Anatomic Terms

Study the following:

TERM	MEANING
epithelium *ep-i-thē' lē-ŭm*	cells covering external and internal surfaces of the body
epidermis *ep-i-derm' is*	thin outer layer of the skin
squamous cell layer *skwā' mŭs sel lā'ĕr*	flat, scale-like epithelial cells comprising the outermost epidermis
basal layer *bā' săl lā'ĕr*	deepest layer of epidermis
melanocyte *mel'ă-nō-sīt*	cell in the basal layer that gives color to the skin
melanin *mel'ă-nin*	dark brown to black pigment contained in melanocytes
dermis *dĕr' mis*	dense, fibrous connective tissue layer of the skin, also known as corium
sebaceous glands *sē-bā' shŭs glanz*	oil glands in the skin
sebum *sē' bŭm*	oily substance secreted by the sebaceous glands
sudoriferous glands *sŭ-dō-rif'ĕr-ŭs glanz*	sweat glands (*sudor* = sweat; *ferre* = to bear)
subcutaneous layer *sŭb-kyū-tā'nē-ŭs lā'er*	connective and adipose tissue layer just under the dermis
collagen *kol'ă-jen*	protein substance in skin and connective tissue (*koila* = glue; *gen* = producing)
hair *hār*	outgrowth of the skin composed of keratin
nail *nāl*	outgrowth of the skin, composed of keratin, at the end of each finger and toe
keratin *ker'ă-tin*	hard protein material found in the epidermis, hair, and nails

 ## Programmed Review: Anatomic Terms

ANSWERS	REVIEW
epithelium upon, -ium	**3.18** The name for the cells covering the external and internal surfaces of the body is the _____. Recall that the prefix *epi-* means _____, and that the suffix _____ means structure or tissue.

ANSWERS	REVIEW
epidermis, epi- skin dermis	**3.19** The thin, outer cellular layer of the skin is called the _____, which is formed from the prefix _____ and the combining form *derm/o*, meaning _____. The middle layer of skin is called the _____ and is where nerves and blood vessels are located.
squamous scale	**3.20** The _____ cell layer is the outermost layer of the epidermis. The combining form *squam/o* means _____, and this layer is so named because the dead skin cells in the outermost layer scale off.
basal pertaining to epidermis	**3.21** Below the squamous cell layer is the _____ cell layer. Recall that the suffix *-al* means _____ ____. This layer is therefore the deepest (or base) layer of the _____.
cyt/o melanin black	**3.22** Recall that the combining form for cell is _____. A melanocyte therefore is a cell containing _____, the dark pigment of the skin. *Melan/o* means _____.
sebum adjective dermis	**3.23** The sebaceous glands produce _____, an oily substance. The suffix *-ous* is added to a combining form to create an _____. These glands are located in the skin layer called the _____.
sudoriferous dermis	**3.24** The sweat glands are called the _____ glands, from *sudor* (sweat) and *ferre* (to bear). They are located in the skin layer called the _____.
subcutaneous sub- skin	**3.25** Beneath the dermis is the _____ layer. The prefix _____ means below or under, and the combining form *cutane/o* means _____.
collagen	**3.26** Formed from the roots *koila* (glue) and *gen* (producing), _____ is a protein substance found in skin and connective tissue.
keratin nails hard	**3.27** Hair is an outgrowth of the skin composed of _____. The _____ on the fingers and toes also are composed of keratin. The combining form *kerat/o* means _____.

Self-Instruction: Symptomatic Terms (Primary and Secondary Lesions)

Study the following:

TERM	MEANING
lesion (Fig. 3-2) *lē'zhŭn*	an area of pathologically altered tissue; the two types of lesions are primary and secondary

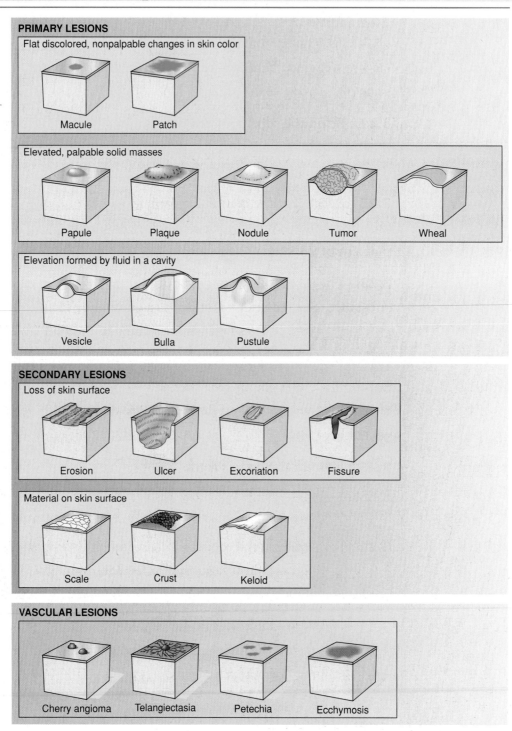

FIGURE 3-2 ■ Types of primary, secondary, and vascular lesions.

TERM	MEANING
PRIMARY LESIONS	
primary lesions *prī'mār-ē lē'zhŭnz*	lesions arising from previously normal skin
Flat, Nonpalpable Changes in Skin Color	
macule or **macula** (Fig. 3-3, A) *mak'yūl*	a flat, discolored spot on the skin up to 1 cm across (e.g., a freckle)
patch (Fig. 3-3, B) *pach*	a flat, discolored area on the skin larger than 1 cm (e.g., vitiligo)
Elevated, Palpable Solid Masses	
papule (Fig. 3-3, C) *pap'yūl*	a solid mass on the skin up to 0.5 cm in diameter (e.g., a nevus [mole])
plaque (Fig. 3-3, D) *plak*	a solid mass greater than 1 cm in diameter and limited to the surface of the skin
nodule (Fig. 3-3, E) *nod'yūl*	a solid mass greater than 1 cm that extends deeper into the epidermis
tumor (Fig. 3-3, F) *tū'mŏr*	a solid mass larger than 1–2 cm

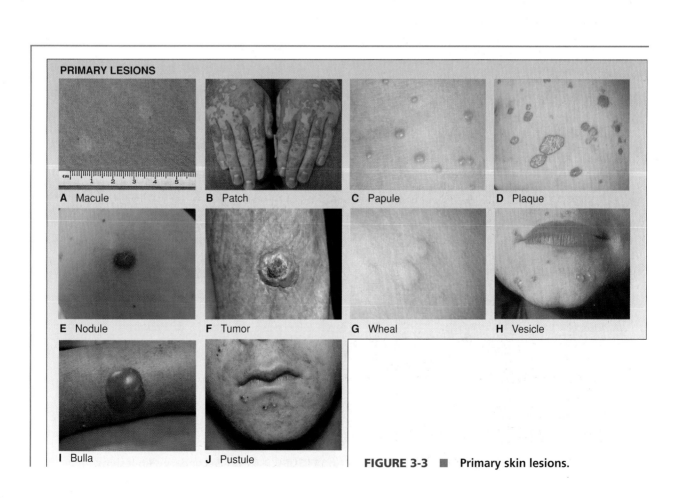

PRIMARY LESIONS

A Macule B Patch C Papule D Plaque
E Nodule F Tumor G Wheal H Vesicle
I Bulla J Pustule

FIGURE 3-3 ■ Primary skin lesions.

TERM	MEANING
wheal (Fig. 3-3, G) *wēl*	an area of localized skin edema (swelling) (e.g., a hive)

Elevations Formed by Fluid Within a Cavity

TERM	MEANING
vesicle (Fig. 3-3, H) *ves'ĭ-kĕl*	little bladder; an elevated, fluid-filled sac (blister) within or under the epidermis up to 0.5 cm in diameter (e.g., a fever blister)
bulla (Fig. 3-3, I) *bul'ă*	a blister larger than 0.5 cm (e.g., a second-degree burn) (*bulla* = bubble)
pustule (Fig. 3-3, J) *pŭs'tyūl*	a pus-filled sac (e.g., a pimple)

SECONDARY LESIONS

TERM	MEANING
secondary lesions *sek'ŏn-dār-ē lē'zhŭnz*	lesions that result in changes in primary lesions

Loss of Skin Surface

TERM	MEANING
erosion (Fig. 3-4, A) *ē-rō'zhŭn*	gnawed away; loss of superficial epidermis, leaving an area of moisture but no bleeding (e.g., area of moisture after rupture of a vesicle)
ulcer (Fig. 3-4, B) *ŭl'sĕr*	an open sore on the skin or mucous membrane that can bleed and scar; sometimes accompanied by infection (e.g., decubitus ulcer)
excoriation (Fig. 3-4, C) *eks-kō'rē-ā'shŭn*	a scratch mark
fissure (Fig. 3-4, D) *fish'ŭr*	a linear crack in the skin

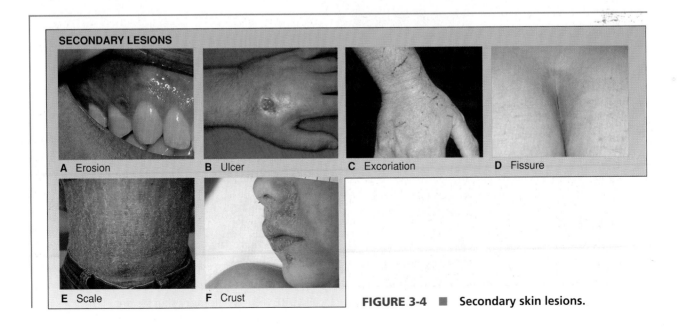

SECONDARY LESIONS

A Erosion B Ulcer C Excoriation D Fissure

E Scale F Crust

FIGURE 3-4 ■ Secondary skin lesions.

TERM	MEANING
Material on Skin Surface	
scale (Fig. 3-4, E) *skāl*	a thin flake of exfoliated epidermis (e.g., dandruff)
crust (Fig. 3-4, F) *krŭst*	a dried residue of serum (body liquid), pus, or blood on the skin (e.g., as seen in impetigo)

VASCULAR LESIONS

TERM	MEANING
vascular lesions *vas'kyūl-lăr lē'zhŭnz*	lesions of a blood vessel
cherry angioma (Fig. 3-5, A) *chār'ē an-jē-ō'mă*	a small, round, bright red blood vessel tumor on the skin, often on the trunk of the elderly
telangiectasia (Fig. 3-5, B) *tel-an'jē-ek-tā'zē-ă* **spider angioma** *spī'dĕr an-jē-ō'mă*	a tiny, red blood vessel lesion formed by the dilation of a group of blood vessels radiating from a central arteriole, most commonly on the face, neck, or chest (*telos* = end)

PURPURIC LESIONS

TERM	MEANING
purpuric lesions *pŭr-pū'rik lē'zhŭnz*	purpura; lesions resulting from hemorrhages into the skin
petechia (Fig. 3-5, C) *pe-tē'kē-ă*	spot; reddish-brown, minute hemorrhagic spots on the skin that indicate a bleeding tendency; a small purpura
ecchymosis (Fig. 3-5, D) *ek-i-mō'sis*	bruise; a black and blue mark; a large purpura (*chymo* = juice)

SCAR FORMATIONS

TERM	MEANING
cicatrix of the skin *sik'ă-triks*	a mark left by the healing of a sore or wound, showing the replacement of destroyed tissue by fibrous tissue (*cicatrix* = scar)
keloid (Fig. 3-6) *kē'loyd*	an abnormal overgrowth of scar tissue that is thick and irregular (*kele* = tumor)

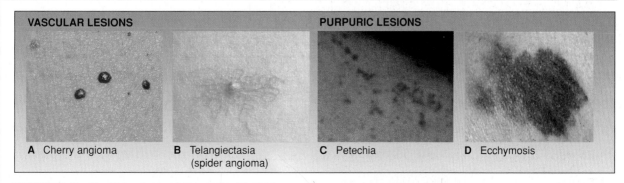

VASCULAR LESIONS   **PURPURIC LESIONS**

A Cherry angioma   B Telangiectasia (spider angioma)   C Petechia   D Ecchymosis

FIGURE 3-5 ■ Vascular and purpuric skin lesions.

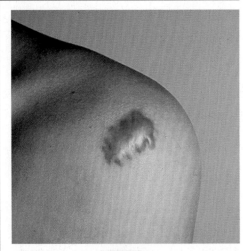

FIGURE 3-6 ▇ 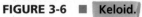 Keloid.

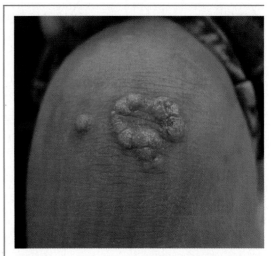

FIGURE 3-7 ▇ Verrucae on a knee.

TERM	MEANING
EPIDERMAL TUMORS	
epidermal tumors *ep-i-dĕr′măl tū′mŏrz*	skin tumors arising from the epidermis
nevus (*see* Fig. 3-1) *nē′vŭs*	a congenital malformation on the skin that can be epidermal or vascular; also called a mole
dysplastic nevus *dis-plas′tik nē′vŭs*	a mole with precancerous changes
verruca (Fig. 3-7) *vĕ-rū′kă*	an epidermal tumor caused by a papilloma virus, also called a wart

Programmed Review: Symptomatic Terms (Primary and Secondary Lesions)

ANSWERS	REVIEW
lesion secondary primary secondary	**3.28** A _____ is an area of pathologically altered tissue. There are primary and _____ types. Lesions that arise from previously normal skin are called _____ lesions, whereas those that result in changes in primary lesions are called _____ lesions.
macule or macula patch, maculae	**3.29** A freckle is an example of a _____, which is a flat, discolored spot on the skin up to 1 cm across. A larger, flat, discolored spot is called a _____. The plural of macula is _____.
solid plaque	**3.30** A papule is a _____ mass on the skin up to 0.5 cm in diameter, such as a mole. A _____ is like a papule but is

ANSWERS	REVIEW
nodule small	greater than 1 cm in diameter and is limited to the surface of the skin. A _____, like a papule, is greater than 1 cm in diameter but extends deeper into the epidermis. Recall that the suffix *-ule* is a diminutive that means _____.
tumor edema	**3.31** Another type of solid mass is a _____, which is larger than 1–2 cm. A wheal is an area of localized skin _____ (swelling).
vesicle bulla -ae pustule	**3.32** There are three types of elevated skin lesions containing fluid within a cavity. A small, elevated blister up to 0.5 cm, such as a fever blister, is a _____. A larger blister (more than 0.5 cm) is a _____, such as may occur with a second-degree burn. The plural form ends in _____. A pus-filled sac, like a pimple, is called a _____.
erosion, sore excoriation, out or away -ation fissure	**3.33** Some secondary lesions result in a loss of skin surface. If skin is lost, leaving an area of moisture but no bleeding, it is called an _____. An ulcer is an open _____ on the skin or mucous membrane that can bleed. A scratch mark is called an _____. Recall that the prefix *ex-* means _____, and that the suffix _____ refers to a process. A crack in the skin is called a _____.
scale crust blood	**3.34** A thin flake of dead epidermis is called a _____. On the other hand, a _____ on the skin is a dried residue of serum, pus, or _____.
cicatrix keloid tumor	**3.35** A healed sore or wound leaves a scar, which is called a _____ of the skin. An abnormal overgrowth of scar tissue, from the root *kele* (tumor), is a _____. Recall that the suffix *-oid* means resembling, which in this case implies that a keloid is not actually a _____.
vascular cherry spider tumor telangiectasia	**3.36** Lesions of a blood vessel are called _____ lesions. A _____ angioma is a small, bright red blood vessel tumor on the skin. A _____ angioma is a tiny, red blood vessel lesion in a group of vessels radiating from a central arteriole. The suffix *-oma* means _____. Another term for a spider angioma is _____.

ANSWERS	REVIEW
Purpuric purple petechia, iae ecchymosis, es	**3.37** _____ lesions look purple because of hemorrhages into the skin. The combining form _purpur/o_ means _____. A small purpura appearing as a tiny, reddish-brown spot on the skin is called a _____. The plural form is petech_____. A bruise is called an _____; the plural form is ecchymos_____.
epidermis, nevus mole painful, difficult, or faulty tumor, wart verrucae	**3.38** Epidermal tumors are skin tumors arising from the _____. A mole is called a _____. A dysplastic nevus is a _____ with precancerous changes. The prefix _dys-_ means _____. A verruca is an epidermal _____ caused by a papilloma virus and is also called a _____. The plural of verruca is _____.

🧊 Self-Instruction: General Symptomatic Terms

Study the following:

TERM	MEANING
alopecia _al-ō-pē'shē-ă_	baldness; natural or unnatural deficiency of hair
comedo (_pl._ **comedos, comedones**) (Fig. 3-8) _kom'ē-dō_	a plug of sebum (oil) within the opening of a hair follicle
closed comedo _klōsd kom'ē-dō_	a comedo below the skin surface, with a white center (whitehead)
open comedo _ō'pĕn kom'ē-dō_	a comedo open to the skin surface, with a black center caused by the presence of melanin exposed to air (blackhead)
eruption _ē-rŭp'shŭn_	appearance of a skin lesion
erythema _er-i-thē'mă_	redness of skin

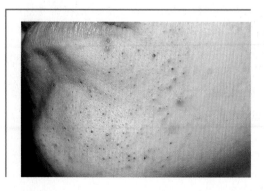

FIGURE 3-8 ▬ Open and closed comedones.

TERM	MEANING
pruritus *prū-rī'tŭs*	severe itching
rash *răsh*	a general term for skin eruption, most often associated with communicable disease
skin pigmentation *skin pig-men-tā'shŭn*	skin color resulting from the presence of melanin
depigmentation *dē-pig-men-tā'shŭn*	loss of melanin pigment in the skin
hypopigmentation *hī'pō-pig-men-tā'shŭn*	areas of skin lacking color because of deficient amounts of melanin
hyperpigmentation *hī'pĕr-pig-men-tā'shŭn*	darkened areas of skin caused by excessive amounts of melanin
suppuration *sŭp'yŭ-rā'shŭn*	production of purulent matter (pus)
urticaria (see Fig. 3-3, G) *ŭr'ti-kar'i-ă*	hives; an eruption of wheals on the skin accompanied by itching (*urtica* = stinging nettle)
xeroderma *zēr'ō-dĕr'mă*	dry skin

◈ Programmed Review: General Symptomatic Terms

ANSWERS	REVIEW
alopecia	**3.39** Baldness, or a deficiency of hair, is called _____.
comedo comedones whitehead blackhead	**3.40** A plug of sebum (oil) within the opening of a hair follicle is called a _____. The plural form is comedos or _____. A comedo below the skin surface with a white center is called a closed comedo or _____. A comedo open to the skin surface with center caused by the presence of melanin exposed to air is called a black _____.
lesion rash urticaria condition of	**3.41** An eruption is the appearance of a skin _____. A _____ is a general term for a skin eruption, often associated with a communicable disease. An eruption of wheals on the skin (hives) accompanied by itching is called _____. Remember that the suffix *-ia* means a _____ ____.
pruritus itching	**3.42** Any severe itching is called _____. Using the adjective form of pruritus, a pruritic eruption is one that is marked by severe _____.

ANSWERS	REVIEW
erthry/o erythema pertaining to	**3.43** The combining form for red is _____. Redness of the skin is called _____. The adjective erythematous means _____ ____ redness of the skin.
black color not deficient, excessive de hypo hyper	**3.44** *Melan/o* is the combining form meaning _____. Melanin is the pigment that gives _____ to the skin. Pigmentation describes the process of skin coloration. Recall the meaning of the following prefixes: *de-* means from, down, or _____; *hypo-* means below or _____; and *hyper-* means above or _____. Each is used to describe a different pigmentation of the skin. Using the prefix meaning from, down, or not, the total loss or absence of melanin is called _____pigmentation. Too little or deficient melanin causes _____pigmentation, and too much or excessive deposits of melanin cause _____pigmentation.
xer/o skin xeroderma	**3.45** The combining form meaning dry is _____. The Greek word derma means _____. Therefore, the term for dry skin is _____.

 ## Self-Instruction: Diagnostic Terms

Study the following:

TERM	MEANING
acne (Fig. 3-9) *ak'nē*	inflammation of the sebaceous glands and hair follicles of the skin, evidenced by comedones (blackheads), pustules, or nodules on the skin (*acne* = point)
albinism *al'bi-nizm*	a hereditary condition characterized by a partial or total lack of melanin pigment (particularly in the eyes, skin, and hair)
burn *bĕrn*	injury to body tissue caused by heat, chemicals, electricity, radiation, or gases
first-degree **(or 1ˢᵗ-degree) burn** *first-dĕ-grē' bĕrn*	a burn involving only the epidermis; characterized by erythema (redness) and hyperesthesia (excessive sensation)
second-degree **(or 2ⁿᵈ-degree) burn** *sek'ŭnd-dĕ-grē' bĕrn*	a burn involving the epidermis and the dermis; characterized by erythema, hyperesthesia, and vesications (blisters)
third-degree **(or 3ʳᵈ-degree) burn** *thĭrd-dĕ-grē' bĕrn*	a burn involving all layers of the skin; characterized by the destruction of the epidermis and dermis, with damage or destruction of subcutaneous tissue

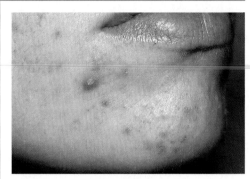

FIGURE 3-9 ■ Acne lesions. Inflammatory papules, pustules, and closed comedones are present on the face of a patient diagnosed with acne vulgaris.

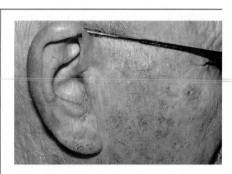

FIGURE 3-10 ■ Actinic (solar) keratoses.

TERM	MEANING
dermatitis *dĕr-mă-tī′tis*	inflammation of the skin characterized by erythema, pruritus (itching), and various lesions
dermatosis *dĕr-mă-tō′sis*	any disorder of the skin
exanthematous viral disease *ek-zan-them′ă-tŭs vī′răl di-zēz′*	an eruption of the skin caused by a viral disease (*exanthema* = eruption)
rubella *rū-bel′ă*	reddish; German measles
rubeola *rū-bē′ō-lă*	reddish; 14-day measles
varicella *var-i-sel′ă*	a tiny spot; chickenpox
eczema *ek′zĕ-mă*	to boil out; often used interchangeably with dermatitis to denote a skin condition characterized by the appearance of inflamed, swollen papules and vesicles that crust and scale, often with sensations of itching and burning
furuncle *fū′rŭng-kel*	boil; a painful nodule formed in the skin by inflammation originating in a hair follicle; caused by staphylococcosis
carbuncle *kar′bŭng-kel*	a skin infection consisting of clusters of furuncles (*carbo* = small, glowing embers)
abscess *ab′ses*	a localized collection of pus in a cavity formed by the inflammation of surrounding tissues, which heals when drained or excised (*abscessus* = a going away)
gangrene *gang′grēn*	an eating sore; death of tissue associated with loss of blood supply
herpes simplex virus type 1 (HSV-1) *hĕr′pēz sim′pleks vī′rŭs*	transient viral vesicles (e.g., cold sores or fever blisters) that infect the facial area, especially the mouth and nose (*herpes* = creeping skin disease)

TERM	MEANING
herpes simplex virus type 2 (HSV-2) (*see* Fig. 15-8) *hĕr'pēz sim'pleks vī'rŭs*	sexually transmitted, ulcer-like lesions of the genital and anorectal skin and mucosa; after initial infection, the virus lies dormant in the nerve cell root and may recur at times of stress
herpes zoster *hĕr'pēz zos'tĕr*	a viral disease affecting the peripheral nerves characterized by painful blisters that spread over the skin following affected nerves, usually unilateral; also known as shingles (*zoster* = girdle)
impetigo *im-pe-tī'gō*	a highly contagious, bacterial skin inflammation marked by pustules that rupture and become crusted, most often around the mouth and nostrils
keratoses *ker-ă-tō'sēz*	thickened areas of epidermis
actinic (or **solar**) **keratoses** (Fig. 3-10) *ak-tin'ik (sō'lăr) ker-ă-tō'sēz*	localized thickening of the skin caused by excessive exposure to sunlight, a known precursor to cancer (*actinic* = ray; *solar* = sun)
seborrheic keratoses (Fig. 3-11) *seb-ō-rē'ik ker-ă-tō'sēz*	benign, wart-like tumors; more common on elderly skin
lupus *lū'pŭs*	a chronic autoimmune disease characterized by inflammation of various parts of the body (*lupus* = wolf)
cutaneous lupus *kyū-tā'nē-ŭs lū'pŭs*	limited to the skin; evidenced by a characteristic rash, especially on the face, neck, and scalp
systemic lupus erythematosus (SLE) *sis-tem'ĭk lū'pŭs ĕr-i-thē'mă-tō'sŭs*	a more severe form of lupus involving the skin, joints, and often vital organs (e.g., lungs or kidneys)
malignant cutaneous neoplasm *mĕ-lig'nănt kyū-tā'nē-ŭs nē'ō-plazm*	skin cancer
squamous cell carcinoma (SCC) (*see* Fig. 3-1) *skwā'mŭs sel kar-si-nō'mă*	malignant tumor of the squamous epithelium

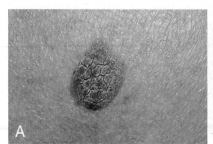 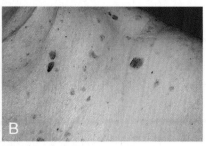

FIGURE 3-11 ■ Seborrheic keratoses. A. Lesion with a warty, stuck-on appearance. B. Multiple lesions showing various colors and sizes.

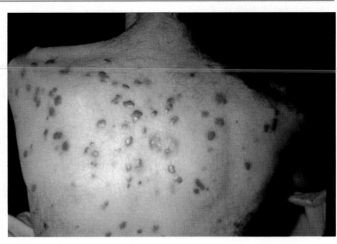

FIGURE 3-12 ■ Lesions of the AIDS-related Kaposi sarcoma.

TERM	MEANING
basal cell carcinoma (BCC) (*see* Fig. 3-1) *bā'săl sel kar-si-nō'mă*	malignant tumor of the basal layer of the epidermis; the most common type of skin cancer
malignant melanoma (*see* Fig. 3-1) *mă-lig'nănt melă-nō'mă*	malignant tumor composed of melanocytes
Kaposi sarcoma (Fig. 3-12) *kă-pō'sē sar-cō'mă*	malignant tumor of the walls of blood vessels, appearing as painless, dark bluish-purple plaques on the skin; often spreads to the lymph nodes and internal organs; commonly seen in patients with HIV/AIDS (human immunodeficiency virus/acquired immunodeficiency syndrome)
onychia *ō-nik'ē-ă*	inflammation of the fingernail or toenail
paronychia (Fig. 3-13) *par-ō-nik'ē-ă*	inflammation of the nail fold
pediculosis (Fig. 3-14) *pĕ-dik'yū-lō'sis*	infestation with lice that causes itching and dermatitis (*pediculo* = louse)
pediculosis capitis *pĕ-dik'yū-lō'sis kap'i-tis*	head lice (*capitis* = head)

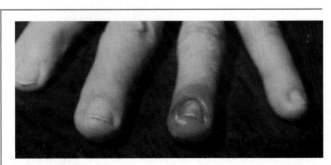

FIGURE 3-13 ■ Chronic paronychia.

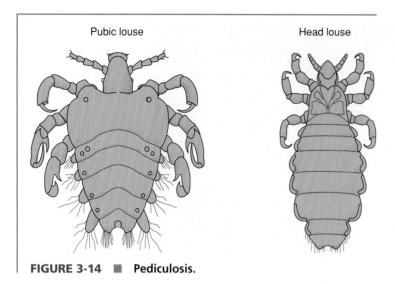

Pubic louse   Head louse

FIGURE 3-14 ■ Pediculosis.

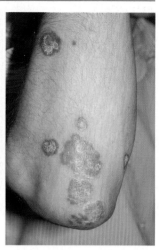

FIGURE 3-15 ■ Psoriasis lesions on arm and elbow.

TERM	MEANING
pediculosis pubis *pĕ-dik'yū-lō'sis pyū'bis*	lice that generally infect the pubic region and sometimes also hair of the axilla, eyebrows, eyelashes, beard, or other hairy body surfaces; also called crabs (*pubis* = groin)
psoriasis (Fig. 3-15) *sō-rī'ă-sis*	itching; a chronic, recurrent skin disease marked by silvery scales covering red patches, papules, and/or plaques on the skin that result from overproduction and thickening of skin cells; common sites of involvement are the elbows, knees, genitals, arms, legs, scalp, and nails
scabies *skā'bēz*	a contagious disease caused by a parasite (mite) that invades the skin, causing an intense itch, most often at articulations between the fingers or toes, elbow, etc. (*scabo* = to scratch)
seborrhea *seb-ō-rē'ă*	a skin condition marked by the hypersecretion of sebum from the sebaceous glands
tinea *tin'ē-ă*	a group of fungal skin diseases identified by the body part affected, including tinea corporis (body), commonly called ringworm, and tinea pedis (foot), also called athlete's foot
vitiligo (*see* Fig. 3-3, B) *vit-i-lī'gō*	a condition caused by the destruction of melanin that results in the appearance of white patches on the skin (commonly the face, hands, legs, and genital areas)

🔷 Programmed Review: Diagnostic Terms

ANSWERS	REVIEW
condition skin dermatosis	**3.46** The suffix *-osis* refers to an increase or _____. *Dermat/o* means _____. Therefore, the general term meaning skin condition is _____. The suffix meaning inflammation is

ANSWERS	REVIEW
-itis dermatitis inflammation, skin eczema	_____. An inflammation of the skin is therefore called _____. There are many forms of dermatitis or _____ of the _____. A term that is interchangeable with dermatitis, characterized by inflamed skin with various lesions accompanied by itching and burning is _____. Eczematous is the adjective form of the term.
comedos or comedones acne	**3.47** An inflammation of the sebaceous glands and hair follicles, often evidenced by _____ (blackheads or whiteheads), pustules, or nodules on the skin, is called _____.
condition of melanin vitiligo	**3.48** The suffix -*ism* refers to a _____ ____. Albinism is a hereditary condition characterized by a partial or total lack of _____ pigment in the body. The condition caused by the destruction of melanin that results in the appearance of white patches on the skin is called _____.
first-degree or 1ˢᵗ-degree epidermis subcutaneous	**3.49** A _____-_____ burn involves only the epidermis. A 2ⁿᵈ-degree burn involves both the _____ and the dermis. A 3ʳᵈ-degree burn involves damage to the _____layer.
viral rubella rubeola chickenpox	**3.50** Exanthematous _____ disease is an eruption of the skin caused by a viral infection. One such viral disease, also called German measles, is _____. A similar-sounding but different form of measles is _____. Varicella, another viral disease, is commonly called _____.
furuncle carbuncle	**3.51** A painful nodule from inflammation in a hair follicle caused by staphylococcosis is called a boil, or a _____. A skin infection consisting of clusters of furuncles is a _____, from *carbo* ("small, glowing embers").
abscess	**3.52** Pus that collects in a cavity formed by the inflammation of surrounding tissues is called an _____. It usually heals when drained or excised.
blood	**3.53** Gangrene is an eating sore in which tissue dies because of a loss of _____ supply.
virus	**3.54** There are several forms of herpes disease, which are caused by a _____. Herpes simplex virus type 1 causes transient

ANSWERS	REVIEW
vesicles or blisters genital or anorectal Herpes vesicles or blisters	_____, such as cold sores or fever blisters. Type 2 is sexually transmitted and causes lesions in _____ skin. _____ zoster affects the peripheral nerves and is characterized by painful _____ that spread over the skin.
Impetigo scabies fungus pediculosis, capitis pubis	**3.55** _____ is a highly contagious, bacterial skin inflammation usually occurring around the mouth and nose. Another contagious skin disease, called _____, is caused by a mite that invades the skin and causes intense itching. Tinea is a different group of contagious skin diseases caused by a _____. Lice also can cause an infestation on the skin, called _____. Head lice are called pediculosis _____, and lice infesting the pubic region are called pediculosis _____.
hard condition of keratosis keratoses actinic sun, seborrheic	**3.56** Putting the combining form *kerat/o*, meaning _____, with the suffix *-osis*, meaning a _____ ____, makes the word _____, a condition of thickened epidermis. The plural form of this term is _____. Solar keratoses, or _____ keratoses, are caused by excessive exposure to the _____. Benign, wart-like tumors are called _____ keratoses.
lupus skin systemic erythematosus	**3.57** An autoimmune disease involving inflammation of various parts of the body was named after the Latin word for wolf, _____. Cutaneous lupus is limited to the _____ and causes a characteristic rash. A more serious form, called _____ lupus _____ (SLE), affects many body organs.
condition of fingernail or toenail, alongside of paronychia	**3.58** In the term onychia, the suffix *-ia* (meaning _____ ____ inflammation), is joined with *onych/o* (meaning a _____). The suffix *para-*, meaning _____ ____, combined with *onych/o* and the suffix *-ia* form the term denoting a condition of inflammation of the nail fold, or _____. (Remember the rules of spelling: drop the final vowel from the prefix before joining it to a combining form that begins with a vowel.)
discharge seborrhea	**3.59** Recall that the suffix *-rrhea* means _____. A skin condition marked by the hypersecretion and discharge of sebum is called _____.

ANSWERS	REVIEW
psoriasis	**3.60** A condition in which the skin has silvery scales covering red patches, papules, and/or plaques is _____.
new malignant benign squamous cell basal cell carcinoma melanoma tumor, sarcoma	**3.61** Neoplasia is a term describing a condition of _____ formation of tissue that is either cancerous (_____) or noncancerous (_____). Several different forms of malignant neoplasia can involve the skin. A _____ _____ carcinoma is a tumor of the squamous epithelium. A malignant tumor of the basal layer of the epidermis is a _____ _____ _____. A tumor composed of melanocytes is a malignant _____. Remember that the suffix *-oma* means _____. Kaposi _____ is a tumor of the walls of blood vessels, commonly seen in patients with HIV/AIDS.

Self-Instruction: Diagnostic Tests and Procedures

Study the following:

TEST OR PROCEDURE	EXPLANATION
biopsy (Bx) (Fig. 3-16) *bī'op-sē*	removal of a small piece of tissue for microscopic pathologic examination
excisional biopsy *ek-sizh'ŭn-al bī'op-sē*	removal of an entire lesion
incisional biopsy *in-sizh'ŭn-ăl bī'op-sē*	removal of a selected portion of a lesion
shave biopsy *shāv bī'op-sē*	a technique using a surgical blade to "shave" tissue from the epidermis and upper dermis

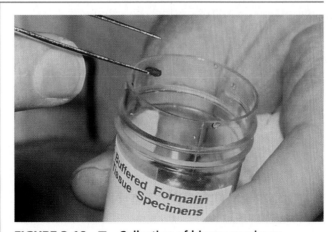

FIGURE 3-16 ■ Collection of biopsy specimen.

TEST OR PROCEDURE	EXPLANATION
culture and sensitivity (C&S) *kŭl'chŭr and sen-si-tiv'i-tē*	a technique of isolating and growing colonies of microorganisms to identify a pathogen and to determine which drugs might be effective for combating the infection it has caused
frozen section (FS) *frō'zen sek'shŭn*	a surgical technique that involves cutting a thin piece of tissue from a frozen specimen for immediate pathologic examination
skin tests *skin testz*	methods for determining the reaction of the body to a given substance by applying it to, or injecting it into, the skin; commonly used in treating allergies
scratch test *skrach test*	a test in which a substance is applied to the skin through a scratch
patch test *pach test*	a test in which a substance is applied topically to the skin on a small piece of blotting paper or wet cloth

◆ Programmed Review: Diagnostic Tests and Procedures

ANSWERS	REVIEW
biopsy lesion out or away, incisional portion shave	**3.62** In many different body systems, small samples of tissue are removed for a diagnostic test involving microscopic examination. This is called a _____ (Bx). An excisional biopsy involves removal of the entire _____. Remember that the prefix *ex-* means _____. An _____ biopsy, in contrast, removes only a _____ of the lesion. Another type, called a _____ biopsy, uses a surgical blade to "shave" tissue from the epidermis and upper dermis.
culture sensitivity	**3.63** A technique for isolating and growing a colony of microorganisms to identify a pathogen is called a _____ and _____ (C&S). This helps to determine which drugs may be effective in fighting the infection.
frozen section FS	**3.64** A tissue specimen may be frozen and cut thin for examination. This is called a _____ _____ and is abbreviated _____.
scratch patch	**3.65** Skin tests are commonly used to identify substances to which a person may be allergic. In the _____ test, a small amount of the substance is applied to the skin through a scratch. Applying the substance topically to the skin with a small piece of paper or cloth is called a _____ test.

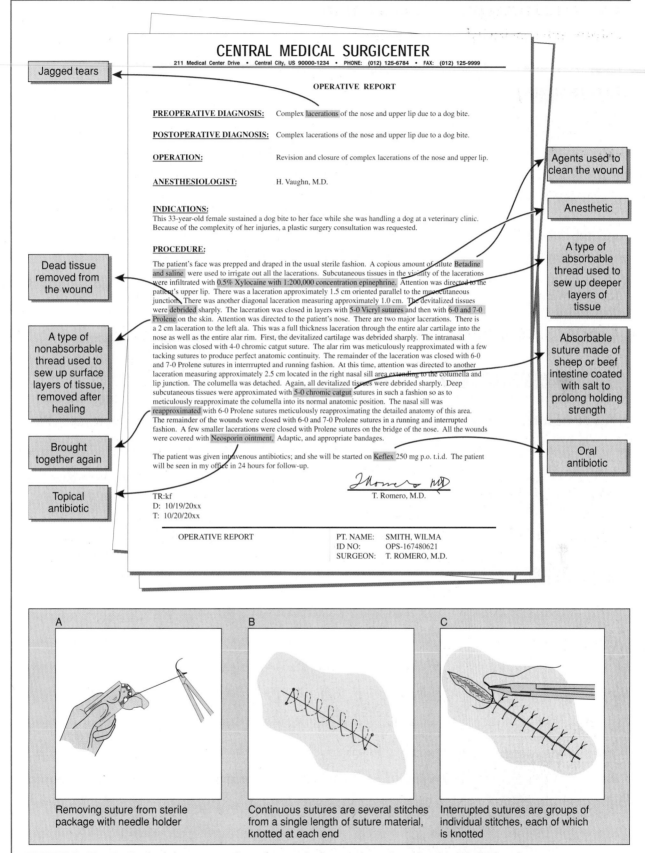

Jagged tears

Agents used to clean the wound

Anesthetic

A type of absorbable thread used to sew up deeper layers of tissue

Absorbable suture made of sheep or beef intestine coated with salt to prolong holding strength

Dead tissue removed from the wound

A type of nonabsorbable thread used to sew up surface layers of tissue, removed after healing

Brought together again

Topical antibiotic

Oral antibiotic

CENTRAL MEDICAL SURGICENTER
211 Medical Center Drive • Central City, US 90000-1234 • PHONE: (012) 125-6784 • FAX: (012) 125-9999

OPERATIVE REPORT

PREOPERATIVE DIAGNOSIS: Complex lacerations of the nose and upper lip due to a dog bite.

POSTOPERATIVE DIAGNOSIS: Complex lacerations of the nose and upper lip due to a dog bite.

OPERATION: Revision and closure of complex lacerations of the nose and upper lip.

ANESTHESIOLOGIST: H. Vaughn, M.D.

INDICATIONS:
This 33-year-old female sustained a dog bite to her face while she was handling a dog at a veterinary clinic. Because of the complexity of her injuries, a plastic surgery consultation was requested.

PROCEDURE:
The patient's face was prepped and draped in the usual sterile fashion. A copious amount of dilute Betadine and saline were used to irrigate out all the lacerations. Subcutaneous tissues in the vicinity of the lacerations were infiltrated with 0.5% Xylocaine with 1:200,000 concentration epinephrine. Attention was directed to the patient's upper lip. There was a laceration approximately 1.5 cm oriented parallel to the mucocutaneous junction. There was another diagonal laceration measuring approximately 1.0 cm. The devitalized tissues were debrided sharply. The laceration was closed in layers with 5-0 Vicryl sutures and then with 6-0 and 7-0 Prolene on the skin. Attention was directed to the patient's nose. There are two major lacerations. There is a 2 cm laceration to the left ala. This was a full thickness laceration through the entire alar cartilage into the nose as well as the entire alar rim. First, the devitalized cartilage was debrided sharply. The intranasal incision was closed with 4-0 chromic catgut suture. The alar rim was meticulously reapproximated with a few tacking sutures to produce perfect anatomic continuity. The remainder of the laceration was closed with 6-0 and 7-0 Prolene sutures in interrupted and running fashion. At this time, attention was directed to another laceration measuring approximately 2.5 cm located in the right nasal sill area extending to the columella and lip junction. The columella was detached. Again, all devitalized tissues were debrided sharply. Deep subcutaneous tissues were approximated with 5-0 chromic catgut sutures in such a fashion so as to meticulously reapproximate the columella into its normal anatomic position. The nasal sill was reapproximated with 6-0 Prolene sutures meticulously reapproximating the detailed anatomy of this area. The remainder of the wounds were closed with 6-0 and 7-0 Prolene sutures in a running and interrupted fashion. A few smaller lacerations were closed with Prolene sutures on the bridge of the nose. All the wounds were covered with Neosporin ointment, Adaptic, and appropriate bandages.

The patient was given intravenous antibiotics; and she will be started on Keflex 250 mg p.o. t.i.d. The patient will be seen in my office in 24 hours for follow-up.

T. Romero, M.D.
T. Romero, M.D.

TR:kf
D: 10/19/20xx
T: 10/20/20xx

OPERATIVE REPORT

PT. NAME: SMITH, WILMA
ID NO: OPS-167480621
SURGEON: T. ROMERO, M.D.

A

B

C

Removing suture from sterile package with needle holder

Continuous sutures are several stitches from a single length of suture material, knotted at each end

Interrupted sutures are groups of individual stitches, each of which is knotted

FIGURE 3-17 ■ **Typical documentation of a surgical procedure. Suturing is also depicted.**

Self-Instruction: Operative Terms (Fig. 3-17)

Study the following:

TERM	MEANING
chemosurgery *kem'ō-sŭr-jĕr-ē*	removal of tissue after it has been destroyed by chemical means
chemical peel *kĕm'i-kăl pēl*	a technique for restoring wrinkled, scarred, or blemished skin by applying an acid solution to "peel" away the top layers of the skin
cryosurgery *krī-ō-sŭr'jĕr-ē*	destruction of tissue by freezing with application of an extremely cold chemical (e.g., liquid nitrogen)
dermabrasion *dĕr-mă-brā'zhŭn*	surgical removal of epidermis frozen by aerosol spray using wire brushes and emery papers to remove scars, tattoos, and/or wrinkles
debridement *dā-brēd-mon'*	removal of dead tissue from a wound or burn site to promote healing and to prevent infection
curettage *kyū-rĕ-tahzh'*	cleaning; scraping a wound using a spoon-like cutting instrument called a curette; used for debridement
electrosurgical procedures *ē-lek-trō-sŭr'ji-căl prō-cē'jŭrz*	use of electric current to destroy tissue; the type and strength of the current and method of application vary
electrocautery (Fig. 3-18) *ē-lek'trō-kaw'tĕr-ē*	use of an instrument heated by electric current (cautery) to coagulate bleeding areas by burning the tissue (e.g., to sear a blood vessel)
electrodesiccation *ē-lek'trō-des-i-kā'shŭn*	use of high-frequency electric currents to destroy tissue by drying it; the active electrode makes direct contact with the skin lesion (*desiccate* = to dry up)
fulguration *ful-gŭ-rā'shŭn*	to lighten; use of long, high-frequency, electric sparks to destroy tissue; the active electrode does *not* touch the skin
incision and drainage (I&D) *in-sizh'ŭn and drān'ăj*	incision and drainage of an infected skin lesion (e.g., an abscess)

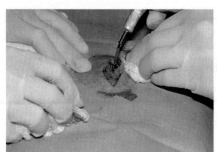

FIGURE 3-18 ■ Electrocautery. A cautery device is used to perform hemostasis during a surgical procedure.

TERM	MEANING
laser *lā'zĕr*	an acronym for *l*ight *a*mplification by *s*timulated *e*mission of *r*adiation; an instrument that concentrates high frequencies of light into a small, extremely intense beam that is precise in depth and diameter; applied to body tissues to destroy lesions or for dissection (cutting of parts for study)
laser surgery *lā'zĕr sŭr'jĕr-ē*	surgery using a laser in various dermatologic procedures to remove lesions, scars, tattoos, etc.
Mohs surgery *mōz sŭr'jĕr-ē*	a technique used to excise tumors of the skin by removing fresh tissue, layer by layer, until a tumor-free plane is reached
skin grafting *skin graft'ing*	transfer of skin from one body site to another to replace skin that has been lost through a burn or injury
autograft *aw'tō-graft*	graft transfer to a new position in the body of the same person (*auto* = self)
heterograft or **xenograft** *het'er-ō-graft, zen'ō-graft*	graft transfer between different species, such as from animal to human (*hetero* = different; *xeno* = strange)
homograft or **allograft** *hō'mō-graft, al'ō-graft*	donor transfer between persons of the same species, such as human to human (*homo* = same)

Programmed Review: Operative Terms

ANSWERS	REVIEW
chemical peel	**3.66** A special form of chemosurgery, called a _____ _____, uses an acid to peel away the top layers of skin.
freezing	**3.67** Cryosurgery destroys tissue by _____ it, usually with an extremely cold chemical, such as liquid nitrogen.
dermabrasion	**3.68** Another way to remove skin tissue, particularly scars, tattoos, or wrinkles, is to surgically scrape off the skin using a wire brush or emery paper. This is called _____.
from, down, or not debridement curettage	**3.69** Recall that the prefix *de-* means _____. When dead tissue is removed from a wound or burn site, this is called _____. This is often done with a cutting instrument called a curette, and the technique is thus called _____.
electrosurgery electrocautery	**3.70** Electricity is used in many dermatologic procedures to destroy unwanted tissue. The general term for such operative procedures is _____. The use of an electrically heated instrument to coagulate a bleeding area by burning the tissue is called _____. Electrodesiccation, in contrast, applies an

ANSWERS	REVIEW
drying fulguration process	electrical current directly to a skin lesion to destroy the tissue by _____ it. A process using electrical sparks to destroy tissue is called _____. In both terms, the suffix -*ation* means a _____.
incision, drainage	**3.71** An infected lesion, such as an abscess, may undergo the surgical procedure called _____ and _____ (I&D).
laser laser	**3.72** An amplified, intense light beam, called a _____, is used to remove various kinds of lesions during an operative procedure called _____ surgery.
layer	**3.73** Mohs surgery is a technique for removing a tumor one _____ at a time until a tumor-free layer is reached.
graft autograft self human allograft species, different xenograft, strange	**3.74** A skin _____ is used to replace skin at a burn or injury site by transferring it from another site. If the graft is transferred from elsewhere on the same person, this is called an _____ (*auto* = _____). A homograft is a graft transferred to one human from another _____ (*homo* = same). This is also called an _____. A heterograft, in contrast, is transferred from a different _____ (*hetero* means _____). The synonym for heterograft is _____ (*xeno* = _____).

◆ Self-Instruction: Therapeutic Terms

Study the following:

TERM	MEANING
chemotherapy *kĕm'ō-thār'ă-pē*	treatment of malignancies, infections, and other diseases with chemical agents that destroy selected cells or impair their ability to reproduce
radiation therapy *rā'dē-ā'shŭn thār'ă-pē*	treatment of neoplastic disease using ionizing radiation to deter the proliferation of malignant cells
sclerotherapy *sklēr'ō-thār'ă-pē*	use of sclerosing agents in treating diseases (e.g., injection of a saline solution into a dilated blood vessel tumor in the skin, resulting in hardening of the tissue within and eventual sloughing away of the lesion)
ultraviolet therapy *ŭl-tră-vī'ō-let thār'ă-pē*	use of ultraviolet light to promote healing of a skin lesion (e.g., an ulcer)

TERM	MEANING
COMMON THERAPEUTIC DRUG CLASSIFICATIONS	
anesthetic *an-es-thet'ik*	a drug that temporarily blocks transmission of nerve conduction to produce a loss of sensations (e.g., pain)
antibiotic *an'tē-bī-ot'ik*	a drug that kills or inhibits the growth of microorganisms
antifungal *an'tē-fŭng'găl*	a drug that kills or prevents the growth of fungi
antihistamine *an-tē-his'tă-mēn*	a drug that blocks the effects of histamine in the body
histamine *his'tă-mēn*	a regulating body substance released in excess during allergic reactions, causing swelling and inflammation of tissues (e.g., in urticaria [hives], hay fever, etc.)
antiinflammatory *an'tē-in-flam'ă-tō'rē*	a drug that reduces inflammation
antipruritic *an'tē-prŭ-rit'ik*	a drug that relieves itching
antiseptic *an-ti-sep'tik*	an agent that inhibits the growth of infectious microorganisms

◈ Programmed Review: Therapeutic Terms

ANSWERS	REVIEW
chemotherapy radiation therapy sclerotherapy light	**3.75** Several different types of therapy are used to treat tumors and other skin lesions. The use of chemical agents as a treatment is called _____. Ionizing _____ is also used on tumors, and this is called radiation _____. In another form of therapy, sclerosing agents are injected into a lesion to harden the tissue within; this is called _____. Finally, ultraviolet therapy is the use of ultraviolet _____ to promote healing of a skin lesion (e.g., an ulcer).
anesthetic	**3.76** An _____ agent (using the suffix *-tic*, which means pertaining to) produces a loss of sensation so that the person undergoing a procedure does not feel pain.

ANSWERS	REVIEW
fungus antifungal against or opposed to	**3.77** Recall that tinea is a group of skin diseases caused by a _____. A drug that kills or prevents the growth of such infections is called an _____, using the prefix *anti-*, which means _____.
antibiotic	**3.78** A different sort of drug kills or inhibits the growth of bacteria. A drug of this class is known as an _____.
antihistamine	**3.79** Histamine is a body substance that is released in excess during an allergic reaction. A drug that blocks the effects of this substance is called an _____. This type of drug is used to combat allergic reactions (e.g., hives or hay fever).
antipruritic antiseptic antiinflammatory	**3.80** Many drug classifications are named according to what they work against, using the prefix *anti-*, meaning against or opposed to. The term for itching is pruritus, and a drug that relieves itching is called an _____. Sepsis is an infection by microorganisms; a drug that inhibits the growth of such microorganisms is called an _____. Similarly, a drug that reduces inflammation is called an _____.

CHAPTER 3 ACRONYMS AND ABBREVIATIONS

ABBREVIATION	EXPANSION
AIDS	acquired immunodeficiency syndrome
BCC	basal cell carcinoma
Bx	biopsy
C&S	culture and sensitivity
FS	frozen section
HIV	human immunodeficiency virus
HSV-1	herpes simplex virus type 1
HSV-2	herpes simplex virus type 2
I&D	incision and drainage
SCC	squamous cell carcinoma
SLE	systemic lupus erythematosus

CHAPTER 3 SUMMARY OF TERMS

The terms introduced in chapter 3 are listed below, followed by the page number on which each term can be found and its written pronunciation. For additional practice and reinforcement, write the definition of each term on a separate piece of paper.

abscess/115
ab′ses

acne/114
ak′nē

actinic keratoses/116
ak-tin′ik ker-ă-tō′sez

albinism/114
al′bi-nizm

allograft/125
al′ō-graft

alopecia/112
al-ō-pē′shē-ă

anesthetic/127
an-es-thet′ik

antibiotic/127
an′tē-bī-ot′ik

antifungal/127
an′tē-fŭng′găl

antihistamine/127
an-tē-his′tă-mēn

antiinflammatory/127
an′tē-in-flam′ă-tō-rē

antipruritic/127
an′tē-prū-rit′ik

antiseptic/127
an-ti-sep′tik

autograft/125
aw′tō-graft

basal cell carcinoma (BCC)/117
bā′săl sel kar-si-nō′mă

basal layer/104
bā′săl lā′er

biopsy (Bx)/121
bī′op-sē

bulla/108
bul′ă

burn/114
bĕrn

carbuncle/115
kar′bŭng-kel

chemical peel/124
kem′i-kăl pēl

chemosurgery/124
kēm′ō-sŭr-jĕr-ē

chemotherapy/126
kēm′ō-thăr-ă-pē

cherry angioma/109
cher′ō an-jē-ō′mă

cicatrix/109
sik′ă-triks

closed comedo/112
klōsd kom′ē-dō

collagen/104
kol′ă-jen

comedo/112
kom′ē-do

crust/109
krŭst

cryosurgery/124
krī-ō-sŭr′jĕr-ē

culture and sensitivity (C&S)/122
kŭl′chŭr and sen-si-tiv′i-tē

curettage/124
kyŭ-rē-tahzh′

cutaneous lupus/116
kyū-tā′nē-ŭs lū′pŭs

debridement/124
dā-brēd-mon′

depigmentation/113
dē-pig-men-tā′shŭn

dermabrasion/124
dĕr-mă-brā′zhŭn

dermatitis/115
dĕr-mă-tī′tis

dermatosis/115
dĕr-mă-tō′sis

dermis/104
dĕrm'is

dysplastic nevus/110
dis-plas' tik nē'vŭs

ecchymosis/109
ek-i-mō'sis

eczema/115
ek'zĕ-mă

electrocautery/124
ē-lek'trō-kaw'tĕr-ē

electrodesiccation/124
ē-lek'trō-des-i-kā'shŭn

electrosurgical procedures/124
ē-lek-trō-sŭr'ji-căl prō-cē'jŭrz

epidermal tumors/110
ep-i-dĕr'măl tū'mŏrz

epidermis/104
ep-i-dĕrm'is

epithelium/104
ep-i-thē' lē-ŭm

erosion/108
ē-rō'zhŭn

eruption/112
ē-rŭp'shŭn

erythema/112
er-i-thē'mă

exanthematous viral disease/115
ek-zan-them'ă-tŭs vī'răl di-zēz'

excisional biopsy/121
ek-sizh'ŭn-ăl bī'op-sē

excoriation/108
eks-kō'rē-ā'shŭn

first-degree (or 1st-degree) burn/114
first-dĕ-grē' bĕrn

fissure/108
fish'ŭr

frozen section (FS)/122
frō'zĕn sek'shŭn

fulguration/124
ful-gŭ-rā'shŭn

furuncle/115
fū'rŭng-kĕl

gangrene/115
gang'grēn

hair/104
hār

herpes simplex virus (HSV)/115–116
her'pēz sim'pleks vī'nŭs

herpes zoster/116
her'pēz zos'tĕr

heterograft/125
het'ĕr-ō-graft

histamine/127
his'tă-mēn

homograft/125
hō'mō-graft

hyperpigmentation/113
hī-pĕr-pig-men-tā'shŭn

hypopigmentation/113
hī'pō-pig-men-tā'shŭn

impetigo/116
im-pe-tī'gō

incisional biopsy/121
in-si'zhŭn-ăl bī'op-sē

incision and drainage (I&D)/124
in-sizh'ŭn and drān'ăj

Kaposi sarcoma/117
ka-pō'sē sar-kō'mă

keloid/109
kē'loyd

keratin/104
ker'ă-tin

keratoses/116
ker-ă-tō'sēz

laser/125
lā'zĕr

laser surgery/125
lā'zĕr sŭr'jĕr-ē

lesion/106
lē'zhŭn

lupus/116
lū'pŭs

macule or **macula**/107
mak'yūl

malignant cutaneous neoplasm/116
mă-lig'nănt kyū-tā'nē-ŭs nē'ō-plazm

malignant melanoma/117
mă-lig'nănt mel'ă-nō'mă

melanin/104
mel'ă-nin

melanocyte/104
mel'ă-nō-sīt

Mohs surgery/125
mōz sŭr'jĕr-ē

nail/104
nāl

nevus/110
nē'vŭs

nodule/107
nod'yūl

onychia/117
ō-nik'ē-ă

open comedo/112
ō'pĕn kom'ē-dō

paronychia/117
par-ō-nik'ē-ă

patch/107
pach

patch test/122
pach test

papule/107
pap'yūl

pediculosis/117
pĕ-dik'yū-lō'sis

pediculosis capitis/117
pĕ-dik'yū-lō'sis kap'i-tis

pediculosis pubis/118
pĕ-dik'yū-lō'sis pyū'bis

petechia/109
pe-tē'kē-ă

plaque/107
plak

primary lesions/107
prī'măr-ē lē'zhŭnz

pruritus/113
prū-rī'tŭs

psoriasis/118
sō-rī'ă-sis

purpuric lesions/109
pŭr-pū'rik lē'zhŭnz

pustule/108
pŭs'tyūl

radiation therapy/126
rā'dē-ā'shŭn thăr'ă-pē

rash/113
rash

rubella/115
rū-bel'ă

rubeola/115
rū-bē'ō-lă

scabies/118
skā'bēz

scale/109
skāl

sclerotherapy/126
sklēr'ō-thăr-ă-pē

scratch test/122
skrach test

sebaceous glands/104
sē-bā'shŭs glanz

seborrhea/118
seb-ō-rē'ă

seborrheic keratoses/116
seb-ō-rē'ik ker-ă-tō'sēz

sebum/104
sē'bŭm

secondary lesions/108
sek'ŏn-dăr-ē lē'zhŭnz

second-degree (or 2ⁿᵈ-degree) burn/114
sek'ŭnd-dĕ-grē' bĕrn

shave biopsy/121
shāv bī'op-sē

skin grafting/125
skin graft'ing

skin pigmentation/113
skin pig-men-tā'shŭn

skin tests/122
skin testz

solar keratoses/116
sō'lăr ker-ă-tō'sez

spider angioma/109
spī'dĕr an-jē-ō'mă

squamous cell carcinoma (SCC)/116
skwā'mŭs sel kar-si-nō'mă

squamous cell layer/104
skwā'mŭs sel lā'ĕr

subcutaneous layer/104
sŭb-kyū-tā'nē-ŭs lā'ĕr

sudoriferous glands/104
sŭ-dō-ri'fĕr-ŭs glanz

suppuration/113
sŭp'yŭ-rā'shŭn

systemic lupus erythematosus (SLE)/116
sis-tem'ik lū'pŭs ĕr-i-thē'mă-tō-sĭs

telangiectasia/109
tel-an'jē-ek-tā'zē-ă

third-degree (or 3ʳᵈ-degree) burn/114
thĭrd-dĕ-grē' bĕrn

tinea/118
tin'ē-ă

tumor/107
tū'mŏr

ulcer/108
ŭl'sĕr

ultraviolet therapy/126
ŭl-tră-vī'ō-let thār'ă-pē

urticaria/113
ŭr-ti-kar'i-ă

varicella/115
var-i-sel'ă

vascular lesions/109
vas'kyū-lăr lē'zhŭnz

verruca/110
vĕ-rū'kă

vesicle/108
ves'i-kĕl

vitiligo/118
vit-i-lī'gō

wheal/108
wēl

xenograft/125
zen'ō-graft

xeroderma/113
zēr'ō-dĕr'mă

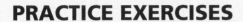

PRACTICE EXERCISES

For each of the following words, write out the term components (prefixes [P], combining forms [CF], roots [R], and suffixes [S]) on the lines below the word. Then define the term according to the meaning of its components.

EXAMPLE

hypodermic

hypo / derm / ic

P   R   S

DEFINITION: below or deficient/skin/pertaining to

1. onychomalacia

_____ / _____

   CF   S

DEFINITION: _____

2. mycotic

_____ / _____

   CF   S

DEFINITION: _____

3. dermatologist

_____ / _____

   CF   S

DEFINITION: _____

4. histotrophic

_____ / _____ / _____

   CF   R   S

DEFINITION: _____

5. paronychia

_____ / _____ / _____

   P   R   S

DEFINITION: _____

6. hyperkeratosis

_____ / _____ / _____

   P   R   S

DEFINITION: _____

7. leukotrichia

_____ / _____ / _____

   CF   R   S

DEFINITION: _____

8. mycology

_____ / _____
    CF   S

DEFINITION: _____

9. epidermal

_____ / _____ / _____
    P   R   S

DEFINITION: _____

10. lipoma

_____ / _____
    R   S

DEFINITION: _____

11. subcutaneous

_____ / _____ / _____
    P   R   S

DEFINITION: _____

12. anhidrosis

_____ / _____ / _____
    P   R   S

DEFINITION: _____

13. histopathology

_____ / _____ / _____
    CF   CF   S

DEFINITION: _____

14. dysplasia

_____ / _____ / _____
    P   R   S

DEFINITION: _____

15. adiposis

_____ / _____
    R   S

DEFINITION: _____

16. squamous

_____ / _____
    R   S

DEFINITION: _____

17. erythrodermatitis

_____ / _____ / _____
      CF   R   S

DEFINITION: _____

18. desquamation

_____ / _____ / _____
      P   R   S

DEFINITION: _____

19. histotoxic

_____ / _____ / _____
      CF   R   S

DEFINITION: _____

20. melanocyte

_____ / _____ / _____
      CF   R   S

DEFINITION: _____

21. xerosis

_____ / _____
      R   S

DEFINITION: _____

22. purpuric

_____ / _____
      R   S

DEFINITION: _____

23. seborrhea

_____ / _____
      CF   S

DEFINITION: _____

24. xanthoma

_____ / _____
      R   S

DEFINITION: _____

25. asteatosis

_____ / _____ / _____
      P   R   S

DEFINITION: _____

Write the correct medical term for each of the following definitions:

26. _____ death of tissue associated with loss of blood supply

27. _____ transfer of skin to a new position in the body of the same person

28. _____ black and blue mark

29. _____ severe itching

30. _____ a cluster of furuncles

31. _____ fungal skin disease

32. _____ hives

33. _____ a graft transfer from one animal species to one of another species

34. _____ pubic lice

35. _____ a boil

36. _____ freckle

37. _____ flake of exfoliated epidermis

38. _____ head lice

39. _____ baldness

40. _____ virus that causes cold sores

41. _____ study of tissue

42. _____ redness of skin

43. _____ a blackhead

44. _____ mark left by a healed wound

45. _____ a linear crack in the skin

46. _____ surgery that freezes tissue

47. _____ excision of tissue for microscopic study

48. _____ appearance of a skin lesion

49. _____ abnormal scar formation

Complete each medical term by writing the missing word or word part:

50. _____ oma = black tumor

51. sebo_____ = discharge of oil

52. _____coriation = scratch mark on skin

53. _____derma = white skin

54. _____ section = type of microscopic study of fresh tissue

55. _____derma = red skin

56. _____derma = hard skin

57. _____ keratoses = thickened skin tumors seen in old age

58. _____oma = fat tumor

59. _____derma = yellow skin

60. _____osis = presence of fungus

61. _____dermic = pertaining to below the skin

62. _____ angioma = bright red, round blood vessel tumor

63. _____derma = dry skin

Give the medical term for the following viral diseases:

64. German measles _____

65. chickenpox _____

66. 14-day measles _____

Write the letter of the matching definition for each of the primary lesions described:

67. vesicle _____   a. a tiny, flat discolored spot on the skin up to 1 cm in diameter

68. pustule _____   b. a large, flat discolored area on the skin larger than 1 cm in diameter

69. papule _____   c. a raised spot on the skin less than 0.5 cm in diameter

70. bulla _____   d. a solid mass greater than 1 cm that extends into the epidermis

71. nodule _____   e. a solid mass greater than 1 cm limited to the skin's surface

72. wheal _____   f. a small blister

73. macule _____   g. an area of localized skin edema, such as a hive

74. tumor _____   h. a large blister

75. patch _____   i. a pus-filled sac

76. plaque _____   j. a solid mass larger than 1–2 cm in diameter

Write out the expanded term for each abbreviation:

77. HSV-2 _____

78. Bx _____

79. FS _____

80. I&D _____

Write the plural for each of the following terms:

81. keratosis _____

82. ecchymosis _____

83. bulla _____

84. macula _____

85. nevus _____

Match the following terms with their meanings:

86. scabies	_____	a.	chemical peel
87. cryosurgery	_____	b.	crabs
88. telangiectasia	_____	c.	mites
89. nevus	_____	d.	freezing treatment
90. cicatrix	_____	e.	intense light
91. actinic keratoses	_____	f.	desiccation
92. radiation therapy	_____	g.	spider angioma
93. petechia	_____	h.	mole
94. liposis	_____	i.	scar
95. verruca	_____	j.	cancer treatment
96. chemosurgery	_____	k.	wart
97. electrosurgery	_____	l.	solar keratoses
98. pediculosis	_____	m.	purpuric lesion
99. laser	_____	n.	adiposis

Circle the correct spelling:

100.	cicatrix	scicatrix	cicatrex
101.	puritis	purritis	pruritus
102.	petechia	patechia	petecchia
103.	veruca	verucca	verruca
104.	eckamosis	ecchymosis	eckemyosis
105.	excission	excisison	excision
106.	soriasis	psoreyeasis	psoriasis
107.	impetigo	infantiego	impatiego
108.	eggszema	eczema	ecczema
109.	debridemant	debridement	debreedment

Give the noun that is used to form each adjective:

110.	keratotic	_____
111.	bullous	_____
112.	nodular	_____
113.	seborrheic	_____
114.	petechial	_____
115.	ecchymotic	_____
116.	urticarial	_____
117.	eczematous	_____
118.	macular	_____
119.	suppurative	_____

Identify the parts of the skin's anatomy by writing the missing words in the spaces provided:

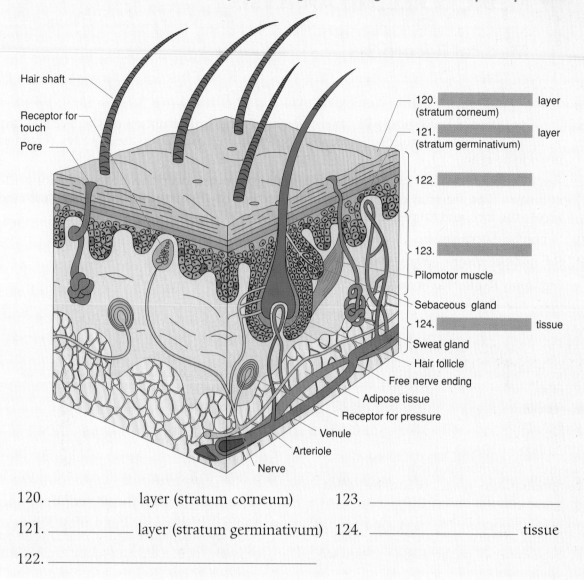

120. _____ layer (stratum corneum)   123. _____

121. _____ layer (stratum germinativum)   124. _____ tissue

122. _____

Circle the combining form that corresponds to the meaning given:

125. **fat**	leuk/o	steat/o	seb/o
126. **black**	necr/o	trich/o	melan/o
127. **fungus**	seb/o	myc/o	onych/o
128. **nail**	onych/o	trich/o	squam/o
129. **red**	xanth/o	purpur/o	erythr/o
130. **hair**	trich/o	histi/o	fibr/o
131. **dry**	kerat/o	xer/o	xanth/o
132. **oil**	py/o	hidr/o	seb/o

MEDICAL RECORD ANALYSIS

Medical Record 3-1

PROGRESS NOTE

S: This is a 30 y.o. ♀ presenting with an erythematous and scaly eruption on the face and ears × 6 mo. Stress and emotional tensions aggravate the rash. Over-the-counter remedies provide no relief.

O: Patchy erythema with greasy, yellowish scaling appears over the nose and along the eyebrows. The external ears are similarly affected. Erythematous papules are scattered across the face, and there is ↑ oiliness around the nose.

A: Seborrheic dermatitis.

P: Rx: hydrocortisone cream, ss̄ oz tube

Sig: apply to affected areas t.i.d.

QUESTIONS ABOUT MEDICAL RECORD 3-1

1. What is the sex of the patient?
   a. male
   b. female
   c. not stated

2. What is the patient's CC?
   a. stress and emotional tension
   b. appearance of raised, yellow, pus-filled lesions on the skin
   c. appearance of red areas on the skin with flaking of the outer layers of the skin
   d. appearance of red areas on the skin with open sores
   e. appearance of a communicable rash on the face and ear

3. What is the diagnosis?
   a. inflammation of the sebaceous glands and hair follicles of the skin, as evidenced by comedones
   b. fungus of the skin
   c. inflammation of the skin with excessive secretion of sebum from the sebaceous glands
   d. highly contagious bacterial skin inflammation marked by pustules that rupture and become crusted
   e. transient, viral cold sores that infect the facial area

4. How much hydrocortisone cream was prescribed?
   a. one ounce
   b. two ounces
   c. one-half dram
   d. one dram
   e. one-half ounce

5. What is the Sig: on the prescription?
   a. apply to affected areas twice a day
   b. apply to affected areas three times a day
   c. apply to affected areas four times a day
   d. apply to affected areas every two hours
   e. apply to affected areas every three hours

Medical Record 3-2

FOR ADDITIONAL STUDY

After ignoring various skin problems for months, Robert Fuller consulted his doctor in October, when he became alarmed by what he saw happening on his right hand. His doctor referred him to Dr. Luong, a dermatologist, who then diagnosed and treated Mr. Fuller. Medical Record 3–2 is a SOAP progress note dictated by Dr. Luong immediately after the treatment of Mr. Fuller and transcribed the next day by his assistant.

Read Medical Record 3–2 (page 142), then write your answers to the following questions in the spaces provided.

QUESTIONS ABOUT MEDICAL RECORD 3-2

1. Below are medical terms used in this record that you have not yet encountered in this text. Underline each where it appears in the record, and define the term below:

   vulgaris _____

   verruciform _____

2. In your own words, not using medical terminology, briefly describe Mr. Fuller's complaint:

   _____

   _____

   _____

3. In your own words, not using medical terminology, briefly describe Dr. Luong's three objective findings:

   a. _____

   b. _____

   c. _____

4. Define the three diagnoses for those three objective findings:

   a. _____

   b. _____

   c. _____

5. Briefly describe the treatments for those three diagnoses:

   a. _____

   b. _____

   c. _____

6. What did Dr. Luong tell Mr. Fuller might occur in the future? Check all that apply:

   _____ scarring where the lesions were

   _____ nausea and possible vomiting from the nitrogen

   _____ red, freckle-like spots appearing on the right hand

   _____ possible regrowth of lesions

   _____ self-desiccating tissue destruction

Medical Record 3-2: For Additional Study

CENTRAL MEDICAL GROUP, INC.
Department of Dermatology

201 Medical Center Drive • Central City, US 90000-1234 • PHONE: (012) 125-8888 • FAX: (012) 125-3434

CHART NOTE

PATIENT: FULLER, ROBERT K.

DATE: October 19, 20xx

SUBJECTIVE: The patient presents with a growth on the right hand, multiple lesions, and other growths.

OBJECTIVE: Ulcerated growth on the right hand, marked A; one verruciform tumor on the left hand; erythematous keratotic patches on the arms.

ASSESSMENT: Basal cell carcinoma, verruca vulgaris, and actinic keratoses.

PLAN: Following full counseling on healing with scarring, keloids, and possible recurrence, the growth from the right hand was excised. The site was anesthetized with Xylocaine 2% without epinephrine, 2 cc. Following excision, the bases of the growths were treated with fulguration and electrodesiccation. Desiccation was also performed on 0.3 cm of normal surrounding skin. The wart was treated with liquid nitrogen, two cycles. Freezing time: 8-10 seconds. Ten erythematous keratotic patches were also treated with liquid nitrogen, two cycles. Freezing time: 10-14 seconds.

D. Luong, M.D.

DL:ti

D: 10/19/20xx
T: 10/20/20xx

ANSWERS TO PRACTICE EXERCISES

1. onycho/malacia
   CF   S
   nail/softening

2. myco/tic
   CF   S
   fungus/pertaining to

3. dermato/logist
   CF   S
   skin/one who specializes in the study or treatment of

4. histo/troph/ic
   CF   R   S
   tissue/nourishment or development/pertaining to

5. par/onych/ia
   P   R   S
   alongside of/nail/condition of

6. hyper/kerat/osis
   P   R   S
   above or excessive/hard/condition or increase

7. leuko/trich/ia
   CF   R   S
   white/hair/condition of

8. myco/logy
   CF   S
   fungus/study of

9. epi/derm/al
   P   R   S
   upon/skin/pertaining to

10. lip/oma
    R   S
    fat/tumor

11. sub/cutane/ous
    P   R   S
    below or under/skin/pertaining to

12. an/hidr/osis
    P   R   S
    without/sweat/condition or increase

13. histo/patho/logy
    CF   CF   S
    tissue/disease/study of

14. dys/plas/ia
    P   R   S
    painful, difficult, or faulty/formation/condition of

15. adip/osis
    R   S
    fat/condition or increase

16. squam/ous
    R   S
    scale/pertaining to

17. erythro/dermat/itis
    CF   R   S
    red/skin/inflammation

18. de/squam/ation
    P   R   S
    from, down, or not/scale/process

19. histo/tox/ic
    CF   R   S
    tissue/poison/pertaining to

20. melano/cyt/e
    CF   R   S
    black/cell/noun marker

21. xer/osis
    R   S
    dry/condition or increase

22. purpur/ic
    R   S
    purple/pertaining to

23. sebo/rrhea
    CF   S
    sebum (oil)/discharge

24. xanth/oma
    R   S
    yellow/tumor

25. a/steat/osis
    P   R   S
    without/fat/condition or increase

26. gangrene
27. autograft
28. ecchymosis
29. pruritus
30. carbuncle
31. tinea

32. urticaria
33. heterograft
34. pediculosis pubis
35. furuncle
36. macule or macula
37. scale
38. pediculosis capitis
39. alopecia
40. herpes simplex virus type 1
41. histology
42. erythema
43. open comedo
44. cicatrix
45. fissure
46. cryosurgery
47. biopsy
48. eruption
49. keloid
50. melanoma
51. seborrhea
52. excoriation
53. leukoderma
54. frozen section
55. erythroderma
56. keratoderma or scleroderma
57. seborrheic keratoses
58. lipoma or steatoma
59. xanthoderma
60. mycosis
61. hypodermic
62. cherry angioma
63. xeroderma
64. rubella
65. varicella
66. rubeola
67. f
68. i
69. c
70. h
71. d
72. g
73. a
74. j
75. b
76. e
77. herpes simplex virus type 2

78. biopsy
79. frozen section
80. incision and drainage
81. keratoses
82. ecchymoses
83. bullae
84. maculae
85. nevi
86. c
87. d
88. g
89. h
90. i
91. l
92. j
93. m
94. n
95. k

96. a
97. f
98. b
99. e
100. cicatrix
101. pruritus
102. petechia
103. verruca
104. ecchymosis
105. excision
106. psoriasis
107. impetigo
108. eczema
109. debridement
110. keratosis
111. bulla
112. nodule
113. seborrhea

114. petechia
115. ecchymosis
116. urticaria
117. eczema
118. macule
119. suppuration
120. squamous
121. basal
122. epidermis
123. dermis
124. subcutaneous
125. steat/o
126. melan/o
127. myc/o
128. onych/o
129. erythr/o
130. trich/o
131. xer/o
132. seb/o

ANSWERS TO MEDICAL RECORD ANALYSIS

Medical Record 3-1: Progress Note

1. b   2. c   3. c   4. e   5. b

Medical Record 3-2: For Additional Study

See CD-ROM for answers.

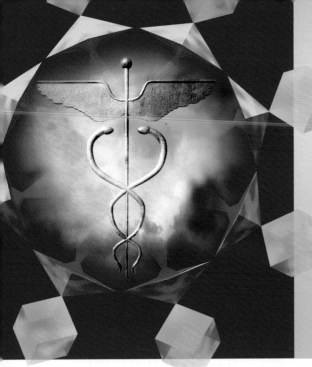

Musculoskeletal System

MUSCULOSKELETAL SYSTEM OVERVIEW

Functions of the skeleton (Fig. 4-1):

* Provides support and shape to the body through a framework of bones and cartilage
* Stores calcium and other minerals
* Produces certain blood cells within bone marrow

Functions of the muscles (Fig. 4-2):

* Supply the forces that make body movements possible
* Provide a protective covering for the internal organs
* Produce body heat

Orthopedics is the specialty most involved with the study and treatment of the musculoskeletal system. The spelling *orthopaedic* (the British form of the term) is frequently used, as in the name of the American Board of Orthopaedic Surgery.

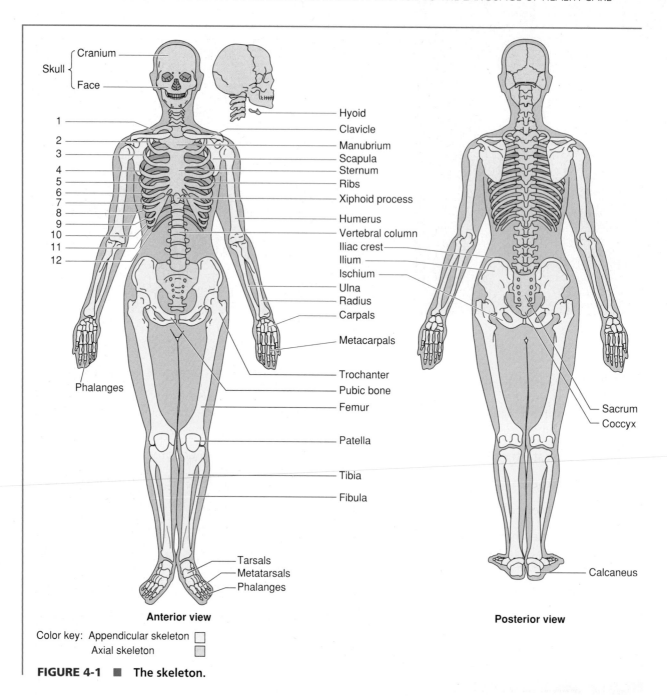

Anterior view

Posterior view

Color key: Appendicular skeleton ☐
Axial skeleton ▨

FIGURE 4-1 ■ **The skeleton.**

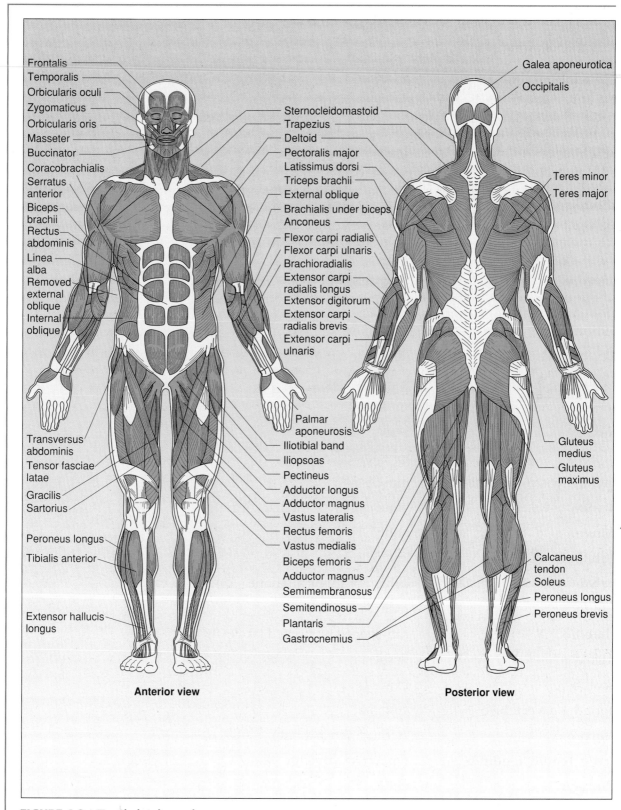

Frontalis
Temporalis
Orbicularis oculi
Zygomaticus
Orbicularis oris
Masseter
Buccinator
Coracobrachialis
Serratus anterior
Biceps brachii
Rectus abdominis
Linea alba
Removed external oblique
Internal oblique

Transversus abdominis
Tensor fasciae latae
Gracilis
Sartorius

Peroneus longus
Tibialis anterior

Extensor hallucis longus

Sternocleidomastoid
Trapezius
Deltoid
Pectoralis major
Latissimus dorsi
Triceps brachii
External oblique
Brachialis under biceps
Anconeus
Flexor carpi radialis
Flexor carpi ulnaris
Brachioradialis
Extensor carpi radialis longus
Extensor digitorum
Extensor carpi radialis brevis
Extensor carpi ulnaris

Palmar aponeurosis
Iliotibial band
Iliopsoas
Pectineus
Adductor longus
Adductor magnus
Vastus lateralis
Rectus femoris
Vastus medialis
Biceps femoris
Adductor magnus
Semimembranosus
Semitendinosus
Plantaris
Gastrocnemius

Galea aponeurotica
Occipitalis

Teres minor
Teres major

Gluteus medius
Gluteus maximus

Calcaneus tendon
Soleus
Peroneus longus
Peroneus brevis

Anterior view

Posterior view

FIGURE 4-2 ■ Skeletal muscles.

Self-Instruction: Combining Forms

Study the following:

COMBINING FORM	MEANING
ankyl/o	crooked or stiff
arthr/o, articul/o	joint
brachi/o	arm
cervic/o	neck
chondr/o	cartilage (gristle)
cost/o	rib
crani/o	skull
dactyl/o	digit (finger or toe)
fasci/o	fascia (a band)
femor/o	femur
fibr/o	fiber
kyph/o	humped-back
lei/o	smooth
lord/o	bent
lumb/o	loin (lower back)
my/o, myos/o, muscul/o	muscle
myel/o	bone marrow or spinal cord
oste/o	bone
patell/o	knee cap
pelv/i	pelvis (basin) or hip bone
radi/o	radius
rhabd/o	rod-shaped or striated (skeletal)
sarc/o	flesh
scoli/o	twisted
spondyl/o, vertebr/o	vertebra
stern/o	sternum (breastbone)
ten/o, tend/o, tendin/o	tendon (to stretch)
thorac/o	chest
ton/o	tone or tension
uln/o	ulna

Programmed Review: Combining Forms

ANSWERS	REVIEW
straight, normal, or correct foot orthopaedic	**4.1** *Orth/o*, meaning _____, and *ped/o*, meaning _____, are combined to form the term orthopedic, meaning pertaining to the medical specialty related to the musculoskeletal system. The British spelling for this specialty is _____.
oste/o -itis myel/o	**4.2** The combining form meaning bone is _____. The suffix _____ means inflammation. Osteitis therefore refers to inflammation of bone. Inside most bones is bone marrow; the combining form meaning bone marrow is _____, as in the adjective myeloid.
myos/o muscle inflammation	**4.3** The three combining forms for muscle are *muscul/o,* *my/o,* and _____. The musculoskeletal system involves both muscles and bones. Recalling that the suffix *-algia* means pain, myalgia must mean _____ pain. Myositis is an _____ of muscle.
skull crani/o cervical neck	**4.4** The cranial bones comprise the _____. The combining form that means skull is _____. Neck bones are referred to as the _____ vertebrae, from the combining form *cervic/o*, meaning _____.
spondyl/o vertebrae twisted condition or increase lord/o kyph/o lumb/o pain, lower	**4.5** The two combining forms for vertebrae, the bones of the spine, are *vertebr/o* and _____. Spondylitis is inflammation of the _____. *Scoli/o* means _____, and when combined with the suffix *-osis*, which means _____, it forms the word scoliosis, which refers to a condition of having a twisted spine. The combining form meaning bent is _____, and a spine that is bent forward is called lordosis. The condition of a humped back is called kyphosis, from the combining form _____, meaning humped-back. The lower back is the lumbar spine, from the combining form _____. Lumbodynia refers to _____ in the _____ back.

ANSWERS	REVIEW
sternum sternum or breastbone, ribs	**4.6** The breastbone is also called the _____, from the combining form *stern/o*. Most of the ribs connect to the breastbone in the front of the body. The combining form *cost/o* means rib. The sternocostal area, therefore, is where the _____ is connected to the _____.
chest thorac/o -ic	**4.7** Thoracic is the adjective referring to the _____, formed from the combining form _____, which means chest, and the adjective-forming suffix _____.
pelvis pelvis measurement	**4.8** Below the ribs and spine are the bones of the _____, from the combining form *pelv/i*. A pelviscope is used to examine the interior of the _____. Pelvimetry is the _____ of the diameters of the pelvis.
femor/o patell/o	**4.9** Below the pelvis is the longest bone in the body, the femur. The combining form for this term is _____. The femur joins the tibia at the knee joint, where a small bone called the kneecap covers the joint. The medical term for the kneecap is patella, from the combining form _____.
ulna, radi/o radius	**4.10** The two bones of the forearm are the radius and the _____, from the combining forms _____ and *uln/o*. Radioulnar is an adjective referring to both the _____ and the ulna.
digit pain	**4.11** The combining form *dactyl/o* refers to _____ (either a finger or a toe). Dactylalgia therefore means _____ of the fingers or toes.
brachi/o arm	**4.12** The combining form for arm is _____. The brachial artery, for example, runs through the _____.
articul/o arthr/o inflammation	**4.13** A joint is where two or more bones join together. This is also called an articulation, from the combining form _____. Another combining term for joint is _____, which is used to form the term arthritis, meaning _____ of a joint.
stiff	**4.14** *Ankyl/o* is a combining form meaning crooked or _____. Ankylosis therefore is a stiffened joint.

ANSWERS	REVIEW
chondr/o	**4.15** Cartilage is a gristle-like substance that covers bones where they articulate at joints. Chondroma is a tumor that arises from cartilage, the combining form for which is _____.
fibr/o smooth tumor, striated	**4.16** Muscle fibers have the ability to contract, allowing them to move bones and, thus, body parts. The combining form for fiber is _____, and a common adjective form is fibrous. Muscles are composed of either smooth (*lei/o*) or striated (*rhabd/o*) muscle tissues. A leiomyoma is a tumor of _____ muscle. A rhabdomyoma is a _____ of _____ (skeletal) muscle.
ton/o muscle tone	**4.17** The combining form for tone is _____. Therefore, myotonia refers to a condition of _____ _____.
tend/o inflammation	**4.18** A tendon connects muscle to bone. Three combining forms for tendon are *ten/o*, _____, and *tendin/o*. Tendinitis is _____ of a tendon.
fasci/o	**4.19** Fascia is a band or sheet of fibrous tissue that encloses muscles or groups of muscles. It comes from the combining form _____.
flesh tumor	**4.20** *Sarc/o* means _____ or a muscular substance. A sarcoma, for example, is a fleshy _____.

Self-Instruction: Anatomic Terms Related to Bones

Study the following:

TERM	MEANING
appendicular skeleton *ap'en-dik'yū-lăr skel'ĕ-tŏn*	bones of the shoulder, pelvis, and upper and lower extremities
axial skeleton *ak'sē-ăl skel'ĕ-tŏn*	bones of the skull, vertebral column (Fig. 4-3), chest, and hyoid bone (U-shaped bone at the base of the tongue)
bone *bōn*	specialized connective tissue composed of osteocytes (bone cells); forms the skeleton
TYPES OF BONE TISSUE	
compact bone *kom'pakt bōn*	tightly solid bone tissue that forms the exterior of bones

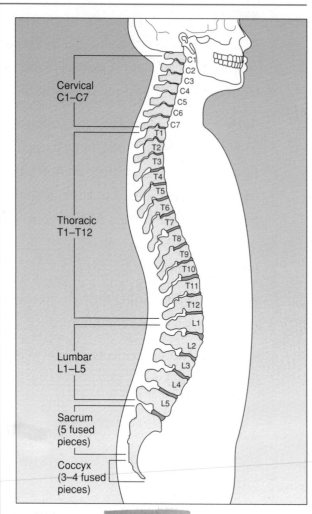

FIGURE 4-3 ■ The vertebrae.

TERM	MEANING
spongy bone *spŏn′ jē bōn* **cancellous bone** *kan′ sĕ-lŭs bōn*	mesh-like bone tissue found in the interior of bones, and surrounding the medullary cavity

CLASSIFICATION OF BONES

long bones *long bōnz*	bones of the arms and legs
short bones *short bōnz*	bones of the wrist and ankles
flat bones *flat bōnz*	bones of the ribs, shoulder blades, pelvis, and skull
irregular bones *ir-reg′ yū-lăr bōnz*	bones of the vertebrae and face
sesamoid bones *ses′ă-moyd bōnz*	round bones found near joints (e.g., the patella)

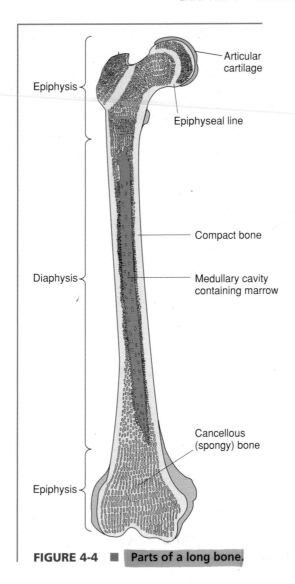

Epiphysis

Articular cartilage

Epiphyseal line

Compact bone

Diaphysis

Medullary cavity containing marrow

Cancellous (spongy) bone

Epiphysis

FIGURE 4-4 ■ Parts of a long bone.

TERM	MEANING
PARTS OF A LONG BONE (Fig. 4-4)	
epiphysis *e-pif′i-sis*	wide ends of a long bone (*physis* = growth)
diaphysis *dī-af′i-sis*	shaft of a long bone
metaphysis *mĕ-taf′i-sis*	growth zone between the epiphysis and the diaphysis during development of a long bone
endosteum *en-dos′tē-ŭm*	membrane lining the medullary cavity of a bone
medullary cavity *med′ŭl-ār-ē kav′i-tē*	cavity within the shaft of the long bones; filled with bone marrow
bone marrow *bōn ma′rō*	soft connective tissue within the medullary cavity of bones

TERM	MEANING
red bone marrow *rĕd bōn ma′rō*	functions to form red blood cells, some white blood cells, and platelets; found in the cavities of most bones in infants and in the flat bones in adults
yellow bone marrow *yel′ō bōn ma′rō*	gradually replaces red bone marrow in adult bones; functions as storage for fat tissue and is inactive in the formation of blood cells
periosteum *per-ē-os′tē-ŭm*	a fibrous, vascular membrane that covers the bone
articular cartilage *ar-tik′yu-lăr kar′ti-lij*	a gristle-like substance on bones where they articulate

◈ Programmed Review: Anatomic Terms Related to Bones

ANSWERS	REVIEW
axial, appendicular skull	**4.21** The skeleton as a whole is divided into the appendicular skeleton and the _____ skeleton. The _____ skeleton includes the shoulders and arms and the pelvis and legs. The axial skeleton includes the spine, chest, and _____.
osteo compact, Cancellous	**4.22** Bone cells, or _____cytes, form the skeleton. The tightly solid bone tissue that forms the exterior of bones is called _____ bone. _____ bone is the spongy, mesh-like bone tissue found in the interior of bones, and surrounding the medullary cavity.
arms, legs Short flat round	**4.23** Long bones are found in the _____ and _____. _____ bones are found in the wrists and ankles. The ribs, shoulder blades, and pelvis are _____ bones. Bones of the vertebrae and face are called irregular bones. Sesamoid bones are _____ bones (e.g., the patella) near joints.
end dia, physis	**4.24** Long bones have several parts. Several of these parts are named with terms from the root *physis* (growth), referring to how the bones grow. The epiphysis is the wide _____ of a long bone. The _____physis is the shaft. The meta_____ is the growth zone between the epiphysis and the diaphysis.

ANSWERS	REVIEW
within bone marrow, Red marrow fat periosteum around	**4.25** The prefix *endo-* means _____. The endosteum is a membrane lining the medullary cavity within a _____. Inside the medullary cavity is bone _____. _____ bone marrow makesred blood cells, whereas yellow bone _____ stores _____ tissue. The membrane that covers a bone is called the _____, from the combining term for bone (*oste/o*) and the prefix *peri-*, meaning _____.
articular	**4.26** The kind of cartilage that is found where bones articulate is called _____ cartilage.

Self-Instruction: Anatomic Terms Related to Joints and Muscles

Study the following:

TERM	MEANING
articulation (Fig. 4-5) *ar'tik-yū-lā'shŭn*	a joint; the point where two bones come together
bursa *bŭr'să*	a fibrous sac between certain tendons and bones that is lined with a synovial membrane that secretes synovial fluid

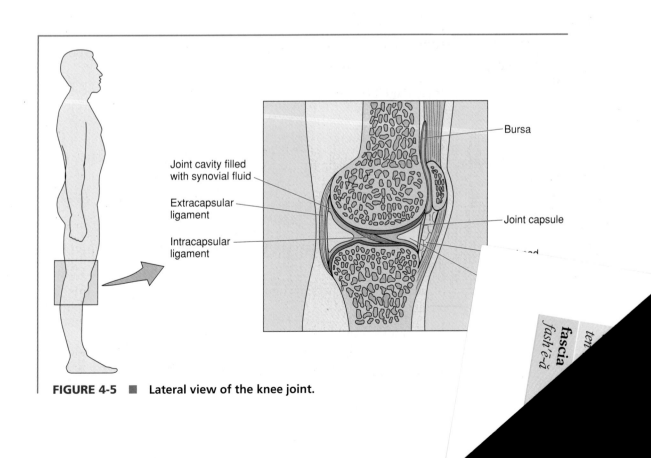

FIGURE 4-5 ■ **Lateral view of the knee joint.**

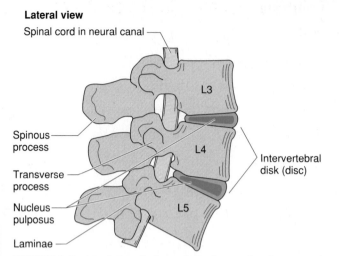

Lateral view
Spinal cord in neural canal

L3

Spinous process

Transverse process

Nucleus pulposus

Laminae

L4

Intervertebral disk (disc)

L5

FIGURE 4-6 ▰ **Lateral view of the lower lumbar vertebrae.**

TERM	MEANING
disk or **disc** (Fig. 4-6) *disk*	a flat, plate-like structure composed of fibrocartilaginous tissue between the vertebrae that reduces friction
nucleus pulposus *nū′klē-ŭs pōl-pō′sŭs*	the soft, fibrocartilaginous, central portion of intervertebral disk
ligament *lig′ă-mĕnt*	a flexible band of fibrous tissue that connects bone to bone
synovial membrane *si-nō′vē-ăl mem′brān*	membrane lining the capsule of a joint
synovial fluid *si-nō′vē-ăl flū′id*	joint-lubricating fluid secreted by the synovial membrane
muscle *mŭs′ĕl*	tissue composed of fibers that can contract, causing movement of an organ or part of the body
striated muscle *strī′āt-ĕd mŭs′ĕl* **skeletal muscle** *skel′e-tăl mŭs′ĕl*	voluntary muscle attached to the skeleton
smooth muscle *smūth mŭs′ĕl*	involuntary muscle found in internal organs
cardiac muscle *kar′dē-ak mŭs′ĕl*	muscle of the heart
origin of a muscle *ōr′i-jin of a mŭs′ĕl*	muscle end attached to the bone that does not move when the muscle contracts
insertion of a muscle *in-sĕr′shŭn of a mŭs′ĕl*	muscle end attached to the bone that moves when the muscle contracts
tendon *′dŏn*	a band of fibrous tissue that connects muscle to bone
	a band or sheet of fibrous connective tissue that covers, supports, and separates muscle

Programmed Review: Anatomic Terms Related to Joints and Muscles

ANSWERS	REVIEW
Muscle Smooth muscle, heart striated	**4.27** _____ tissue can contract, causing movement of an organ or body part. There are three types of muscle tissue. _____ muscle is found in internal organs and is also called involuntary muscle, because you cannot will it to contract. Cardiac _____ is an involuntary muscle found only in the _____. Skeletal muscle, or _____ muscle, is under voluntary control.
origin insertion tendons fascia	**4.28** Skeletal muscle is attached to bone at both ends of the muscle. The end attached to the bone that does not move when the muscle contracts is called the _____ of the muscle. The other end, which is attached to the bone and that moves with contraction, is called the _____ of the muscle. Muscles are connected to bones by _____. The band or sheet of fibrous tissue that covers muscles is called _____.
articulation ligament synovial fluid	**4.29** The point where two muscles come together is called a joint or an _____. A fibrous band that connects bone to bone is a _____. The joint capsule is lined with a _____ membrane, which secretes a lubricating fluid called synovial _____.
bursa inflammation	**4.30** The fibrous sac between certain tendons and bones is a _____; an inflammation of this tissue is called bursitis. The suffix *-itis* means _____.
disks, discs pulposus	**4.31** The flat, plate-like structures between the vertebrae are called _____, which sometimes is also spelled _____. The nucleus _____ is a soft fibrocartilaginous tissue in the center of intervertebral disks.

Self-Instruction: Anatomic Position and Terms of Reference

Study the following:

TERM	MEANING
anatomic or **anatomical position** *an-ah-tŏm′ik or an-ah-tŏm′ik-ăl pō-zĭ′shŭn*	a term of reference that health professionals use when noting body planes, positions, or directions: the person is assumed to be standing upright (erect), facing forward, feet pointed forward and slightly apart, with arms at the sides and palms facing forward; the patient is visualized in this pose when applying any other term of reference
body planes (Fig. 4-7) *bod′ē plānz*	reference planes for indicating the location or direction of body parts

BODY PLANES

coronal plane *kōr′ŏ-năl plān* **frontal plane** *frŏn′tăl plān*	vertical division of the body into front (anterior) and back (posterior) portions
sagittal plane *saj′i-tăl plān*	vertical division of the body into right and left portions
transverse plane *trans-vĕrs′ plān*	horizontal division of the body into upper and lower portions

DIRECTIONAL TERMS

anterior (A) *an-tēr′ē-ŏr* **ventral** *ven′trăl*	front of the body

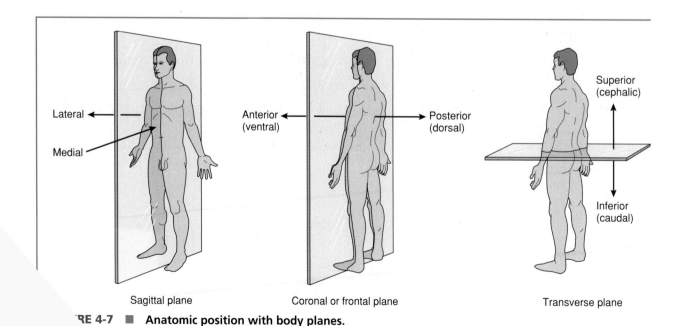

FIGURE 4-7 ■ **Anatomic position with body planes.**

TERM	MEANING
posterior (P) *pos-tēr′ē-ŏr* **dorsal** *dōr′săl*	back of the body
anterior-posterior (AP)	from front to back, as in reference to the direction of an x-ray beam
posterior-anterior (PA)	from back to front, as in reference to the direction of an x-ray beam
superior *sū-pĕr′ē-ŏr* **cephalic** *se-fal′ik*	situated above another structure, toward the head
inferior *in-fēr′ē-ŏr* **caudal** *kaw′dăl*	situated below another structure, away from the head
proximal *prok′si-măl*	toward the beginning or origin of a structure; for example, the proximal aspect of the femur (thigh bone) is the area closest to where it attaches to the hip
distal *dis′tăl*	away from the beginning or origin of a structure; for example, the distal aspect of the femur (thigh bone) is the area at the end of the bone near the knee
medial *mē′dē-ăl*	toward the middle (midline)
lateral *lat′er-ăl*	toward the side
axis *ak′sis*	the imaginary line that runs through the center of the body or a body part

BODY POSITIONS

erect *ē-rĕkt′*	normal standing position
decubitus *dē-kyū′bi-tŭs*	lying down, especially in a bed; lateral decubitus is lying on the side (*decumbo* = to lie down)
prone *prōn*	lying face down and flat
recumbent *rē-kŭm′bĕnt*	lying down
supine (Fig. 4-8) *sū-pīn′*	horizontal recumbent; lying flat on the back ("on the spine")

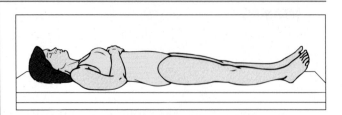

FIGURE 4-8 ■ Supine (horizontal recumbent) position. Patient lies on back with the legs extended.

TERM	MEANING
BODY MOVEMENTS (Fig. 4-9)	
flexion *flek'shŭn*	bending at the joint so that the angle between the bones is decreased

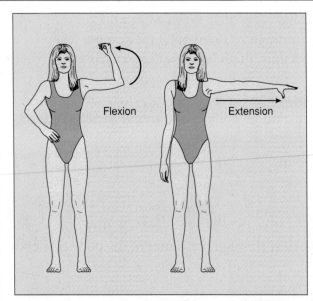

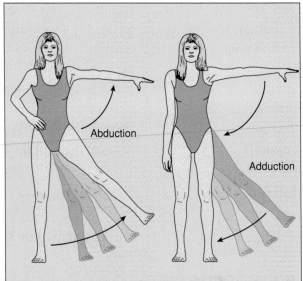

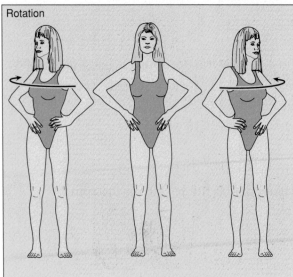

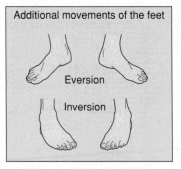

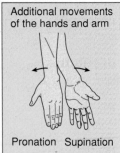

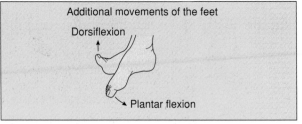

FIGURE 4-9 ■ Body movements.

TERM	MEANING
extension *eks-ten'shŭn*	straightening at the joint so that the angle between the bones is increased
abduction *ab-dŭk'shŭn*	movement away from the body
adduction *ă-dŭk'shŭn*	movement toward the body
rotation *rō-tā'shŭn*	circular movement around an axis
eversion *ē-ver'zhŭn*	turning outward, i.e., of a foot
inversion *in-vĕr'zhŭn*	turning inward, i.e., of a foot
supination *sū'pi-nā'shŭn*	turning of the palmar surface (palm of the hand) or plantar surface (sole of the foot) upward or forward
pronation *prō-nā'shŭn*	turning of the palmar surface (palm of the hand) or plantar surface (sole of the foot) downward or backward
dorsiflexion *dōr-si-flek'shŭn*	bending of the foot or the toes upward
plantar flexion *plan'tăr flek'shŭn*	bending of the sole of the foot by curling the toes toward the ground
range of motion (ROM) *rānj of mō'shŭn*	total motion possible in a joint, described by the terms related to body movements (i.e., ability to flex, extend, abduct, or adduct); measured in degrees

goniometer
    (Fig. 4-10)
    gō-nē-om'ĕ-tĕr
	instrument used to measure joint angles (*gonio* = angle)

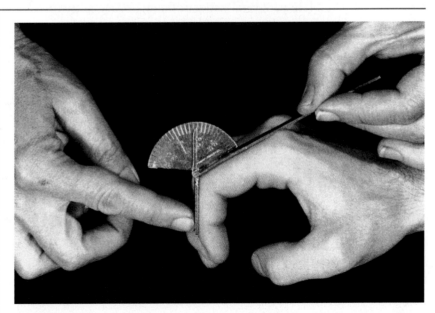

FIGURE 4-10 ■ Dorsal placement of goniometer used when measuring digital motion.

Programmed Review: Anatomic Position and Terms of Reference

ANSWERS	REVIEW
anatomic erect, forward sides forward	**4.32** Health professionals describe body part locations relative to the _____ position, in which one is standing upright, or _____, and is facing _____, with the feet pointed forward and slightly apart, the arms at the _____, and the palms facing _____.
planes coronal sagittal horizontally	**4.33** Body _____ help one to understand directional and positional terms. The body is vertically divided into front (anterior) and back (posterior) portions by the _____, or frontal, plane. The _____ plane divides the body vertically into right and left portions. The transverse plane divides the body _____ into upper and lower portions.
before after anterior posterior	**4.34** Recall that the prefix *ante-* means _____ and the prefix *post-* means _____. Using these word parts, the front of the body is _____ (also called ventral), and the back of the body is _____ (also called dorsal).
anterior-posterior posterior-anterior	**4.35** The direction of an x-ray beam from front to back is designated _____-_____, whereas the direction from back to front is designated _____-_____.
superior inferior	**4.36** The head is _____ to, or above, the shoulders, whereas the feet are _____ to, or below, the knees.
closest distal proximal end	**4.37** The proximal aspect of a structure is the area _____ to its origin or attachment. The _____ aspect of a structure is the area away from its origin or attachment. The _____ aspect of the femur (thigh bone) is the area closest to where it attaches to the hip. The distal aspect of the femur (thigh bone) is the area at the _____ of the bone near the knee.
medial side	**4.38** Toward the middle or midline is called _____, whereas lateral means toward the _____.
axis	**4.39** An imaginary line that runs through the center of the body or a body part is called an _____. For example, you can rotate your wrist on its axis.

ANSWERS	REVIEW
erect	**4.40** The normal standing position is _____ (as in the anatomic position). Several terms describe different ways the body lies down.
recumbent decubitus lateral face, supine	The general term for lying down is _____. Lying down, especially in bed, is called _____. A patient lying on one side in bed is in a _____ decubitus position. Prone means lying _____ down and flat, and _____ means lying face up, flat on the back.
decreases extension, away away from adduction toward	**4.41** Many different terms are used to describe body movements at joints. Flexing a joint (flexion) _____ the angle between the bones; the opposite movement (increasing the angle) is _____. Movement _____ from the body is called abduction (the prefix *ab-* means _____ _____); the opposite movement is called _____ (the prefix *ad-* means _____).
rotation eversion	**4.42** A circular movement around an axis is called _____. For example, you can rotate your feet inward and outward. The term for inward rotation is inversion; the term for outward rotation begins with the prefix *e-* (out or away): _____.
supination, pronation	**4.43** Turning the palm of the hand upward or forward is called _____; the opposite movement is called _____. Note the relationship of these terms to the terms for the body lying supine or prone.
dorsiflexion plantar flexion	**4.44** The foot and toes bend upward in _____ and downward in _____ _____.
range goniometer	**4.45** The total amount of motion in a joint is called its _____ of motion. In certain musculoskeletal conditions, the range of motion may decrease. The instrument used to measure a joint _____ _____.

Self-Instruction: Symptomatic Terms

Study the following:

TERM	MEANING
arthralgia *ar-thral′jē-ă*	joint pain
atrophy *at′rō-fē*	shrinking of muscle size
crepitation *krep-i-tā′shŭn* **crepitus** *krep′i-tŭs*	grating sound sometimes made by the movement of a joint or broken bones
exostosis *eks-os-tō′sis*	a projection arising from a bone that develops from cartilage
flaccid *flas′ĭd*	flabby, relaxed, or having defective or absent muscle tone
hypertrophy *hī-pĕr′trō-fē*	increase in the size of tissue, such as muscle
hypotonia *hī′pō-tō′nē-ă*	reduced muscle tone or tension
myalgia *mī-al′jē-ă* **myodynia** *mī′ō-din′ē-ă*	muscle pain
ostealgia *os-tē-al′jē-ă* **osteodynia** *os-tē-ō-din′ē-ă*	bone pain
rigor *rig′ŏr* **rigidity** *ri-jid′i-tē*	stiffness; stiff muscle
spasm *spazm*	drawing in; involuntary contraction of muscle
spastic *spas′tik*	uncontrolled contractions of skeletal muscles, causing stiff and awkward movements (resembles spasm)
tetany *ĕt′ă-nē*	tension; prolonged, continuous muscle contraction
...or	shaking; rhythmic muscular movement

Programmed Review: Symptomatic Terms

ANSWERS	REVIEW
crepitation	**4.46** Broken bones rubbing together may produce a grating sound, which is called crepitus or _____. This sound may also occur in a joint.
outside exostosis	**4.47** Recall that the prefix *exo-* means _____. A term for a cartilage projection growing outside a bone is _____.
-algia osteodynia, ostealgia myodynia, myalgia arthralgia	**4.48** Two suffixes for pain are *-dynia* and _____. Using the combining form for bone, two terms for bone pain are _____ and _____. Two similarly formed terms for muscle pain are _____ and _____. Using the combining form *arthr/o*, the term for joint pain is _____.
above or excessive increased atrophy	**4.49** The prefix *hyper-* means _____. Hypertrophy refers to _____ muscle size. Shrinking muscle size is called _____.
deficient hypotonia flaccid	**4.50** The prefix *hypo-* means below or _____. A condition of reduced muscle tension or tone is called _____. In such a case, the muscle can be said to be flabby or _____.
rhythmic	**4.51** Tremor, from the Latin word for shaking, is a _____ muscular movement. This may result from certain neurologic conditions.
rigor	**4.52** A stiff muscle is called _____ or rigidity.
spasm tetany, condition	**4.53** An involuntary contraction of a muscle is called a _____. A prolonged, continuous muscle contraction is a condition called _____. Recall that the suffix *-y* means a _____ or process.

Self-Instruction: Diagnostic Terms

Study the following:

TERM	MEANING
ankylosis *ang′ki-lō′sis*	stiff joint condition
arthritis *ar-thrī′tis*	inflammation of the joints chara____ redness, warmth, and limitation ____ 100 different types of arthritis

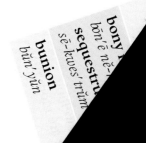

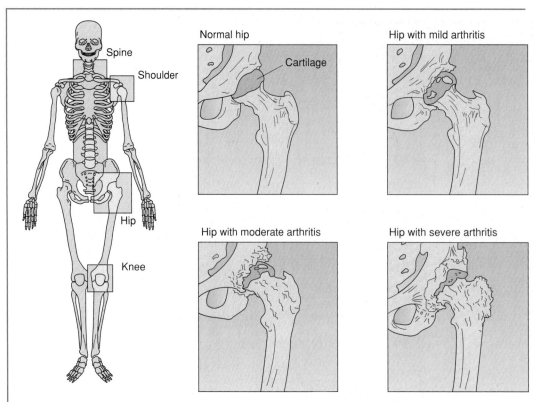

FIGURE 4-11 ■ Osteoarthritis. A. Common sites of osteoarthritis. B. How osteoarthritis affects the hip.

TERM	MEANING
osteoarthritis (OA) (Fig. 4-11) *os'tē-ō-ar-thrī'tis* **degenerative arthritis** *dē-jen'ĕr-ă-tiv ar-thrī'tis* **degenerative joint disease (DJD)** *dē-jen'ĕr-ă-tiv joynt di-zēz'*	most common form of arthritis, especially affecting the weight-bearing joints (e.g., knee or hip), characterized by the erosion of articular cartilage
rheumatoid arthritis (RA) (Fig. 4-12) *rū'mă-toyd ar-thrī'tis*	most crippling form of arthritis; characterized by chronic, systemic inflammation, most often affecting joints and synovial membranes (especially in the hands and feet) and causing ankylosis and deformity
gouty arthritis *gow'tē ar-thrī'tis*	acute attacks of arthritis, usually in a single joint (especially the great toe), caused by hyperuricemia (an excessive level of uric acid in the blood)
necrosis *krō'sis*	bone tissue that has died from loss of blood supply, such as can occur after a fracture (*sequestrum* = something laid aside)
	swelling of the joint at the base of the great toe caused by inflammation of the bursa

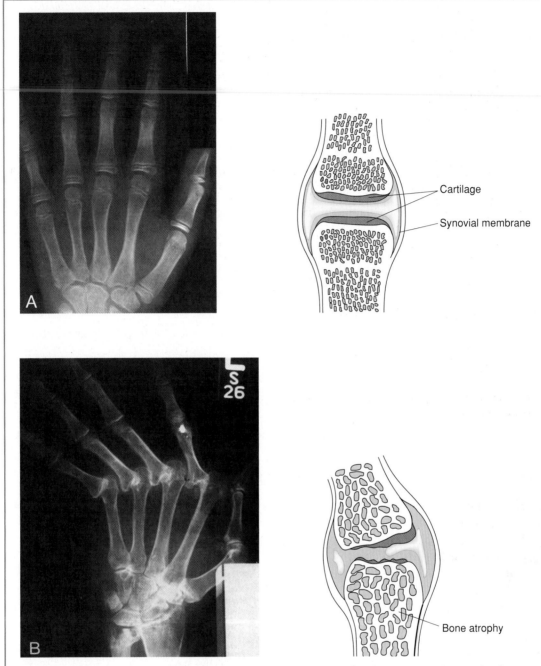

FIGURE 4-12 ■ Joints of the hand affected by rheumatoid arthritis. A. Radiograph of a normal hand. B. Radiograph of a hand with rheumatoid arthritis.

TERM	MEANING
bursitis *ber-sī′ tis*	inflammation of a bursa
chondromalacia *kon′ drō-mă-lā′ shē-ă*	softening of cartilage
epiphysitis *e-pif-i-sī′ tis*	inflammation of the epiphyseal regions of the long bone

TERM	MEANING
fracture (Fx) (Fig. 4-13) *frak′chūr*	broken or cracked bone
closed fracture *klōsd frak′chūr*	broken bone with no open wound
open fracture *ō′pen frak′chūr*	compound fracture; broken bone with an open wound
simple fracture *sim′pĕl frak′chūr*	nondisplaced fracture with one fracture line that does not require extensive treatment to repair (e.g., hairline fracture, stress fracture, or a crack)
complex fracture *kom′pleks frak′chūr*	displaced fracture that requires manipulation or surgery to repair
fracture line *frak′chūr līn*	the line of the break in a broken bone (e.g., oblique, spiral, or transverse)
comminuted fracture *kom′i-nyū-tĕd frak′chūr*	broken in many small pieces
greenstick fracture *grēn′stik frak′chūr*	bending and incomplete break of a bone; most often seen in children
herniated disk *hĕr′nē-ā-tĕd disk*	protrusion of a degenerated or fragmented intervertebral disk so that the nucleus pulposus protrudes, causing compression on the nerve root (*see* Chapter 8, Fig. 8-8)
myeloma *mī-ĕ-lō′mă*	bone marrow tumor
myositis *mī-ō-sī′tis*	inflammation of muscle
myoma *mī-ō′mă*	muscle tumor
leiomyoma *lī′ō-mī-ō′mă*	smooth muscle tumor
leiomyosarcoma *lī′ō-mī′ō-sar-kō′mă*	malignant smooth muscle tumor
rhabdomyoma *rab′dō-mī-ō′mă*	skeletal muscle tumor
rhabdomyosarcoma *rab′dō-mī′ō-sar-kō′mă*	malignant skeletal muscle tumor
muscular dystrophy *mŭs′kyū-lăr dis′trō-fē*	a category of genetically transmitted diseases characterized by progressive atrophy of skeletal muscles; Duchenne type is most common
osteoma *os-tē-ō′mă*	bone tumor
osteosarcoma *os′tē-ō-sar-kō′mă*	type of malignant bone tumor
osteomalacia *os′tē-ō-mă-lā′shē-ă*	disease marked by softening of the bone caused by calcium and vitamin D deficiency

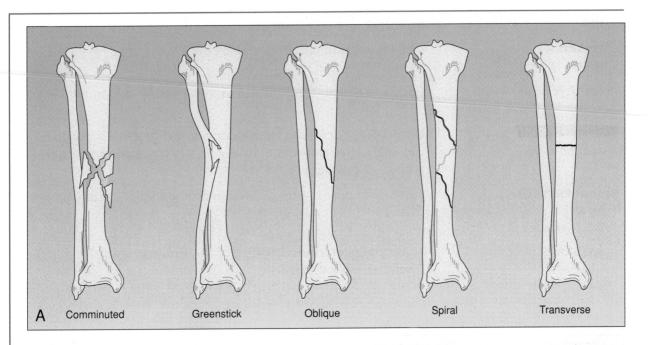

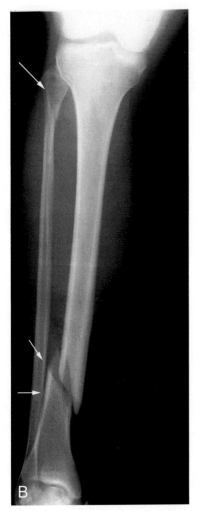

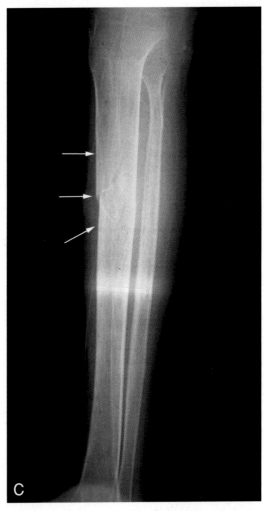

FIGURE 4-13 ■ A. Types of common fractures. B. Anterior-posterior radiograph of a lower leg demonstrating open fractures of the tibia and fibula (*arrows*). C. Lateral-view radiograph demonstrating a closed spiral fracture of the tibia (*arrows*).

TERM	MEANING
rickets *rik′ets*	osteomalacia in children; causes bone deformity
osteomyelitis *os′tē-ō-mī-ĕ-lī′tis*	infection of bone and bone marrow, causing inflammation
osteoporosis (Fig. 4-14) *os′tē-ō-pō-rō′sis*	condition of decreased bone density and increased porosity, causing bones to become brittle and to fracture more easily (*porosis* = passage)
spinal curvatures (Fig. 4-15) *spī′năl ker′vă-chŭrz*	curvatures of the spine (backbone) or spinal column (vertebral column)
kyphosis *kī-fō′sis*	abnormal posterior curvature of the thoracic spine (humped-back condition)

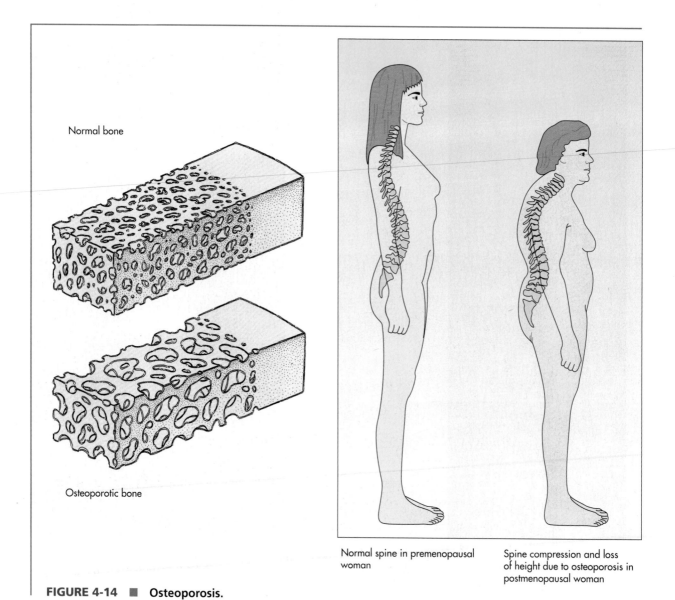

Normal bone

Osteoporotic bone

Normal spine in premenopausal woman

Spine compression and loss of height due to osteoporosis in postmenopausal woman

FIGURE 4-14 ■ Osteoporosis.

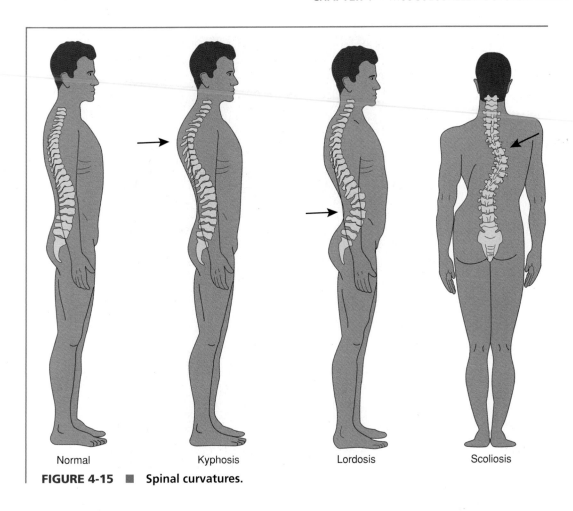

Normal   Kyphosis   Lordosis   Scoliosis

FIGURE 4-15 ■ **Spinal curvatures.**

TERM	MEANING
lordosis *lōr-dō′sis*	abnormal anterior curvature of the lumbar spine (sway-back condition)
scoliosis (Fig 4-16) *skō-lē-ō′sis*	abnormal lateral curvature of the spine (S-shaped curve)
spondylolisthesis (Fig. 4-17) *spon′di-lō-lis-thē′sis*	forward slipping of a lumbar vertebra (*listhesis* = slipping)
spondylosis *spon-di-lō′sis*	stiff, immobile condition of vertebrae caused by joint degeneration
sprain *sprān*	injury to a ligament caused by joint trauma but without joint dislocation or fracture
subluxation *sŭb-lŭk-sā′shŭn*	partial dislocation (*luxation* = dislocation)
tendinitis or **tendonitis** *ten-di-nī′tis or ten-dŏ-nī′tis*	inflammation of a tendon

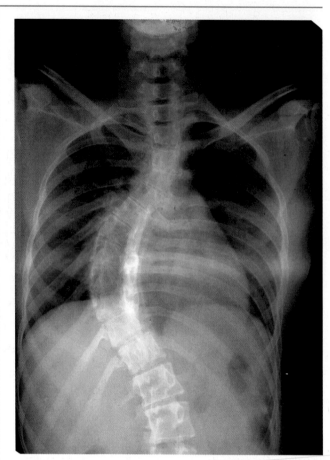

FIGURE 4-16 ■ **Anterior-posterior thoracic spine radiograph demonstrating scoliosis.**

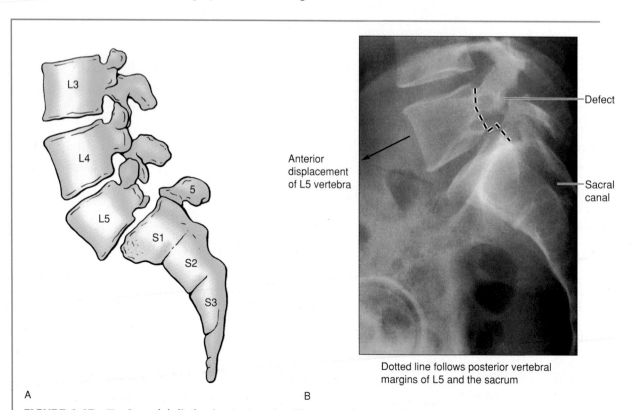

A   B

FIGURE 4-17 ■ **Spondylolisthesis. A. Drawing illustrates forward slipping of L5 vertebra. B. X-ray showing displacement.**

Programmed Review: Diagnostic Terms

ANSWERS	REVIEW
condition or increase ankylosis	**4.54** Formed from the combining form for stiff and the suffix -osis, meaning _____, a stiff joint condition is called _____.
inflammation arthritis osteoarthritis joint rheumatoid, Gouty hyper	**4.55** Formed from the combining form for joint and the suffix -itis, meaning _____, the term for inflammation of joints characterized by pain and swelling is _____. The most common form of arthritis, which is formed using the combining form for bone, is _____. This is also called degenerative arthritis or degenerative _____ disease. The most crippling type of arthritis, which is characterized by chronic systemic inflammation, is _____ arthritis. _____ arthritis attacks a single joint (e.g., the great toe) because of too much uric acid in the blood, or _____ uricemia.
-itis bursa epiphysitis muscle tendonitis or tendinitis bone marrow	**4.56** Recall that the suffix _____ refers to inflammation. Bursitis is inflammation of a _____. Inflammation of the epiphyseal regions of a long bone is called _____. Myositis is inflammation of a _____. Inflammation of a tendon is called _____. Osteomyelitis is an infection and inflammation of bone and _____ _____.
swelling	**4.57** A bunion is a _____ at the joint at the base of the great toe caused by inflammation of the bursa.
death condition, increase necrosis, sequestrum	**4.58** The combining form necr/o means _____, and the suffix -osis means _____ or _____. The term for the condition or increase of dead bone tissue caused by a loss of blood supply is bony _____, which is also called _____.
chrondr/o cartilage	**4.59** Recall that the combining form for cartilage is _____. The term chondromalacia refers to a softening of _____.
fracture closed open simple complex, Fx	**4.60** A broken bone, or _____, can happen in various ways. The skin is not broken in a _____ fracture, wh____ there is an open wound with an _____ fracture. If the fract__ one fracture line and the bones are not displaced, this i__ _____ fracture, whereas a displaced fracture t__ manipulation to put the bone pieces in correct positi__ _____ fracture. The abbreviation for fract__

ANSWERS	REVIEW
comminuted greenstick	**4.61** A fracture involving a bone that is broken in many small pieces is a _____ fracture. An incomplete fracture, which usually is seen in children and is named for how a living tree branch may break when you bend it, is a _____ fracture.
herniated	**4.62** A degenerated or fragmented intervertebral disk that protrudes and compresses a nerve is called a _____ disk.
tumor myoma, osteoma bone marrow malignant	**4.63** Recall that the suffix -*oma* means _____. Using the combining forms for muscle and bone, a muscle tumor is a _____, and a bone tumor is an _____. A myeloma is a tumor of the _____ _____. An osteosarcoma is a type of _____ bone tumor.
leiomyoma rhabdomyoma rhabdomyosarcoma	**4.64** There are several types of muscle tumors. The suffix -*oma* refers to any tumor, but a sarcoma is a malignant tumor. Recall the meanings of the combining forms *lei/o* and *rhabd/o*. A smooth muscle tumor is a _____, whereas a skeletal muscle tumor is a _____. A malignant smooth muscle tumor is a leiomyosarcoma, and a malignant skeletal muscle tumor is a _____.
dystrophy shrinking painful or faulty	**4.65** Muscular _____ is a group of diseases that are characterized by progressive atrophy of skeletal muscles. Recall that atrophy means _____ of muscle size, and the prefix *dys-* means _____.
osteomalacia rickets	**4.66** Recall that chondromalacia means softening of cartilage. The term for softening of bone is _____. This is caused by a deficiency of calcium and vitamin D. In children, this is called _____.
condition or increase osteoporosis	**4.67** The suffix -*osis* means _____. The condition in which bones become less dense and more porous is called _____.
subluxation sprain	**4.68** Joints can be injured by trauma in various ways. If the bones are partially dislocated from their usual position in a joint, this is called _____. An injury to a ligament without a dislocation or fracture is called a _____.

ANSWERS	REVIEW
posterior lordosis scoliosis	**4.69** Several abnormal spinal curvatures are common. Kyphosis is an abnormal _____ curvature of the thoracic region. From the combining form meaning bent, an abnormal anterior curvature of the lumbar region is called _____. From the combining form meaning twisted, an abnormal lateral curvature is called _____.
vertebra spondylosis spondylolisthesis	**4.70** Recall that *spondyl/o* is the combining form for _____. The term for a stiff, immobile condition of the vertebrae is _____. The term for forward slipping of lumbar vertebra is _____.

◆ Self-Instruction: Diagnostic Tests and Procedures

Study the following:

TEST OR PROCEDURE	EXPLANATION
electromyogram (EMG) *ē-lek-trō-mī′ō-gram*	a neurodiagnostic, graphic record of the electrical activity of muscle both at rest and during contraction; used to diagnose neuromusculoskeletal disorders (e.g., muscular dystrophy); usually performed by a neurologist
magnetic resonance imaging (MRI) *mag-net′ik rez′ō-nănts im′ă-jing*	a nonionizing (no x-ray) imaging technique using magnetic fields and radiofrequency waves to visualize anatomic structures; useful in orthopedic studies to detect joint, tendon, and vertebral disk disorders (*see* MRI of knee in Chapter 2, Fig. 2-13)
nuclear medicine imaging *nū′klē-ăr med′i-sin im′ă-jing* **radionuclide organ imaging** *rā′dē-ō-nū′klīd ōr′găn im′ă-jing*	an ionizing imaging technique using radioactive isotopes
bone scan *bōn skan*	a nuclear scan (radionuclide image) of bone tissue to detect a tumor, malignancy, etc. (*see* Fig. 2-12B, whole body bone scan)
radiography *rā′dē-og′ră-fē*	an imaging modality using x-rays (ionizing radiation); commonly used in orthopedics to visualize the extremities, ribs, back, shoulders, and joints (*see* Fig. 2-10)
arthrogram *ar′thrō-gram*	a radiograph of a joint taken after the injection of a contrast medium

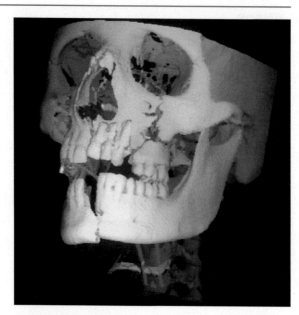

FIGURE 4-18 ■ **Three-dimensional computed tomographic reconstruction of a skull showing traumatic injury to facial bones suffered as the result of a motor vehicle accident.**

TEST OR PROCEDURE	EXPLANATION
computed tomography (CT) (Fig. 4-18) *kom-pyū'těd tō-mog'ră-fē* **computed axial tomography (CAT)** *kom-pyū'těd ak'sē-ăl tō-mog'ră-fē*	a specialized x-ray procedure producing a series of cross-sectional images that are processed by a computer into a two-dimensional or three-dimensional image (*see* Fig. 2-11 for an explanation of the principles of CT technology)
sonography *sŏ-nog'ră-fē*	ultrasound imaging; a nonionizing technique that is useful in orthopedics to visualize muscles, ligaments, displacements, and dislocations or to guide a therapeutic intervention, such as that performed during arthroscopy

Programmed Review: Diagnostic Tests and Procedures

ANSWERS	REVIEW
record electromyogram	**4.71** The combining form *electr/o* refers to electricity, and the suffix *-gram* means a _____. Join these word parts with the combining form for muscle to create the word for the diagnostic record of the electrical activity of a muscle: _____.
magnetic resonance imaging	**4.72** The imaging technique using magnetic fields and radiofrequency waves to visualize bone and joint structures is called _____ _____ _____ (MRI).

ANSWERS	REVIEW
process recording radiography record arthrogram	**4.73** The suffix *-graphy* refers to the _____ of _____. *Radi/o* is the combining term for radiation, from the Latin word for ray. The general imaging modality that records images produced by x-rays is called _____. Recall that the suffix *-gram* means a _____. Using the combining form for joint, an x-ray of a joint, usually taken using a contrast medium, is an _____.
computed tomography, axial	**4.74** A special imaging modality using an x-ray scanner and a computer to produce cross-sectional images is called _____ _____ (CT). This is also called computed _____ tomography (CAT), because the scanner rotates around the axis of the body to make the image.
radionuclide bone scan	**4.75** The Latin word nucleus refers to a little nut, or the inside of a thing. In modern physics, nucleus refers to the inside of an atom and radiation using subatomic particles. Nuclear medicine imaging, also called _____ organ imaging, is a diagnostic technique using radioactive isotopes instead of x-rays. A _____ _____ is a nuclear scan of bone tissue to detect abnormalities.
sonography	**4.76** The combining form meaning sound is *son/o*. The imaging modality using high-frequency sound (ultrasound) is called _____.

 ## Self-Instruction: Operative Terms

Study the following:

TERM	MEANING
amputation *am-pyū-tā′shŭn*	partial or complete removal of a limb (AKA = above-knee amputation; BKA = below-knee amputation)
arthrocentesis *ar′thrō-sen-tē′sis*	puncture for aspiration of a joint
arthrodesis *ăr-thrō-dē′sĭs*	binding or fusing of joint surfaces
arthroplasty *ar′thrō-plas-tē*	repair or reconstruction of a joint
arthroscopy (Fig. 4-19) *ar-thros′kŏ-pē*	procedure using an arthroscope to examine, diagnose, ar[ ] joint from within

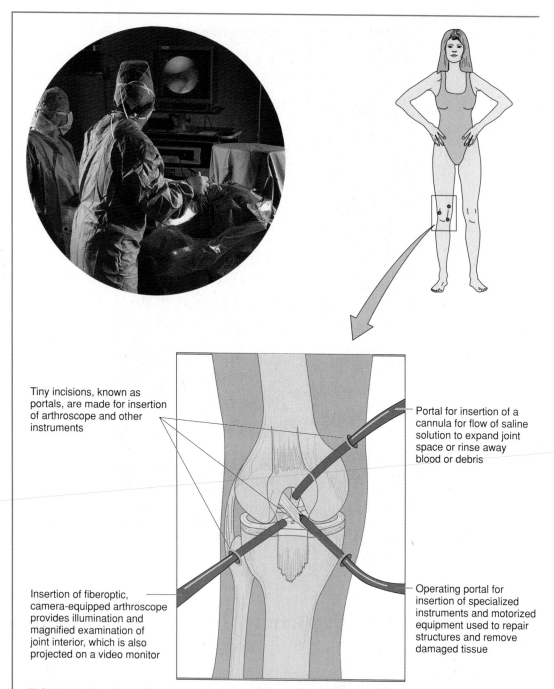

Tiny incisions, known as portals, are made for insertion of arthroscope and other instruments

Portal for insertion of a cannula for flow of saline solution to expand joint space or rinse away blood or debris

Insertion of fiberoptic, camera-equipped arthroscope provides illumination and magnified examination of joint interior, which is also projected on a video monitor

Operating portal for insertion of specialized instruments and motorized equipment used to repair structures and remove damaged tissue

FIGURE 4-19 ■ **Arthroscopic knee surgery, showing projection of surgeon's view on video monitor.**

TERM	MEANING
bone grafting *bōn graft′ing*	transplantation of a piece of bone from one site to another to repair a skeletal defect
bursectomy *ber-sek′tō-mē*	excision of a bursa
myoplasty *mī′ō-plas-tē*	repair of muscle

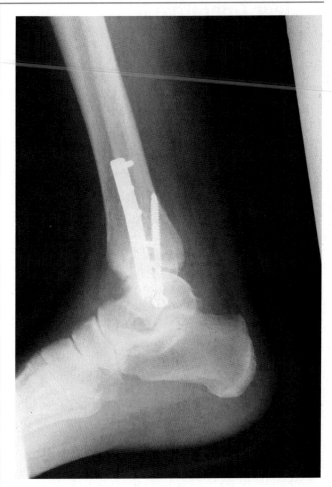

FIGURE 4-20 ■ Radiograph taken after open reduction, internal fixation (ORIF) of right ankle (see Medical Record 4-1).

TERM	MEANING
open reduction, internal fixation (ORIF) of a fracture (Fig. 4-20) *ō′pen rē-duk′shŭn, in-tĕr′năl fik-sā′shŭn of a frak′chŭr*	internal surgical repair of a fracture by bringing bones back into alignment and fixing them in place with devices such as plates, screws, and pins
osteoplasty *os′tē-ō-plas-tē*	repair of bone
osteotomy *os-tē-ot′ŏ-mē*	an incision into bone
spondylosyndesis *spon′di-lō-sin-dē′sis*	spinal fusion
tenotomy *te-not′ŏ-mē*	division of a tendon by incision to repair a deformity caused by shortening of a muscle

Programmed Review: Operative Terms

ANSWERS	REVIEW
joint arthrodesis -centesis arthrocentesis arthroscopy repair arthroplasty	**4.77** Several different operative procedures are performed on joints. Often, the term for these procedures is formed using the combining form *arthr/o*, meaning _____. Recall that the suffix *-desis* means binding; the term for binding or fusing of joint surfaces is therefore _____. The suffix meaning a puncture for aspiration is _____; the term for puncture of a joint for aspiration is therefore _____. The procedure using an instrument to examine a joint from within is called _____. The suffix *-plasty* means surgical _____ or reconstruction, and the repair or reconstruction of a joint is called _____.
amputation	**4.78** A partial or complete removal of a limb is an _____.
excision or removal bursectomy	**4.79** Recall that the suffix *-ectomy* means a surgical _____. The excision of a bursa is therefore called a _____.
grafting	**4.80** Transplantation of a piece of bone from one site to another is called bone _____. This is done, for example, to repair a skeletal defect.
-plasty myoplasty osteoplasty	**4.81** The suffix for surgical repair or reconstruction is _____. The repair of a muscle is therefore called _____. The repair of a bone is called _____.
incision osteotomy tenotomy	**4.82** The suffix *-tomy* refers to a surgical _____. An incision into bone is therefore called _____, and an incision into a tendon is called _____.
binding spondylosyndesis	**4.83** The suffix *-desis* means _____ or fusing. From the combining form for vertebrae, the term for surgical spinal fusion is _____.
open reduction, internal fixation	**4.84** Some fractures, particularly comminuted fractures, must be surgically repaired by internal (open) surgery using devices such as screws and pins to hold the bone fragments in place. This procedure is called _____ _____, _____ _____ (ORIF).

ANSWERS	REVIEW
nonsteroidal antiinflammatory	**4.92** There are several types of analgesic and antiinflammatory drugs. The group that includes aspirin and ibuprofen is called _____ _____ drugs (NSAIDs).

CHAPTER 4 ACRONYMS AND ABBREVIATIONS

ABBREVIATION	EXPANSION
A	anterior
AKA	above-knee amputation
AP	anterior-posterior
BKA	below-knee amputation
CAT	computed axial tomography
CT	computed tomography
DJD	degenerative joint disease
EMG	electromyogram
Fx	fracture
MRI	magnetic resonance imaging
NSAID	nonsteroidal antiinflammatory drug
OA	osteoarthritis
ORIF	open reduction, internal fixation
P	posterior
PA	posterior-anterior
PT	physical therapy
RA	rheumatoid arthritis
ROM	range of motion
Tx	traction

CHAPTER 4 SUMMARY OF TERMS

The terms introduced in chapter 4 are listed below, followed by the page number on which each term can be found and its written pronunciation. For additional practice and reinforcement, write the definition of each term on a separate piece of paper.

abduction/161
ab-dŭk′shŭn

adduction/161
ă-duk′shŭn

amputation/177
am-pyū-tā′shŭn

analgesic/182
an-ăl-jē′zik

anatomic or **anatomical position**/158
an-ăh-tom′ik or an-ăh-tom′ik-ăl pō-zĭ′shŭn

ankylosis/165
ang′ki-lō′sis

anterior (A)/158
an-tēr′ē-ŏr

anterior-posterior (AP)/159
an-tēr′ē-ŏr-pos-tēr′ē-ŏr

antiinflammatory/182
an′tē-in-flam′ă-tō-rē

antipyretic/182
an′tē-pī-ret′ik

appendicular skeleton/151
ap′en-dik′yū-lăr skel′ĕ-tŏn

arthralgia/164
ar-thral′jē-ă

arthritis/165
ar-thrī′tis

arthrocentesis/177
ar′thrō-sen-tē′sis

arthrodesis/177
ăr-thrō-dē′sĭs

arthrogram/175
ar′thrō-gram

arthroplasty/177
ar′thrō-plas-tē

arthroscopy/177
ar-thros′kŏ-pē

articular cartilage/154
ar-tik′yū-lăr kar′ti-lij

articulation/155
ar′tik-yū-lā′shŭn

atrophy/164
at′rō-fē

axial skeleton/151
ak′sē-ăl skel′ĕ-tŏn

axis/159
ak′sis

body planes/158
bod′ē plānz

bone/151
bōn

bone grafting/178
bōn graft′ing

bone marrow/153
bōn ma′rō

bone scan/175
bōn skan

bony necrosis/166
bōn′ē nĕ-krō′sis

bunion/166
bŭn′yŭn

bursa/155
bŭr′să

bursectomy/178
ber-sek′tō-mē

bursitis/167
ber-sī′tis

cancellous bone/152
kan′sĕ-lŭs bōn

cardiac muscle/156
kar′dē-ak mŭs′ĕl

casting/181
kast′ing

caudal/159
kaw′dăl

cephalic/159
se-fal′ik

chondromalacia/167
kon′drō-mă-lā′shē-ă

closed fracture/168
klōsd frak′chŭr

closed reduction, external fixation of a fracture/181
klōsd rē-dŭk′shŭn, eks-tĕr′năl fik-sā′shŭn of a frak′chŭr

closed reduction, percutaneous fixation of a fracture/181
klōsd rē-dŭk′shŭn, per-kyū-tā′nē-ŭs fik-sā′shŭn of a frak′chŭr

comminuted fracture/168
kom′i-nyū-tĕd frak-chŭr

compact bone/151
kom′pakt bōn

complex fracture/168
kom′pleks frak′chŭr

computed axial tomography (CAT)/176
kom-pyū′tĕd ak′sē-ăl tō-mog′ră-fē

computed tomography (CT)/176
kom-pyū′ted tō-mog′ră-fē

coronal plane/158
kōr′ŏ-năl plān

crepitation/164
krep-i-tā'shŭn

crepitus/164
krep'i-tŭs

decubitus/159
dē-kyū'bi-tŭs

degenerative arthritis/166
dē-jen'ĕr-ă-tiv ar-thrī'tis

degenerative joint disease (DJD)/166
dē-jen'ĕr-ă-tiv joynt di-zēz'

diaphysis/153
dī-af'i-sis

disk or **disc**/156
disk

distal/159
dis'tăl

dorsal/159
dōr'săl

dorsiflexion/161
dōr-si-flek'shŭn

electromyogram (EMG)/175
ē-lek-trō-mī'ō-gram

endosteum/153
en-dos'tē-ŭm

epiphysis/153
e-pif'i-sis

epiphysitis/167
e-pif-i-sī'tis

erect/159
ĕ-rĕkt'

eversion/161
ē-ver'zhŭn

exostosis/164
eks-os-tō'sis

extension/161
eks-ten'shŭn

fascia/156
fash'ē-ă

flaccid/164
flas'ĭd

flat bones/152
flat bōnz

flexion/160
flek'shŭn

fracture (Fx)/168
frak'chūr

fracture line/168
frak'chūr līn

frontal plane/158
frŏn'tăl plān

goniometer/161
gō-nē-om'ĕ-ter

gouty arthritis/166
gow'tē ar-thrī'tis

greenstick fracture/168
grēn'stik frak'chūr

herniated disk/168
hĕr'nē-ā-tĕd disk

hypertrophy/164
hī-pĕr'trō-fē

hypotonia/164
hī'pō-tō'nē-ă

inferior/159
in-fēr'ē-ŏr

insertion of a muscle/156
in-sĕr'shŭn of a mŭs'ĕl

inversion/161
in-vĕr'zhŭn

irregular bones/152
ir-reg'yū-lăr bōnz

kyphosis/170
kī-fō'sis

lateral/159
lat'er-ăl

leiomyoma/168
lī'ō-mī-ō'mă

leiomyosarcoma/168
lī'ō-mī'o-sar-kō'mă

ligament/156
lig'ă-mĕnt

long bones/152
long bōnz

lordosis/171
lōr-dō'sis

magnetic resonance imaging (MRI)/175
mag-net'ik rez'ō-nănts im'ă-jing

medial/159
mē'dē-ăl

medullary cavity/153
med′ul-ăr-ē kav′i-tē

metaphysis/153
mĕ-taf′i-sis

muscle/156
mŭs′ĕl

muscular dystrophy/168
mŭs′kyū-lăr dis′trō-fē

myalgia/164
mī-al′jē-ă

myeloma/168
mī-ĕ-lō′mă

myodynia/164
mī′ō-din′ē-ă

myoma/168
mī-ō′mă

myoplasty/178
mī′ō-plas-tē

myositis/168
mī-ō-sī′tis

narcotic/182
nar-kot′ik

**nonsteroidal antiinflammatory drug
  (NSAID)**/182
non-stēr-oy′dăl an′tē-in-flam′ă-tōr-ē drŭg

nuclear medicine imaging/175
nū′klē-ăr med′i-sin im′ă-jing

nucleus pulposus/156
nu′klē-ŭs pŭl-pō′sŭs

open fracture/168
ō′pen frak′chūr

**open reduction, internal fixation (ORIF)
  of a fracture**/179
*ō′pen rē-dŭk′shŭn, in-tĕr′năl fik-sā′shŭn of a
  frak′chūr*

origin of a muscle/156
ōr′i-jin of a mŭs′ĕl

orthosis/181
ōr-thō′sis

ostealgia/164
os-tē-al′jē-ă

osteoarthritis (OA)/166
os′tē-ō-ar-thrī′tis

osteodynia/164
os-tē-ō-din′ē-ă

osteoma/168
os′tē-ō′mă

osteomalacia/168
os′tē-ō-mă-lā′shē-ă

osteomyelitis/170
os′tē-ō-mī-ĕ-lī′tis

osteoplasty/179
os′tē-ō-plas-tē

osteoporosis/170
os′tē-ō-pō-rō′sis

osteosarcoma/168
os′tē-ō-sar-kō′mă

osteotomy/179
os-tē-ot′ō-mē

periosteum/154
per-ē-os′tē-ŭm

physical therapy (PT)/181
fiz′i-kăl ther′ă-pē

plantar flexion/161
plan′tăr flek′shŭn

posterior (P)/159
pos-tēr′ē-ŏr

posterior-anterior (PA)/159
pos-tēr′ē-ŏr-an-tēr′ē-ŏr

pronation/161
prō-nā′shŭn

prone/159
prōn

prosthesis/182
pros′thē-sis

proximal/159
prok′si-măl

radiography/175
rā′dē-og′ră-fē

radionuclide organ imaging/175
rā′dē-ō-nū′klīd ōr′găn im′ă-jing

range of motion (ROM)/161
rănj of mō′shŭn

recumbent/159
rē-kŭm′bĕnt

red bone marrow/154
red bōn mar′ō

rhabdomyoma/168
rab′dō-mī-ō′mă

rhabdomyosarcoma/168
rab′dō-mī′ō-sar-kō′mă

rheumatoid arthritis (RA)/166
rū′mă-toyd ar-thrī′tis

rickets/170
rik′ets

rigidity/164
ri-jid′i-tē

rigor/164
rig′ŏr

rotation/161
rō-tā′shŭn

sagittal plane/158
saj′i-tăl plān

scoliosis/171
skō-lē-ō′sis

sequestrum/166
sē-kwes′trŭm

sesamoid bones/152
ses′ă-moyd bōnz

short bones/152
short bōnz

simple fracture/168
sĭm′pel frak′chŭr

skeletal muscle/156
skel′e-tăl mŭs′ĕl

smooth muscle/156
smūth mŭs′ĕl

sonography/176
sŏ-nog′ră-fĭ

spasm/164
spazm

spastic/164
spas′tik

spinal curvatures/170
spī′năl ker′vă-chŭrz

splinting/181
splint′ing

spondylolisthesis/171
spon′di-lō-lis-thē′sis

spondylosis/171
spon-di-lō′sis

spondylosyndesis/179
spon′di-lō-sin-dē′sis

spongy bone/152
spŏn′jē bōn

sprain/171
sprān

striated muscle/156
strī′ă-ted mŭs′ĕl

subluxation/171
sŭb-lŭk-sā′shŭn

superior/159
sū-pēr′ē-ŏr

supination/161
sū′pi-nā′shŭn

supine/159
sū-pīn′

synovial fluid/156
si-nō′vē-ăl flū′id

synovial membrane/156
si-nō′vē-ăl mem′brān

tendinitis or **tendonitis**/171
ten-di-nī′tis or ten-dŏ-nī′tis

tendon/156
ten′dŏn

tenotomy/179
te-not′ō-mē

tetany/164
tet′ă-nē

traction (Tx)/181
trak′shŭn

transverse plane/158
trans-vĕrs′ plān

tremor/164
trem′ŏr

ventral/158
ven′trăl

yellow bone marrow/154
yel′ō bōn mar′ō

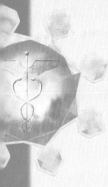

PRACTICE EXERCISES

For each of the following words, write out the term components (prefixes [P], combining forms [CF], roots [R], and suffixes [S]) on the lines below the word. Then define the term according to the meaning of its components.

EXAMPLE:

hypertrophy

$$\underline{\frac{hyper}{P}} / \underline{\frac{troph}{R}} / \underline{\frac{y}{S}}$$

DEFINITION: above or excessive/nourishment or development/condition or process of

1. hemipelvectomy

   _____ / _____ / _____

       P   R   S

   DEFINITION: _____

2. thoracic

   _____ / _____

       R   S

   DEFINITION: _____

3. myofascial

   _____ / _____ / _____

       CF   R   S

   DEFINITION: _____

4. arthropathy

   _____ / _____ / _____

       CF   R   S

   DEFINITION: _____

5. spondylolysis

   _____ / _____

       CF   S

   DEFINITION: _____

6. osteogenic

   _____ / _____ / _____

       CF   R   S

   DEFINITION: _____

7. chondrectomy

   _____ / _____

       R   S

   DEFINITION: _____

8. myonecrosis

   _____ / _____ / _____

       CF   R   S

   DEFINITION: _____

9. ostealgia

_____ / _____
   R   S

DEFINITION: _____

10. periosteitis

_____ / _____ / _____
   P   R   S

DEFINITION: _____

11. leiomyosarcoma

_____ / _____ / _____ / _____
   CF   CF   R   S

DEFINITION: _____

12. myelocyte

_____ / _____ / _____
   CF   R   S

DEFINITION: _____

13. costovertebral

_____ / _____ / _____
   CF   R   S

DEFINITION:_____

14. spondylomalacia

_____ / _____
   CF   S

DEFINITION: _____

15. osteoarthritis

_____ / _____ / _____
   CF   R   S

DEFINITION: _____

16. intercostal

_____ / _____ / _____
   P   R   S

DEFINITION: _____

17. orthosis

_____ / _____
   R   S

DEFINITION:_____

18. myotonia

_____ / _____ / _____
   CF   R   S

DEFINITION: _____

19. kyphosis

_____ / _____
    R   S

DEFINITION:_____

20. craniectomy

_____ / _____
    R   S

DEFINITION:_____

21. arthrodesis

_____ / _____
    CF   S

DEFINITION:_____

22. fibromyalgia

_____ / _____ / _____
    CF   R   S

DEFINITION: _____

23. rhabdomyoma

_____ / _____ / _____
    CF   R   S

DEFINITION: _____

24. sternocostal

_____ / _____ / _____
    CF   R   S

DEFINITION: _____

25. intraarticular

_____ / _____ / _____
    P   R   S

DEFINITION: _____

26. syndactylism

_____ / _____ / _____
    P   R   S

DEFINITION: _____

27. lumbodynia

_____ / _____
    CF   S

DEFINITION:_____

28. cervicobrachial

_____ / _____ / _____
    CF   R   S

DEFINITION: _____

29. arthroscopy

_____ / _____
   CF   S

DEFINITION: _____

30. lordosis

_____ / _____
   R   S

DEFINITION: _____

Write the correct medical term for each of the following definitions:

31. _____ lateral curvature of the spine

32. _____ joint pain

33. _____ bone tumor

34. _____ muscle tumor

35. _____ grating sound made by the movement of broken bones

36. _____ bone pain

37. _____ x-ray of a joint

38. _____ plane that divides the body into right and left halves

39. _____ surgical reconstruction of bone

40. _____ plane that divides the body into front and back portions

41. _____ opposite of hypertrophy

42. _____ striated (skeletal) muscle tumor

43. _____ test to record muscle response to electrical stimulation

44. _____ smooth muscle tumor

45. _____ application of a pulling force to a fractured or dislocated joint to maintain proper position during healing

46. _____ flabby or relaxed muscle

47. _____ lying flat on the back

48. _____ bone marrow tumor

49. _____ arthritis caused by hyperuricemia

50. _____ horizontal plane that divides the body into superior and inferior portions

51. _____ turning the palm of the hand or sole of the foot downward or backward

52. _____ stiff joint condition

53. _____ a partial dislocation

54. _____ toward the beginning or origin of a structure

55. _____ lying face down and flat

56. _____ an artificial replacement for a missing body part

57. _____ diagnostic test that uses nuclear imaging techniques to visualize bone tissue

58. _____ above another structure or toward the head

59. _____ bending of the foot or the toes upward

60. _____ internal surgical repair of a fracture by bringing bones into alignment

61. _____ osteomalacia in children

62. _____ diagnostic imaging technique using high-frequency sound waves to visualize body tissues and structures

63. _____ physician specializing in x-ray technology

64. _____ stiff muscle

Complete each medical term by writing the missing word or word part:

65. inter_____al = pertaining to between the ribs

66. _____myosarcoma = malignant striated or skeletal muscle tumor

67. hyper_____ = excessive nourishment or development; increase in the size of a muscle

68. myo_____ = suture of a muscle

69. spondylosyn_____ = binding together of vertebrae

70. _____myoma = smooth muscle tumor

71. osteo_____ = softening of bone

72. _____listhesis = slipping of vertebra

73. arthro_____ = radiograph of a joint

74. _____tomy = incision into bone

75. epiphys_____ = inflammation of the ends of the long bones

76. _____al = pertaining to the neck

77. bony _____osis = dead bone tissue

78. _____oma = tumor of cartilage

79. arthro_____ = puncture for aspiration of a joint

Write the letter of the matching definition for each body movement:

80. flexion   _____   a. movement toward the body

81. inversion   _____   b. straightening

82. adduction   _____   c. bending

83. extension   _____   d. to turn inward

84. abduction   _____   e. to turn outward

85. eversion   _____   f. movement away from the body

Write out the expanded term or meaning for each abbreviation:

86. CT _____

87. PT _____

88. Tx _____

89. ROM _____

90. Fx _____

Circle the correct spelling:

91. spondelosis	spandalosis	spondylosis
92. scholiosis	scoliosis	scoleosis
93. arthrodynia	arthradynia	arthrodenia
94. osteoalgia	ostealgia	osstealgia
95. sagital	saggittal	sagittal
96. flaccid	flacid	flascid
97. sekquestrum	sequestrom	sequestrum
98. anklylosis	ankylosis	anklosis
99. chondral	chrondral	chondrel
100. dorsaflexion	dorsiflexion	dorsflexion
101. osteoparosis	osteoporosis	osteophorosis
102. rabdomyoma	rrhabdomyoma	rhabdomyoma

Identify the planes of the body by writing the missing words in the spaces provided:

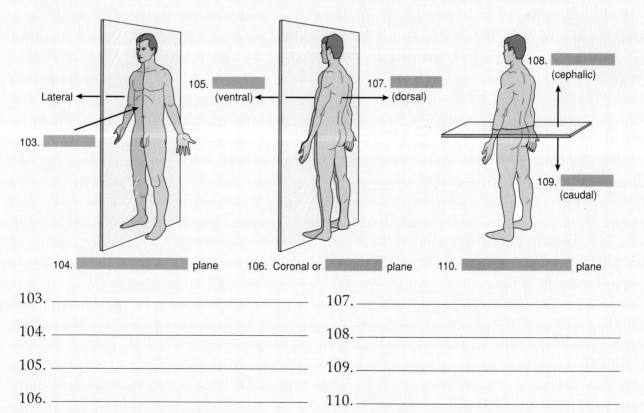

Lateral ←

103. ▨▨▨▨▨

104. ▨▨▨▨▨ plane

105. ▨▨▨▨▨ (ventral) ←

106. Coronal or ▨▨▨▨▨ plane

107. ▨▨▨▨▨ → (dorsal)

108. ▨▨▨▨▨ (cephalic)

109. ▨▨▨▨▨ (caudal)

110. ▨▨▨▨▨ plane

103. _____

104. _____

105. _____

106. _____

107. _____

108. _____

109. _____

110. _____

Identify the movements of the body by writing the missing words in the spaces provided:

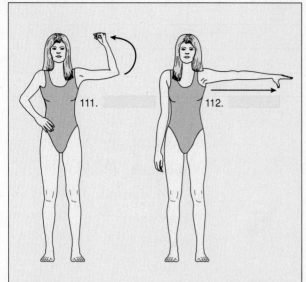

111. _____

112. _____

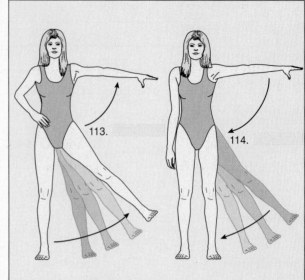

113. _____

114. _____

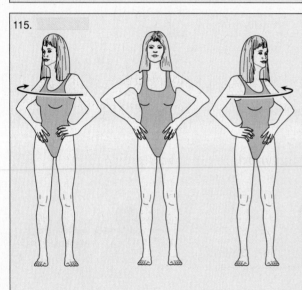

115. _____

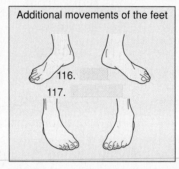

Additional movements of the feet

116. _____

117. _____

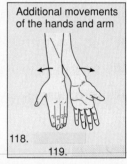

Additional movements of the hands and arm

118. _____

119. _____

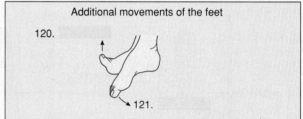

Additional movements of the feet

120. _____

121. _____

111. _____

112. _____

113. _____

114. _____

115. _____

116. _____

117. _____

118. _____

119. _____

120. _____

121. _____

Identify the parts of the skeleton by writing the missing words in the spaces provided:

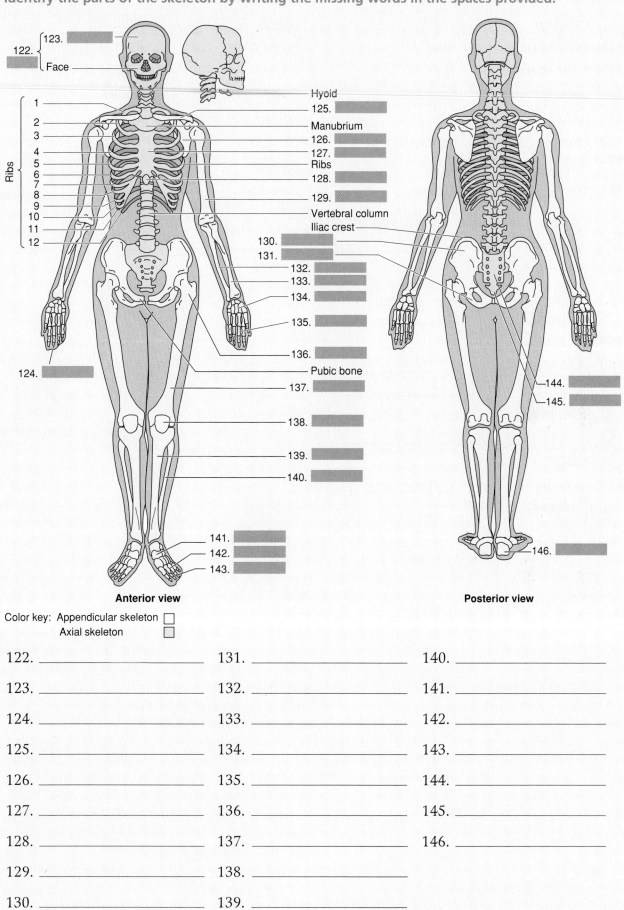

Anterior view

Posterior view

Color key: Appendicular skeleton ☐
Axial skeleton ☐

122. _____

123. _____

124. _____

125. _____

126. _____

127. _____

128. _____

129. _____

130. _____

131. _____

132. _____

133. _____

134. _____

135. _____

136. _____

137. _____

138. _____

139. _____

140. _____

141. _____

142. _____

143. _____

144. _____

145. _____

146. _____

Circle the combining form that corresponds to the meaning given:

147. **cartilage**	crani/o	cost/o	chondr/o
148. **vertebra**	myel/o	spondyl/o	lumb/o
149. **bone marrow**	my/o	myel/o	muscul/o
150. **neck**	thorac/o	crani/o	cervic/o
151. **joint**	oste/o	arthr/o	ankyl/o
152. **chest**	thorac/o	cervic/o	spondyl/o
153. **muscle**	my/o	myel/o	lei/o
154. **rib**	stern/o	chondr/o	cost/o

Give the noun that is used to form each adjective:

155. orthotic _____

156. hypertrophic _____

157. radial _____

158. kyphotic _____

159. bursal _____

160. dystrophic _____

161. necrotic _____

162. osteoporotic _____

163. lordotic _____

164 ulnar _____

165. scoliotic _____

166. prosthetic _____

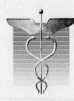

MEDICAL RECORD ANALYSIS

Medical Record 4-1

HISTORY AND PHYSICAL EXAMINATION

CC: "attacks" of right knee discomfort and instability

HPI: This 19 y/o ♂ presents with "attacks" of right knee pain and instability. Three years ago, while playing basketball, he turned sharply and felt his kneecap pop in and out. It was acutely swollen and painful and required manipulation to reduce it. He had a course of PT and did reasonably well for a few months until resuming athletic activities. Since then, he has had recurrent episodes of the knee slipping in and out, all related to twisting and turning while surfing and playing basketball. His primary complaint is the episodic discomfort and the inability to trust the knee. He is asymptomatic at this time.

PMH: NKDA. Hx of right ankle Fx in 20xx. Meds: none. Operations: none.

SH: Alcohol rarely used. FH: Father, age 49, Mother, age 43, both L&W.

ROS: Noncontributory.

PE: The patient is a cooperative male in NAD.

VS: T 97.2° F, P 64, R 14, BP 118/66
HEENT: WNL. Neck: supple, no tenderness, full ROM, no adenopathy.
Lungs, heart, abdomen: WNL. Back: no tenderness or deformity.
Extremities: unremarkable except for involved knee. Knee ROM is 0–45 degrees equally. There is no parapatellar tenderness.
Neurologic: Negative.
Radiographs show subluxation of the right knee.

IMP: RECURRENT RIGHT KNEE PATELLAR INSTABILITY

RECOMMENDATION: Patelloplasty is being discussed, and the risks and benefits of the procedure have been explained. The patient will return with his parents for further consultation before deciding whether to proceed with treatment.

QUESTIONS ABOUT MEDICAL RECORD 4-1

1. Which describes the patient's symptoms at the time of the initial injury?
   a. severe pain over a short course
   b. pain that comes and goes
   c. pain that progressively gets worse
   d. pain that develops slowly over time
   e. no pain

2. What treatment was provided 3 years ago?
   a. puncture for aspiration of a joint
   b. transplantation of a piece of bone from one site to another

   c. examination of a joint from within
   d. physical rehabilitation including exercise
   e. binding or fusing joint surfaces

3. Which best describes the patient's symptoms at the time of this visit?
   a. severe pain
   b. moderate pain
   c. progressive pain
   d. mild pain
   e. no pain

4. Describe the orthopedic condition noted in the past history:
   a. forward slipping of a vertebra
   b. broken bone
   c. arthritis
   d. bone pain
   e. dislocation

5. What does full ROM indicate?
   a. swelling
   b. spasm
   c. inflammation
   d. bruising
   e. mobility

6. What did the radiographs indicate?
   a. no radiographs were mentioned
   b. patellar instability
   c. partial dislocation
   d. inflammation
   e. joint stiffness

7. What treatment did the physician recommend?
   a. surgical reconstruction of the kneecap
   b. physical therapy
   c. surgical repair of bone
   d. excision of the patella
   e. examination and repair of a joint from within using an endoscope

Medical Record 4-2

FOR ADDITIONAL STUDY

As Alice Toohey was playing with her young granddaughter, she stepped on a toy dump truck and fell down her porch steps, wrenching her ankle violently. Because of the sharp pain and immediate swelling, Ms. Toohey was taken immediately to the hospital. After being seen by the emergency room physician, she was admitted and scheduled for surgery. Medical Record 4-2 is the operative report dictated by the surgeon, Dr. Ricardo Rodriguez, immediately after the operation and processed by a medical transcriptionist.

Read Medical Record 4-2 (page 203), then write your answers to the following questions in the spaces provided.

QUESTIONS ABOUT MEDICAL RECORD 4-2

1. Below are medical terms used in this record that you have not yet encountered in this text. Underline each term where it appears in the record, and define the term below.

   malleolus _____

   oblique _____

   sterile _____

2. In your own words, not using medical terminology, briefly describe the preoperative diagnosis for Ms. Toohey:

   _____

   _____

   _____

3. Put the following operative steps in correct order by numbering them from 1 to 10:

   _____   radiograph of the screws that were too long

   _____   incision on the outer side of the ankle

   _____   plate placed onto fibula

   _____   sewing the incisions

   _____   radiograph of satisfactory screw position

   _____   towel clip positioned

   _____   removal of medial hematoma

   _____   removal of lateral hematoma

   _____   placement of screw into lower tibia

   _____   incision on the inner side of the right ankle

4. In this operation, the surgeon redid one step after using a diagnostic procedure to check whether that step was as effective as possible. In your own words, explain what Dr. Rodriguez changed and why:

   _____

   _____

   _____

5. Describe the fracture line: _____

6. When Dr. Rodriguez examined the ankle after making the first incision, he found a problem he could not and did not repair. In your own words, what had been destroyed in Ms. Toohey's injury?

_____

_____

7. Which of the following actions did *not* occur in this operation?

   a. washing the wound with antibiotic

   b. taping the fracture line

   c. drilling holes in the bone

   d. stapling the skin closed

8. Describe Ms. Toohey's condition when transferred to postanesthesia recovery (PAR) after the operation:

_____

_____

_____

Medical Record 4-2

CENTRAL MEDICAL CENTER

211 Medical Center Drive • Central City, US 90000-1234 • PHONE: (012) 125-6784 • FAX: (012) 125-9999

OPERATIVE REPORT

PREOPERATIVE DIAGNOSIS: Trimalleolar fracture, right ankle/fracture dislocation.

POSTOPERATIVE DIAGNOSIS: Trimalleolar fracture, right ankle/fracture dislocation.

OPERATION PERFORMED: Open reduction and internal fixation of medial malleolus and lateral malleolus, right ankle.

ANESTHESIOLOGIST: K. Teglam, M.D.

ANESTHESIA: General.

DESCRIPTION OF OPERATION: After successful general anesthesia, the right lower extremity was prepped and draped in a sterile fashion. A pneumatic tourniquet was used in the case at 300 mm Hg (mercury) for 51 minutes. The medial side was opened first; the skin was incised, and this was carried down through the subcutaneous tissue down to the periosteum which was incised enough at the fracture site for visualization of a large transverse medial malleolar fracture. A hematoma was evacuated by curettage and irrigation. Unfortunately, there was some debris within the joint which was articular cartilage destruction and damage on the talus.

Attention was then directed laterally where an incision was made and carried through the skin and subcutaneous tissue. The fracture was brought into full view very easily. The fracture was long and oblique. This was curetted of hematoma and irrigated, and using a bone clamp, it was clamped in a reduced position. A 6-hole semitubular fibular-type plate was then bent to position and placed onto the fibula; and after predrilling, premeasuring, and pretapping, six cortical 3.5 mm diameter screws were used to hold the plate to the fractured fibula.

Attention was then directed medially. The fracture was reduced and held in place with a towel clip, and a 60 mm long malleolar screw was then inserted into the fragment into the distal tibia. X-rays revealed that three of the screws laterally were too long, and these were changed. The medial malleolus screw was also tightened down further. Repeat film revealed very satisfactory position of all the screws. The posterior malleolar fragment was felt to be adequately positioned. All the wounds were then irrigated with goodly amounts of antibiotic solution. Vicryl sutures, 0 and 2-0, were used to close the subcutaneous tissue on both sides; and staples were used for the skin. A bulky Jones dressing was applied with splints anteriorly and posteriorly.

The patient tolerated the procedure well and was transferred to the recovery room with stable vital signs.

R. Rodriguez, M.D.

RR:mb

D: 10/19/20xx
T: 10/20/20xx

OPERATIVE REPORT	PT. NAME:	TOOHEY, ALICE M.
	ID NO:	IP-236701
	ROOM NO:	729
	ATT. PHYS:	R. RODRIGUEZ, M.D.

ANSWERS TO PRACTICE EXERCISES

1. hemi / pelv / ectomy
   P   R   S
   half/pelvis (basin) or hip bone/excision (removal)

2. thorac / ic
   R   S
   chest/pertaining to

3. myo / fasci / al
   CF   R   S
   muscle/fascia (a band)/pertaining to

4. arthro / path / y
   CF   R   S
   joint/disease/condition or process of

5. spondylo / lysis
   CF   S
   vertebra/breaking down or dissolution

6. osteo / gen / ic
   CF   R   S
   bone/origin or production/pertaining to

7. chondr / ectomy
   R   S
   cartilage/excision (removal)

8. myo / necr / osis
   CF   R   S
   muscle/death/condition or increase

9. oste / algia
   R   S
   bone/pain

10. peri / oste / itis
    P   R   S
    around/bone/inflammation

11. leio / myo / sarc / oma
    CF   CF   R   S
    smooth/muscle/flesh/tumor

12. myelo / cyt / e
    CF   R   S
    bone marrow or spinal cord/cell/noun marker

13. costo / vertebr / al
    CF   R   S
    rib/vertebra/pertaining to

14. spondylo / malacia
    CF   S
    vertebra/softening

15. osteo / arthr / itis
    CF   R   S
    bone/joint/inflammation

16. inter / cost / al
    P   R   S
    between/rib/pertaining to

17. orth / osis
    R   S
    straight, normal, or correct/condition or increase

18. myo / ton / ia
    CF   R   S
    muscle/tone/condition of

19. kyph / osis
    R   S
    humped-back/condition or increase

20. crani / ectomy
    R   S
    skull/excision (removal)

21. arthro / desis
    CF   S
    joint/binding

22. fibro / my / algia
    CF   R   S
    fiber/muscle/pain

23. rhabdo / my / oma
    CF   R   S
    rod-shaped or striated (skeletal)/muscle/tumor

24. sterno / cost / al
    CF   R   S
    sternum (breastbone)/rib/pertaining to

25. intra / articul / ar
    P   R   S
    within/joint/pertaining to

26. syndactylism
    syn / dactyl / ism
    P   R   S
    together or with/digit (finger or toe)/condition of

27. lumbo / dynia
    CF   S
    loin (lower back)/pain

28. cervico / brachi / al
    CF   R   S
    neck/arm/pertaining to

29. arthro / scopy
    CF   S
    joint/process of examination

30. lord / osis
    R   S
    bent/condition or increase

31. scoliosis

32. arthralgia or arthrodynia

33. osteoma

34. myoma

35. crepitation or crepitus

36. ostealgia or osteodynia

37. arthrogram

38. sagittal

39. osteoplasty

40. coronal or frontal

41. atrophy

42. rhabdomyoma

43. electromyogram

44. leiomyoma

45. traction

46. flaccid

47. horizontal recumbent or supine

48. myeloma

49. gouty arthritis

50. transverse

51. pronation

52. ankylosis

53. subluxation

54. proximal
55. prone
56. prosthesis
57. bone scan
58. superior or cephalic
59. dorsiflexion
60. open reduction, internal fixation (ORIF) of a fracture
61. rickets
62. sonography
63. radiologist
64. rigor or rigidity
65. intercostal
66. rhabdomyosarcoma
67. hypertrophy
68. myorrhaphy
69. spondylosyndesis
70. leiomyoma
71. osteomalacia
72. spondylolisthesis
73. arthrogram
74. osteotomy
75. epiphysitis
76. cervical
77. bony necrosis
78. chondroma
79. arthrocentesis
80. c
81. d
82. a
83. b
84. f
85. e
86. computed tomography
87. physical therapy
88. traction or treatment
89. range of motion
90. fracture (broken bone)

91. spondylosis
92. scoliosis
93. arthrodynia
94. ostealgia
95. sagittal
96. flaccid
97. sequestrum
98. ankylosis
99. chondral
100. dorsiflexion
101. osteoporosis
102. rhabdomyoma
103. medial
104. sagittal
105. anterior
106. frontal
107. posterior
108. superior
109. inferior
110. transverse
111. flexion
112. extension
113. abduction
114. adduction
115. rotation
116. eversion
117. inversion
118. pronation
119. supination
120. dorsiflexion
121. plantar flexion
122. skull
123. cranium
124. phalanges
125. clavicle
126. scapula
127. sternum
128. xiphoid process
129. humerus

130. ilium
131. ischium
132. ulna
133. radius
134. carpals
135. metacarpals
136. trochanter
137. femur
138. patella
139. tibia
140. fibula
141. tarsals
142. metatarsals
143. phalanges
144. sacrum
145. coccyx
146. calcaneus
147. chondr/o
148. spondyl/o
149. myel/o
150. cervic/o
151. arthr/o
152. thorac/o
153. my/o
154. cost/o
155. orthosis
156. hypertrophy
157. radius
158. kyphosis
159. bursa
160. dystrophy
161. necrosis
162. osteoporosis
163. lordosis
164. ulna
165. scoliosis
166. prosthesis

ANSWERS TO MEDICAL RECORD ANALYSIS

Medical Record 4-1: History and Physical Examination

1. a   2. d   3. e   4. b   5. e   6. c   7. a

Medical Record 4-2: For Additional Study

See CD-ROM for answers.

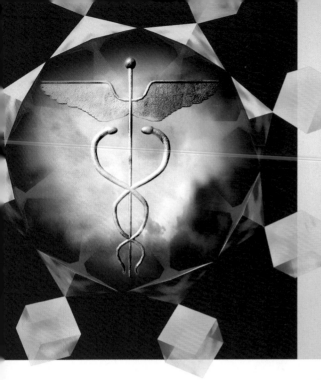

Cardiovascular System

✓ Chapter 5 Checklist

CARDIOVASCULAR SYSTEM OVERVIEW

The cardiovascular system consists of the heart (Fig. 5-1) and blood vessels, which work together to transport blood throughout the body.

- The heart is a muscular organ that pumps blood throughout the body.
- The heart consists of four chambers: the **right atrium** and **left atrium** (upper chambers), and the **right ventricle** and **left ventricle** (lower chambers).
- The heart is divided into right and left portions by the **interatrial septum** and the **interventricular septum**.
- Heart valves open and close to maintain the one-way flow of blood through the heart.
- The heart has three layers: the **endocardium**, which lines the interior cavities of the heart; the **myocardium**, which is the thick, muscular layer; and the **epicardium**, which is the outer membrane.
- Enclosing the heart is a loose, protective sac called the **pericardium**.

STRUCTURES OF THE HEART (arrows indicate path of blood flow)

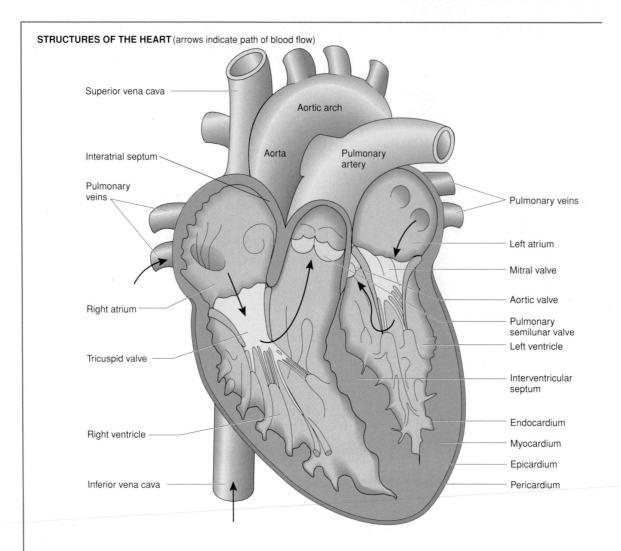

Superior vena cava

Aortic arch

Aorta

Pulmonary artery

Interatrial septum

Pulmonary veins

Pulmonary veins

Left atrium

Mitral valve

Aortic valve

Pulmonary semilunar valve

Left ventricle

Right atrium

Tricuspid valve

Interventricular septum

Endocardium

Myocardium

Epicardium

Pericardium

Right ventricle

Inferior vena cava

ECHOCARDIOGRAM
Normal, two-dimensional, apical four-chamber view

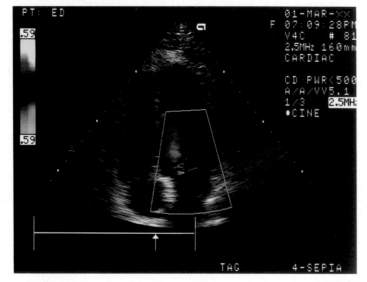

BLOOD CIRCULATION

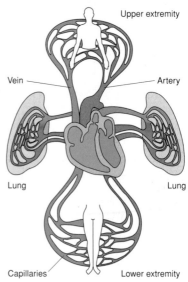

Upper extremity

Vein

Artery

Lung

Lung

Capillaries

Lower extremity

FIGURE 5-1 ■ **Structures of the heart.**

Blood, which transports essential elements within the body, flows through the heart as follows:

- **Deoxygenated** blood from the body enters the heart through the **superior vena cava** and **inferior vena cava** into the right atrium.
- During atrial contraction, the tricuspid valve opens to allow blood to flow into the right ventricle.
- Contraction of the ventricle pushes blood through the pulmonary semilunar valve into the pulmonary artery.
- The **pulmonary artery** carries the blood to the lungs and through the **pulmonary circulation** (a network of arteries, capillaries, air sacs, and veins in the lung), where it is oxygenated.
- Oxygenated blood returns to the heart via the **pulmonary veins** into the left atrium.
- With atrial contraction, the mitral (or bicuspid) valve opens to allow blood to flow into the left ventricle.
- Contraction of the left ventricle pushes blood through the aortic valve into the aorta and on to all parts of the body through the **systemic circulation** (a network of arteries, arterioles, capillaries, and veins throughout the body).
- The heart is the first to receive oxygenated blood via the right and left coronary arteries, which distribute blood throughout the entire heart (Fig. 5-2).

Self-Instruction: Combining Forms

Study the following:

COMBINING FORM	MEANING
angi/o, vas/o, vascul/o	vessel
aort/o	aorta
arteri/o	artery
ather/o	fatty (lipid) paste
atri/o	atrium
cardi/o	heart
coron/o	circle or crown
my/o	muscle
pector/o, steth/o	chest
sphygm/o	pulse
thromb/o	clot
ven/o, phleb/o	vein
varic/o	swollen, twisted vein
ventricul/o	ventricle (belly or pouch)

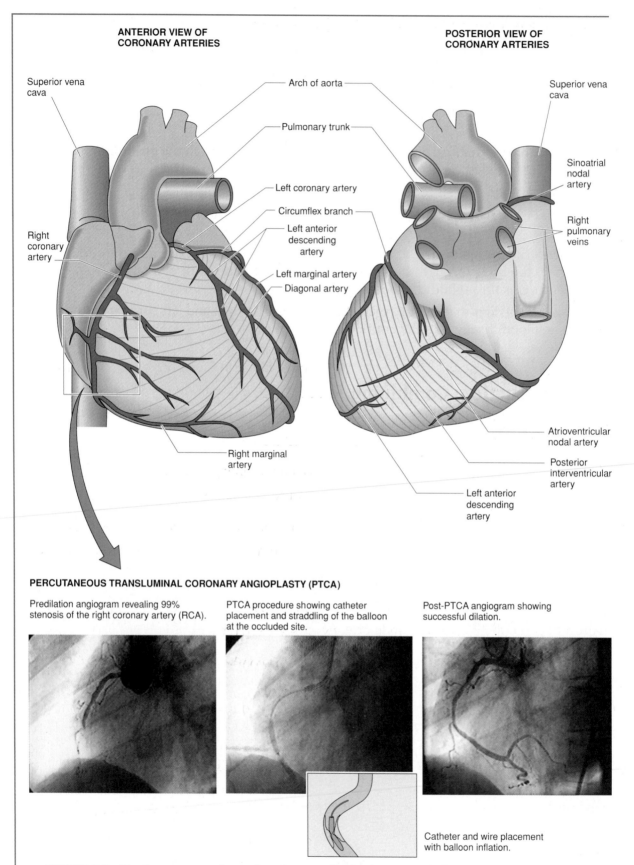

PERCUTANEOUS TRANSLUMINAL CORONARY ANGIOPLASTY (PTCA)

Predilation angiogram revealing 99% stenosis of the right coronary artery (RCA).

PTCA procedure showing catheter placement and straddling of the balloon at the occluded site.

Post-PTCA angiogram showing successful dilation.

Catheter and wire placement with balloon inflation.

FIGURE 5-2 ■ **Coronary arteries and angiograms illustrating angioplasty.**

Programmed Review: Combining Forms

ANSWERS	REVIEW
heart	**5.1** A cardiologist is a physician who specializes in the study of the _____.
angiogram	**5.2** Formed from *angi/o*, an _____ is an x-ray record of a blood vessel.
vessel	**5.3** A vasospasm is an involuntary contraction of a blood _____.
Cardiology	**5.4** _____ is the medical specialty dealing with the study of the heart.
Thromb/o breaking down or dissolution	**5.5** _____, the combining form meaning clot, is the subject of thrombolysis, a term referring to the _____ _____ of a clot or clots.
ventricle ventricul/o cardiologist	**5.6** Someone with a congenital ventricular defect is born with an imperfection of a _____ in the heart. (The combining form in this term is _____.) That person would likely be under the care of a _____.
fatty or lipid paste	**5.7** Atherosclerosis is a condition in which hardened _____ _____ builds up inside blood vessels.
veins phleb/o, vein	**5.8** A phlebotomist is someone trained to draw blood samples from the _____. This term comes from the combining form _____, meaning _____.
varic/o	**5.9** Varicose veins, from the combining form _____, are so named because they are swollen and twisted.
ven/o arteries	**5.10** Veins (named from the combining form _____) return blood to the heart from all around the body. Based on the root *arteri/o*, _____ carry blood in the other direction (from the heart to the body or lungs).
pector/o steth/o	**5.11** The heart is located in the chest, behind the area of the pectoral muscle. The pectoral muscles get their name from the combining form _____, which means chest. Another combining form that means chest is _____, which is the subject of the term stethoscope, an instrument used to listen to the heart or to breathing within the chest.

ANSWERS	REVIEW
atria atri/o ventricul/o	**5.12** The heart has four chambers: two ventricles and two _____, which is the plural form of atrium. Atrium comes from the combining form _____, and ventricle comes from the combining form _____.
aorta myocardium circle or crown coronary	**5.13** The _____, from the combining form *aort/o*, is the large blood vessel through which blood leaves the heart for delivery to all parts of the body. The coronary arteries branch from the aorta and supply the heart's muscular tissue, or the _____, with blood. The original meaning of *coron/o* refers to a _____. The _____ arteries are so named because they seem to encircle the heart like a crown.
sphygm/o veins vascul/o	**5.14** Each beat of the heart produces a pulse. The combining form that means pulse is _____. This is the key combining form in the term sphygmomanometer, an instrument that measures blood pressure (BP) based on its pressurized pulse through an artery. Arteries and _____ are the two types of larger blood vessels. Along with the capillaries, they are sometimes referred to collectively as the vasculature, from the combining form _____, meaning vessel.

🔷 Self-Instruction: Anatomic Terms

Study the following:

TERM	MEANING
SEPTA AND LAYERS OF THE HEART (*see* Fig. 5-1)	
atrium *ā′ trē-ŭm*	upper right or left chamber of the heart
endocardium *en-dō-kar′ dē-ŭm*	membrane lining the cavities of the heart
epicardium *ep-i-kar′ dē-ŭm*	membrane forming the outer layer of the heart
interatrial septum *in-tĕr-ā′ trē-ăl sep′ tŭm*	partition between the right and left atria
interventricular septum *in-tĕr-ven-trik′ yū-lăr sep′ tŭm*	partition between the right and left ventricles

TERM	MEANING
myocardium *mī′ō-kar′dē-ŭm*	heart muscle
pericardium *per-i-kar′dē-ŭm*	protective sac enclosing the heart composed of two layers with fluid between
visceral pericardium *vis′ĕr-ăl per-i-kar′ dē-ŭm*	layer closest to the heart (*visceral* = pertaining to organ)
parietal pericardium *pă-rī′ĕ-tăl per-i-kar′ dē-ŭm*	outer layer (*parietal* = pertaining to wall)
pericardial cavity *per-i-kar′ dē-ăl kav′i-tē*	fluid-filled cavity between the pericardial layers
ventricle *ven′tri-kĕl*	lower right or left chamber of the heart

VALVES OF THE HEART AND VEINS (*see* Fig. 5-1)

heart valves *hart valvz*	structures within the heart that open and close with the heartbeat to regulate the one-way flow of blood
aortic valve *ā-ōr′tik valv*	heart valve between the left ventricle and the aorta
mitral valve *mī′trăl valv* **bicuspid valve** *bī-kŭs′pid valv*	heart valve between the left atrium and the left ventricle (*cuspis* = point)
pulmonary semilunar valve *pul′mō-nār-ē sem-ē-lū′năr valv*	heart valve opening from the right ventricle to the pulmonary artery (*luna* = moon)
tricuspid valve *trī-kŭs′pid valv*	valve between the right atrium and the right ventricle
valves of the veins *valvz of the vānz*	valves located at intervals within the lining of veins, especially in the legs, which constrict with muscle action to move the blood returning to the heart

BLOOD VESSELS (Fig. 5-3)

arteries (Fig. 5-4) *ar′tĕr-ēz*	vessels that carry blood from the heart to the arterioles
aorta *ā-ōr′tă*	large artery that is the main trunk of the arterial system branching from the left ventricle
arterioles *ar-tēr′ē-ōlz*	small vessels that receive blood from the arteries
capillaries *kap′i-lār-ēz*	tiny vessels that join arterioles and venules
venules *ven′ūlz*	small vessels that gather blood from the capillaries into the veins
veins (Fig. 5-5) *vānz*	vessels that carry blood to the heart from the venules

TERM	MEANING
CIRCULATION	
systemic circulation *sis-tem'ik sĭr-kyū-lā'shŭn*	circulation of blood throughout the body via arteries, arterioles, capillaries, venules, and veins to deliver oxygen and nutrients to body tissues
coronary circulation *kōr'ŏ-nār-ē sĭr-kyū-lā'shŭn*	circulation of blood through the coronary blood vessels to deliver oxygen and nutrients to the heart muscle tissue (*see* Fig. 5-2)
pulmonary circulation *pul'mō-nār-ē sĭr-kyū-lā'shŭn*	circulation of blood from the pulmonary artery through the vessels in the lungs and back to the heart via the pulmonary vein, providing for the exchange of gases

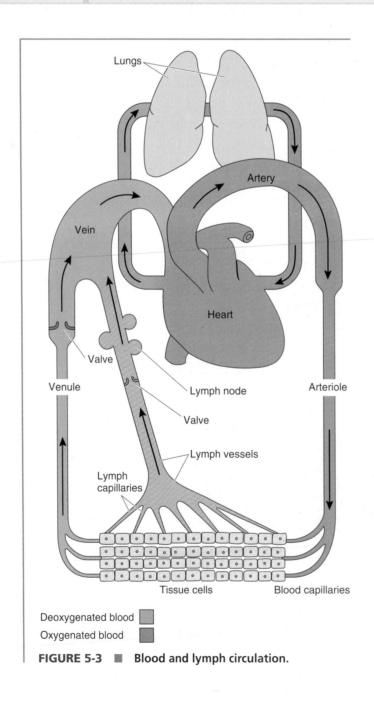

FIGURE 5-3 ■ **Blood and lymph circulation.**

ARTERIAL BLOOD CIRCULATION

Arteries (carry blood from the heart)

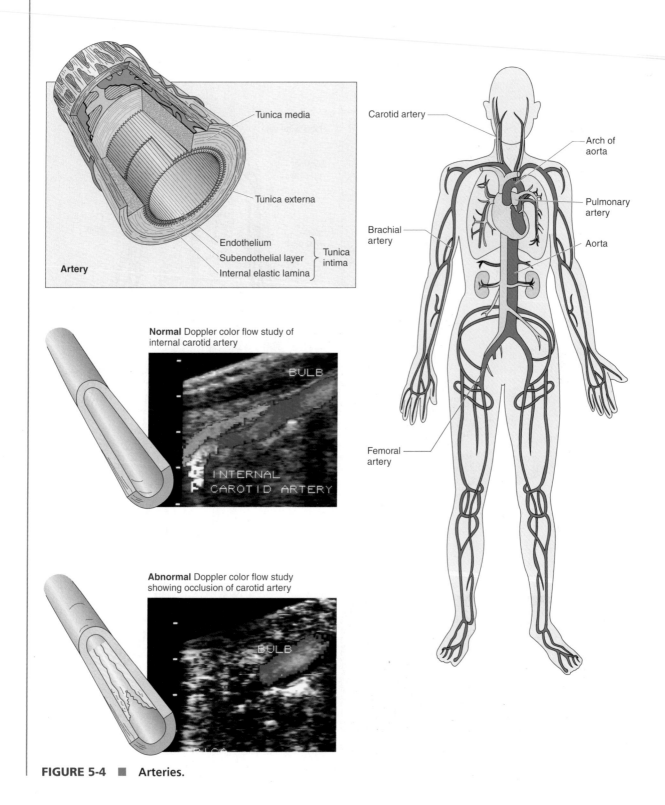

Tunica media

Tunica externa

Endothelium
Subendothelial layer
Internal elastic lamina

} Tunica intima

Artery

Carotid artery

Arch of aorta

Pulmonary artery

Brachial artery

Aorta

Femoral artery

Normal Doppler color flow study of internal carotid artery

BULB

INTERNAL CAROTID ARTERY

Abnormal Doppler color flow study showing occlusion of carotid artery

BULB

FIGURE 5-4 ■ Arteries.

VENOUS CIRCULATION

Veins (carry blood to the heart)

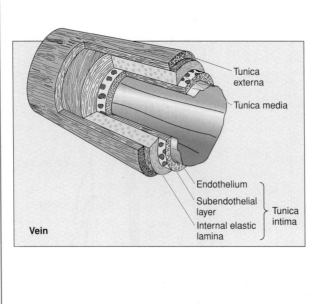

Tunica
externa

Tunica media

Endothelium

Subendothelial
layer

Internal elastic
lamina

Tunica
intima

Vein

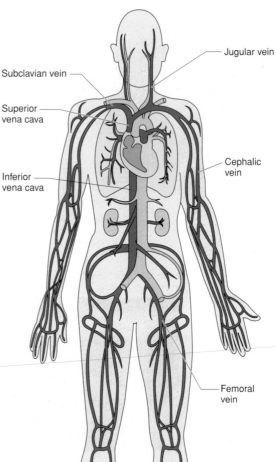

Jugular vein

Subclavian vein

Superior
vena cava

Inferior
vena cava

Cephalic
vein

Femoral
vein

FEMORAL THROMBUS

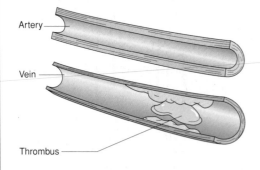

Artery

Vein

Thrombus

Color flow Doppler showing femoral vein thrombus

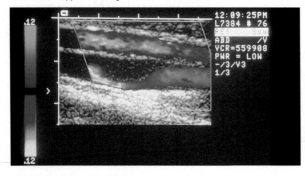

FIGURE 5-5 ■ **Veins.**

Programmed Review: Anatomic Terms

ANSWERS	REVIEW
atri/o atria upper	**5.15** The term atrium is from the combining form _____. The plural form of this word is _____. The right and left atria are the _____ chambers of the heart.
within heart tissue -ium	**5.16** Recall that the prefix *endo-* means _____. Combined with *cardi/o*, it refers to something within the _____. The endocardium is the structure or _____ that lines the cavities of the heart. The suffix denoting structure or tissue is _____.
epi- suffix structure, tissue	**5.17** A common prefix that means upon is _____. Combined with *cardi/o* and the _____ *-ium*, it forms the term epicardium, which is the _____ or _____ forming the outer layer of the heart.
muscle myocardium	**5.18** *My/o* is a combining form meaning _____. The term for heart muscle tissue is _____.
around heart pericardium pericardial	**5.19** *Peri-* is a prefix that means _____. The pericardium is a protective sac that encloses the _____. It has two layers with fluid between. Using the term that means pertaining to organ, the layer closest to the heart is called the visceral pericardium. The outer layer uses the term that means pertaining to wall and is called the parietal _____. Using the term that means pertaining to the pericardium, the fluid-filled space between these two layers is called the _____ cavity.
ventricul/o lower	**5.20** The ventricles of the heart are so named from the combining form _____, meaning belly or pouch. The ventricles are the two _____ chambers of the heart.
between atria interventricular chambers	**5.21** The term septum refers to an anatomic partition. The interatrial septum is the partition _____ the left and right _____. Between the left and right ventricles is the _____ septum. The two atria and two ventricles are the four _____ of the heart.

ANSWERS	REVIEW
valves aortic	**5.22** The one-way blood flow from one heart chamber to another, or from a heart chamber to an artery, is regulated by heart _____, which open and close as the heart beats. The valve between the left ventricle and the aorta is called the _____ valve.
bicuspid right, right	**5.23** The mitral, or _____, valve is between the left atrium and the left ventricle. The tricuspid valve is between the _____ atrium and the _____ ventricle.
pulmonary	**5.24** The pulmonary semilunar valve is between the right ventricle and the _____ artery.
veins	**5.25** Other valves that open and close with muscle action to move blood back to the heart are known as the valves of the _____.
arteries ven/o	**5.26** The names of blood vessels are easy to remember because they are similar to the combining forms. The _____, which carry blood from the heart, get their name from the combining form *arteri/o*. The veins, which carry blood to the heart, are so named from the combining form _____.
arterioles capillaries venules small	**5.27** The _____, also from the combining form *arteri/o*, are the small vessels that receive blood from the arteries. The blood then flows to the _____, the tiniest vessels. Next, the blood is gathered from the capillaries into the _____, which are small vessels that connect to the veins. The suffixes *-ole* and *-ule* are used to indicate something _____.
aorta	**5.28** As blood leaves the heart to be distributed to the rest of the body, it first passes through the _____, a large artery that leads to the arteries that will carry the blood throughout the body.
systemic lungs coronary	**5.29** The term circulation refers to the flow of blood through the vessels. Blood flow through the body (except the lungs) is called _____ circulation. Pulmonary circulation is blood flow through the _____. Blood flow to the heart muscle, based on the combining form *coron/o*, is called _____ circulation.

Self-Instruction: Blood Pressure Terms

Study the following:

TERM	MEANING
diastole *dī-as′tō-lē*	to expand; period during the cardiac cycle when blood enters the relaxed ventricles from the atria
systole *sis′tō-lē*	to contract; period during the cardiac cycle when the heart is in contraction and blood is ejected through the aorta and the pulmonary artery
normotension *nōr-mō-ten′shŭn*	normal blood pressure
hypotension *hī′pō-ten′shŭn*	low blood pressure
hypertension (HTN) *hī′pĕr-ten′shŭn*	high blood pressure

 ## Programmed Review: Blood Pressure Terms

ANSWERS	REVIEW
BP	**5.30** Blood pressure, which is abbreviated as _____, is a measurement of the pressure on the walls of the arteries during
systole, diastole	contraction (_____) and relaxation (_____) of the heart (Fig. 5-6).

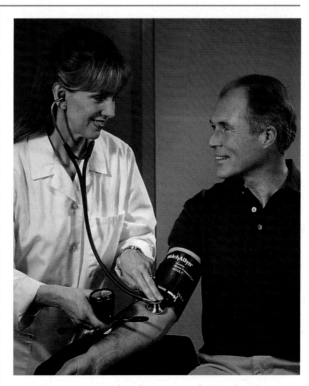

FIGURE 5-6 ■ **Blood pressure determination.**

ANSWERS	REVIEW
blood pressure systole diastole suffix, pertaining to systolic diastolic	**5.31** When BP, or _____ _____, is recorded, the contraction phase, or _____, is written first, followed by a slash, followed by the relaxation phase, or _____. The _____ -ic is used to modify the terms to mean _____ ___. The term that means pertaining to the contraction phase is _____, and the term that means pertaining to the relaxation phase is _____.
normo 120, 80 hyper hypo	**5.32** A blood pressure of 120/80 or below is considered to be a normal blood pressure and is termed _____tension. The numbers reflect a systolic reading of _____ and a diastolic reading of _____. High blood pressure is called _____tension, and low blood pressure is called _____tension.

Systole
Diastole

CARDIAC CONDUCTION

Cardiac conduction provides the electrical stimulus that is necessary to cause the heart muscle to pump blood by the continual contraction (systole) and relaxation (diastole) of myocardial cells (Fig. 5-7).

Repeated electrical impulses are conducted:

from the sinoatrial (SA) node (the pacemaker of the heart)
↓
to the atrioventricular (AV) node
↓
to the bundle of His
↓
to the left and right bundle branches
↓
to the Purkinje fibers

The impulses cause each myocardial cell to change:

from a resting state (polarized)
↓
to a state of contraction (depolarized)
↓
then back to a resting state by recharging (repolarizing)

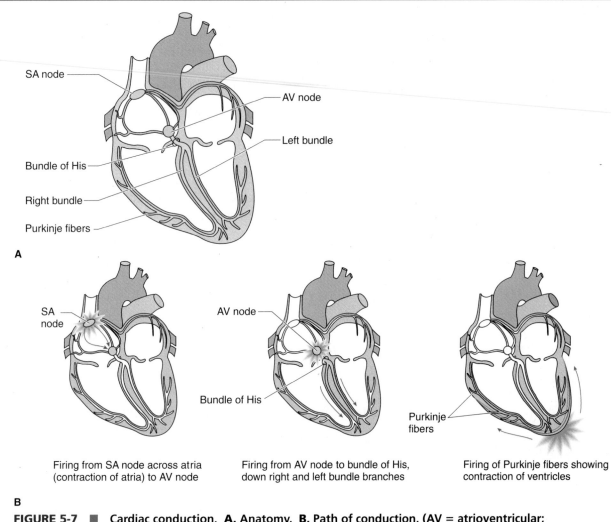

FIGURE 5-7 ■ **Cardiac conduction. A. Anatomy. B. Path of conduction. (AV = atrioventricular; SA = sinoatrial.)**

Self-Instruction: Cardiac Conduction Terms

Study the following:

TERM	MEANING
sinoatrial (SA) node *sī′ nō-ā′ trē-ăl nōd*	the pacemaker; highly specialized, neurological tissue impeded in the wall of the right atrium; responsible for initiating electrical conduction of the heartbeat, causing the atria to contract and firing conduction of impulses to the AV node
atrioventricular (AV) node *ā′ trē-ō-ven-trik′ yū-lăr nōd*	neurological tissue in the center of the heart that receives and amplifies the conduction of impulses from the SA node to the bundle of His
bundle of His *bŭn′ dĕl of hiz*	neurological fibers extending from the AV node to the right and left bundle branches that fire the impulse from the AV node to the Purkinje fibers

TERM	MEANING
Purkinje fibers *pĕr-kin'jĕ fī'bĕrz* **Purkinje network** *pĕr-kin'jĕ net'wŏrk*	fibers in the ventricles that transmit impulses to the right and left ventricles, causing them to contract
polarization *pō'lăr-i-ză'shŭn*	resting; resting state of a myocardial cell
depolarization *dē-pō'lăr-i-zā'shŭn*	change of a myocardial cell from a polarized (resting) state to a state of contraction (*de* = not; *polarization* = resting)
repolarization *rē'pō-lăr-i-zā'shŭn*	recharging of the myocardial cell from a contracted state back to a resting state (*re* = again; *polarization* = resting)
normal sinus rhythm (NSR) *nŏr'măl sī'nŭs rith'ŭm*	regular rhythm of the heart cycle stimulated by the SA node (average rate of 60–100 beats/minute) (*see* Fig. 5-11)

🔷 Programmed Review: Cardiac Conduction Terms

ANSWERS	REVIEW
sinoatrial AV, atri/o ventricul/o	**5.33** Review Figure 5-7. The term SA node refers to the _____ node, which is where the heart's electrical impulse originates. This impulse is conducted to the atrioventricular, or _____, node, a term made from the combining forms _____ and _____.
Purkinje contract	**5.34** The impulse then moves from the bundle of His down the right and left bundle branches to the _____ fibers, which transmit impulses to the ventricles and cause them to _____. This rhythmic contraction is the heartbeat.
muscle heart heart muscle	**5.35** The combining form *my/o* means _____, and the combining form *cardi/o* means _____. Myocardial cells comprise the _____ _____.
depolarization repolarization	**5.36** The resting state of the myocardial cells is called polarization. When each cell contracts, it changes to a state of _____. The stage of _____ is the change back to a resting state.
sinoatrial, normal sinus	**5.37** The normal regular heart rhythm produced by this continued simulation of heart muscle by electrical impulses originating in the _____, or SA, node is called _____ _____ rhythm, or NSR.

Self-Instruction: Symptomatic Terms

Study the following:

TERM	MEANING
aneurysm (Fig. 5-8) *an'yū-rizm*	a widening; a bulging of the wall of the heart, aorta, or artery caused by a congenital defect or acquired weakness
saccular aneurysm *sak-yū-lăr an'yū-rizm*	a sac-like bulge on one side
fusiform aneurysm *fyū'si-fōrm an'yū-rizm*	a spindle-shaped bulge
dissecting aneurysm *di-sek'ting an'yū-rizm*	a split or tear of the vessel wall
angina pectoris *an'ji-nă pek'tō-ris*	chest pain caused by a temporary loss of oxygenated blood to heart muscle; often caused by narrowing of the coronary arteries (*angina* = to choke)
arteriosclerosis *ar-tēr'ē-ō-skler-ō'sis*	thickening, loss of elasticity, and calcification (hardening) of arterial walls
atherosclerosis *ath'er-ō-skler-ō'sis*	a form of arteriosclerosis characterized by the buildup of fatty substances that harden within the walls of arteries
atheromatous plaque (Fig. 5-9, A) *ath-ĕr-ō'mă-tŭs plak*	a swollen area within the lining of an artery caused by the buildup of fat (lipids)
claudication *klaw-di-kā'shŭn*	to limp; pain in a limb (especially the calf) while walking that subsides after rest; caused by inadequate blood supply
constriction (*see* Fig. 5-9, A) *kon-strik'shŭn*	compression of a part that causes narrowing (stenosis)
diaphoresis *dī'ă-fō-rē'sis*	profuse sweating (perspiration)

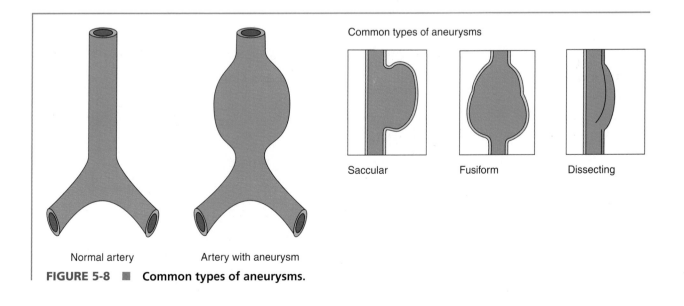

Common types of aneurysms

Saccular   Fusiform   Dissecting

Normal artery   Artery with aneurysm

FIGURE 5-8 ■ **Common types of aneurysms.**

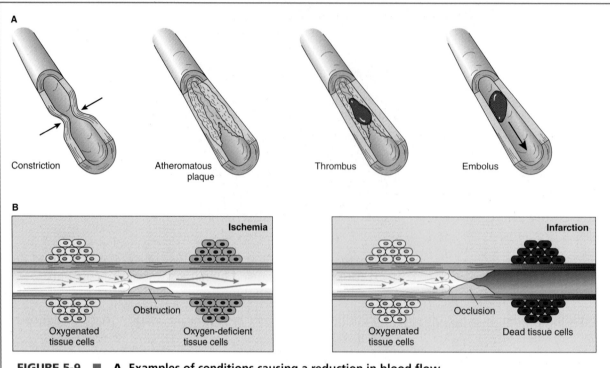

FIGURE 5-9 ■ **A. Examples of conditions causing a reduction in blood flow. B. Effects of reduced blood flow.**

TERM	MEANING
embolus (*see* Fig. 5-9, A) *em′bō-lŭs*	a clot (e.g., air, fat, or a foreign object) carried in the bloodstream that obstructs the flow of blood when it lodges (*embolus* = a stopper)
heart murmur *hart mŭr′mŭr*	an abnormal sound from the heart produced by defects in the chambers or valves
infarct (*see* Fig. 5-9, B) *in′farkt*	to stuff; a localized area of necrosis (condition of tissue death) caused by ischemia resulting from occlusion of a blood vessel
ischemia (*see* Fig. 5-9, B) *is-kē′mē-ă*	to hold back blood; decreased blood flow to tissue caused by constriction or occlusion of a blood vessel
perfusion deficit *pĕr-fyū′zhŭn def′i-sit*	lack of flow through a blood vessel caused by narrowing, occlusion, etc.
occlusion (*see* Fig. 5-9, B) *ŏ-klū′zhŭn*	plugging; an obstruction or a closing off
palpitation *pal-pi-tā′shŭn*	subjective experience of pounding, skipping, or racing heartbeats
stenosis *ste-nō′sis*	condition of narrowing of a part
thrombus (*see* Fig. 5-9, A) *throm′bŭs*	a stationary blood clot
vegetation (Fig. 5-10) *vej-ĕ-tā′shŭn*	to grow; an abnormal growth of tissue around a valve, generally as a result of infection

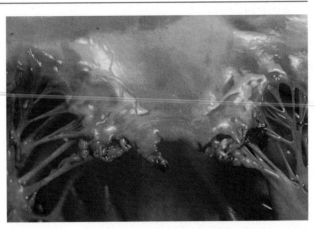

FIGURE 5-10 ■ The mitral valve shows destructive vegetations, which have eroded through the free margins of the valve leaflets in a patient with bacterial endocarditis.

Programmed Review: Symptomatic Terms

ANSWERS	REVIEW
hard	**5.38** *Scler/o*, a combining form meaning _____, is a key component in the term arteriosclerosis, which refers to thickening,
artery or arterial	loss of elasticity, and hardening of _____ walls. *Ather/o*, a
fatty or lipid	combining form meaning _____ paste, is used in the term that specifically describes a condition or increase of hardened fatty
atherosclerosis	substances built up within the walls of arteries: _____.
embolus	**5.39** An _____ is a clot of any sort carried in the bloodstream that obstructs the flow of blood when it lodges. A thrombus, on the
stationary	other hand, is a _____ blood clot.
	5.40 Blood flow through a vessel can be affected by various kinds of restrictions. A condition or increase of narrowing is called
stenosis	_____. Stenotic conditions can be the result of a compression
constriction	or _____ of a vessel. A buildup of atherosclerotic substances
narrowing	can also cause stenosis, a condition of _____. An
plugging or obstruction	occlusion, which is the _____ of a vessel, also might occur.
ischemia	**5.41** If blood flow is reduced to tissue, _____ occurs. When diagnostic tests detect the lack of blood flow from a vessel to tissue
deficit	cells, it is called a perfusion _____. Perfusion refers to tissues with an adequate circulation of blood.

ANSWERS	REVIEW
angina pector/o	**5.42** A heart condition of chest pain may occur when a temporary or transient restriction of blood flow to heart muscle occurs, which is called _____ pectoris. Recall that the combining form _____ refers to the chest. Therefore, this chest pain is called angina pectoris.
death infarct	**5.43** When prolonged or total ischemia occurs in an area, tissue necrosis or _____ results. The area of scarring from necrosis is called an _____.
bulge or widen saccular dissecting, fusiform	**5.44** An aneurysm can occur in the heart or a blood vessel because of a weakness in the wall. This causes the wall to _____. The type of aneurysm with a sac-like bulge is called a _____ aneurysm. If the bulge causes a split or tear of the vessel wall, it is called a _____ aneurysm. The bulge of a _____ aneurysm is spindle-shaped.
pain	**5.45** Various symptoms help cardiologists to determine what condition a patient is experiencing. Claudication is _____ in a limb, sometimes causing a limp, that results during movement because of an inadequate blood supply to the limb.
palpitation	**5.46** The subjective symptom of the heart pounding, skipping, or racing is called _____. Be careful not to confuse this term with palpation, the word meaning to touch or feel.
diaphoresis	**5.47** Sweating brought on by physical activity or a high-temperature environment is perfectly normal; however, profuse sweating, known as _____, accompanied by chest pain, shortness of breath, or heart palpitations, is a significant symptom of heart disease.
murmur	**5.48** The physician, when listening to the heart through a stethoscope, might hear an abnormal sound, called a heart _____, which is produced by a defect in the heart chambers or valves.

Self-Instruction: Diagnostic Terms

Study the following:

TERM	MEANING
RELATED TO THE HEART AND ARTERIES	
acute coronary syndrome (ACS) *ă-kyūt′ kōr′ŏ-nār-ē sin′drōm*	signs and symptoms indicating an active process of atherosclerotic plaque buildup or formation of a thrombus, or spasm within a coronary artery, causing a reduction or loss of blood flow to myocardial tissue; includes unstable angina and other pathological events leading to myocardial infarction (MI); early diagnosis and rapid treatment are critical to avoid or minimize damage to heart muscle
arrhythmia (Fig. 5-11) *ă-rith′mē-ă* **dysrhythmia** *dis-rith′mē-ă*	any of several kinds of irregularity or loss of rhythm of the heartbeat
bradycardia *brad-ē-kar′dē-ă*	slow heart rate (less than 60 beats/minute)
fibrillation *fi-bri-lā′shŭn*	chaotic, irregular contractions of the heart, as in atrial or ventricular fibrillation
premature ventricular contraction (PVC) *prē-mă-tūr′ ven-trik′ū-lăr kon-trak′shŭn*	a ventricular contraction preceding the normal impulse initiated by the SA node (pacemaker)
tachycardia *tak-i-kar′dē-ă*	fast heart rate (greater than 100 beats/minute)
bacterial endocarditis *bak-tēr′ē-ăl en′dō-kar-dī′tis*	a bacterial inflammation that affects the endocardium or the heart valves
cardiac tamponade *kar′dē-ak tam-pŏ-nād′*	compression of the heart produced by the accumulation of fluid in the pericardial sac, as results from pericarditis or trauma, causing rupture of a blood vessel within the heart (*tampon* = a plug)
cardiomyopathy *kar′dē-ō-mī-op′ă-thē*	a general term for disease of the heart muscle, such as alcoholic cardiomyopathy (damage to the heart muscle caused by excessive consumption of alcohol)
congenital anomaly of the heart *kon-jen′ĭ-tăl ah-nom′ah-lē of the hart*	malformations of the heart that are present at birth (*congenital* = born with; *anomaly* = irregularity)
atrial septal defect (ASD) *ā′trē-ăl sep′tăl dē′fekt*	an opening in the septum separating the atria
coarctation of the aorta *kō-ark-tā′shŭn of the ā-ōr′tă*	narrowing of the descending portion of the aorta, resulting in a limited flow of blood to the lower part of the body

Normal sinus rhythm (NSR)

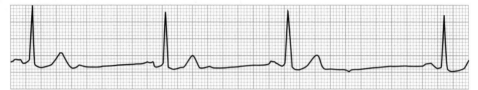

Bradycardia

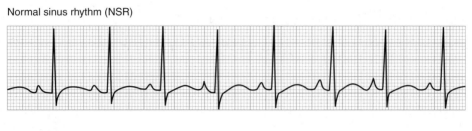

Fibrillation (ventricular)

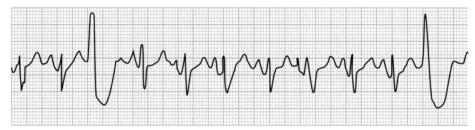

Flutter (atrial)

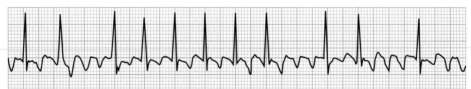

Premature ventricular contraction (PVC)

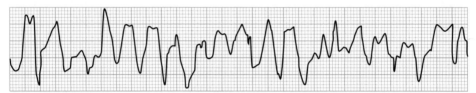

Tachycardia (sinus)

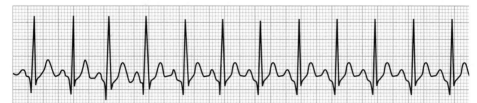

FIGURE 5-11 ■ **Electrocardiogram (ECG or EKG) tracings showing common types of arrhythmia.**

TERM	MEANING
patent ductus arteriosus (PDA) *pā′tent dŭk′tŭs ar-tē′rē-ō′sŭs*	an abnormal opening between the pulmonary artery and the aorta caused by failure of the fetal ductus arteriosus to close after birth (*patent* = open)
ventricular septal defect (VSD) *ven-trik′yū-lăr sep′tăl dē′fekt*	an opening in the septum separating the ventricles
congestive heart failure (CHF) *kon-jes′tiv hart fāl′yūr* **left ventricular failure** *left ven-trik′yū-lăr fāl′yūr*	failure of the left ventricle to pump an adequate amount of blood to meet the demands of the body, resulting in a "bottleneck" of congestion in the lungs that may extend to the veins, causing edema in lower portions of the body
cor pulmonale *kōr pul-mō-nā′lē* **right ventricular failure** *rīt ven-trik′yū-lăr fāl′yūr*	enlargement of the right ventricle, resulting from chronic disease within the lungs, that causes congestion within the pulmonary circulation and resistance of blood flow to the lungs (*cor* = heart)
coronary artery disease (CAD) (Fig. 5-12) *kōr′ŏ-nār-ē ar′tĕr-ē di-zēz′*	a condition affecting arteries of the heart that reduces the flow of blood and the delivery of oxygen and nutrients to the myocardium; most often caused by atherosclerosis
hypertension (HTN) *hī′pĕr-ten′shŭn*	persistently high blood pressure
essential hypertension *ĕ-sen′shăl hī′pĕr-ten′shŭn* **primary hypertension** *prī′mār-ē hī′pĕr-ten′shŭn*	high blood pressure attributed to no single cause; risks include smoking, obesity, increased salt intake, hypercholesterolemia, and hereditary factors
secondary hypertension *sĕk′ŏn-dār′ē hī′pĕr-ten′shŭn*	high blood pressure caused by the effects of another disease (e.g., kidney disease)

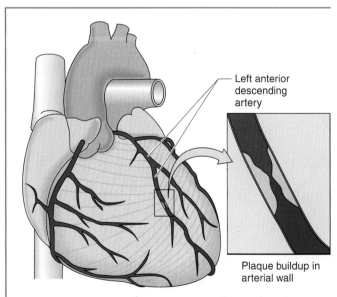

Left anterior descending artery

Plaque buildup in arterial wall

FIGURE 5-12 ■ Coronary artery disease (CAD).

TERM	MEANING
mitral valve prolapse (MVP) *mī′trăl valv prō′lapz*	protrusion of one or both cusps of the mitral valve back into the left atrium during ventricular contraction, resulting in incomplete closure and backflow of blood
myocardial infarction (MI) (Fig. 5-13) *mī-ō-kar′dē-ăl in-fark′shŭn*	heart attack; death of myocardial tissue (infarction) caused by ischemia (loss of blood flow) as a result of an occlusion (plugging) of a coronary artery; usually caused by atherosclerosis; symptoms include pain in the chest or upper body (shoulders, neck, and jaw), shortness of breath, diaphoresis, and nausea
myocarditis *mī′ō-kar-dī′tis*	inflammation of myocardium; most often caused by viral or bacterial infection
pericarditis *per′i-kar-dī′tis*	inflammation of the pericardium
rheumatic heart disease *rū-mat′ik hart di-zēz′*	damage to heart muscle and heart valves by rheumatic fever (a streptococcal infection)
sudden cardiac arrest (SCA) *sŭd′dĕn kar′dē-ak ă-rest′*	the abrupt cessation of any cardiac output (CO), most commonly as the result of ventricular fibrillation; causes sudden death unless defibrillation is initiated immediately

RELATED TO THE VEINS

TERM	MEANING
deep vein thrombosis (DVT) *dēp vān throm-bō′sis*	formation of a clot in a deep vein of the body, occurring most often in the femoral and iliac veins
phlebitis *fle-bī′tis*	inflammation of a vein
thrombophlebitis *throm′bō-fle-bī′tis*	inflammation of a vein associated with a clot formation
varicose veins (Fig. 5-14) *var′ĭ-kōs vāns*	abnormally swollen, twisted veins with defective valves; most often seen in the legs

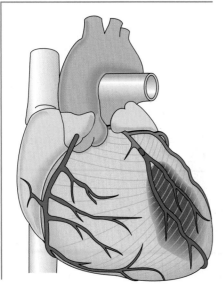

FIGURE 5-13 ■ Anterolateral myocardial infarction (MI) (*darkened area*), caused by occlusion of anterior descending branch of the left coronary artery.

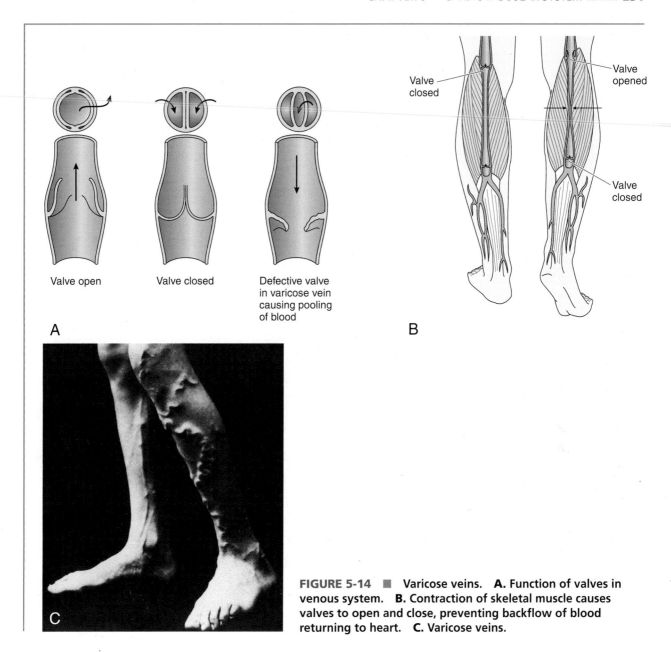

Valve open

Valve closed

Defective valve in varicose vein causing pooling of blood

A

Valve closed

Valve opened

Valve closed

B

C

FIGURE 5-14 ■ **Varicose veins. A. Function of valves in venous system. B. Contraction of skeletal muscle causes valves to open and close, preventing backflow of blood returning to heart. C. Varicose veins.**

Programmed Review: Diagnostic Terms

ANSWERS	REVIEW
inflammation	**5.49** The suffix -*itis* refers to an _____. Myocarditis
myocardium	therefore means an inflammation of the _____.
pericarditis	Inflammation of the pericardium is called _____.
	Bacterial endocarditis is a bacterial inflammation affecting the
endocardium	_____ and heart valves.

ANSWERS	REVIEW
coronary artery disease atherosclerosis	**5.50** The condition of reduced blood flow through the arteries that supply the heart muscle is called _____ _____ _____ (CAD). It most commonly results from a hardened buildup of fatty substances within the lining of the arteries, a condition known as _____.
occlusion ischemia death myocardial infarction heart attack chest pain diaphoresis acute coronary syndrome	**5.51** Atherosclerotic buildup within the wall of one or more coronary arteries can lead to a partial or total obstruction, which is called an _____. The resulting loss of blood flow, or _____, deprives the affected heart muscle of the oxygen it needs to survive. Prolonged ischemia leads to necrosis, the _____ of myocardial tissue. The term describing the death of myocardial tissue is _____ _____ (MI), which is commonly known as a _____ _____. Symptoms of myocardial infarction include angina (_____ _____), shortness of breath, nausea, and profuse sweating (_____). The abbreviation ACS, which stands for _____ _____ _____, includes the signs and symptoms that indicate an active process of the pathological events leading to myocardial infarction.
muscle cardiomyopathy	**5.52** Myopathy refers to a condition of diseased _____. The general term for a condition of diseased heart muscle is _____.
tamponade	**5.53** The word root *tampon* means a plug (obstruction), and the term tamponade refers to an obstruction. A compression of the heart produced by accumulated fluid in the pericardial sac is called a cardiac _____.
pulmonale enlarged	**5.54** Another word root that means heart is *cor*. The condition called cor _____ is caused by congestion in the pulmonary circulation that results in right ventricular failure. The right ventricle becomes _____ because of the increased effort to pump blood to the diseased lungs.
heart failure	**5.55** Congestive _____ failure (CHF) is a failure of the left ventricle to pump enough blood to the body. This condition is also called left ventricular _____.

ANSWERS	REVIEW
with partition atria, ventricular	**5.56** The term anomaly means irregularity (not normal). The term congenital pertains to something a person is born _____. There are several congenital anomalies of the heart. An atrial septal defect (ASD) is an irregularity in the septum, or _____, which separates the _____. A _____ septal defect (VSD) is an opening in the septum separating the ventricles.
coarctation	**5.57** A narrowing of the descending portion of the aorta that restricts blood flow to the lower body is called a _____ of the aorta.
close	**5.58** Patent ductus arteriosus (PDA) is an abnormal opening between the pulmonary artery and the aorta. The term patent means open. PDA results if the fetal ductus arteriosus fails to _____ after birth.
without dysrhythmia brady- slow fast, tachycardia	**5.59** The prefix *a-* means without. An arrhythmia is a heartbeat _____ a normal rhythm. The synonym for arrhythmia, which is formed using the prefix describing painful, difficult, or faulty, is _____. There are several types of heart arrhythmias or dysrhythmias. The prefix meaning slow is _____. Therefore, bradycardia is a condition of _____ heart rate. *Tachy-* is the prefix meaning _____, so _____ is a condition of fast heart rate.
fibrillation	**5.60** Fast, chaotic, irregular contractions of the heart occur in a condition called _____.
contraction node	**5.61** Another common arrhythmia is a premature ventricular _____ (PVC). In this case, the contraction precedes the normal impulse initiated by the sinoatrial (SA) _____.
sudden cardiac arrest	**5.62** Ventricular fibrillation is a lethal arrhythmia that causes the ventricles to quiver rapidly (to fibrillate) instead of contracting and to be unable to pump blood. The term describing the abrupt cessation of any cardiac output (CO) as caused by ventricular fibrillation is _____ _____ _____ (SCA).

ANSWERS	REVIEW
hypertension, HTN essential Secondary	**5.63** The condition of persistently high blood pressure is called _____ and is abbreviated as _____. Primary, or _____, hypertension cannot be attributed to a single cause. _____ hypertension, however, is caused by another condition, such as kidney disease.
rheumatic	**5.64** Rheumatic fever can cause damage to heart muscle and valves. This is called _____ heart disease.
vein phlebitis thrombophlebitis	**5.65** *Phleb/o* is a combining form for _____. Combined with the suffix for inflammation, this forms the term _____, which means inflammation of a vein. If that inflammation is associated with a clot formation, the condition is called _____.
deep vein thrombosis thrombus embolus	**5.66** The condition of a formed clot in a deep vein of the body is called _____ _____ _____ (DVT). The danger of any clot (_____) formation in a vein is that it can break loose to become a traveling _____.

◆ Self-Instruction: Diagnostic Tests and Procedures

Study the following:

TEST OR PROCEDURE	EXPLANATION
auscultation (Fig. 5-15) *aws-kŭl-tā′shŭn*	physical examination method of listening to sounds within the body with a stethoscope (e.g., auscultation of the chest for heart and lung sounds)
gallop *gal′ŏp*	abnormal heart sound that mimics the gait of a horse; related to abnormal ventricular contraction

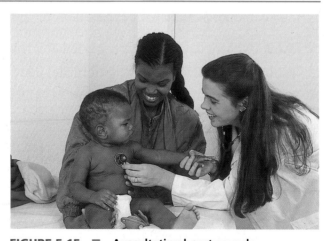

FIGURE 5-15 ■ **Auscultating heart sounds.**

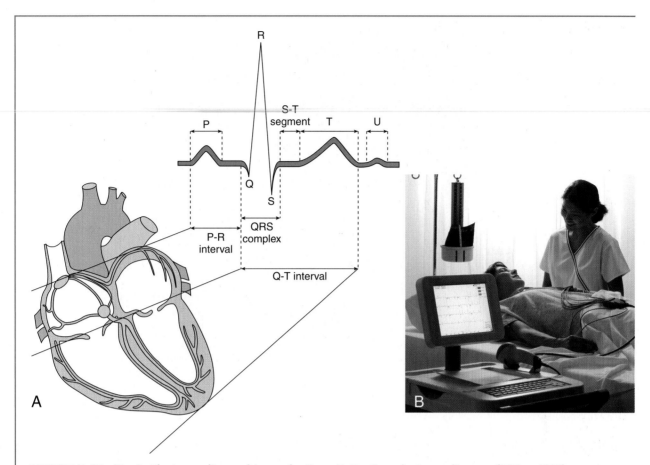

FIGURE 5-16 ■ **A.** Electrocardiographic conduction. **B.** Resting electrocardiogram (ECG or EKG).

TEST OR PROCEDURE	EXPLANATION
electrocardiogram (ECG or EKG) (Fig. 5-16; *see* Fig. 5-11) *ē-lek-trō-kar′ dē-ō-gram*	an electrical picture of the heart represented by positive and negative deflections on a graph labeled with the letters P, Q, R, S, and T, which correspond to events of the cardiac cycle
stress electrocardiogram (stress ECG or EKG) (Fig. 5-17) *stres ē-lek-trō-kar′ dē-ō-gram*	electrocardiogram (ECG or EKG) of the heart recorded during the induction of controlled physical exercise using a treadmill or ergometer (bicycle); useful in detecting heart conditions (e.g., ischemia or infarction)
Holter ambulatory monitor *hōl′ ter am′ byū-lă-tōr-ē mon′ i-tŏr*	portable electrocardiograph worn by the patient that monitors electrical activity of the heart over 24 hours; useful in detecting periodic abnormalities
intracardiac electrophysiological study (EPS) *in′ tră-kar′ dē-ak ē-lek′ trō-fiz′ē-ō-loj′ i-kăl stŭd′ē*	invasive procedure involving placement of catheter-guided electrodes within the heart to evaluate and map the electrical conduction of cardiac arrhythmias; intracardiac catheter ablation may be performed at the same time to treat the arrhythmia
intracardiac catheter ablation *in′ tră-kar′ dē-ak kath′ē-tĕr ab-lā′ shŭn*	use of radiofrequency waves sent through a catheter within the heart to treat arrhythmias by selectively destroying myocardial tissue at sites that generate abnormal electrical pathways

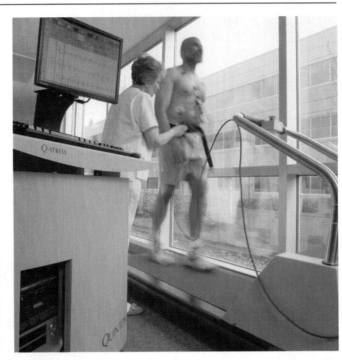

FIGURE 5-17 ■ Stress electrocardiography.

TEST OR PROCEDURE	EXPLANATION
magnetic resonance angiography (MRA) *mag-net′ik rez′ŏ-nănts an-jē-og′ră-fē*	magnetic resonance imaging of the heart and blood vessels for evaluation of pathology (*see* Fig. 8-15)
nuclear medicine imaging *nū′klē-ăr med′i-sin im′ă-jing*	radionuclide organ imaging of the heart after administration of radioactive isotopes to visualize structures and to analyze functions
myocardial radionuclide perfusion scan *mī-ō-kar′ dē-ăl rā′ dē-ō-nū′klīd pĕr-fyū′zhŭn skan*	scan of the heart made after an intravenous (IV) injection of an isotope (e.g., thallium) as it is absorbed by myocardial cells in proportion to blood flow throughout the heart; useful in evaluating coronary artery disease (CAD)
myocardial radionuclide perfusion stress scan *mī-ō-kar′dē-ăl rā′dē-ō-nū′klīd pĕr-fyū′zhŭn stres skan*	nuclear perfusion scan of the heart that is made before and after the induction of controlled physical exercise (treadmill or bicycle) or a pharmaceutical agent that produces the effect of exercise stress in patients who are unable to ambulate
multiple-gated acquisition (MUGA) scan *mŭl′ti-pul-gāt′ĕd ak-wi-zish′ŭn skan*	nuclear image of the beating heart in motion made as radioactive isotopes are injected in the bloodstream and traced through the heart's chambers; useful in evaluating the pumping function of the ventricles

TEST OR PROCEDURE	EXPLANATION
positron-emission tomography (PET) scan of the heart *poz'i-tron-ē-mish'ŭn tō-mog'ră-fē skan of the hart*	use of specialized nuclear isotopes and computed tomographic techniques to produce perfusion (blood flow) images and to study the cellular metabolism of the heart; can be performed at rest or with stress
radiology *rā-dē-ol'ŏ-jē*	x-ray imaging
angiography *an-jē-og'ră-fē*	process of x-ray imaging a blood vessel after injection of contrast medium, most commonly after catheter placement
angiogram *an'jē-ō-gram*	record obtained by angiography
coronary angiogram *kōr'ŏ-nār-ē an'jē-ō-gram*	x-ray image of the blood vessels of the heart using a catheter to inject contrast (*see* Fig. 5-2)
arteriogram *ar-tēr'ē-ō-gram*	x-ray image of a particular artery (e.g., coronary arteriogram or renal arteriogram)
aortogram *ā-ōr'tō-gram*	x-ray image of the aorta
venogram *vē'nō-gram*	x-ray image of a vein
cardiac catheterization (Fig. 5-18) *kar'dē-ak kath'ĕ-ter-ĭ-zā'shŭn*	introduction of a flexible, narrow tube (or catheter) through a vein or artery into the heart to withdraw samples of blood, to measure pressures within the heart chambers or vessels, and to inject contrast media for fluoroscopic radiography and cine film (motion picture) imaging of the chambers of the heart and coronary arteries; often includes interventional procedures, such as angioplasty and atherectomy (*see* percutaneous coronary intervention [PCI] procedures listed under *Self-Instruction: Operative Terms*)
left heart catheterization *left hart kath'ĕ-ter-ĭ-zā'shŭn*	x-ray imaging of the left ventricular cavity and coronary arteries
right heart catheterization *rīt hart kath'ĕ-ter-ĭ-zā'shŭn*	measurement of oxygen saturation and pressure readings of the right side of the heart
ventriculogram *ven-trik'ū-lō-gram*	x-ray image of the ventricles
stroke volume (SV) *strōk vol'yŭm*	measurement of the amount of blood ejected from a ventricle in one contraction
cardiac output (CO) *kăr'dē-ak owt'put*	measurement of the amount of blood ejected per minute from either ventricle of the heart
ejection fraction *ē-jek'shŭn frak'shŭn*	measurement of the volume percentage of left ventricular contents ejected with each contraction

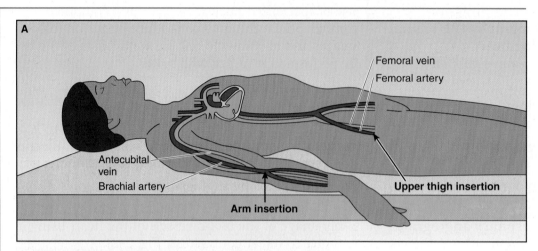

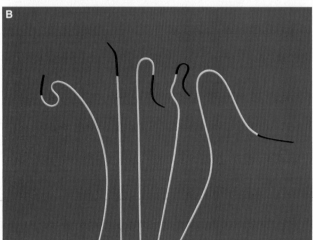

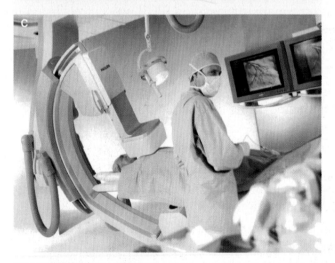

FIGURE 5-18 ■ **Cardiac catheterization. A. Possible insertion sites for cardiac catheterization. B. Angiographic catheters. (Photo courtesy of Cook Incorporated, Bloomington, IN.) C. Cardiac catheterization laboratory.**

TEST OR PROCEDURE	EXPLANATION
computed tomographic angiography (CTA) (Fig. 5-19) *kom-pyŭ'tĕd tō-mo-grăf'ik an-jē-og'ră-fē*	specialized, noninvasive, three-dimensional (3-D) computed tomographic scan of the heart and circulation of the "greater" blood vessels, such as the coronary arteries, aorta, and pulmonary veins; performed with or without contrast
sonography *sŏ-nog'ră-fē*	sonographic imaging
echocardiography (echo) (Fig. 5-20) *ek'ō-kar-dē-og'ră-fē*	recording of sound waves through the heart to evaluate structure and motion (*see* Fig. 5-1)
stress echocardiogram (stress echo) *stres ek-ō-kar'dē-ō-gram*	echocardiogram of the heart recorded during the induction of controlled physical exercise (treadmill or bicycle) or a pharmaceutical agent that produces the effect of exercise stress in patients who are unable to ambulate; useful in detecting conditions such as ischemia or infarction
transesophageal echocardiogram (TEE) *trans-e-sof'ăj-ē-ăl ek-ō-kar'dē-ō-gram*	echocardiogram of the heart after placement of an ultrasonic transducer at the end of an endoscope inside the esophagus
Doppler sonography *dop'lĕr sŏ-nog'ră-fē*	ultrasound technique used to evaluate blood flow to determine the presence of a deep vein thrombosis (DVT) or carotid insufficiency, or to determine flow through the heart, chambers, valves, and so on (*see* Figs. 5-4 and 5-5)

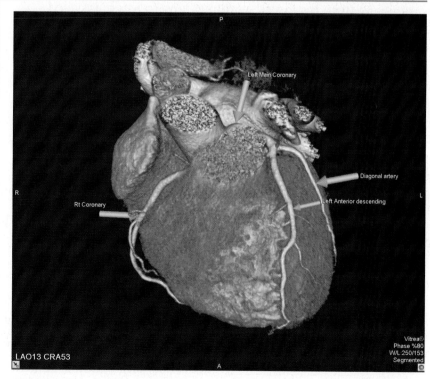

FIGURE 5-19 ■ Computed tomographic angiography (CTA) of normal heart. Arrows point to right coronary artery (RCA), left main coronary artery, diagonal artery, and left anterior descending artery (LAD)

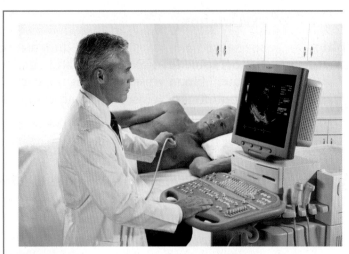

FIGURE 5-20 ■ Echocardiography (echo).

Programmed Review: Diagnostic Tests and Procedure

ANSWERS	REVIEW
chest stethoscope auscultation	**5.67** Recall that the combining form *steth/o* means _____, and that a _____ is an instrument for listening to sounds within the chest or elsewhere in the body. This procedure, from the Greek word meaning to listen, is called _____.
gallop	**5.68** Auscultation can be used to detect a heart murmur or other abnormal heart sound, such as that which mimics the gait of a horse, called a _____.
record heart electrocardiogram stress electrocardiogram	**5.69** The suffix *-gram* refers to a _____. The combining form *cardi/o* refers to the _____. A record of the electrical conductivity of the heart is called an _____ (ECG or EKG). A special kind of electrocardiogram obtained during the physical stress of exercise is called a _____ _____.
vessel angiography angiogram heart	**5.70** The combining form *angi/o* refers to a _____. The suffix *-graphy* refers to the diagnostic process of making a record, such as by x-ray imaging. The process of x-ray imaging a blood vessel is called _____, and the record itself is called an _____. A coronary angiogram is an x-ray image of the blood vessels encircling the _____.

ANSWERS	REVIEW
aortogram venogram	**5.71** An x-ray of a particular artery is called an arteriogram. An x-ray image of the aorta is called an _____. An x-ray image of a vein is called a _____.
cardiac catheterization right oxygen	**5.72** A catheter can be introduced into the heart for diagnostic purposes. This process is called _____ _____. Left heart catheterization is usually done to obtain a radiograph of the left ventricular cavity and coronary arteries, and _____ heart catheterization is usually done to measure _____ saturation and pressure.
ventriculogram -gram	**5.73** An x-ray image of the ventricles is called a _____, from the combining form *ventricul/o* and the suffix _____.
contraction, output left ejected	**5.74** Cardiac catheterization also allows for measurement of stroke volume (SV), or how much blood is ejected from a ventricle in one _____. Cardiac _____ (CO) measures the amount of blood ejected per minute from either ventricle; ejection fraction measures the volume percentage of the _____ ventricular contents _____ with each contraction.
magnetic resonance imaging angiography computed tomography three-dimensional or 3-D heart	**5.75** The abbreviation MRI stands for _____ _____ _____. The abbreviation MRA stands for magnetic resonance _____, which is specialized imaging of the heart and blood vessels. The abbreviation CT stands for _____ _____. The process abbreviated as CTA provides a specialized _____-_____ x-ray image of the _____ and greater vessels.
radionuclide organ imaging function radionuclide heart, intravenous myo, blood motion, pumping positron emission tomography	**5.76** Nuclear medicine imaging, or _____ _____ _____, uses radioactive isotopes to visualize body structures and to analyze _____. A myocardial _____ perfusion scan is made of the _____ after _____ (IV) injection of an isotope is absorbed by _____cardial cells in proportion to _____ flow. A MUGA scan provides a nuclear image of the beating heart in _____ and is useful in evaluating the _____ function of the ventricles. The abbreviation PET stands for _____ _____ _____, which is a nuclear scan that

ANSWERS	REVIEW
isotopes stress	uses radioactive _____ and computed tomographic (CT) technology. PET is used in cardiology to study the cellular metabolism of the heart. These scans can be made with the patient at rest or after exercise or _____.
ultrasound sound echo	**5.77** Sonography, or diagnostic _____, is the imaging modality using high-frequency _____ waves to visualize body tissues. The recording of sound waves through the heart to evaluate structure and motion is called _____cardiography.
echocardiogram stress transesophageal	**5.78** A record of the heart made with echocardiography (echo) is called an _____. If made during controlled exercise, it is called a _____ echocardiogram. If made after passing the transducer through the esophagus, it is called a _____ echocardiogram (TEE).
Doppler	**5.79** The type of sonography that uses ultrasound to evaluate blood flow is called _____ sonography.
within, heart arrhythmias electrophysiological study intracardiac, ablation	**5.80** Intracardiac means pertaining to _____ the _____. Physiological means pertaining to function. The invasive procedure involving the placement of a catheter within the heart to map the electrical conduction of cardiac dysrhythmias, or _____, is abbreviated as EPS, which stands for intracardiac _____ _____. The myocardial tissue generating abnormal electrical pathways can be treated at the time of an intracardiac electrophysiological study by using high-frequency waves sent through a catheter to ablate or destroy myocardial tissue responsible for generating the abnormal conduction. This treatment is called _____ catheter _____.

◆ **Self-Instruction: Operative Terms**

Study the following:

TERM	MEANING
PROCEDURES PERFORMED IN THE TRADITIONAL OPERATING ROOM	
coronary artery bypass graft (CABG) (Fig. 5-21) *kōr'ŏ-nār-ē ar'tĕr-ē bī'pas graft*	grafting a portion of a blood vessel retrieved from another part of the body (e.g., a length of saphenous vein from the leg or mammary artery from the chest wall) to bypass an occluded

A. Common sites for bypass grafts

B. Bypass process

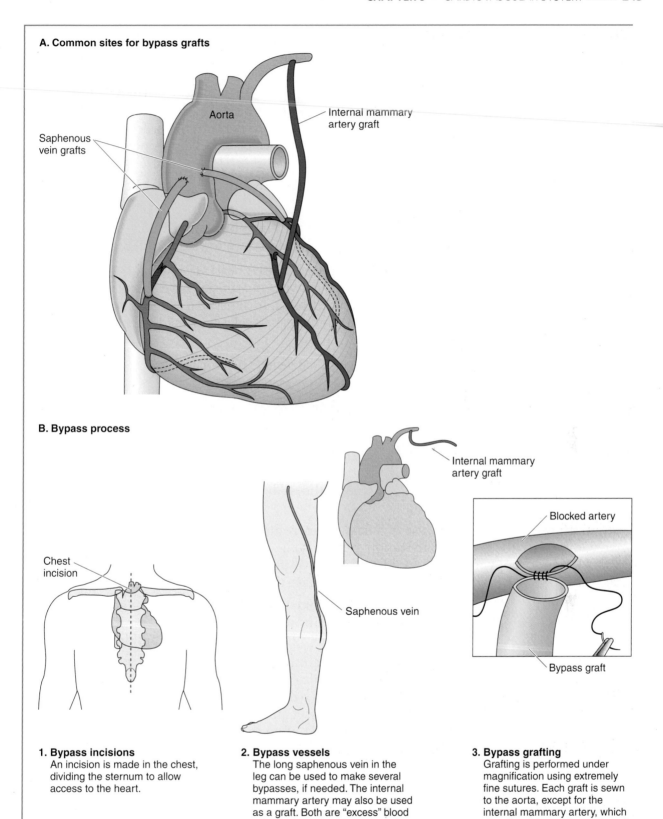

1. Bypass incisions
An incision is made in the chest, dividing the sternum to allow access to the heart.

2. Bypass vessels
The long saphenous vein in the leg can be used to make several bypasses, if needed. The internal mammary artery may also be used as a graft. Both are "excess" blood vessels the body does not need.

3. Bypass grafting
Grafting is performed under magnification using extremely fine sutures. Each graft is sewn to the aorta, except for the internal mammary artery, which already originates from a branch of the aorta. The other end is sewn to the artery below the blockage.

FIGURE 5-21 ■ **Traditional method of coronary artery bypass graft (CABG).** **A. Common sites for bypass grafts.** **B. Bypass grafting.**

TERM	MEANING
	coronary artery, restoring circulation to myocardial tissue; the traditional method includes temporary arrest of the heart with circulation (bypass) of the patient's blood through a heart-lung machine during the procedure; an alternative, off-pump approach uses a stabilizer to perform the procedure on the beating heart; the abbreviation CABG is pronounced "cabbage"
anastomosis *ă-nas′tō-mō′sis*	opening; the joining of two blood vessels to allow flow from one to the other
endarterectomy *end′ar-tĕr-ek′tŏ-mē*	surgical removal of the lining of an artery to clear a blockage caused by a clot or atherosclerotic plaque buildup
valve replacement *valv rē-plās′ment*	surgery to replace a diseased heart valve with an artificial valve; there are two types of artificial valves: tissue valves, most commonly made from animal tissue (e.g., porcine [pig] or bovine [cow]), and mechanical valves, made from synthetic material
valvuloplasty *val′vyū-lō-plas-tē*	surgical repair of a defective heart valve

PROCEDURES PERFORMED IN A CATHETERIZATION LABORATORY

percutaneous coronary intervention (PCI) (Fig. 5-22) *pĕr-kyū-tā′nē-yŭs kōr′ŏ-nār′ē in′tĕr-ven′shŭn*	interventional procedures used to treat coronary artery disease (CAD) performed at the time of cardiac catheterization in a specialized laboratory setting (or "cath lab") instead of the traditional operating room

angioscopy
   an-jē-os′kō-pē
   vascular endoscopy
   vas′kyū-lăr en-dos′kŏ-pē
	use of a flexible fiberoptic angioscope (accompanied by an irrigation system, camera, video recorder, and monitor) that is guided through a specific blood vessel to visually assess a lesion and to select the mode of therapy

atherectomy
   (see Fig. 5-22, A)
   ath-e-rek′tō-mē
	excision of atheromatous plaque from within an artery utilizing a device housed in a flexible catheter that selectively cuts away or pulverizes tissue buildup

percutaneous transluminal coronary angioplasty (PTCA)
   (see Fig. 5-2)
   pĕr-kyū-tā′nē-ŭs tranz′lū-men′ăl kōr′ŏ-nār-ē an′jē-ō-plas-tē
	a method for treating the narrowing of a coronary artery by inserting a specialized catheter with a balloon attachment, then inflating the balloon to dilate and open the narrowed portion of the vessel and restore blood flow to the myocardium; most often includes the placement of a stent

intravascular stent placement
     (see Fig. 5-22, B)
     in′tră-vas′kyū-lăr stent plās′ment
	implantation of a device used to reinforce the wall of a vessel and assure its patency (openness); most often used to treat a stenosis or a dissection (a split or tear in the wall of a vessel) or to reinforce patency of a vessel after angioplasty

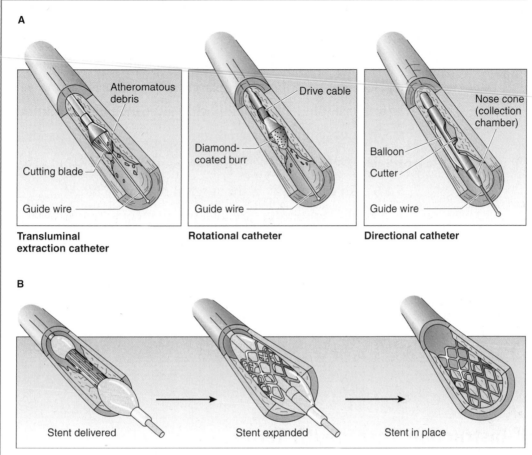

FIGURE 5-22 ■ Examples of devices used in percutaneous coronary interventional procedures. **A.** Atherectomy devices. **B.** Intravascular stent.

Programmed Review: Operative Terms

ANSWERS	REVIEW
vessel angioscope	**5.81** The suffix *-scopy* refers to the process of examination. Angioscopy is the examination of a blood _____ using a fiberoptic _____.
-ectomy atherectomy endarterectomy	**5.82** The suffix _____ refers to removal or excision. Removal of an atheromatous plaque is called an _____. Using the prefix *endo-,* the term for the surgical removal of the lining of an artery is an _____.
bypass graft	**5.83** CABG is the abbreviation for a coronary artery _____ _____, in which a portion of a blood vessel is grafted in place to bypass an occluded coronary artery.
vessels	**5.84** An anastomosis is the joining of two blood _____ to allow flow from one to the other.

ANSWERS	REVIEW
valvuloplasty tissue pig, cow	**5.85** The suffix *-plasty* refers to a surgical repair or reconstruction. A _____ is the repair of a defective heart valve. Valve replacement describes the replacement of a diseased heart valve with an artificial valve. Types of artificial valves include mechanical ones, made from synthetic material, and _____ valves made from animal tissue, such as porcine (_____) or bovine (_____).
vessel coronary angioplasty	**5.86** An angioplasty is the surgical repair of a blood _____. A specialized procedure called a percutaneous transluminal _____ _____ (PTCA) is a treatment for a narrowed coronary artery.
stent	**5.87** An intravascular _____ is implanted to keep a blood vessel open and to reinforce the vessel's wall.

 ## Self-Instruction: Therapeutic Terms

Study the following:

TERM	MEANING
defibrillation (Fig. 5-23) *dē-fib-ri-lā'shŭn*	termination of ventricular fibrillation by delivering an electrical stimulus to the heart; most commonly, this is done by applying the electrodes of the defibrillator externally to the chest wall, but it can also be performed internally, such as during open heart surgery or via an implanted device
defibrillator *dē-fib'ri-lā-tŏr*	device that delivers the electrical stimulus in defibrillation
cardioversion *kar'dē-ō-ver'zhŭn*	restoration of a fast or irregular heart rate to a normal rhythm, either by pharmaceutical means or by delivery of electrical energy
implantable cardioverter defibrillator (ICD) *im-plan'tă-bĕl* *kar'dē-ō-ver'ter* *dē-fib'ri-lā-tŏr*	an implanted, battery-operated device with rate-sensing leads; the device monitors cardiac impulses and initiates an electrical stimulus as needed to stop ventricular fibrillation or tachycardia
pacemaker (Fig. 5-24) *pās'mā-kĕr*	a device used to treat slow heart rates (bradycardia) by electrically stimulating the heart to contract; most often, it is implanted with lead wires and battery circuitry under the skin, but it can also be placed on a temporary basis externally with lead wires inserted into the heart via a vein

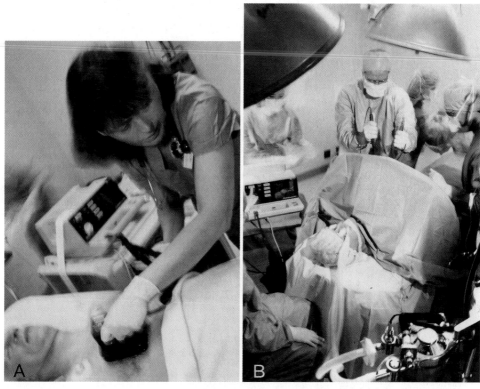

FIGURE 5-23 ■ **A.** External defibrillation. **B.** Internal defibrillation performed in the operating room.

TERM	MEANING
COMMON THERAPEUTIC DRUG CLASSIFICATIONS	
angiotensin-converting enzyme (ACE) inhibitor *an-jē-ō-ten'sin-kon-vert'ing en'zīm in-hib'i-tŏr*	drug that suppresses the conversion of angiotensin in the blood by the angiotensin-converting enzyme (ACE); used in the treatment of hypertension
antianginal *an'tē-an'ji-năl*	drug that dilates coronary arteries, restoring oxygen to the tissues to relieve the pain of angina pectoris
antiarrhythmic *an'tē-ă-rith'mik*	drug that counteracts cardiac arrhythmia
anticoagulant *an'tē-kō-ag'yū-lant*	drug that prevents clotting of the blood; commonly used in the treatment of thrombophlebitis and myocardial infarction
antihypertensive *an'tē-hī-per-ten'siv*	drug that lowers blood pressure
beta-adrenergic blocking agents *bā'tă-ad-rĕ-nĕr'jik blok'ing ā'jentz* **beta-blockers** *bā'tă-blok'ĕrz*	agents that inhibit responses to sympathetic adrenergic nerve activity, causing a slowing of electrical conduction and heart rate and a lowering of the pressure within the walls of the vessels; used to treat angina pectoris and hypertension; the Greek small letter *beta* is commonly used in the names of these agents (i.e., β-blockers)

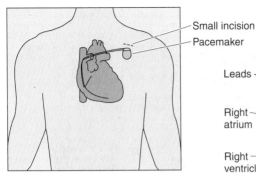

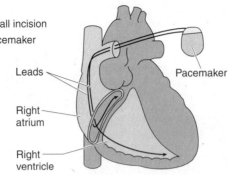

A small incision is made in the upper chest, below the clavicle, to access a large vein nearby.

A

The pacemaker leads are then guided through the vein and into the heart. After proper placement is determined, the leads are secured in position.

A small "pocket" to house the pacemaker is created just under the skin at the incision site. The leads are connected to the pacemaker that is secured in the "pocket." Finally, the incision is closed with a few sutures.

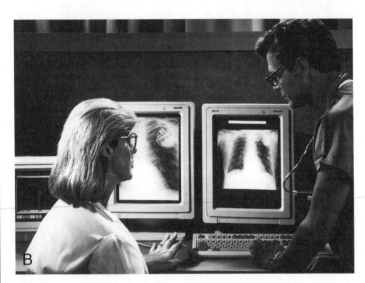

FIGURE 5-24 ■ **Pacemaker.** **A.** Endocardial pacemaker. **B.** Teleradiology/critical care workstation chest radiographs on screen show pacemaker placement.

TERM	MEANING
calcium-channel blockers *kal' sē-ŭm-chan'ĕl blok'ĕrz*	agents that inhibit the entry of calcium ions into heart muscle cells, causing a slowing of the heart rate, a lessening of the demand for oxygen and nutrients, and a relaxing of the smooth muscle cells of the blood vessels to cause dilation; used to prevent or treat angina pectoris, some arrhythmias, and hypertension
cardiotonic *kar' dē-ō-ton'ik*	drug that increases the force of myocardial contractions in the heart; commonly used to treat congestive heart failure (CHF)
diuretic *dī-yū-ret'ik*	drug that increases the secretion of urine; commonly prescribed in treating hypertension
hypolipidemic *hī-pō-lip'i-dē'mik*	drug that reduces serum fat and cholesterol

TERM	MEANING
thrombolytic agents *throm-bō-lit′ik ā′jentz*	drugs used to dissolve thrombi (blood clots) (e.g., streptokinase or tissue plasminogen activator [TPA or tPA]); used in acute management of myocardial infarction (MI) and ischemic stroke; commonly called "clot busters"
vasoconstrictor *vă′sō-kon-strik′tŏr*	drug that causes a narrowing of the blood vessels, thereby decreasing blood flow
vasodilator *vă′sō-dī-lă′tŏr*	drug that causes dilation of the blood vessels, thereby increasing blood flow

🔷 Programmed Review: Therapeutic Terms

ANSWERS	REVIEW
bradycardia pacemaker	**5.88** The term for a condition of slow heart is _____. A device that is surgically implanted to make a slow heart maintain an adequate pace is called a _____.
fast cardioversion	**5.89** Tachycardia is a condition of _____ heart rate. Version is a process of turning. The method of turning an abnormally fast or irregular heart rate back to normal by use of a drug or delivery of electrical energy is called _____.
fibrillation, not defibrillator	**5.90** Chaotic, irregular contractions of the heart are called _____. The prefix *de-* means from, down, or _____. A device used on a patient to stop ventricular fibrillation is called a _____. The process of doing so is called defibrillation.
implantable cardioverter defibrillator	**5.91** An implantable device that initiates an electrical stimulus to stop ventricular fibrillation or tachycardia is called an _____ _____ (ICD).
against or opposed to coagulation or clotting hypertensive	**5.92** The prefix *anti-* means _____. Drugs in the class known as anticoagulants work to prevent _____. A drug that lowers high blood pressure is called an anti_____.
chest pain antianginal dilator myocardium	**5.93** Recall that angina pectoris is _____ _____. Drugs that treat this pain are classified as _____ drugs. Nitroglycerin is a common antianginal medication. It acts as a vaso_____, causing the coronary arteries to expand and, thereby, increasing the flow of blood to the heart muscle tissue, also known as the _____.

ANSWERS	REVIEW
arrhythmic	**5.94** A drug that counteracts a cardiac arrhythmia is called an anti_____.
beta-blockers	**5.95** A number of different drug classifications are used to treat hypertension. Beta-adrenergic blocking agents, also called, more simply, _____-_____, work by inhibiting responses to a nerve activity and slowing electrical conduction and heart rate.
calcium-channel	**5.96** Another type of antihypertensive drug works by inhibiting the entry of calcium ions into heart muscle cells, thereby slowing the heart and causing other changes. These are called _____-_____ blockers.
urine	**5.97** Another antihypertensive drug, called a diuretic, works by increasing the secretion of _____ from the body.
tonic	**5.98** Congestive heart failure (CHF) is often treated with drugs that increase the force of ventricular contractions. These drugs are called cardio_____ agents.
hypolipid	**5.99** Recall that lipids are fats. Using the prefix *hypo-*, the term for a drug that lowers the amount of fat in the blood is a _____emic agent.
breaking down or dissolution clots thrombo clot busters myocardial infarction	**5.100** The suffix *-lysis* means _____ _____. Drugs that work to dissolve thrombi or _____ in the blood are called _____lytic agents. Thrombolytics, commonly known as _____ _____, are used in acute management of ischemic stroke and _____ _____ (MI).

CHAPTER 5 ACRONYMS AND ABBREVIATIONS

ABBREVIATION	EXPANSION
ACE	angiotensin-converting enzyme
ACS	acute coronary syndrome
ASD	atrial septal defect
AV	atrioventricular
BP	blood pressure
CABG	coronary artery bypass graft
CAD	coronary artery disease

ABBREVIATION	EXPANSION
CHF	congestive heart failure
CO	cardiac output
CTA	computed tomographic angiography
DVT	deep vein thrombosis
ECG or EKG	electrocardiogram
ECHO	echocardiography
EPS	electrophysiological study
HTN	hypertension
ICD	implantable cardioverter defibrillator
IV	intravenous
MI	myocardial infarction
MRA	magnetic resonance angiography
MUGA	multiple-gated acquisition (scan)
MVP	mitral valve prolapse
NSR	normal sinus rhythm
PCI	percutaneous coronary intervention
PDA	patent ductus arteriosus
PET	positron-emission tomography
PTCA	percutaneous transluminal coronary angioplasty
PVC	premature ventricular contraction
SA	sinoatrial
SCA	sudden cardiac arrest
SV	stroke volume
TEE	transesophageal echocardiogram
tPA or TPA	tissue plasminogen activator
VSD	ventricular septal defect

CHAPTER 5 SUMMARY OF TERMS

The terms introduced in chapter 5 are listed below, followed by the page number on which each term can be found and its written pronunciation. For additional practice and reinforcement, write the definition of each term on a separate piece of paper.

acute coronary syndrome (ACS)/227
ă-kyūt′ kōr′ŏ-nār-ē sin′drŏm

aneurysm/223
an′yū-rizm

anastomosis/244
ă-nas′tō-mō′sis

angina pectoris/223
an′ji-nă pek′tō-ris

angiogram/237
an'jē-ō-gram

angiography/237
an-jē-og'ră-fē

angioscopy/244
an-jē-os'kō-pē

**angiotensin-converting enzyme (ACE)
  inhibitor**/247
an-jē-ō-ten'sin-kon-ver'ting en'zīm in-hib'i-tŏr

antianginal/247
an'tē-an'ji-năl

antiarrhythmic/247
an'tē-ă-rith'mik

anticoagulant/247
an'tē-kō-ag'yū-lant

antihypertensive/247
an'tē-hī-per-ten'siv

aorta/213
ā-ōr'tă

aortic valve/213
ă-ōr'tik valv

aortogram/237
ā-ōr'tō-gram

arrhythmia/227
ă-rith'mē-ă

arteries/213
ar'tĕr-ēz

arteriogram/237
ar-tĕr'ē-ō-gram

arterioles/213
ar-tĕr'ē-ōlz

arteriosclerosis/223
ar-tĕr'ē-ō-skler-ō'sis

atherectomy/244
ath-e-rek'tō-mē

atheromatous plaque/223
ath-ĕr-ō'mă-tŭs plak

atherosclerosis/223
ath'er-ō-skler-ō'sis

atrial septal defect (ASD)/227
ā'trē-ăl sep'tăl dē'fekt

atrioventricular (AV) node/221
ă'trē-ō-ven-trik'yū-lăr nōd

atrium/212
ā'trē-ŭm

auscultation/234
aws-kŭl-tā'shŭn

bacterial endocarditis/227
bak-tēr'ē-ăl en'dō-kar-dī'tis

beta-adrenergic blocking agents/247
bā'tă-ad-rĕ-nĕr'jik blok'ing ā'jentz

beta-blockers/247
bā'tă-blok'ĕrz

bicuspid valve/213
bī-kŭs'pid valv

bradycardia/227
brad-ē-kar'dē-ă

bundle of His/221
bŭn'dĕl of hiz

calcium-channel blockers/248
kal'sē-ŭm-chan'ĕl blok'ĕrz

capillaries/213
kap'i-lār-ēz

cardiac catheterization/237
kar'dē-ak kath'ĕ-ter-ī-zā'shŭn

cardiac output (CO)/237
kăr'dē-ak owt'put

cardiac tamponade/227
kar'dē-ak tam-pŏ-nād'

cardiomyopathy/227
kar'dē-ō-mī-op'ă-thē

cardiotonic/248
kar'dē-ō-ton'ik

cardioversion/246
kar'dē-ō-ver'zhŭn

claudication/223
klaw-di-kā'shŭn

coarctation of the aorta/227
kō-ark-tā'shŭn of the ā-ōr'tă

**computed tomographic angiography
  (CTA)**/239
kom-pyū'tĕd tō-mo-graf'ik an-jē-og'ră-fē

congenital anomaly of the heart /227
kon-jen'ĭ-tăl ah-nom'ah-lē of the hart

congestive heart failure (CHF)/229
kon-jes'tiv hart fāl'yūr

constriction/223
kon-strik′shŭn

cor pulmonale/229
kŏr pul-mō-nā′lē

coronary angiogram/237
kŏr′ŏ-năr-ē an′jē-ō-gram

coronary artery bypass graft (CABG)/242
kŏr′ŏ-năr-ē ar′tĕr-ē bī′pas graft

coronary artery disease (CAD)/229
kŏr′ŏ-năr-ē ar′tĕr-ē di-zēz′

coronary circulation/214
kŏr′ŏ-năr-ē ser-kyū-lā′shŭn

deep vein thrombosis (DVT)/230
dēp vān throm-bō′sis

defibrillation/246
dē-fib-ri-lā′shŭn

defibrillator/246
dē-fib′ri-lā-tŏr

depolarization/222
dē-pō′lăr-i-zā′shŭn

diaphoresis/223
dī′ă-fō-rē′sis

diastole/219
dī-as′tō-lē

dissecting aneurysm/223
di-sek′ting an′yū-rizm

diuretic/248
dī-yū-ret′ik

Doppler sonography/239
dop′lĕr sŏ-nog′ră-fē

dysrhythmia/227
dis-rith′mē-ă

echocardiography (echo)/239
ek′ō-kar-dē-og′ră-fē

ejection fraction/237
ē-jek′shŭn frak′shŭn

electrocardiogram (ECG or EKG)/235
ē-lek-trō-kar′dē-ō-gram

embolus/224
em′bō-lŭs

endarterectomy/244
end′ar-tĕr-ek′tŏ-mē

endocardium/212
en-dō-kar′dē-ŭm

epicardium/212
ep-i-kar′dē-ŭm

essential hypertension/229
ĕ-sen′shăl hī′pĕr-ten′shŭn

fibrillation/227
fi-bri-lā′shŭn

fusiform aneurysm/223
fyū′si-form an′yū-rizm

gallop/234
gal′ŏp

heart murmur/224
hart mŭr′mŭr

heart valves/213
hart valvz

Holter ambulatory monitor/235
hōl′ter am′byū-lă-tōr-ē mon′i-tŏr

hypertension (HTN)/219, 229
hī′pĕr-ten′shŭn

hypolipidemic/248
hī-pō-lip′i-dē′mik

hypotension/219
hī′pō-ten′shŭn

implantable cardioverter defibrillator (ICD)/246
im-plan′tă-bel kar′dē-ō-ver′ter dē-fib′ri-lā-tŏr

infarct/224
in′farkt

interatrial septum/212
in′tĕr-ā′trē-ăl sep′tŭm

interventricular septum/212
in′tĕr-ven-trik′yū-lăr sep′tŭm

intracardiac catheter ablation/235
in′tră-kar′dē-ak kath′ĕ-tĕr ab-lā′shun

intracardiac electrophysiological study (EPS)/235
in′tră-kar′dē-ak ē-lek′trō-fiz′ē-ō-loj′i-kăl stŭd′ē

intravascular stent placement/244
in′tra-vas′kyū-lăr stent plās′ment

ischemia/224
is-kē′mē-ă

left heart catheterization/237
left hart kath′ĕ-ter-ĭ-zā′shŭn

left ventricular failure/229
left ven-trik′yū-lăr fāl′yūr

magnetic resonance angiography (MRA)/236
mag-net′ik rez′ŏ-nănts an-jē-og′ră-fē

mitral valve/213
mī′trăl valv

mitral valve prolapse (MVP)/230
mī′trăl valv prō′laps

multiple-gated acquisition (MUGA) scan/236
mŭl′ti-pul-gāt′ĕd ak-wi-zish′ŭn skan

myocardial infarction (MI)/230
mī-ō-kar′dē-ăl in-fark′shŭn

myocardial radionuclide perfusion scan/236
mī-ō-kar′dē-ăl rā′dē-ō-nū′klīd pĕr-fyū′zhŭn skan

myocardial radionuclide perfusion stress scan/236
mī-ō-kar′dē-ăl rā′dē-ō-nū′klīd pĕr-fyū′zhŭn stres skan

myocarditis/230
mī′ō-kar-dī′tis

myocardium/213
mī′ō-kar′dē-ŭm

normal sinus rhythm (NSR)/222
nōr′măl sī′nŭs rith′ŭm

normotension/219
nōr-mō-ten′shŭn

nuclear medicine imaging/236
nū′klē-ăr med′i-sin im′ă-jing

occlusion/224
ŏ-klū′zhŭn

pacemaker/246
pās′mā-kĕr

palpitation/224
pal-pi-tā′shŭn

parietal pericardium/213
pă-rī′ĕ-tăl per-i-kar′dē-ŭm

patent ductus arteriosus (PDA)/229
pā′tent dŭk′tŭs ar-tē′rē-ō′sus

percutaneous coronary intervention (PCI)/244
pĕr-kyū-tā′nē-yŭs kōr′ŏ-nār-ē in′tĕr-ven′shŭn

percutaneous transluminal coronary angioplasty (PTCA)/244
pĕr-kyū-tā′nē-yŭs tranz′lū-men′ăl kōr′ŏ-nār-ē an′jē-ō-plas-tē

perfusion deficit/224
pĕr-fyū′zhŭn def′i-sit

pericardial cavity/213
per-i-kar′dē-ăl kav′i-tē

pericarditis/230
per′i-kar-dī′tis

pericardium/213
per-i-kar′dē-ŭm

phlebitis/230
fle-bī′tis

polarization/222
pō′lăr-i-zā′shŭn

positron-emission tomography (PET) scan of the heart/237
poz′i-tron ē-mish′ŭn tō-mog′ră-fē skan of the hart

premature ventricular contraction (PVC)/227
prē-mă-tūr′ ven-trik′ū-lăr kon-trak′shŭn

primary hypertension/229
prī′măr-ē hī′pĕr-ten′shŭn

pulmonary circulation/214
pul′mō-nār-ē sĭr-kyū-lā′shŭn

pulmonary semilunar valve/213
pul′mō-năr-ē sem-ē-lū′năr valv

Purkinje fibers/222
pĕr-kin′jē fī′bĕrz

Purkinje network/222
pĕr-kin′jē net′wŏrk

radiology/237
rā-dē-ol′ŏ-jē

repolarization/222
rē′pō-lăr-i-zā′shŭn

rheumatic heart disease/230
rū-mat′ik hart di-zēz′

right heart catheterization/237
rīt hart kath′ĕ-ter-ĭ-zā′shŭn

right ventricular failure/229
rīt ven-trik′yū-lăr fāl′yūr

saccular aneurysm/223
sak-yū-lăr an′yū-rizm

secondary hypertension/229
se′kŏn-dār′ē hī′pĕr-ten′shŭn

sinoatrial (SA) node/221
sī′nō-ă′trē-ăl nōd

sonography/239
sŏ-nog′ră-fē

stenosis/224
ste-nō′sis

stress echocardiogram (stress echo)/239
stres ek′ō-kar′dē-ō-gram

**stress electrocardiogram (stress ECG
    or EKG)**/235
stres ē-lek-trō-kar′dē-ō-gram

stroke volume (SV)/237
strōk vol′yŭm

sudden cardiac arrest (SCA)/230
sŭd′dĕn kar′dē-ak ă-rest′

systemic circulation/214
sis-tem′ik sĭr-kyū-lā′shŭn

systole/219
sis′tō-lē

tachycardia/227
tak-i-kar′dē-ă

thrombolytic agents/249
throm-bō-lit′ik ā′jentz

thrombophlebitis/230
throm′bō-fle-bī′tis

thrombus/224
throm′bŭs

**transesophageal echocardiogram
    (TEE)**/239
trans-e-sof′ăj-ē-ăl ek-o-kar′dē-ō-gram

tricuspid valve/213
trī-kŭs′pid valv

valve replacement/244
valv rē-plās′ment

valves of the veins/213
valvz of the vānz

valvuloplasty/244
val′vyū-lō-plas-tē

varicose veins/230
var′i-kōs vānz

vascular endoscopy/244
vas′kyū-lăr en-dos′kŏ-pē

vasoconstrictor/249
vā′sō-kon-strik′tŏr

vasodilator/249
vā′sō-dī-lā′tŏr

vegetation/224
vej-ĕ-tā′shŭn

veins/213
vānz

venogram/237
vē′nō-gram

ventricle/213
ven′tri-kĕl

**ventricular septal defect
    (VSD)**/229
ven-trik′yū-lăr sep′tăl dē′fekt

ventriculogram/237
ven-trik′yū-lō-gram

venules/213
ven′yūlz

visceral pericardium/213
vis′ĕr-ăl per-i-kar′dē-ŭm

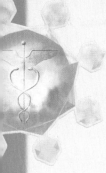

PRACTICE EXERCISES

For each of the following words, write out the term components (prefixes [P], combining forms [CF], roots [R], and suffixes [S]) on the lines below the word. Then define the term according to the meaning of its components.

EXAMPLE:

pericardial

peri / _cardi_ / _al_

P   R   S

DEFINITION: around/heart/pertaining to

1. angiography

_____ / _____

CF   S

DEFINITION: _____

2. varicosis

_____ / _____

R   S

DEFINITION: _____

3. pectoral

_____ / _____

R   S

DEFINITION: _____

4. vasospasm

_____ / _____

CF   S

DEFINITION: _____

5. venous

_____ / _____

R   S

DEFINITION: _____

6. thrombophlebitis

_____ / _____ / _____

CF   R   S

DEFINITION: _____

7. vasculopathy

_____ / _____ / _____

CF   R   S

DEFINITION: _____

8. atherogenesis

_____ / _____

CF   S

DEFINITION: _____

9. stethoscope

_____ / _____
    CF   S

DEFINITION: _____

10. myocardium

_____ / _____ / _____
    CF   R   S

DEFINITION: _____

11. aortoplasty

_____ / _____
    CF   S

DEFINITION: _____

12. venostomy

_____ / _____
    CF   S

DEFINITION: _____

13. phlebotomy

_____ / _____
    CF   S

DEFINITION: _____

14. ventriculography

_____ / _____
    CF   S

DEFINITION: _____

15. phlebitis

_____ / _____
    R   S

DEFINITION: _____

16. angioplasty

_____ / _____
    CF   S

DEFINITION: _____

17. endovascular

_____ / _____ / _____
    P   R   S

DEFINITION: _____

18. arteriogram

_____ / _____
    CF   S

DEFINITION: _____

19. atherectomy

_____ / _____
　　　R　　　　　S

DEFINITION:_____

20. intracardiac

_____ / _____ / _____
　　　P　　　　　R　　　　　S

DEFINITION: _____

Write the letter of the matching meaning in the space after the term.

21. atherosclerosis _____   a. high blood pressure

22. infarct _____   b. bulging of a vessel

23. hypotension _____   c. stationary clot

24. vegetation _____   d. cramp in leg muscle

25. embolus _____   e. normal blood pressure

26. occlusion _____   f. hard, nonelastic condition of arterial walls

27. hypertension _____   g. traveling clot that obstructs when it lodges

28. thrombus _____   h. buildup of fat

29. constriction _____   i. growth of tissue

30. normotension _____   j. a plugging

31. angina _____   k. loss of blood flow

32. claudication _____   l. compression that causes narrowing

33. ischemia _____   m. cramp in heart muscle

34. arteriosclerosis _____   n. low blood pressure

35. aneurysm _____   o. scar left by necrosis

Write the correct medical term for each of the following definitions:

36. _____ malformations of the heart present at birth

37. _____ thickening, loss of elasticity, and calcification (hardening) of arterial walls

38. _____ irregularity or loss of rhythm of the heartbeat

39. _____ a general term for disease of the heart muscle

40. _____ joining of two blood vessels to allow flow from one vessel to the other

41. _____ an abnormal heart sound that mimics the gait of a horse

42. _____ a recording of sound waves directed through the heart to evaluate structure and motion

43. _____ a condition of enlargement of the right ventricle as a result of chronic disease within the lungs

44. _____ an x-ray image of the blood vessels of the heart made with the introduction of a catheter and the release of a contrast medium

45. _____ electrocardiogram of the heart recorded during controlled physical exercise

Identify the structures of the heart by writing the missing words in the spaces provided:

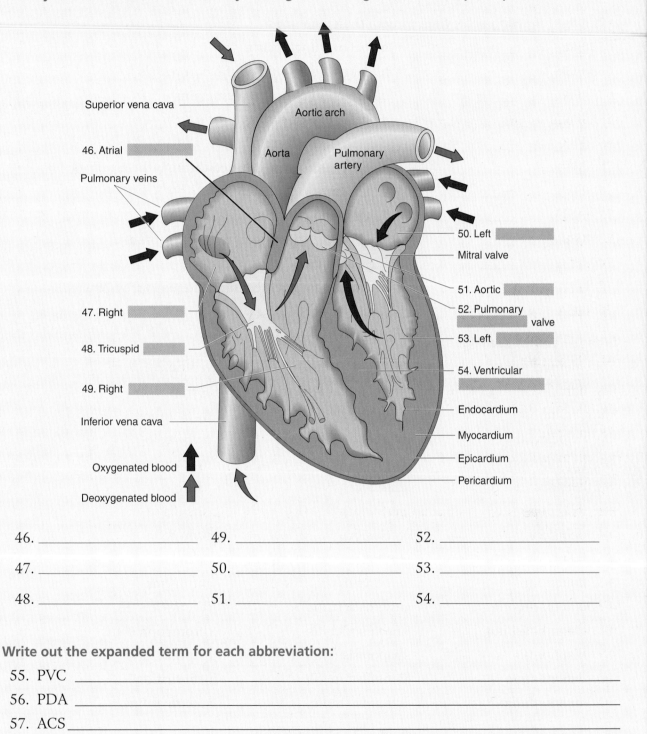

Superior vena cava

Aortic arch

46. Atrial

Aorta

Pulmonary artery

Pulmonary veins

50. Left

Mitral valve

51. Aortic

47. Right

52. Pulmonary
_____ valve

48. Tricuspid

53. Left

49. Right

54. Ventricular

Inferior vena cava

Endocardium

Myocardium

Epicardium

Pericardium

Oxygenated blood

Deoxygenated blood

46. _____	49. _____	52. _____
47. _____	50. _____	53. _____
48. _____	51. _____	54. _____

Write out the expanded term for each abbreviation:

55. PVC _____

56. PDA _____

57. ACS _____

58. ICD _____

59. CHF _____

60. CAD _____

61. HTN _____

62. MVP _____

63. PCI _____

64. VSD _____

Match the following abbreviations with their meanings:

65. EPS _____   a. balloon angioplasty

66. ECG _____   b. magnetic resonance of blood vessels

67. tPA _____   c. cessation of heart contractions

68. MRA _____   d. heart bypass surgery

69. PTCA _____   e. electrical picture of heart

70. MI _____   f. echocardiogram directed through the esophagus

71. DVT _____   g. left ventricular failure

72. ASD _____   h. thrombolytic drug

73. CABG _____   i. abnormal opening in the atrial septum

74. TEE _____   j. heart attack

75. CHF _____   k. cardiac catheter technique to map arrhythmias

76. SCA _____   l. clot in vein

Circle the correct spelling:

77. ventricel	ventrical	ventricle
78. aorta	aorto	aorrta
79. thrombos	thrombus	thrommbus
80. myocardial	mycardial	myocardiol
81. hypatension	hyptension	hypotension
82. diastolie	diastoly	diastole
83. ischemia	ishchemia	ishemia
84. oclusion	occlusion	ocllusion
85. infart	enfarct	infarct
86. anuerysm	aneurysm	annurysm
87. atherosclerotic	atherosclerrotic	atherasclerotic
88. thromboflebitus	thromboflebitis	thrombophlebitis
89. diaphoresis	diaporesis	diephoresis
90. defibrillation	defibillation	defibrilation
91. antarhythmic	antiarrhythmic	antiarhythmic

Write the term that means the opposite of the term given:

92. vasoconstriction _____

93. coagulant _____

94. hypotension _____

95. bradycardia   _____

96. diastole   _____

Circle the combining form that corresponds to the meaning given:

97.	**chest**	phleb/o	sphygm/o	pector/o
98.	**vein**	aort/o	phleb/o	varic/o
99.	**vessel**	angi/o	arteri/o	coron/o
100.	**heart**	ven/o	coron/o	cardi/o
101.	**fatty paste**	aort/o	ather/o	atri/o
102.	**circle**	cardi/o	coron/o	sphygm/o
103.	**pulse**	sphygm/o	steth/o	thromb/o
104.	**clot**	atri/o	angi/o	thromb/o
105.	**artery**	arteri/o	angi/o	aort/o

MEDICAL RECORD ANALYSIS

Medical Record 5-1

PROGRESS NOTE

S: This 54 y.o. ♂ was admitted to CCU with onset of acute anterior chest pain radiating to the left shoulder and SOB; pt underwent a CABG × 4 six months ago.

O: BP 190/110, P 100, R 72, T 38°C
On PE, pt was in moderate to severe distress. An ECG showed sinus tachycardia, and a CXR revealed left ventricular hypertrophy.

A: R/O MI

P: Order blood enzyme measurement STAT
Echocardiogram
CT scan of chest

QUESTIONS ABOUT MEDICAL RECORD 5-1

1. What is the patient's CC?
   a. severe angina
   b. angina developing slowly over time
   c. enlargement of the heart
   d. fast heart rate
   e. slow heart rate

2. Describe the procedure that the patient underwent 6 months ago:
   a. surgery to dilate and open narrowed portions of coronary arteries
   b. diversion of blood flow around occluded coronary arteries
   c. replacement of a diseased heart valve
   d. coring of the lining of an artery to remove a clot
   e. heart transplant

3. Where was the patient treated?
   a. outpatient medical office
   b. outpatient emergency room
   c. inpatient intensive care
   d. inpatient coronary care
   e. outpatient cardiology department

4. What type of physician is most appropriate to provide initial care and assessment of this patient?
   a. ER physician
   b. internist
   c. gerontologist
   d. cardiovascular surgeon
   e. cardiologist

5. What did the electrical picture of the heart reveal?
   a. extremely rapid but regular contractions of the heart
   b. slow heart rate
   c. chaotic, irregular contractions of the heart
   d. fast heart rate
   e. interference with normal electrical conduction of the heart known as a block

6. What was the assessment?
   a. patient may have had a heart attack
   b. patient may be suffering from right heart failure
   c. patient has congestive heart failure
   d. patient may have high blood pressure
   e. patient may have an enlarged heart

7. What were the objective findings of the chest radiograph?
   a. unknown
   b. increase in size of left ventricle
   c. vessel disease
   d. dead heart muscle
   e. fast heart rate

8. Identify the x-ray imaging procedure ordered in the plan:
   a. sonogram of heart
   b. chest radiography
   c. blood pressure
   d. computed tomography
   e. biochemistry panel

Medical Record 5-2

FOR ADDITIONAL STUDY

Richard Stratten has had serious heart problems for more than 10 years and has undergone two operations. During the past six months, he has developed increasing pain in the chest and is having more trouble breathing. His cardiologist, Dr. Charles Feingold, has now admitted him to Central Medical Center for further tests. Medical Record 5-2 is the history and physical examination report dictated by Dr. Feingold after his examination of Mr. Stratten.

Read Medical Record 5-2 (pages 266–269), then write your answers to the following questions in the spaces provided.

QUESTIONS ABOUT MEDICAL RECORD 5-2

1. Below are medical terms used in this record that you have not yet encountered in this text. Underline each where it appears in the record, and define the term below:

   obtuse _____

   dyspnea (dyspneic) _____

   hiatal hernia _____

   basilar rales _____

   visceromegaly _____

   clubbing _____

2. In your own words (not using medical terminology), briefly describe why Mr. Stratten has been admitted to the hospital and what test he will be undergoing:

   _____

   _____

   _____

3. Name the diagnosis that underlies the nature of Mr. Stratten's heart conditions:

   _____

   _____

   _____

   Briefly describe this diagnosis using nonmedical language:

   _____

   _____

   _____

4. Identify the surgical procedure noted in the history that was performed initially to treat Mr. Stratten's heart disease:

   a. dilation of narrow occluded coronary arteries

   b. replacement of occluded arteries with transplanted portion of vein

   c. replacement of a diseased heart valve

   d. coring of the lining of an artery to remove a thrombus

   e. heart transplant

5. What were the patient's symptoms 8 years later on May 15, 20xx?

_____

Using nonmedical language, briefly describe the diagnosis made at that time:

_____

_____

_____

6. Describe the test that showed changes consistent with the diagnosis:

_____

_____

7. Spell out TPA, and identify the reason why the drug was given to Mr. Stratten:

_____

_____

_____

8. Which of the following were findings of the radiographic tests performed after the May 15th hospitalization? (Mark all that are appropriate.)

   a. hemorrhage of insertion site of obtuse marginal artery graft

   b. thromboembolism in the left anterior descending artery

   c. occluded circumflex artery

   d. torn sutures of the circumflex artery graft

   e. stenosis of the left anterior descending artery graft

   f. total occlusion of the left internal mammary vein graft

   g. dilated right coronary artery graft

9. List the arteries that were grafted in *both* bypass operations:

_____

_____

10. Using nonmedical language, list the three symptoms Mr. Stratten is now experiencing:

   a. _____

   b. _____

   c. _____

11. Mr. Stratten is taking eight different medications. Translate the medication instructions for each one:

Drug Name	Dose	Frequency of Dose
_____	_____	_____
_____	_____	_____
_____	_____	_____
_____	_____	_____
_____	_____	_____
_____	_____	_____
_____	_____	_____
_____	_____	_____

12. What family members have had a medical history of problems in the same body system?

_____

_____

13. In addition to Mr. Stratten's heart problems, Dr. Feingold's physical examination revealed abnormal findings in what other areas?

a. head

b. abdomen

c. extremities

d. all of the above

e. none of the above

14. What does "probable end-stage cardiomyopathy" mean? What treatment seemed possible to Dr. Feingold, even though he had not yet performed the diagnostic tests for which he hospitalized Mr. Stratten?

_____

_____

_____

_____

Medical Record 5-2: For Additional Study

CENTRAL MEDICAL CENTER
211 Medical Center Drive • Central City, US 90000-1234 • PHONE: (012) 125-6784 • FAX: (012) 125-9999

HISTORY

CHIEF COMPLAINT:
The patient is admitted for heart catheterization and coronary arteriography with a view of possible cardiac transplantation.

HISTORY OF PRESENT ILLNESS:
The patient is a 53-year-old Caucasian male who has had a known history of coronary artery disease. The patient had initial 4-vessel bypass surgery 10 years ago on July 18, 20xx, at which time the patient had a saphenous vein bypass graft to the left anterior descending, diagonal, obtuse marginal, and right coronary artery.

Eight years later, on May 15, 20xx, the patient was rehospitalized at Central Medical Center because of acute chest pain with electrocardiogram changes consistent with acute inferior wall infarction for which the patient was given TPA. Following that, the patient had dramatic improvement in terms of electrocardiogram changes and symptoms and subsequently underwent reevaluation, including heart catheterization and coronary arteriography. This revealed the following findings:

> Native right coronary artery, left anterior descending, and circumflex were all totally occluded. The bypass graft to the left anterior descending had an 80% stenosis proximally and was totally occluded distally. Circumflex was previously totally occluded. Bypass graft to the obtuse marginal had a 70% occlusion followed by 90% occlusion at the insertion site of the graft. The right coronary artery graft had 95-98% stenosis. This diagonal graft was previously demonstrated to be totally occluded.

Because of this, the patient underwent a second bypass surgery on May 25, 20xx, at which time the patient had a left internal mammary graft to the left anterior descending and right internal mammary graft to the diagonal. The patient also had a saphenous vein bypass graft to the obtuse marginal and right coronary artery.

Since that time, the patient has continued to have intermittent angina, particularly within the last six months or so. In addition, the patient has gotten progressively weaker and dyspneic.

(continued)

HISTORY AND PHYSICAL PAGE 1	PT. NAME: STRATTEN, R. ID NO: ROOM NO: ADM. DATE: October 15, 20xx ATT. PHYS: C. FEINGOLD, M.D.

Medical Record 5-2: For Additional Study (Continued)

CENTRAL MEDICAL CENTER
211 Medical Center Drive • Central City, US 90000-1234 • PHONE: (012) 125-6784 • FAX: (012) 125-9999

HISTORY

At the present time, the patient is taking Prinivil 5 mg daily in a.m., Procainamide 500 mg q 6 h, Lasix 80 mg b.i.d., Lipitor 10 mg daily, Lanoxin 0.25 mg daily, Aspirin 81 mg daily, Atenolol 10 mg daily, and Nitro-Dur 0.4 mg/hr patch, apply daily q a.m. and remove h.s.

Because of increasing symptoms, the patient is being evaluated for cardiac transplant. The patient is undergoing heart catheterization for evaluation.

PAST MEDICAL HISTORY:
PAST ILLNESSES: There is no prior history of hypertension or diabetes. See above regarding previous coronary bypass surgery and myocardial infarctions. •

The patient has a known hiatal hernia, but it is asymptomatic at this time.

ALLERGIES: None known.

MEDICATIONS: See above.

PREVIOUS OPERATIONS: See above.

FAMILY HISTORY:
Father died of coronary artery disease at age 50. Paternal uncle also died of coronary artery disease. Maternal uncle and grandfather are both diabetic. The patient has no siblings. The remainder of family history is noncontributory.

SOCIAL HISTORY:
MARITAL HISTORY: Single.

HABITS: The patient is a nonsmoker and denies drinking ethanolic beverages.

INVENTORY BY SYSTEMS:
Noncontributory. There is no prior history of transient ischemic attack or claudication.

(continued)

HISTORY AND PHYSICAL PAGE 2	PT. NAME: STRATTEN, R. ID NO: ROOM NO: ADM. DATE: October 15, 20xx ATT. PHYS: C. FEINGOLD, M.D.

Medical Record 5-2: For Additional Study (Continued)

CENTRAL MEDICAL CENTER
211 Medical Center Drive • Central City, US 90000-1234 • PHONE: (012) 125-6784 • FAX: (012) 125-9999

PHYSICAL EXAMINATION

GENERAL:
The patient is a well-developed, well-nourished Caucasian male who is not in acute distress.

VITAL SIGNS:
Blood Pressure: 120/80. Pulse: 70 and regular.

HEENT:
HEAD: Normocephalic, atraumatic.

NECK: Neck veins are essentially normal. There are no carotid bruits.

CHEST:
HEART: Revealed cardiomegaly. There is no murmur. There is an equivocal third heart sound.

LUNGS: There are a few basilar rales.

ABDOMEN:
No visceromegaly. The bowel sounds are normal. No masses or tenderness.

RECTAL:
Deferred.

EXTREMITIES:
No clubbing, cyanosis, or peripheral edema. The peripheral pulses are intact.

NEUROLOGIC:
Physiologic.

IMPRESSION:
CORONARY ARTERY DISEASE WITH PREVIOUS ANTERIOR AND INFERIOR WALL
INFARCTION STATUS POST PREVIOUS CORONARY BYPASS SURGERY x 2 WITH
PROGRESSIVE INCREASE IN SYMPTOMATOLOGY IN TERMS OF ANGINA AND
DYSPNEA WITH PROBABLE END-STAGE CARDIOMYOPATHY.

(continued)

HISTORY AND PHYSICAL PAGE 3	PT. NAME: STRATTEN, R. ID NO: ROOM NO: ADM. DATE: October 15, 20xx ATT. PHYS: C. FEINGOLD, M.D.

Medical Record 5-2: For Additional Study (Continued)

CENTRAL MEDICAL CENTER
211 Medical Center Drive • Central City, US 90000-1234 • PHONE: (012) 125-6784 • FAX: (012) 125-9999

HISTORY AND PHYSICAL

The details of heart catheterization and coronary angiography have been discussed with the patient, including the risks and potential complications. The patient understands and wishes to proceed. This will be performed on October 16, 20xx.

C. Feingold, M.D.

CF:ti

D: 10/19/20xx
T: 10/20/20xx

HISTORY AND PHYSICAL
Page 4

PT. NAME: STRATTEN, R.
ID NO:
ROOM NO:
ADM. DATE: October 15, 20xx
ATT. PHYS: C. FEINGOLD, M.D.

ANSWERS TO PRACTICE EXERCISES

1. angio/graphy
   CF   S
   vessel/process of
      recording
2. varic/osis
   R   S
   swollen, twisted
      vein/condition or
      increase
3. pector/al
   R   S
   chest/pertaining to
4. vaso/spasm
   CF   S
   vessel/involuntary
      contraction
5. ven/ous
   R S
   vein/pertaining to
6. thrombo/phleb/itis
   CF   R   S
   clot/vein/inflammation
7. vasculo/path/y
   CF   R S
   vessel/disease/condition
      or process of
8. athero/genesis
   CF   S
   fatty paste (lipids)/origin
      or production
9. stetho/scope
   CF   S
   chest/instrument for
      examination
10. myo/card/ium
    CF R S
    muscle/heart/structure
       or tissue
11. aorto/plasty
    CF   S
    aorta/surgical repair or
       reconstruction
12. veno/stomy
    CF   S
    vein/creation of an
       opening

13. phlebo/tomy
    CF   S
    vein/incision
14. ventriculo/graphy
    CF   S
    ventricle/process of
       recording
15. phleb/itis
    R S
    vein/inflammation
16. angio/plasty
    CF   S
    vessel/surgical repair
       or reconstruction
17. endo/vascul/ar
    P   R   S
    within/vessel/
       pertaining to
18. arterio/gram
    CF   S
    artery/record
19. ather/ectomy
    R   S
    fat (lipids)/excision
       or removal
20. intra/cardi/ac
    P   R   S
    within/heart/
       pertaining to
21. h
22. o
23. n
24. i
25. g
26. j
27. a
28. c
29. l
30. e
31. m
32. d
33. k
34. f
35. b
36. congenital anomalies
37. arteriosclerosis

38. arrhythmia or
    dysrhythmia
39. cardiomyopathy
40. anastomosis
41. gallop
42. echocardiogram
43. cor pulmonale or right
    ventricular failure
44. coronary angiogram
45. stress electrocardiogram
46. atrial septum
47. right atrium
48. tricuspid valve
49. right ventricle
50. left atrium
51. aortic valve
52. pulmonary semilunar
    valve
53. left ventricle
54. ventricular septum
55. premature ventricular
    contraction
56. patent ductus arteriosus
57. acute coronary
    syndrome
58. implantable cardioverter
    defibrillator
59. congestive heart failure
60. coronary artery disease
61. hypertension
62. mitral valve prolapse
63. percutaneous coronary
    intervention
64. ventricular septal defect
65. k
66. e
67. h
68. b
69. a
70. j
71. l
72. i
73. d
74. f
75. g
76. c
77. ventricle
78. aorta

79. thrombus
80. myocardial
81. hypotension
82. diastole
83. ischemia
84. occlusion
85. infarct
86. aneurysm
87. atherosclerotic

88. thrombophlebitis
89. diaphoresis
90. defibrillation
91. antiarrhythmic
92. vasodilation
93. anticoagulant
94. hypertension
95. tachycardia
96. systole

97. pector/o
98. phleb/o
99. angi/o
100. cardi/o
101. ather/o
102. coron/o
103. sphygm/o
104. thromb/o
105. arteri/o

ANSWERS TO MEDICAL RECORD ANALYSIS

Medical Record 5-1: Progress Note

1. a   2. b   3. d   4. e   5. d   6. a   7. b   8. d

Medical Record 5-2: For Additional Study

See CD-ROM for answers.

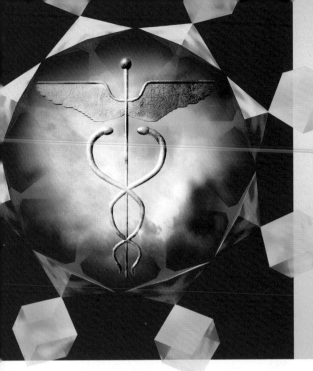

Blood and Lymphatic Systems

✓ Chapter 6 Checklist

BLOOD AND LYMPHATIC SYSTEMS OVERVIEW

The blood is responsible for:

❋ Transporting oxygen, nutrients, and hormones to body cells

❋ Carrying wastes away from the cells

The lymphatic system functions to:

❋ Protect the body by filtering microorganisms and foreign particles from the lymph, a clear fluid collected from body tissues

❋ Support the activities of the lymphocytes in the immune response

❋ Maintain the body's internal fluid environment as an intermediary between the blood in the capillaries and tissue cells

❋ Carry fats away from the digestive organs

Self-Instruction: Combining Forms

Study the following:

COMBINING FORM	MEANING
blast/o (also a suffix, -*blast*)	germ or bud
chrom/o, chromat/o	color
chyl/o	juice
cyt/o	cell
hem/o, hemat/o	blood
immun/o	safe
lymph/o	clear fluid
morph/o	form
myel/o	bone marrow or spinal cord
phag/o	eat or swallow
plas/o	formation
reticul/o	a net
splen/o	spleen
thromb/o	clot
thym/o	thymus gland

 ## Programmed Review: Combining Forms

ANSWERS	REVIEW
blast/o	**6.1** The combining form meaning germ or bud is _____, as in the term blastogenesis, which refers to the origin or production of
-blast	cells by budding. The suffix from this combining form is _____. Hemocytoblasts (a term formed from the combination of -*blast* with
cell, blood	*cyt/o,* meaning _____, and *hem/o* meaning _____) are the primitive stem cells in the bone marrow that develop into blood cells.
red	An erythroblast develops into an erythrocyte, or a _____ blood cell.
chromat/o	**6.2** The combining form *chrom/o* or _____ means
color	_____. For example, chromone refers to plant pigments. Recall
condition of	that the suffix -*ism* means _____ _____; therefore, chromatism is a condition of abnormal pigmentation.

ANSWERS	REVIEW
juice blood chyle	**6.3** The combining form *chyl/o* means _____ or fluid. Chyle is a pale yellow fluid from the intestine that is carried by the lymphatic system. The suffix *-emia* refers to a _____ condition; thus, chylemia means the presence of _____ in the blood.
hemat/o hem/o formation blood	**6.4** Hematology, a term made from the combining form _____, meaning blood, is the medical study of the blood. Another combining form for blood is _____, as in hemostat, which is an agent or device that stops the flow of blood from a vessel. Recall that the suffix *-poiesis* means _____. Therefore, hemopoiesis refers to the process of formation and development of various types of _____ cells.
immun/o immunocompromised	**6.5** The combining form meaning safe is _____. The immune system helps to keep the body safe from infectious disease. Both the blood and lymphatic systems are involved in the immune system. Someone whose immune system has been compromised by disease is said to be _____.
clear lymphoma	**6.6** The combining form *lymph/o* means _____ fluid. Lymph is a clear fluid, collected from body tissues, that flows through lymphatic vessels and, eventually, into the venous blood circulation. Using the suffix that means tumor, a neoplasm of the lymphatic system is called a _____.
eat cell eats condition of	**6.7** The combining form *phag/o* means _____ or swallow. The suffix *-cyte* refers to a _____. A phagocyte therefore is a cell that _____ bacteria, foreign particles, and other cells. Using the suffix *-osis*, which generally means increase or _____ _____, phagocytosis is the process or condition of phagocytes ingesting other solid substances.
formation without condition of	**6.8** *Plas/o* is a combining form meaning _____. Using the prefix *a-*, meaning _____, and the suffix *-ia*, meaning _____ _____, aplasia is a condition in which a formation (tissue or organ) is absent or defective.

ANSWERS	REVIEW
form study of	**6.9** *Morph/o* is a combining form meaning _____. Combined with *-logy*, the suffix meaning _____ ____, morphology is the study of form, including the size and shape of a specimen, such as blood cells.
myel/o cell bone marrow	**6.10** The combining form referring to either bone marrow or the spinal cord is _____. Bone marrow is the tissue within the cavities of bones, where many types of blood cells are produced. Combined with *cyt/o*, which is the combining form meaning _____, a myelocyte is an immature blood cell in the _____ _____.
net erythro reticulo red	**6.11** *Reticul/o* is a combining form meaning a _____. A network of substances influences the development of red blood cells from a primitive _____blast (red bud or germ) to a _____cyte (from the combining form meaning a net). Reticulocytes are immature _____ blood cells, or erythrocytes.
splen/o enlargement spleen splenectomy	**6.12** The spleen is a key organ of the lymphatic system. It filters the blood and performs other functions. The combining form for spleen is _____. Recalling that the suffix *-megaly* means _____, splenomegaly is an enlarged _____. Use the common suffix for excision or removal to construct the word that means the removal of the spleen: _____.
cells thromb/o clot	**6.13** Thrombocytes are blood _____ that function to clot the blood. The combining form meaning clot is _____. A thrombus is a blood _____ inside a blood vessel.
thym/o thymoma	**6.14** The thymus is a gland in the lymphatic system; the term comes from the combining form _____. A tumor of thymus tissue is called a _____.

Self-Instruction: Anatomic Terms in the Blood System

Study the following:

TERM	MEANING
TERMS RELATED TO BLOOD FLUID (Fig. 6-1)	
plasma *plaz′mă*	liquid portion of the blood and lymph; contains water, proteins, and cellular components (i.e., leukocytes, erythrocytes, and platelets)
serum *sēr′ŭm*	liquid portion of the blood that remains after clotting
CELLULAR COMPONENTS OF THE BLOOD (Fig. 6-2)	
erythrocyte *ĕ-rith′rō-sīt*	red blood cell; transports oxygen and carbon dioxide
hemoglobin *hē-mō-glō′bin*	the protein-iron compound in erythrocytes that transports oxygen and carbon dioxide
leukocyte *lū′kō-sīt*	white blood cell; protects the body from harmful invading substances
granulocytes *gran′yū-lō-sītz*	a group of leukocytes containing granules in their cytoplasm
neutrophil *nū′trō-fil*	a granular leukocyte, named for the neutral stain of its granules, that fights infection by swallowing bacteria (phagocytosis) (*neutr* = neither; *phil* = attraction for)

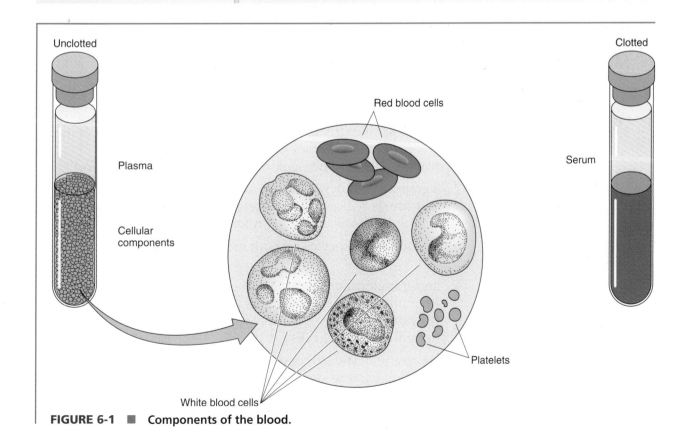

FIGURE 6-1 ■ **Components of the blood.**

CELLULAR COMPONENTS OF THE BLOOD

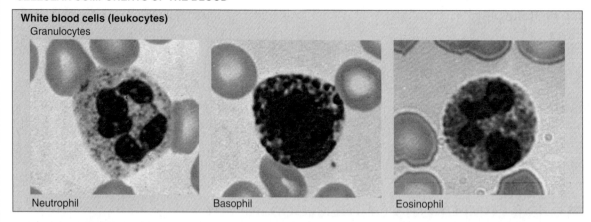

White blood cells (leukocytes)
Granulocytes

Neutrophil   Basophil   Eosinophil

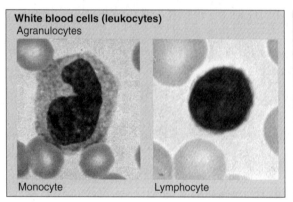

White blood cells (leukocytes)
Agranulocytes

Monocyte   Lymphocyte

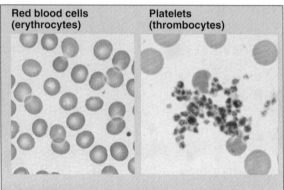

Red blood cells (erythrocytes)   **Platelets (thrombocytes)**

FIGURE 6-2 ▬ Cellular components of the blood.

TERM	MEANING
polymorphonuclear (PMN) leukocyte *pol'ē-mōr'fō-nū'klē-ăr lū'kō-sīt*	another term for neutrophil, referring to the many segments in its nucleus (*poly* = many; *morpho* = form; *nucleus* = kernel)
eosinophil *ē-ō-sin'ō-fil*	a granular leukocyte, named for the rose-colored stain of its granules, that increases in allergic and some infectious reactions (*eos* = dawn-colored [rosy]; *phil* = attraction for)
basophil *bā'sō-fil*	a granular leukocyte, named for the dark stain of its granules, that brings anticoagulant substances to inflamed tissues (*baso* = base; *phil* = attraction for)
agranulocytes *ā-grăn'ū-lō-sītz*	a group of leukocytes without granules in their nuclei
lymphocyte *lim'fō-sīt*	an agranulocytic leukocyte that is active in the process of immunity; the three categories of lymphocytes are T cells (thymus-dependent), B cells (bone marrow–derived), and natural killer (NK) cells
monocyte *mon'ō-sīt*	an agranulocytic leukocyte that performs phagocytosis to fight infection (*mono* = one)
platelets *plāt'lets*	thrombocytes; cell fragments in the blood that are essential for blood clotting (coagulation)

Programmed Review: Anatomic Terms in the Blood System

ANSWERS	REVIEW
plasma serum	**6.15** The liquid portion of the blood and lymph is called _____. The plasma contains proteins, cells, and other substances. After blood clots, the liquid portion that remains is called _____.
cell red red, cell hemoglobin blood	**6.16** Recall that *-cyt/o* is a combining form meaning _____, and that *erythr/o* is a combining form meaning _____. Therefore, an erythrocyte is a _____ blood _____. Erythrocytes transport oxygen and carbon dioxide. Oxygen and carbon dioxide bond to the protein-iron compound contained in the erythrocytes, which is called _____ (from the combining form *hem/o*, meaning _____).
white leukocyte granulocytes without agranulocytes	**6.17** The combining form *leuk/o* means _____; thus, a white blood cell is a _____. There are many types of leukocytes in the blood, but they can be divided into two general categories: those with granules in their cytoplasm and those without granules in their cytoplasm. Leukocytes with granules are called _____. Because the prefix *a-* means _____, the term for leukocytes without granules is _____.
eosinophil basophil	**6.18** Several types of leukocytes are named according to how they appear when stained, or by which stain they attract (*phil* = attraction for). A neutrophil is a leukocyte in which the granules stain neutrally or without color; a neutrophil has an attraction for neither (*neutr*) color stain. An _____ is a leukocyte in which the granules stain (attract) a rose color (*eos* = rosy color). Finally, another type of leukocyte has granules that stain (attract) a dark base color (*baso* = base); this type is called a _____.
polymorphonuclear	**6.19** Another term for a neutrophil is _____ (PMN) leukocyte. This term comes from the many segments in the nucleus.
lymphocyte infection	**6.20** An agranulocytic leukocyte in the lymphatic system that is active in the process of immunity is called a _____. A monocyte, which is another agranulocytic leukocyte, performs phagocytosis to fight _____.

ANSWERS	REVIEW
platelet	**6.21** Another term for a thrombocyte is _____. The
clot	combining form *thromb/o* means _____; therefore, platelets
clotting	function in blood _____.

Self-Instruction: Anatomic Terms in the Lymphatic System (Fig. 6-3)

Study the following:

TERM	MEANING
ORGANS OF THE LYMPHATIC SYSTEM	
thymus *thī′ mŭs*	primary gland of the lymphatic system, located within the mediastinum, that helps to maintain the body's immune response by producing T lymphocytes
spleen *splēn*	organ between the stomach and the diaphragm that filters out aging blood cells, removes cellular debris by performing phagocytosis, and provides an environment for lymphocytes to initiate immune responses
STRUCTURES OF THE LYMPHATIC SYSTEM	
lymph *limf*	fluid that is circulated through the lymph vessels
lymph capillaries *limf kap′ i-lār-ēz*	microscopic vessels that draw lymph from tissues to the lymph vessels
lymph vessels *limf ves′ĕlz*	vessels that receive lymph from the lymph capillaries and circulate it to the lymph nodes
lacteals *lak′ tē-ălz*	specialized lymph vessels in the small intestine that absorb fat into the bloodstream (*lacteus* = milky)
chyle *kīl*	white or pale yellow substance in lymph that contains fatty substances absorbed by the lacteals
lymph nodes *limf nōdz*	many small, oval structures that filter lymph from the lymph vessels; major locations include the cervical, axillary, and inguinal regions
lymph ducts *limf dŭktz*	collecting channels that carry lymph from the lymph nodes to the veins
right lymphatic duct *rīt lim-fat′ ik dŭkt*	receives lymph from the right upper part of the body
thoracic duct *thō-ras′ ik dŭkt*	receives lymph from the left side of the head, neck, chest, abdomen, left arm, and lower extremities
IMMUNITY	
immunity *i-myū′ ni-tē*	process of disease protection induced by exposure to an antigen

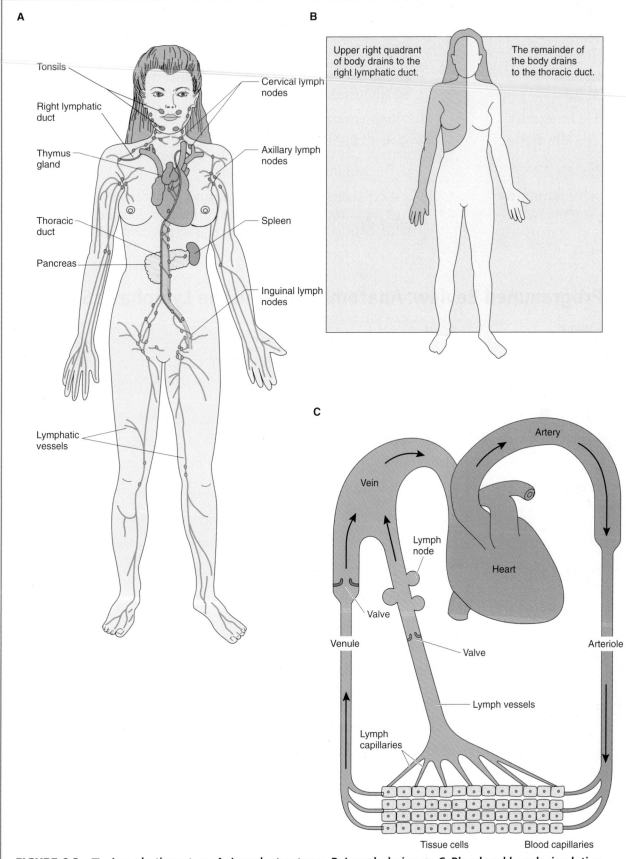

FIGURE 6-3 ■ **Lymphatic system. A. Lymph structures. B. Lymph drainage. C. Blood and lymph circulation.**

TERM	MEANING
antigen *an'ti-jen*	a substance that, when introduced into the body, causes the formation of antibodies against it
antibody *an'tē-bod-ē*	a substance produced by the body that destroys or inactivates an antigen that has entered the body
active immunity *ak'tiv i-myū'ni-tē*	a long-lasting immunity that results from stimulating the body to produce its own antibodies; developed either *naturally*, in response to an infection, or *artificially*, in response to the administration of a vaccine
passive immunity *pas'iv i-myū'ni-tē*	a short-lasting immunity that results from foreign antibodies that are conveyed either *naturally*, through the placenta to a fetus, or *artificially*, by injection of a serum containing antibodies

🔷 Programmed Review: Anatomic Terms in the Lymphatic System

ANSWERS	REVIEW
thymus thym/o	**6.22** Located in the mediastinum, the _____ gland produces T lymphocytes for the body's immune response. This term comes from the combining form _____.
spleen splenectomy	**6.23** Aging blood cells are filtered out in the _____, which also removes cellular debris by performing phagocytosis. The removal of this organ is called a _____.
lymph clear	**6.24** The fluid circulating through the lymph vessels is called _____. The meaning of the combining form *lymph/o* reminds us that this fluid is _____.
capillaries	**6.25** The microscopic vessels that draw lymph from body tissues to the lymph vessels are called lymph _____. The same term is used in the circulatory system for the tiny vessels connecting arteries and veins.
lacteals chyle	**6.26** In addition to lymph capillaries, which collect lymph from body tissues, special lymph vessels in the intestine, called _____, absorb fat. This liquid in lymph absorbed by the lacteals is called _____.
nodes ducts, lymphatic	**6.27** Lymph vessels carry lymph to the lymph _____, which filter the lymph. Lymph is then carried from the lymph nodes to the veins via lymph _____. The right _____ duct receives lymph from the right upper part of the body, and the

ANSWERS	REVIEW
thoracic extremities	_____ duct receives lymph from the left side of the head, neck, chest, left arm, and lower _____.
antibody immunity antigen, antibody	**6.28** The body protects itself from infectious disease in several ways. An antigen is a substance that, when introduced into the body, causes formation of an _____ against it. This process of disease protection is called _____. Exposure to an _____ starts the process, and the _____ destroys or inactivates the antigen.
active immunity	**6.29** Antibodies that develop naturally, after contracting an infection, or artificially, after administering a vaccine, result in _____ immunity. Antibodies that are conveyed naturally through the placenta to a fetus result in passive _____. The difference between active and passive in this case is whether the body itself actively makes the antibodies or passively receives them from outside.

Self-Instruction: Symptomatic Terms

Study the following:

TERM	MEANING
RELATED TO BLOOD	
microcytosis (Fig. 6-4, B) mī′krō-sī-tō′sis	presence of small red blood cells
macrocytosis (Fig. 6-5) mak′rō-sī-tō′sis	presence of large red blood cells

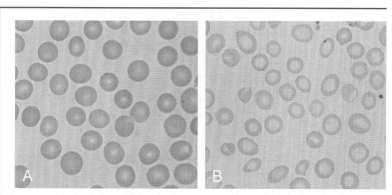

FIGURE 6-4 ■ A blood smear showing normal erythrocytes (A) compared with a blood smear revealing microcytic-hypochromic erythrocytes in a patient with iron deficiency anemia (B).

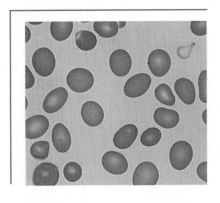

FIGURE 6-5 ■ Photomicrograph of a blood smear from a patient with pernicious anemia reveals macrocytosis, anisocytosis, and poikilocytosis.

TERM	MEANING
anisocytosis (*see* Fig. 6-5) *an-ī′sō-sī-tō′sis*	presence of red blood cells of unequal size (*an* = not, without; *iso* = equal)
poikilocytosis (*see* Fig. 6-5) *poy′ki-lō-sī-tō′sis*	presence of large, irregularly shaped red blood cells (*poikilo* = irregular)
reticulocytosis *re-tik′ū-lō-sī-tō′sis*	an increased number of immature erythrocytes in the blood
erythropenia *ĕ-rith-rō-pē′nē-ă*	an abnormally reduced number of red blood cells
lymphocytopenia *lim′fō-sī-tō-pē′nē-ă*	an abnormally reduced number of lymphocytes
neutropenia *nū′trō-pē′nē-ă*	a decreased number of neutrophils
pancytopenia *pan′sī-tō-pē′nē-ă*	an abnormally reduced number of all cellular components in the blood
thrombocytopenia *throm′bō-sī-tō-pē′nē-ă*	an abnormally decreased number of platelets in the blood, impairing the clotting process
hemolysis *hē-mol′i-sis*	breakdown of the red blood cell membrane

RELATED TO THE LYMPHATIC SYSTEM

immunocompromised *im′yū-nō-kom′prō-mīzd*	impaired immunologic defenses caused by an immunodeficiency disorder or by therapy with immunosuppressive agents
immunosuppression *im′yū-nō-sŭ-presh′ŭn*	impaired ability to provide an immune response
lymphadenopathy *lim-fad′ĕ-nop′ă-thē*	enlarged (diseased) lymph nodes
splenomegaly *splē-nō-meg′ă-lē*	enlargement of the spleen

Programmed Review: Symptomatic Terms

ANSWERS	REVIEW
increase cytosis macrocytosis	**6.30** The suffix *-osis* can mean either a condition of or an _____. In either case, the suffix is used with symptomatic terms to indicate an abnormal or unusual condition. The presence of small red blood cells is called micro_____, and the presence of large red blood cells is called _____.
anisocytosis poikilocytosis	**6.31** Red blood cells also may be present in unequal sizes. The presence of red blood cells of unequal size (*aniso* = unequal) is termed _____. The presence of large, irregularly shaped (*poikilo* = irregular) red blood cells is called _____.
net reticulocytosis	**6.32** The combining form *reticul/o* means _____. As mentioned previously, a reticulocyte is a young red blood cell (so named because of the network of substances in the cell). The condition of an increased number of immature erythrocytes in the blood is called _____.
reduction lymphocytopenia thrombocytopenia erythropenia	**6.33** Recall that the suffix *-penia* means an abnormal _____. Several symptomatic terms involving blood cells are formed with this suffix. An abnormally reduced number of lymphoctyes is called _____. An abnormal reduction in the number of platelets (thrombocytes) is termed _____. An abnormally reduced number of erythrocytes can be termed erythrocytopenia, but the shorter term, _____, generally is used.
all pancytopenia neutropenia	**6.34** The prefix *pan-* means _____. An abnormally reduced number of all types of blood cells is therefore called _____. Like the shorter term erythropenia, the term for a reduced number of neutrophils uses just one combining form with the suffix *-penia*: _____.
-lysis hemolysis	**6.35** The suffix meaning breakdown or dissolution is _____. The term for the breakdown of the red blood cell membrane uses the combining form for blood (in effect, the blood itself breaks down): _____.
immunosuppression	**6.36** Some drugs or disease states suppress the body's ability to provide an immune response; this is called _____.

ANSWERS	REVIEW
immunocompromised	A patient with impaired immunologic defenses caused by a disorder or by immunosuppressive agents is said to be _____.
lymphadenopathy	**6.37** The combining form *path/o* simply means disease, as in the term pathology. The combining form *aden/o* means gland or node. A disease state in which lymph nodes are enlarged is called _____.
enlargement	**6.38** The symptomatic suffix *-megaly* refers to an _____. An enlarged spleen, which may result from several different diseases,
splenomegaly	is called _____.

Self-Instruction: Diagnostic Terms

Study the following:

TERM	MEANING
acquired immunodeficiency syndrome (AIDS) *ă-kwĭrd' im'yŭ-nō-dē-fish'en-sē sin'drōm*	a syndrome caused by the human immunodeficiency virus (HIV) that renders immune cells ineffective, permitting opportunistic infections, malignancies, and neurologic diseases to develop; transmitted sexually or through contaminated blood
anemia *ă-nē'mē-ă*	a condition of reduced numbers of red blood cells, hemoglobin, or packed red cells in the blood, resulting in a diminished ability of red blood cells to transport oxygen to the tissues
aplastic anemia *ā-plas'tik ă-nē'mē-ă*	a normocytic-normochromic type of anemia characterized by the failure of bone marrow to produce red blood cells
iron deficiency anemia (*see* Fig. 6-4, B) *ī'ĕrn de-fish'en-sē ă-nē'mē-ă*	a microcytic-hypochromic type of anemia characterized by a lack of iron that affects the production of hemoglobin and is characterized by small red blood cells containing low amounts of hemoglobin
pernicious anemia (*see* Fig. 6-5) *pĕr-nish'ŭs ă-nē'mē-ă*	a macrocytic-normochromic type of anemia characterized by an inadequate supply of vitamin B_{12}, causing red blood cells to become large, varied in shape, and reduced in number
autoimmune disease *aw-tō-i-myūn' di-zēz'*	any disorder characterized by abnormal function of the immune system that causes the body to produce antibodies against itself, resulting in tissue destruction or loss of function; rheumatoid arthritis and lupus are examples of autoimmune diseases (*auto* = self)
erythroblastosis fetalis *ĕ-rith'rō-blas-tō'sis fē-tă'lis*	a disorder that results from the incompatibility of a fetus with Rh-positive blood and a mother with Rh-negative blood, causing red blood cell destruction in the fetus; a blood transfusion is necessary to save the fetus

TERM	MEANING
Rh factor *r-h fak′tōr*	presence or lack of antigens on the surface of red blood cells, which causes a reaction between Rh-positive blood and Rh-negative blood
Rh positive *r-h poz′i-tiv*	presence of antigens
Rh negative *r-h neg′ă-tiv*	absence of antigens
hemochromatosis *hē′mō-krō-mă-tō′sis*	hereditary disorder with an excessive buildup of iron deposits in the body
hemophilia *hē-mō-fil′ē-ă*	a group of hereditary bleeding disorders caused by a defect in clotting factors necessary for the coagulation of blood
leukemia *lū-kē′mē-ă*	chronic or acute malignant (cancerous) disease of the blood-forming organs, characterized by abnormal leukocytes in the blood and bone marrow
myelodysplasia *mī′ĕ-lō-dis-plā′zē-ă*	disorder within the bone marrow characterized by a proliferation of abnormal stem cells (cells that give rise to different types of blood cells); usually develops into a specific type of leukemia
lymphoma *lim-fō′mă*	any neoplastic disorder of lymph tissue, usually malignant, as in Hodgkin disease
metastasis *mĕ-tas′tă-sis*	process by which cancer cells are spread by blood or lymph circulation to a distant organ; the plural form, metastases, indicates spreading to two or more distant sites
mononucleosis *mon′ō-nū-klē-ō′sis*	condition caused by the Epstein-Barr virus and characterized by an increase in mononuclear cells (monocytes and lymphocytes) in the blood along with enlarged lymph nodes (lymphadenopathy), fatigue, and sore throat (pharyngitis)
polycythemia *pol′ē-sī-thē′mē-ă*	increased number of erythrocytes and hemoglobin in the blood
septicemia *sep-ti-sē′mē-ă*	systemic disease caused by infection with microorganisms and their toxins in circulating blood

◆ Programmed Review: Diagnostic Terms

ANSWERS	REVIEW
acquired immunodeficiency syndrome	**6.39** AIDS is the acronym for _____ _____ _____, which is caused by the human immunodeficiency virus (HIV).

ANSWERS	REVIEW
without anemia iron deficiency pernicious aplastic	**6.40** The prefix *an-* means _____ or reduction. The general term for a blood condition in which there is a reduction in the number of red blood cells, hemoglobin, or the volume of packed red blood cells is _____. Several types of anemia are common. Anemia characterized by a lack of iron, affecting the production of hemoglobin, is called _____ _____ anemia. Anemia characterized by an inadequate supply of vitamin B_{12} is called _____ anemia. Another type is described by the term formed in part by *a-* (without) and *plas/o* (formation): _____ anemia.
safe autoimmune	**6.41** *Auto-*, a prefix meaning self, is used in combination with *immun/o*, the combining form meaning _____, to name the disorder characterized by abnormal function of the immune system that causes the body to produce antibodies against itself: _____ disease.
erythroblastosis fetalis factor Rh negative	**6.42** A disorder resulting from incompatibility of a fetus with Rh-positive blood and a mother with Rh-negative blood, named in part because of the large number of erythroblasts that are found in the fetal blood, is called _____ _____. The Rh _____ is said to be positive when Rh antigens are present on the surface of red blood cells. The absence of such antigens is called _____ _____.
hemochromatosis	**6.43** One hereditary blood disorder results in an excessive buildup of iron deposits in the body. Because skin pigmentation may change because of this condition, the term used to describe it uses the combining form meaning color and the combining form meaning blood. This condition is called _____.
clotting	**6.44** Hemophilia is a group of hereditary bleeding disorders with a defect in _____ factors necessary for coagulation.

ANSWERS	REVIEW
blood	**6.45** The diagnostic suffix *-emia* refers to a _____ condition. A malignant blood disease marked by abnormal
leukemia	white blood cells (leukocytes) is called _____. A disorder in the bone marrow that usually develops into leukemia is built from the combining form *myel/o*, meaning bone marrow; the prefix *dys-*, meaning faulty; and the
formation	suffix *-plasia*, meaning a condition of _____.
myelodysplasia	This disorder is called _____.
	6.46 Also built with the suffix *-emia*, the term for an increase in hemoglobin and the number of erythrocytes in the blood begins with the prefix *poly-*, which means
many, polycythemia	_____. This disorder is called _____.
-oma	**6.47** Recall that the suffix meaning tumor is _____.
lymphoma	A tumor of lymph tissue is called a _____.
beyond	**6.48** The prefix *meta-* means _____, after, or change. The term for the spread of cancer cells beyond the original site of the tumor through blood or lymph is
metastasis	_____.
	6.49 Monocytes and lymphocytes are mononuclear cells. The viral condition characterized by an increase in both
mononucleosis	types is called _____. The suffix *-osis*
increase	means condition of or _____.
	6.50 Sepsis is from the Greek word for putrefaction, indicating infection. A systemic condition caused by
septicemia	infection in the blood is therefore termed _____.

 ## Self-Instruction: Diagnostic Tests and Procedures

Study the following:

TEST OR PROCEDURE	EXPLANATION
BLOOD STUDIES	
phlebotomy *fle-bot'ŏ-mē* **venipuncture** *ven'i-pŭnk-chūr*	incision into or puncture of a vein to withdraw blood for testing

TEST OR PROCEDURE	EXPLANATION
blood chemistry *blŭd kem'is-trē*	test of the fluid portion of blood to measure the amounts of its chemical constituents (e.g., glucose and cholesterol)
blood chemistry panels *blŭd kem'is-trē păn'lz*	specialized batteries of automated blood chemistry tests performed on a single sample of blood; used as a general screen for disease or to target specific organs or conditions (e.g., metabolic panel, lipid panel, and arthritis panel)
basic metabolic panel (BMP) *bā'sik met-ă-bol'ik păn'l*	battery of tests used as a general screen for disease; includes tests for calcium, carbon dioxide (CO_2), chloride, creatinine, glucose, potassium, sodium, and blood urea nitrogen (BUN)
comprehensive metabolic panel (CMP) (Fig. 6-6) *kom-prē-hen'siv met-ă-bol'ik păn'l*	tests performed in addition to the basic panel for expanded screening: albumin, bilirubin, alkaline phosphatase, protein, alanine aminotransferase (ALT), and aspartate aminotransferase (AST)
blood culture *blŭd kŭl'chĕr*	test to determine if infection is present in the bloodstream by isolating a specimen of blood in an environment that encourages the growth of microorganisms; the specimen is observed, and the organisms that grow in the culture are identified
CD4 cell count *c-d-fōr sel kownt*	a measure of the number of CD4 cells (a subset of T lymphocytes) in the blood; used in monitoring the course of HIV and in timing the treatment of AIDS; the normal adult range is 600–1500 cells in a given volume of blood
erythrocyte sedimentation rate (ESR) *ĕ-rith'rō-sīt sed'i-men-tā'shŭn rāt*	timed test that measures the rate at which red blood cells settle through a volume of plasma
partial thromboplastin time (PTT) *par'shăl throm-bō-plas'tin tīm*	test to determine coagulation defects, such as platelet disorders
thromboplastin *throm-bō-plas'tin*	substance present in tissues, platelets, and leukocytes that is necessary for coagulation
prothrombin time (PT) *prō-throm'bin tīm*	test to measure activity of prothrombin in the blood
prothrombin *prō-throm'bin*	protein substance in the blood that is essential to the clotting process
complete blood count (CBC) (Fig. 6-7) *kom-plēt' blŭd kownt*	a common laboratory blood test performed as a screen of general health or for diagnostic purposes and typically includes the component tests that follow; test results are usually reported along with normal values so that the clinician can interpret the results based on the instrumentation used by the laboratory; normal ranges also may vary depending on the region and climate
white blood count (WBC) *wīt blŭd kownt*	a count of the number of white blood cells in a given volume of blood obtained via manual or automated laboratory methods

CENTRAL MEDICAL CENTER
211 Medical Center Drive • Central City, US 90000-1234 • PHONE: (012) 125-6784 • FAX: (012) 125-9999

11/02/20xx
14:27

NAME   : TEST, PATIENT   LOC: TEST   DOB: 02/03/xx   AGE: 38Y
MR#   : TEST-221   SEX: M
ACCT#   : H111111111

M63561 COLL: 11/02/20xx 13:24   REC: 11/02/20xx 13:25

COMPREHENSIVE METABOLIC PANEL

Blood Urea Nitrogen (BUN)	*30	[5 - 25]	mg/dl
Sodium	139	[135 - 153]	mEq/L
Potassium	4.2	[3.5 - 5.3]	mEq/L
Chloride	105	[101 - 111]	mEq/L
Carbon Dioxide (CO_2)	27	[24 - 31]	mmol/L
Glucose, Random	*148	[70 - 110]	mg/dl
Creatinine	*1.5	[< 1.5]	mg/dl
SGOT (AST)	18	[10 - 42]	U/L
SGPT (ALT)	*8	[10 - 60]	U/L
Alkaline Phosphatase	58	[42 - 121]	U/L
Total Protein	6.5	[6.0 - 8.0]	G/dl
Albumin	3.7	[3.5 - 5.0]	G/dl
Amylase	33	[< 129]	U/L
Bilirubin, Total	0.7	[< 1.5]	mg/dl
Calcium, Total	9.7	[8.6 - 10.6]	mg/dl

TEST, PATIENT   TEST-221   END OF REPORT   PAGE 1
11/02/20xx 14:27

INTERIM REPORT COMPLETED

FIGURE 6-6 ■ Comprehensive metabolic panel report. Normal ranges are in brackets [ ].

TEST OR PROCEDURE	EXPLANATION
red blood count (RBC) *rĕd blŭd kownt*	a count of the number of red blood cells in a given volume of blood obtained via manual or automated laboratory methods
hemoglobin (HGB or Hgb) *hē-mō-glō′bin*	a test to determine the blood level of hemoglobin (expressed in grams)
hematocrit (HCT or Hct) *hē′mă-tō-krit*	a measurement of the percentage of packed red blood cells in a given volume of blood
blood indices *blŭd in′di-sēz*	calculations of RBC, HGB, and HCT results to determine the average size, hemoglobin concentration, and content of red blood cells to classify an anemia (Note: in the entries below, the term corpuscular pertains to a blood cell)
mean corpuscular (cell) volume (MCV) *mēn kōr-pŭs′kū-lăr (sel) vol′yŭm*	calculation of the volume (size) of individual red blood cells using HCT and RBC results: MCV = HCT/RBC

CENTRAL MEDICAL CENTER
211 Medical Center Drive • Central City, US 90000-1234 • PHONE: (012) 125-6784 • FAX: (012) 125-9999

11/02/20xx
14:27

NAME   : TEST, PATIENT   LOC: TEST   DOB: 2/2/xx   AGE: 27Y
MR#   : TEST-221   SEX: M
ACCT#   : H111111111

M63558 COLL: 11/2/20xx 13:23   REC: 11/2/20xx 13:24

HEMOGRAM
CBC
  WBC   *11.5   [4.5 - 10.5]   K/UL
  RBC   5.84   [4.6 - 6.2]   M/UL
  HGB   17.2   [14.0 - 18.0]   G/DL
  HCT   50.8   [42.0 - 52.0]   %
  MCV   87   [82 - 92]   FL
  MCH   29.5   [27 - 31]   PG
  MCHC   33.9   [32 - 36]   G/DL
  PLT   202   [150 - 450]   K/UL

  Auto Lymph %   15   [20 - 40]   %
  Auto Mono %   2   [1 - 11]   %
  Auto Neutro %   82   [50 - 75]   %
  Auto Eos %   1   [0 - 6]   %
  Auto Baso %   0   [0 - 2]   %
  Auto Lymph #   1.7   [1.5 - 4.0]   K/UL
  Auto Mono #   0.2   [0.2 - 0.9]   K/UL
  Auto Neutro #   9.4   [1.0 - 7.0]   K/UL
  Auto Eos #   0.1   [0 - 0.7]   K/UL
  Auto Baso #   0.0   [0 - 0.2]   K/UL

TEST, PATIENT   TEST-221   END OF REPORT   PAGE 1
11/02/20xx   14:27   INTERIM REPORT

INTERIM REPORT COMPLETE

FIGURE 6-7 ■ Complete blood count (CBC) report. Normal ranges are in brackets [ ].

TEST OR PROCEDURE	EXPLANATION
mean corpuscular (cell) hemoglobin (MCH) *mēn kōr-pŭs′kū-lăr (sel) hē-mō-glō′bin*	calculation of the content (weight) of hemoglobin in the average red blood cell using HGB and RBC results: MCH = HGB/RBC
mean corpuscular (cell) hemoglobin concentration (MCHC) *mēn kōr-pŭs′kū-lăr (sel) hē-mō-glō′bin kon-sen-trā′shŭn*	calculation of the average hemoglobin concentration in each red blood cell using HGB and HCT results: MCHC = HGB/HCT
differential count *dif-ĕr-en′shăl kownt*	determination of the number of each type of white blood cell (leukocyte) in a stained blood smear; each type is counted and reported as a percentage of the total examined

TEST OR PROCEDURE	EXPLANATION
	Type of Leukocyte *Normal Range* lymphocytes 25–33% monocytes 3–7% neutrophils 54–75% eosinophils 1–3% basophils 0–1%
red cell morphology *rĕd sel mōr-fol'ŏ-jē*	as part of identifying and counting the white blood cells, the condition, size, and shape of red blood cells in the background of the smeared slide are noted (e.g., anisocytosis, poikilocytosis)
platelet count (PLT) *plāt'let kownt*	calculation of the number of thrombocytes in the blood; the normal adult range is 150,000–450,000 platelets in a given volume of blood

BONE AND LYMPH STUDIES

bone marrow aspiration (Fig. 6-8) *bōn mar'ō as-pi-rā'shŭn*	needle aspiration of bone marrow tissue for pathologic examination
bone marrow biopsy *bōn mar'ō bī'op-sē*	pathologic examination of bone marrow tissue
lymphangiogram *lim-fan'jē-ō-gram*	an x-ray image of a lymph node or vessel obtained after injection of a contrast medium

DIAGNOSTIC IMAGING

computed tomography (CT) *kom-pyū'tĕd tō-mog'ra-fē*	full body x-ray CT images are used to detect tumors and cancers such as lymphoma
positron-emission tomography (PET) *pŏz'i-tron ē-mish'ŭn tō-mog'ră-fē*	scanning technique combining nuclear medicine and computed tomography technology to produce images of anatomy and metabolic function within the body; useful in determining the recurrence of cancers or to measure response to therapy; commonly used in evaluating lymphoma

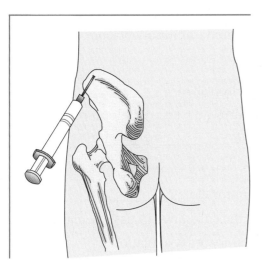

FIGURE 6-8 ▬ **Bone marrow aspiration. Posterior view of the pelvic region showing a common site for bone marrow aspiration.**

Programmed Review: Diagnostic Tests and Procedures

ANSWERS	REVIEW
venipuncture, phlebotomy incision	**6.51** Blood studies are tests performed with samples of blood. The blood sample, often drawn by a phlebotomist, is obtained through a needle puncture (or incision) of a vein, which is called a _____ or a _____. Recall that the suffix *-tomy* refers to an _____.
chemistry, panel metabolic comprehensive metabolic panel	**6.52** Blood studies generally examine the chemical constituents of the blood or the physical properties of different kinds of blood cells. A test of the fluid portion of blood for the presence of chemical constituents is called a blood _____. A blood chemistry _____ includes a battery of chemistry tests using a single sample of blood. Some panels target specific organs or conditions, such as a lipid or arthritis panel. Two panels of chemistry tests are used as a general or expanded screen for disease: a basic _____ panel (BMP), and a _____ _____ _____ (CMP).
culture	**6.53** To determine the presence and type of an infection in the blood, a blood sample may be put in an environment that encourages the growth of microorganisms. This test is called a blood _____.
CD4 AIDS	**6.54** CD4 cells are a subset of T lymphocytes in the blood that are increased in patients who are positive for HIV. The measure of these cells, which is known as a _____ cell count, is used in monitoring the course of HIV infection and in timing the treatment of acquired immunodeficiency syndrome (_____).
erythrocytes erythrocyte sedimentation	**6.55** Red blood cells are also called _____. A diagnostic test that measures how fast red blood cells settle through plasma is called the _____ _____ rate.
thromb/o	**6.56** The combining form for clot is _____. That root is part of the term for the substance in tissues, platelets, and leukocytes that is necessary for coagulation:

ANSWERS	REVIEW
thromboplastin partial thromboplastin	_____. The test for coagulation defects is called a _____ _____ time (PTT). The term for a protein substance in blood that is essential for
prothrombin prothrombin time	clotting comes from a prefix meaning before and the combining form for clot: _____. The diagnostic test that measures the activity of this protein is called a _____ _____ (PT).
blood count red blood white cells HGB, Hgb hematocrit	**6.57** A complete _____ _____ (CBC) is a diagnostic test that is often performed as a general screen. It includes several component tests. The RBC is a count of the number of _____ _____ cells in a given volume of blood. A WBC is a count of the number of _____ blood _____ in a given volume of blood. The test of the blood level of hemoglobin is often simply called a hemoglobin, and it is abbreviated as _____ or _____. The measurement of the percentage of packed red blood cells in a given volume of blood is called the _____ (HCT or Hct).
indices mean corpuscular (cell) mean hemoglobin hemoglobin concentration	**6.58** Different values in the CBC are used to calculate the size, makeup, and content of red blood cells to classify an anemia. These calculations are called blood _____. The calculation of the volume (size) of individual cells is called the _____ _____ volume (MCV). The term mean refers to average. The calculation of the weight of hemoglobin in an average red blood cell is called the _____ corpuscular (cell) _____ (MCH). The calculation of the mean hemoglobin concentration in each cell is called the mean corpuscular (cell) _____ _____ (MCHC).
platelet platelet count	**6.59** Thrombocytes are counted as part of a CBC. Another term for thrombocyte is _____. Thus, this measure is simply called a _____ _____ (PLT).
white, cytes phils differential count	**6.60** Recall that there are several kinds of leukocytes (_____ blood cells), such as lymphocytes, mono_____, neutrophils, eosino_____, and basophils. The study that determines the percentage of each type present in a smear of blood is called a _____ _____.

ANSWERS	REVIEW
morphology	**6.61** When the differential count is done, the size and shape of red blood cells in the sample are also noted. This is called the red cell _____.
aspiration bone marrow biopsy	**6.62** The removal of bone marrow tissue by a needle for pathologic examination is called a bone marrow _____. Pathologic examination of bone marrow tissue is called a _____ _____ _____.
-gram lymphangiogram	**6.63** The combining form *angi/o* refers to either blood or lymph vessels. The suffix meaning a record is _____. Using these two components along with the combining form for lymph, the term _____ is an x-ray of a lymph node or vessel.
computed tomography cancers positron-emission tomography	**6.64** Full body CT (_____ _____), a specialized ionizing x-ray image of the whole body, is commonly used to detect tumors and _____, such as lymphoma. Another ionizing imaging modality is the use of whole body PET (_____-_____ _____) to determine the recurrence of cancers or to measure the response to therapy.

 ## Self-Instruction: Operative Terms

Study the following:

TERM	MEANING
bone marrow transplant *bōn mar'ō tranz'plant*	transplantation of healthy bone marrow from a compatible donor to a diseased recipient to stimulate blood cell production
lymphadenectomy *lim-fad'ĕ-nĕk'tŏ-mē*	removal of a lymph node
lymphadenotomy *lim-fad'ĕ-not'ŏ-mē*	incision into a lymph node
lymph node dissection *limf nōd di-sek'shŭn*	removal of possible cancer-carrying lymph nodes for pathologic examination
splenectomy *splē-nek'tŏ-mē*	removal of the spleen
thymectomy *thī-mek'tŏ-mē*	removal of the thymus gland

Programmed Review: Operative Terms

ANSWERS	REVIEW
removal splenectomy thymectomy lymphadenectomy	**6.65** The suffix *-ectomy* means _____ or excision. The removal of the spleen is called a _____. The removal of the thymus gland is called a _____. The removal of a lymph node is called a _____.
incision lymphadenotomy	**6.66** The suffix *-tomy*, on the other hand, means _____. An incision into a lymph node is called a _____.
dissection	**6.67** Removal of possible cancer-carrying lymph nodes for pathologic examination is called a lymph node _____.
bone marrow	**6.68** To stimulate blood cell production inside bones, a _____ _____ transplant is made from a compatible donor to a diseased recipient.

 ## Self-Instruction: Therapeutic Terms

Study the following:

TERM	MEANING
blood transfusion *blŭd trans-fyū'zhŭn*	introduction of blood products into the circulation of a recipient whose blood volume is reduced or deficient in some manner
autologous blood *aw-tol'ŏ-gŭs blŭd*	blood donated by and stored for a patient for future personal use (e.g., upcoming surgery) (*auto* = self)
homologous blood *hŏ-mol'ō-gŭs blŭd*	blood voluntarily donated by any person for transfusion to a compatible recipient (*homo* = same)
blood component therapy *blŭd kom-pō'nent thār'ă-pē*	transfusion of a specific blood component, such as packed red blood cells, platelets, or plasma
cross-matching *kros-match'ing*	method of matching a donor's blood to the recipient by mixing a sample in a test tube to determine compatibility
chemotherapy *kem'ō-thār-ă-pē*	treatment of malignancies, infections, and other diseases with chemical agents to destroy selected cells or to impair their ability to reproduce
immunotherapy *im'ū-nō-thār'ă-pē*	use of biologic agents to prevent or treat disease by stimulating the body's own defense mechanisms, as seen in the treatment of AIDS, cancer, or allergy
plasmapheresis *plaz'mă-fĕ-rē'sis*	removal of plasma from the body with separation and extraction of specific elements (e.g., platelets) followed by reinfusion (*apheresis* = a withdrawal)

TERM	MEANING
COMMON THERAPEUTIC DRUG CLASSIFICATIONS	
anticoagulant *an′ tē-kō-ag′ yū-lant*	a drug that prevents clotting of the blood
hemostatic *hē-mō-stat′ ik*	a drug that stops the flow of blood within the vessels
vasoconstrictor *vā′ sō-kon-strik′ tŏr*	a drug that causes a narrowing of blood vessels, thereby decreasing blood flow
vasodilator *vā′ sō-dī-lā′ tŏr*	a drug that causes dilation of blood vessels, thereby increasing blood flow

◆ Programmed Review: Therapeutic Terms

ANSWERS	REVIEW
transfusion autologous homologous	**6.69** The general term for giving blood or blood products to a recipient whose blood is in some way deficient is blood _____. There are several types of blood transfusions. A patient's own blood removed for his or her own personal use in a later transfusion is called _____ blood (*auto* = self). Blood from a compatible donor (i.e., a donor with the same blood type) is called _____ blood (*homo* = same).
component	**6.70** The transfusion of specific blood components, such as platelets or plasma, is called blood _____ therapy.
cross-matching	**6.71** The process of determining compatibility between donated blood and the recipient's blood is called _____-_____. This must be done to ensure the recipient does not suffer a potentially fatal transfusion reaction.
chemotherapy	**6.72** The treatment of neoplasms and other diseases with chemical agents that destroy the targeted cells is called _____. Chemotherapy is used for many forms of cancer in virtually all body systems.
safe, immunotherapy	**6.73** The term describing the use of biologic agents to prevent or treat disease by stimulating the body's own defense mechanisms was coined by combining -*therapy* with *immun/o*, the combining form meaning _____. Therefore, the term is _____.

ANSWERS	REVIEW
plasmapheresis	**6.74** The root *apheresis* means withdrawal. The withdrawal of blood plasma from the body to separate out specific components before reinfusing the plasma is called _____.
against anticoagulant	**6.75** Recall that the prefix *anti-* means _____. Drug classes are frequently named by their actions against something. A drug that prevents blood clotting or coagulation is an _____.
vasoconstrictor vasodilator	**6.76** Drug classes are also named for their specific actions. The combining form for blood vessel is *vas/o*. A drug that narrows or constricts blood vessels is a _____. A drug that widens or dilates blood vessels is a _____.
-stasis hem/o hemostatic	**6.77** Recall that the suffix that means stop or stand is _____. The combining form for blood is *hemat/o* or _____. A type of drug that stops blood from flowing within a vessel is called a _____ drug.

CHAPTER 6 ACRONYMS AND ABBREVIATIONS

ABBREVIATION	EXPANSION
AIDS	acquired immunodeficiency syndrome
ALT	alanine aminotransferase (enzyme)
AST	aspartate aminotransferase (enzyme)
BMP	basic metabolic panel
BUN	blood urea nitrogen
CBC	complete blood count
CMP	comprehensive metabolic panel
CO_2	carbon dioxide
CT	computed tomography
ESR	erythrocyte sedimentation rate
HCT or Hct	hematocrit
HGB or Hgb	hemoglobin
HIV	human immunodeficiency virus
MCH	mean corpuscular (cell) hemoglobin
MCHC	mean corpuscular (cell) hemoglobin concentration
MCV	mean corpuscular (cell) volume
NK	natural killer (cell)
PET	positron-emission tomography

ABBREVIATION	EXPANSION
PLT	platelet count
PMN	polymorphonuclear (leukocyte)
PT	prothrombin time
PTT	partial thromboplastin time
RBC	red blood cell; red blood count
WBC	white blood cell; white blood count

CHAPTER 6 SUMMARY OF TERMS

The terms introduced in chapter 6 are listed below, followed by the page number on which each term can be found and its written pronunciation. For additional practice and reinforcement, write the definition of each term on a separate piece of paper.

acquired immunodeficiency syndrome (AIDS)/286
ă-kwīrd' im-yū-nō-dē-fish'en-sē sin'drŏm

active immunity/282
ak'tiv i-myū'ni-tē

agranulocytes/278
ā-grăn'ū-lō-sītz

anemia/286
ă-nē'mē-ă

anisocytosis/284
an-ī'sō-sī-tō'sis

antibody/282
an'tē-bod-ē

anticoagulant/298
an'tē-kō-ag'yū-lant

antigen/282
an'ti-jen

aplastic anemia/286
ā-plas'tik ă-nē'mē-ă

autoimmune disease/286
aw-tō-i-myūn' di-zēz'

autologous blood/297
aw-tol'ŏ-gŭs blŭd

basic metabolic panel (BMP)/290
bā'sik met-ă-bol'ik păn'l

basophil/278
bā'sō-fil

blood chemistry/290
blŭd kem'is-trē

blood chemistry panels/290
blŭd kem'is-trē păn'lz

blood component therapy/297
blŭd kom-pō'nent thār'ă-pē

blood culture/290
blŭd kŭl'chŭr

blood indices/291
blŭd in'di-sēz

blood transfusion/297
blŭd trans-fyū'zhŭn

bone marrow aspiration/293
bōn mar'ō as-pi-rā'shŭn

bone marrow biopsy/293
bōn mar'ō bī'op-sē

bone marrow transplant/296
bōn mar'ō tranz'plant

CD4 cell count/290
c-d-fōr sel kownt

chemotherapy/297
kem'ō-thār-ă-pē

chyle/280
kīl

complete blood count (CBC)/290
kom-plēt blŭd kownt

comprehensive metabolic panel (CMP)/290
kom-prē-hen'siv met-ă-bol'ik păn'l

computed tomography (CT)/293
kom-pyū'těd tō-mog'ră-fē

cross-matching/297
kros-match'ing

differential count/292
dif-ĕr-en'shăl kownt

eosinophil/278
ē-ō-sin'ō-fil

erythroblastosis fetalis/286
ĕ-rith'rō-blas-tō'sis fē-tă'lis

erythrocyte/277
ĕ-rith'rō-sīt

erythrocyte sedimentation rate (ESR)/290
ĕ-rith'rō-sīt sed'i-men-tā'shŭn răt

erythropenia/284
ĕ-rith-rō-pē'nē-ă

granulocytes/277
gran'yū-lō-sītz

hematocrit (HCT or Hct)/291
hē'mă-tō-krit

hemochromatosis/287
hē'mō-krō-mă-tō'sis

hemoglobin (HGB or Hgb)/277, 291
hē-mō-glō'bin

hemolysis/284
hē-mol'i-sis

hemophilia/287
hē-mō-fil'ē-ă

hemostatic/298
hē-mō-stat'ik

homologous blood/297
hŏ-mol'ō-gŭs blŭd

immunity/280
i-myū'ni-tē

immunocompromised/284
im'yū-nō-kom'prō-mīzd

immunosuppression/284
im'yū-nō-sŭ-presh'ŭn

immunotherapy/297
im'ū-nō-thār'ă-pē

iron deficiency anemia/286
i'ĕrn de-fish'en-sē ă-nē'mē-ă

lacteals/280
lak'tē-ălz

leukemia/287
lū-kē'mē-ă

leukocyte/277
lū'kō-sīt

lymph/280
limf

lymph capillaries/280
limf kap'i-lăr-ēz

lymph ducts/280
limf dŭktz

lymph node dissection/296
limf nōd di-sek'shŭn

lymph nodes/280
limf nōdz

lymph vessels/280
limf ves'ĕlz

lymphadenectomy/296
lim-fad'ĕ-nek'tō-mē

lymphadenopathy/284
lim-fad'ĕ-nop'ă-thē

lymphadenotomy/296
lim-fad'ĕ-not'ŏ-mē

lymphangiogram/293
lim-fan'jē-ō-gram

lymphocyte/278
lim'fō-sīt

lymphocytopenia/284
lim'fō-sī-tō-pē'nē-ă

lymphoma/287
lim-fō'mă

macrocytosis/283
mak'rō-sī-tō'sis

mean corpuscular (cell) hemoglobin (MCH)/292
mēn kōr-pŭs'kyū-lăr (sel) hē-mō-glō'bin

mean corpuscular (cell) hemoglobin concentration (MCHC)/292
mēn kōr-pŭs'kyū-lăr (sel) hē-mō-glō'bin kon-sen-trā'shŭn

mean corpuscular (cell) volume (MCV)/291
mēn kōr-pŭs'kyū-lăr (sel) vol'yūm

metastasis/287
mĕ-tas'tă-sis

microcytosis/283
mī'krō-sī-tō'sis

monocyte/278
mon'ō-sīt

mononucleosis/287
mon'ō-nū-klē-ō'sis

myelodysplasia/287
mī'ě-lō-dis-plā'zē-ă

neutropenia/284
nū-trō-pē'nē-ă

neutrophil/277
nū'trō-fil

pancytopenia/284
pan'sī-tō-pē'nē-ă

partial thromboplastin time (PTT)/290
par'shăl throm-bō-plas'tin tīm

passive immunity/282
pas'iv i-myū'ni-tē

pernicious anemia/286
pěr-nish'ŭs ă-nē'mē-ă

phlebotomy/289
fle-bot'ŏ-mē

plasma/277
plaz'mă

plasmapheresis/297
plaz'mă-fě-rē'sis

platelet count (PLT)/293
plāt'let kownt

platelets/278
plāt'letz

poikilocytosis/284
poy'ki-lō-sī-tō'sis

polycythemia/287
pol'ē-sī-thē'mē-ă

**polymorphonuclear (PMN)
 leukocyte**/278
pol'ē-mōr-fō-nū'klē-ăr lū'kō-sīt

**positron-emission tomography
 (PET)**/293
pŏz'i-tron ē-mish'ŭn tō-mog'ră-fē

prothrombin/290
prō-throm'bin

prothrombin time (PT)/290
prō-throm'bin tīm

red blood count (RBC)/291
rěd blŭd kownt

red cell morphology/293
rěd sel mōr-fol'ŏ-jē

reticulocytosis/284
re-tik'ū-lō-sī-tō'sis

Rh factor/287
r-h fak'tōr

Rh negative/287
r-h neg'ă-tiv

Rh positive/287
r-h poz'i-tiv

right lymphatic duct/280
rīt lim-fat'ik dŭkt

septicemia/287
sep-ti-sē'mē-ă

serum/277
sēr'ŭm

spleen/280
splēn

splenectomy/296
splē-nek'tŏ-mē

splenomegaly/284
splē-nō-meg'ă-lē

thoracic duct/280
thō-ras'ik dŭkt

thrombocytopenia/284
throm'bō-sī-tō-pē'nē-ă

thromboplastin/290
throm-bō-plas'tin

thymectomy/296
thī-mek'tŏ-mē

thymus/280
thī'mŭs

vasoconstrictor/298
vā'sō-kon-strik'tŏr

vasodilator/298
vā'sō-dī-lā'tŏr

venipuncture/289
ven'i-pŭnk-chūr

white blood count (WBC)/290
wīt blŭd kownt

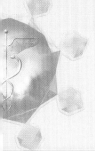

PRACTICE EXERCISES

For each of the following words, write out the term components (prefixes [P], combining forms [CF], roots [R], and suffixes [S]) on the lines below the word. Then define the term according to the meaning of its components.

EXAMPLE

dyshematopoiesis

<u>dys</u> / <u>hemato</u> / <u>poiesis</u>

P   CF   S

DEFINITION: painful, difficult, or faulty/blood/formation

1. erythroblastosis

_____ / _____ / _____

  CF   R   S

DEFINITION: _____

2. chylopoiesis

_____ / _____

  CF   S

DEFINITION: _____

3. hemocytometer

_____ / _____ / _____

  CF   CF   S

DEFINITION: _____

4. splenorrhagia

_____ / _____

  CF   S

DEFINITION: _____

5. lymphadenitis

_____ / _____ / _____

   R   R   S

DEFINITION: _____

6. immunotoxic

_____ / _____ / _____

  CF   R   S

DEFINITION: _____

7. reticulocytosis

_____ / _____ / _____

  CF   R   S

DEFINITION: _____

8. thymopathy

_____ / _____ / _____
    CF   R   S

DEFINITION: _____

9. leukocytic

_____ / _____ / _____
    CF   R   S

DEFINITION: _____

10. lymphangiogram

_____ / _____ / _____
    R   CF   S

DEFINITION: _____

11. splenomegaly

_____ / _____
    CF   S

DEFINITION: _____

12. promyelocyte

_____ / _____ / _____ / _____
    P   CF   R   S

DEFINITION: _____

13. leukocytopenia

_____ / _____ / _____
    CF   CF   S

DEFINITION: _____

14. splenectomy

_____ / _____
    R   S

DEFINITION: _____

15. dialysis

_____ / _____
    P   S

DEFINITION: _____

16. lymphoma

_____ / _____
    R   S

DEFINITION: _____

17. cytomorphology

    _____ / _____ / _____
    　　　CF　　　　　　CF　　　　　　S

    DEFINITION: _____

18. hemolysis

    _____ / _____
    　　　CF　　　　　　S

    DEFINITION: _____

19. anemia

    _____ / _____
    　　　P　　　　　　S

    DEFINITION: _____

20. metastasis

    _____ / _____
    　　　P　　　　　　S

    DEFINITION: _____

Name the three calculations that are part of the blood indices:

21. _____

22. _____

23. _____

Fill in the blanks with the correct medical terms and abbreviations:

24. The procedure of counting the number of leukocytes in the blood is called a _____ _____ _____ and is abbreviated as _____.

25. The blood study that determines the amount of pigment in red blood cells is called a _____ and is abbreviated as _____ or _____.

26. The blood study that determines packed red blood cell volume is called a _____ and is abbreviated as _____ or _____.

27. The classification of white blood cells is performed in a _____ _____.

Write out the expanded term for each abbreviation:

28. PT _____

29. ESR _____

30. PTT _____

31. CBC _____

Write the letter of the matching definition in the space after the term:

32. microcytosis	_____	a.	large RBCs
33. poikilocytosis	_____	b.	thrombocyte
34. neutrophil	_____	c.	WBC with rose-stained granules
35. monocyte	_____	d.	RBC
36. eosinophil	_____	e.	an agranulocyte active in immunity
37. lymphocyte	_____	f.	WBC with dark-stained granules
38. basophil	_____	g.	WBC termed "one cell"
39. platelet	_____	h.	RBCs of unequal size
40. erythrocyte	_____	i.	WBC with granules
41. granulocyte	_____	j.	large, irregular RBCs
42. anisocytosis	_____	k.	a polymorphonuclear WBC
43. macrocytosis	_____	l.	small RBCs

Write the correct medical term for each of the following definitions:

44. _____ a decrease in the number of neutrophils

45. _____ blood donated by a person and stored for his or her future use

46. _____ impaired ability to provide an immune response

47. _____ test tube method of matching a donor's blood to the recipient

48. _____ syndrome caused by HIV

49. _____ removal of plasma from the body, extraction of specific elements, and then reinfusion

50. _____ blood voluntarily donated by any person for transfusion

Circle the combining form that corresponds to the meaning given:

51.	**eat or swallow**	phas/o	phag/o	plas/o
52.	**clot**	thromb/o	thym/o	lymph/o
53.	**juice**	lymph/o	hemat/o	chyl/o
54.	**formation**	plas/o	troph/o	thromb/o
55.	**color**	hem/o	chrom/o	cyan/o
56.	**blood**	erythr/o	hem/o	lymph/o
57.	**safe**	toxic/o	reticul/o	immun/o
58.	**germ or bud**	blast/o	gen/o	crin/o

Circle the correct spelling:

59.	hematopoesis	hematopoiesis	hematoepoisis
60.	platelets	plattelets	plateletts
61.	anissocytosis	aniscocytosis	anisocytosis
62.	polkulocytosis	poikilocytosis	poiekilocytosis
63.	hemalysis	hemoliesis	hemolysis
64.	lymphadenpathy	lymphadenopathy	lymphoadenopathy

65. myelodysplasia	mylodysplaszia	myelodysphazia
66. thrombocytopnea	thrombocytopenia	throbocytpenia
67. hematocrit	hemacrit	hematocrete
68. splenecktomy	splenectomy	spleenectomy
69. plasmapheresis	plazmaphoresis	plasmophoresis
70. vasodialator	vasodilater	vasodilator

Give the noun used to form each adjective:

71. leukemic   _____

72. immunosuppressive _____

73. plasmapheretic   _____

74. thymic   _____

75. hematopoietic   _____

76. splenic   _____

77. septicemic   _____

78. hemophilic   _____

79. myelodysplastic   _____

80. thrombocytopenic _____

Write in the missing words on lines in the following illustrations of the components of blood:

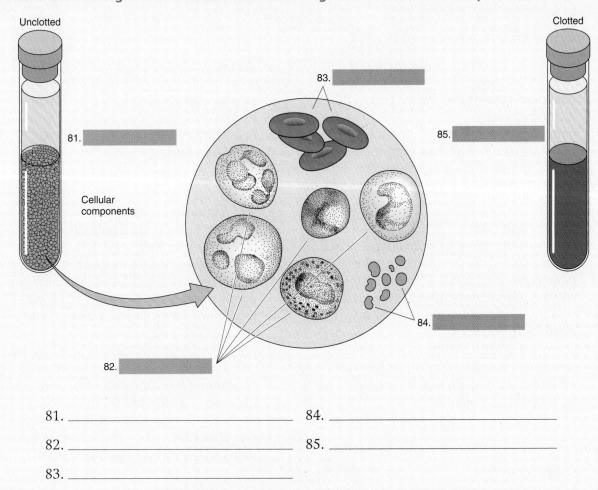

81. _____   84. _____

82. _____   85. _____

83. _____

MEDICAL RECORD ANALYSIS

Medical Record 6-1

PROGRESS NOTE

CC: Fatigue

S: This 43 y/o female c/o feeling run down with lack of energy x 1 mo. Pt denies fever, chills, nausea, vomiting, diarrhea, constipation and reports no weight loss. She has had very heavy menstrual periods lasting 5 days since DC of birth control pills 1 year ago.

PMH: mononucleosis at age 14, NKDA. FH: father, age 68, died of MI; mother, age 74, has myelodysplasia; sister, age 45, L&W

SH: married x 8 yr, no children; ETOH–wine with dinner, denies smoking.

O: VS: T 98.8°, P 81, R 15, BP 136/62. WDWN female in NAD. HEENT—WNL

Neck: supple s̄ lymphadenopathy. Lungs: clear. Heart: RRR s̄ murmur

Abdomen: soft and tender s̄ organomegaly. Extremities: no edema.

A: Etiology of fatigue and decreased energy unclear. Possible iron deficiency anemia in light of heavy menstrual periods.

P: Blood studies to include comprehensive metabolic panel, CBC c̄ differential.

RTO in 1 wk for lab results.

QUESTIONS ABOUT MEDICAL RECORD 6-1

1. Which of the following is not mentioned in the history?
   a. type of treatment the patient received for mononucleosis
   b. patient's consumption of alcohol
   c. how long the patient has been married
   d. health status of the patient's sister

2. Describe the condition of the patient's mother:
   a. she has leukemia
   b. she has a bleeding disorder characterized by an abnormally decreased number of platelets in the blood
   c. she has a hereditary disorder characterized by an excessive buildup of iron deposits in the body
   d. she has a disorder within the bone marrow characterized by a proliferation of abnormal stem cells, which usually develops into leukemia

3. Which of the following describes the findings of the physical examination?
   a. swollen lymph glands
   b. normal examination
   c. fast heart rate
   d. heart murmur

4. What is the possible cause of the patient's fatigue?
   a. viral condition characterized by an increase in mononuclear cells (monocytes and lymphocytes) in the blood
   b. macrocytic-normochromic type of anemia characterized by an inadequate supply of vitamin B_{12}, causing red blood cells to become large, varied in shape, and reduced in number
   c. microcytic-hypochromic type of anemia characterized by small red blood cells containing low amounts of hemoglobin because of a lack of iron in the body
   d. normocytic-normochromic type of anemia characterized by the failure of bone marrow to produce red blood cells

5. Identify the subjective information most significantly linked to the assessment:
   a. enlarged lymph glands
   b. heavy menstrual periods
   c. fatigue
   d. the patient quit taking birth control pills

6. Which of the following tests is part of the plan?
   a. test to determine coagulation defects, such as platelet disorders
   b. test to diagnose an infection in the bloodstream by culturing a specimen of blood
   c. needle aspiration of bone marrow tissue for pathologic examination
   d. expanded battery of automated blood chemistry tests used as a general screen for disease

Medical Record 6-2 A and B

FOR ADDITIONAL STUDY

Henry Lin went to his personal physician after an extended period of feeling weak and tired and starting to lose weight. His doctor then admitted him to Central Medical Center hospital for additional tests after conducting a physical examination and blood tests. He is now being treated as an outpatient by his internist, Dr. Bradley, and an oncologist, Dr. Ellison, to whom he was referred for consultation and concurrent care. Medical Record 6-2A is the oncology/hematology progress note dictated by Dr. Ellison, the oncologist treating Mr. Lin, at the time of a follow-up visit two weeks after Mr. Lin's hospitalization. The second document, Medical Record 6-2B, is a hematology lab report, submitted before a second follow-up with Dr. Ellison two weeks later.

Read Medical Record 6-2 (pages 312–313), then write your answers to the following questions in the spaces provided.

QUESTIONS ABOUT MEDICAL RECORD 6-2

1. Below are medical terms used in the progress note that you have not yet encountered in this text. Underline each where it appears in the record, and define the term below.

   edema _____

   scaphoid _____

   anorexia _____

2. In your own words, not using medical terminology, translate Mr. Lin's diagnosis:

   _____

3. Name the diagnostic test that confirmed this diagnosis:

   _____

4. Write the medical term for Mr. Lin's enlarged spleen: _____

5. Dr. Ellison's March 31 record includes the results of two CBC component tests from the earlier March 23 lab report as well as results from the same tests for March 31. The April 15 lab report also contains the CBC component tests. In the spaces below, write the name of the tests and their results at these three times. Do not use abbreviations. Be sure to include units of measure.

Test	Result		
	March 23	March 31	April 15
_____	_____	_____	_____
_____	_____	_____	_____

6. What are the three elements Dr. Ellison includes in Mr. Lin's treatment plan?

   a. _____

   b. _____

   c. _____

7. Study the April 15 laboratory report carefully, and complete the following table of selected test results. Write out the full name of the abbreviated measurement; circle *N* (normal) if the result for Mr. Lin is within the normal range or *A* (abnormal) if the result is outside the normal range.

Test Name		Result Range	
a. WBC	_____	N	A
b. RBC	_____	N	A
c. HGB	_____	N	A
d. HCT	_____	N	A
e. MCV	_____	N	A
f. MCH	_____	N	A
g. MCHC	_____	N	A
h. PLT	_____	N	A
i. lymph	_____	N	A
j. mono	_____	N	A
k. neutro	_____	N	A
l. eos	_____	N	A
m. baso	_____	N	A

Medical Record 6-2A: For Additional Study

CENTRAL MEDICAL GROUP, INC.

Department of Oncology/Hematology

201 Medical Center Drive • Central City, US 90000-1234 • PHONE: (012) 125-8888 • FAX: (012) 125-3434

PROGRESS NOTE

PATIENT: LIN, HENRY N.

DATE: March 31, 20xx

Mr. Lin is a 69-year-old man seen for myelodysplasia while hospitalized on March 17, 20xx. He was transfused with 4.0 U of packed cells during that hospitalization. A bone marrow biopsy revealed histology consistent with chronic myelomonocytic leukeumia (myelodysplasia).

A follow-up blood count was obtained through Dr. Bradley's office on March 23, 20xx, and revealed a hemoglobin of 11.0 G/DL and a hematocrit of 31.0%.

There have been no fevers, sweats, or anorexia; but he has noted some weight loss. There has been no bleeding. There has been no nausea, vomiting, or dark and bloody stools.

Exam: Weight: 172 lb. Blood Pressure: 120/50. Temperature: 98.6°F. Pulse: 88. Respirations: 18.

HEENT: Mild gum atrophy and inflammation. NECK: Supple. LYMPH NODES: There is no cervical or supraclavicular adenopathy. LUNGS: Clear. CARDIOVASCULAR: Normal. ABDOMEN: Scaphoid, soft, and nontender. The spleen is enlarged. EXTREMITIES: Without edema or petechiae.

TODAY'S LAB: Complete blood count reveals a total leukocyte count of 6600/cu mm, a hemoglobin of 8.0 G/DL, a hematocrit of 23.0%, and a platelet count of 149,000/cu mm.

CLINICAL DIAGNOSIS:

Chronic myelomonocytic leukemia (myelodysplastic syndrome). The patient is transfusion dependent.

The patient will be typed and crossmatched today and will be transfused with 2.0 U of packed red blood cells through the Oncology Day Facility tomorrow on April 1, 20xx

I have asked the patient to follow up with Dr. Bradley next week and with me in two weeks.

A. Ellison, M.D.

AE:gds
cc: Blair Bradley, M.D.

D: 3/31/20xx
T: 4/3/20xx

Medical Record 6-2B: For Additional Study

CENTRAL MEDICAL CENTER
211 Medical Center Drive • Central City, US 90000-1234 • PHONE: (012) 125-6784 • FAX: (012) 125-9999

04/15/20xx
14:27

NAME : Lin, Henry   LOC: TEST   DOB: 2/2/xx   AGE: 69Y
MR# : TEST-226   SEX: M
ACCT# :168946701

M63558 COLL: 04/15/20xx 13:23   REC: 04/15/20xx 13:25

HEMOGRAM

CBC

WBC	4.1	[4.5 - 10.5]	K/UL
RBC	2.93	[4.6 - 6.2]	M/UL
HGB	9.1	[14.0 - 18.0]	G/DL
HCT	25.3	[42.0 - 52.0]	%
MCV	86.2	[82 - 92]	FL
MCH	31.1	[27 - 31]	PG
MCHC	36.0	[32 - 36]	G/DL
PLT	90	[150 - 450]	K/UL
Auto Lymph %	8.3	[20 - 40]	%
Auto Mono %	32.6	[1 - 11]	%
Auto Neutro %	57.8	[50 - 75]	%
Auto Eos %	1.0	[0 - 6]	%
Auto Baso %	0.3	[0 - 2]	%
Auto Lymph #	0.3	[1.5 - 4.0]	K/UL
Auto Mono #	1.3	[0.2 - 0.9]	K/UL
Auto Neutro #	2.4	[1.0 - 7.0]	K/UL
Auto Eos #	0.0	[0 - 0.7]	K/UL
Auto Baso #	0.0	[0 - 0.2]	K/UL

TEST, PATIENT   TEST-221   END OF REPORT   PAGE 1
04/15/20xx 14:27   INTERIM REPORT

INTERIM REPORT COMPLETE

ANSWERS TO PRACTICE EXERCISES

1. erythro/blast/osis
   CF   R   S
   red/germ or bud/condi-
   tion or increase
2. chylo/poiesis
   CF   S
   juice/formation
3. hemo/cyto/meter
   CF   CF   S
   blood/cell/instrument
   for measuring
4. spleno/rrhagia
   CF   S
   spleen/to burst forth
5. lymph/aden/itis
   R   R   S
   clear fluid/gland/inflam-
   mation
6. immuno/tox/ic
   CF   R   S
   safe/poison/pertaining
   to
7. reticulo/cyt/osis
   CF   R   S
   a net/cell/condition or
   increase
8. thymo/path/y
   CF   R   S
   thymus gland/disease/
   condition or process of
9. leuko/cyt/ic
   CF   R   S
   white/cell/pertaining to
10. lymph/angio/gram
    R   CF   S
    clear fluid/vessel/record
11. spleno/megaly
    CF   S
    spleen/enlargement
12. pro/myelo/cyt/e
    P   CF   R   S
    before/bone marrow/
    cell/noun marker
13. leuko/cyto/penia
    CF   CF   S
    white/cell/abnormal
    reduction

14. splen/ectomy
    R   S
    spleen/excision
    (removal)
15. dia/lysis
    P   S
    across or through/
    breaking down or
    dissolution
16. lymph/oma
    R   S
    clear fluid/tumor
17. cyto/morpho/logy
    CF   CF   S
    cell/form/study of
18. hemo/lysis
    CF   S
    blood/breaking down or
    dissolution
19. an/emia
    P   S
    without/blood condition
20. meta/stasis
    P   S
    beyond, after, or
    change/stop or stand
21. mean corpuscular (cell)
    volume (MCV)
22. mean corpuscular (cell)
    hemoglobin (MCH)
23. mean corpuscular (cell)
    hemoglobin concentra-
    tion (MCHC)
24. white blood count,
    WBC
25. hemoglobin, HGB, Hgb
26. hematocrit, HCT, Hct
27. differential count
28. prothrombin time
29. erythrocyte sedimenta-
    tion rate
30. partial thromboplastin
    time
31. complete blood count
32. l
33. j
34. k

35. g
36. c
37. e
38. f
39. b
40. d
41. i
42. h
43. a
44. neutropenia
45. autologous blood
46. immunosuppression
47. cross-matching
48. acquired immunodefi-
    ciency syndrome (AIDS)
49. plasmapheresis
50. homologous blood
51. phag/o
52. thromb/o
53. chyl/o
54. plas/o
55. chrom/o
56. hem/o
57. immun/o
58. blast/o
59. hematopoiesis
60. platelets
61. anisocytosis
62. poikilocytosis
63. hemolysis
64. lymphadenopathy
65. myelodysplasia
66. thrombocytopenia
67. hematocrit
68. splenectomy
69. plasmapheresis
70. vasodilator
71. leukemia
72. immunosuppression
73. plasmapheresis
74. thymus
75. hematopoiesis
76. spleen
77. septicemia
78. hemophilia
79. myelodysplasia
80. thrombocytopenia

81. plasma
82. leukocytes or white blood cells
83. erythrocytes or red blood cells
84. thrombocytes or platelets
85. serum

ANSWERS TO MEDICAL RECORD ANALYSIS

Medical Record 6-1: Progress Note

1. a   2. d   3. b   4. c   5. b   6. d

Medical Record 6-2: For Additional Study

See CD-ROM for answers.

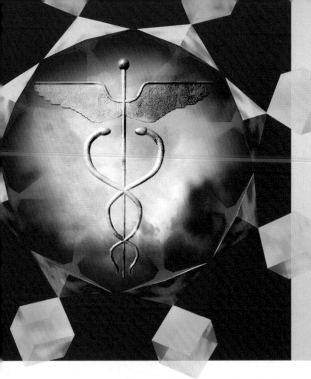

7

Respiratory System

✓ *Chapter 7 Checklist*	LOCATION
☐ Read Chapter 7: Respiratory System and complete all programmed review segments.	pages 317-349
☐ Review the starter set of flash cards and term components related to Chapter 7.	back of book
☐ Complete the Chapter 7 Practice Exercises and Medical Record Analysis 7-1.	pages 355-363
☐ Complete Medical Record Analysis 7-2 For Additional Study.	pages 364-368
☐ Complete the Chapter 7 Exercises by Chapter.	CD-ROM
☐ Complete the Chapter 7 Review and Test Modes.	CD-ROM
☐ Review the Pronunciation Drill for the Chapter 7 terms.	CD-ROM

RESPIRATORY SYSTEM OVERVIEW

The respiratory system has two primary functions (Fig. 7-1):

❋ Brings oxygen into the body as air is inhaled into the lungs (inspiration) and passes the oxygen into the blood

❋ Rids the body of carbon dioxide through exhalation (expiration) as the lungs receive carbon dioxide diffused out of the blood

THE RESPIRATORY SYSTEM

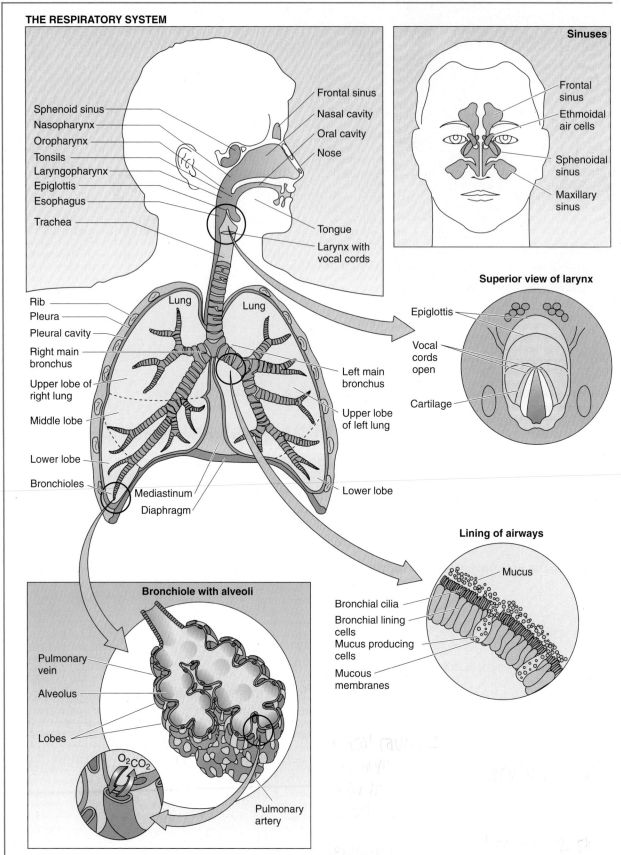

Sinuses

Frontal sinus
Ethmoidal air cells
Sphenoidal sinus
Maxillary sinus

Sphenoid sinus
Nasopharynx
Oropharynx
Tonsils
Laryngopharynx
Epiglottis
Esophagus
Trachea

Frontal sinus
Nasal cavity
Oral cavity
Nose

Tongue
Larynx with vocal cords

Superior view of larynx

Epiglottis
Vocal cords open
Cartilage

Rib
Pleura
Pleural cavity
Right main bronchus
Upper lobe of right lung
Middle lobe
Lower lobe
Bronchioles

Lung
Lung

Left main bronchus
Upper lobe of left lung
Lower lobe

Mediastinum
Diaphragm

Lining of airways

Mucus
Bronchial cilia
Bronchial lining cells
Mucus producing cells
Mucous membranes

Bronchiole with alveoli

Pulmonary vein
Alveolus
Lobes
O_2 CO_2
Pulmonary artery

FIGURE 7-1 ■ **Respiratory tract.**

Self-Instruction: Combining Forms

Study the following:

COMBINING FORM	MEANING
alveol/o	alveolus (air sac)
bronch/o, bronchi/o	bronchus (airway)
bronchiol/o	bronchiole (little airway)
capn/o, carb/o	carbon dioxide
laryng/o	larynx (voice box)
lob/o	lobe (a portion)
nas/o, rhin/o	nose
or/o	mouth
ox/o	oxygen
palat/o	palate
pharyng/o	pharynx (throat)
phren/o	diaphragm (also mind)
pleur/o	pleura (lining of lungs)
pneum/o, pneumon/o	air or lung
pulmon/o	lung
sinus/o	sinus (cavity)
spir/o, -pnea (suffix)	breathing
thorac/o, pector/o, steth/o	chest
tonsill/o	tonsil
trache/o	trachea (windpipe)
uvul/o	uvula

 ## Programmed Review: Combining Forms

ANSWERS	REVIEW
	7.1 The lungs are the primary organs of the respiratory system. A pulmonologist is a medical specialist who is concerned with the lungs. The combining form for lung is
pulmon/o	_____. The two combining forms that can refer
pneum/o, pneumon/o	to either air or lung are _____ and _____. For example, pneumothorax describes air in the chest (pleural
inflammation	cavity). Pneumonitis is an _____ of the lung.

ANSWERS	REVIEW
lob/o excision lobectomy	**7.2** The combining form for lobe (as in a lung lobe) is _____. Because the suffix *-ectomy* means an _____ or removal, the removal of a lung lobe is called a _____.
incision thorac/o steth/o pain pector/o	**7.3** Several different combining forms refer to the chest and are the basis of terms related to the respiratory system. A thoracotomy is an _____ into the chest; the term uses the combining form _____. A stethoscope, from the combining form _____, is an instrument used to listen to lung sounds through the chest wall. Because the suffix *-algia* refers to _____, pectoralgia, from the combining form _____, means chest pain.
ox/o deficient or below condition of hypoxia blood hypoxemia	**7.4** The combining form meaning oxygen is _____. Using the prefix *hypo-*, which means _____, and the suffix *-ia*, which means _____ _____, the term for a condition of deficient oxygen levels is _____. (Note that occasionally, when a prefix ends in a vowel and the root begins with a vowel, the final vowel is dropped from the prefix.) Because the suffix *-emia* refers to a _____ condition, the term for a condition of deficient oxygen in the blood is _____.
capn/o, carb/o much hypocapnia, hypocarbia	**7.5** The lungs move oxygen into the blood and carbon dioxide out of the blood. The combining forms for carbon dioxide are _____ and _____. Hypercapnia, for example, is a condition of too _____ carbon dioxide in the blood; hypercarbia is a synonym. The term for a condition of too little carbon dioxide in the blood is _____ or _____.
breathing measuring spirometry -pnea difficult, painful, or faulty	**7.6** The combining form *spir/o* means _____. Because *-metry* refers to the process of _____ something, the term for the measuring of breathing is _____. A suffix related to breathing is _____, as in the term dyspnea, meaning _____ breathing.

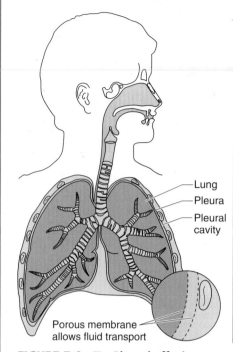

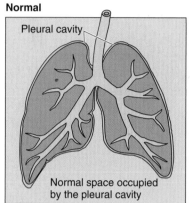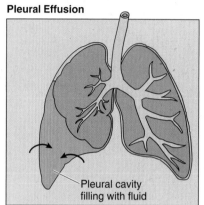

Normal

Pleural cavity

Normal space occupied
by the pleural cavity

Pleural Effusion

Pleural cavity
filling with fluid

Lung
Pleura
Pleural
cavity

Porous membrane
allows fluid transport

FIGURE 7-6 ■ **Pleural effusion.**

TERM	MEANING
pneumonia (Fig. 7-7) *nū-mō′nē-ă*	inflammation in the lung resulting from infection by bacteria, viruses, fungi, or parasites or from aspiration of chemicals
***Pneumocystis* pneumonia** *nū-mō-sis′tis nū-mō′nē-ă*	pneumonia caused by the *Pneumocystis carinii* organism, a common opportunistic infection in those who are positive for the human immunodeficiency virus (HIV)
pneumothorax (Fig. 7-8) *nū-mō-thōr′aks*	air in the pleural cavity caused by a puncture of the lung or chest wall

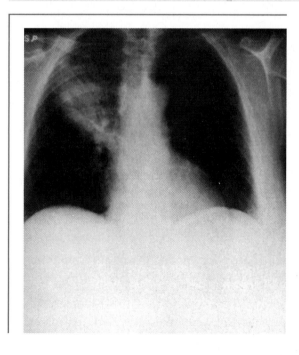

FIGURE 7-7 ■ **Chest x-ray image showing pulmonary infiltrates in right upper lobe consistent with lobar pneumonia. Dense material (inflammatory exudate) absorbs radiation, whereas normal alveoli do not.**

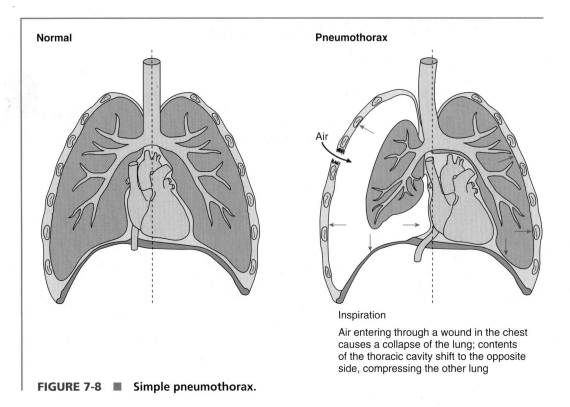

FIGURE 7-8 ■ **Simple pneumothorax.**

TERM	MEANING
pneumohemothorax *nū'mō–hē–mō–thōr'aks*	air and blood in the pleural cavity
pneumonitis *nū–mō–nī'tis*	inflammation of the lung, often caused by hypersensitivity to chemicals or dusts
pulmonary embolism (PE) *pul'mō–nār–ē em'bō–lizm*	occlusion in the pulmonary circulation, most often caused by a blood clot
pulmonary tuberculosis (TB) *pul'mō–nār–ē tū–bĕr–kyū–lō'sis*	disease caused by the presence of *Mycobacterium tuberculosis* in the lungs; characterized by the formation of tubercles, inflammation, and necrotizing caseous lesions (caseous necrosis)
sinusitis *sī–nŭ–sī'tis*	inflammation of the sinuses
sleep apnea *slēp ap'nē–ă*	periods of breathing cessation (10 seconds or more) that occur during sleep, often resulting in snoring
tonsillitis *ton–si–lī'tis*	acute or chronic inflammation of the tonsils
upper respiratory infection (URI) *up'er rĕs–par'uh–tōr–ē in–fek'shŭn*	infectious disease of the upper respiratory tract involving the nasal passages, pharynx, and bronchi

Programmed Review: Diagnostic Terms

ANSWERS	REVIEW
upper respiratory infection	**7.44** URI is the abbreviation for _____ _____ _____, an infection of the upper respiratory tract involving the nasal passages, pharynx, and bronchi.
-itis sinusitis tonsillitis pharyngitis laryngitis bronchitis	**7.45** Recall that the suffix for inflammation is _____. Many individual structures of the respiratory system can become inflamed, often by an infection. Inflammation of the sinuses is called _____. Inflammation of the tonsils is called _____. Inflammation of the pharynx is called _____. Inflammation of the larynx is called _____. Inflammation of the bronchi is called _____.
pleuritis pleurisy	**7.46** Inflammation of the pleura is called _____. Another term for this condition is _____.
pneumonitis laryngotracheobronchitis croup	**7.47** The term for inflammation of the lung is built from the combining form meaning either air or lung. This term is _____. Another "itis" inflammation involving the larynx, trachea, and bronchi causes a distinctive, seal-like bark. The longer term for this condition, _____, uses all three combining forms; the shorter term for this condition is _____.
pneumonia Pneumocystis pneumoconiosis	**7.48** Several other diagnostic terms are built from the combining form meaning air or lung. Using a suffix indicating a condition of, the term for an inflammation of the lung caused by infection with bacteria or viruses, or by exposure to chemicals, is _____. A particular kind of pneumonia caused by the *Pneumocystis carinii* organism is called _____ pneumonia. A chronic restrictive disease resulting from inhaling dust (*conio* = dust) is called _____.
pneumothorax	**7.49** This same combining form for air is used to build the terms referring to air in a body cavity. Air in the thorax caused by a puncture of the lung or chest wall is called _____. The term for both air and blood

ANSWERS	REVIEW
pneumohemothorax hemothorax	(*hem/o* = blood) in the thorax is _____. The presence of blood alone in the pleural cavity of the chest is called _____.
bronchitis -spasm bronchospasm -ectasis bronchiectasis, carcinoma bronchogenic carcinoma	**7.50** In addition to inflammation of the bronchi, called _____, several other diagnostic conditions can occur in the bronchi. Recall that the suffix for an involuntary contraction is _____. A constriction of the bronchi caused by contraction of the smooth muscle around the bronchi is called _____. Recall that the diagnostic suffix for expansion or dilation is _____; thus, the condition of abnormal dilation of the bronchi with an accumulation of mucus is called _____. Recall that _____ means cancer tumor. Lung cancer originating in the bronchi is called _____ _____.
-spasm laryngospasm	**7.51** Again, the suffix for an involuntary contraction is _____. A contraction of laryngeal muscles, causing a constriction, is termed _____.
-ectasis atelectasis	**7.52** Recall that the suffix for expansion or dilation is _____. Therefore, the term for a collapse of lung tissue uses this suffix combined with the root *atele* (meaning imperfect): _____.
asthma emphysema chronic obstructive pulmonary disease	**7.53** There are several types of obstructive pulmonary disease. Caused by a spasm of the bronchial tubes or by swelling of their mucous membrane, _____ is characterized by sudden attacks of wheezing, dyspnea, and cough. Another condition, characterized by overexpansion of the alveoli with air and destructive changes in their walls, is called _____. The permanent destructive pulmonary disorder that is a combination of emphysema and chronic bronchitis is called _____ _____ _____ _____ (COPD).
condition nasal polyposis	**7.54** The diagnostic suffix *-osis* means _____ or increase. The condition of numerous polyps in the nose is called _____ _____.

ANSWERS	REVIEW
cystic fibrosis	**7.55** Another use for *-osis* is in the term describing the hereditary condition of exocrine gland malfunction that causes secretion of abnormally thick mucus in the lungs, obstructing the airways and leading to infection and damage to lung tissue: _____ _____.
hemothorax pyothorax pleural effusion	**7.56** Fluid, pus, blood, or air can accumulate in the pleural cavity. The term for blood in this cavity in the thorax is _____. The combining form meaning pus is *py/o*; thus, the accumulation of pus in the pleural cavity is called _____, or empyema. An accumulation of fluid in the pleural cavity is called a _____ _____.
apnea sleep apnea	**7.57** Recall that the term for an inability to breathe is _____. The condition in which this happens for short periods during sleep is called _____ _____.
pulmonary tuberculosis	**7.58** The bacteria *Mycobacterium tuberculosis* causes the lung disease _____ _____.
pulmonary embolism	**7.59** A blood clot that lodges in the pulmonary circulation, causing an occlusion, is called a _____ _____.

 ## Self-Instruction: Diagnostic Tests and Procedures

Study the following:

TEST OR PROCEDURE	EXPLANATION
arterial blood gas (ABG) *ar-tē'rē-ăl blŭd gas*	analysis of arterial blood to determine the adequacy of lung function in the exchange of gases
pH	abbreviation for the potential of hydrogen; measurement of blood acidity or alkalinity
PaO₂	abbreviation for partial pressure of oxygen; measurement of the amount of oxygen in the blood
PaCO₂	abbreviation for partial pressure of carbon dioxide; measurement of the amount of carbon dioxide in the blood
endoscopy *en-dos'kŏ-pē*	examination inside a body cavity with a flexible endoscope for diagnostic or treatment purposes

TEST OR PROCEDURE	EXPLANATION
bronchoscopy (Fig. 7-9) *brong-kos'kŏ-pē*	use of a flexible endoscope, called a bronchoscope, to examine the airways
nasopharyngoscopy *nā'zō-far-in-gos'kŏ-pē*	use of a flexible endoscope to examine the nasal passages and the pharynx (throat) to diagnose structural abnormalities, such as obstructions, growths, and cancers
examination methods *ek-zam-i-nā'shŭn meth'ŏdz*	techniques used during physical examination to objectively evaluate the respiratory system
auscultation *aws-kŭl-tā'shŭn*	to listen; a physical examination method of listening to the sounds within the body with the aid of a stethoscope, such as auscultation of the chest for heart and lung sounds
percussion *pĕr-kŭsh'ŭn*	a physical examination method of tapping the body to elicit vibrations and sounds to estimate the size, border, or fluid content of a cavity, such as the chest
lung biopsy (Bx) *lŭng bī'op-sē*	removal of a small piece of lung tissue for pathologic examination
lung scan (Fig. 7-10) *lŭng skan* **ventilation-perfusion (V/Q) scan** *ven-ti-lā'shŭn-per-fyū'zhŭn skan*	a two-part nuclear (radionuclide) scan of the lungs to detect abnormalities of ventilation (respiration) or perfusion (blood flow) made 1) after radioactive material is injected in the patient's blood, and 2) as the patient breathes radioactive material into the airways; comparison of the two scans indicates whether an abnormality exists in the airways or the pulmonary circulation
magnetic resonance imaging (MRI) *mag-net'ic rez'ō-nănts im'ă-jing*	nonionizing image of the lung to visualize lung lesions
polysomnography (PSG) *pol'ē-som-nog'ră-fē*	recording of various aspects of sleep (i.e., eye and muscle movements, respiration, and brain-wave patterns) for diagnosis of sleep disorders (*somn/o* = sleep) (*see* Chapter 8, Figure 8-14)
pulmonary function testing (PFT) *pŭl'mō-nār-ē fŭnk'shŭn test'ing*	direct and indirect measurements of lung volumes and capacities
spirometry (Fig. 7-11) *spī-rom'ĕ-trē*	direct measurement of lung volume and capacity
tidal volume (TV or V_T) *tī'dăl vol'yŭm*	amount of air exhaled after a normal inspiration
vital capacity (VC) *vīt-ăl kă-pas'i-tē*	amount of air exhaled after a maximal inspiration
peak flow (PF) *pēk flō* **peak expiratory flow rate (PEFR)** *pēk ek-spī'ră-tō-rē flō rāt*	measure of the fastest flow of exhaled air after a maximal inspiration

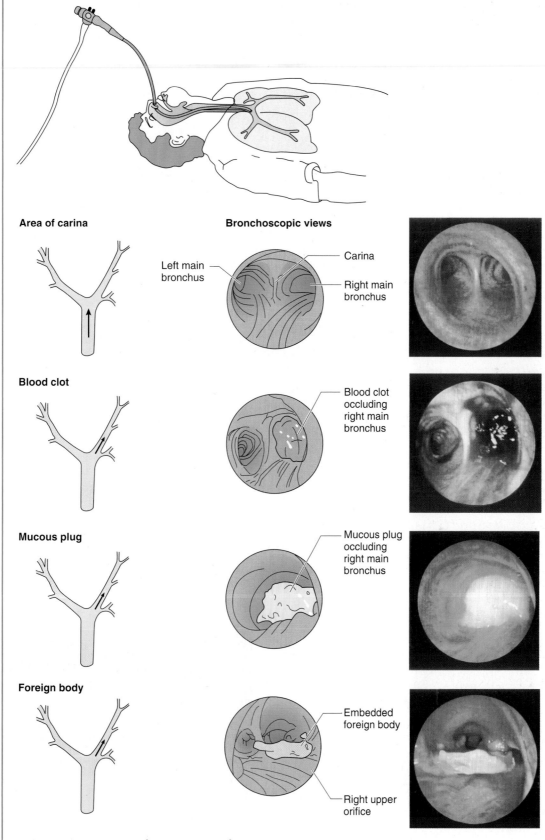

Area of carina

Bronchoscopic views

Left main bronchus

Carina

Right main bronchus

Blood clot

Blood clot occluding right main bronchus

Mucous plug

Mucous plug occluding right main bronchus

Foreign body

Embedded foreign body

Right upper orifice

FIGURE 7-9 ■ **Bronchoscopy procedure.**

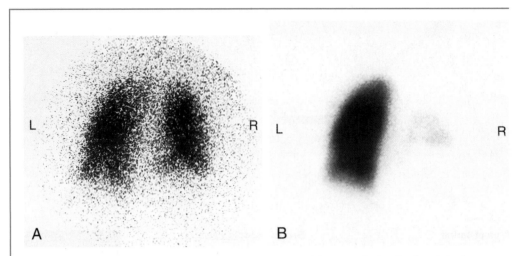

FIGURE 7-10 ■ **Posterior lung scan in a patient with an embolus in the right lung. A. Ventilation image shows a normal pattern. B. Absence of blood flow to the right lung is apparent on perfusion scan.** *L*, left; *R*, right.

TEST OR PROCEDURE	EXPLANATION
pulse oximetry (Fig. 7-12) *pŭls ok-sim'ă-trē*	noninvasive method of estimating the percentage of oxygen saturation in the blood using an oximeter with a specialized probe attached to the skin at a site of arterial pulsation, commonly the finger; used to monitor hypoxemia
radiology *rā-dē-ol'ŏ-jē*	x-ray imaging

chest x-ray (CXR)
    chest x-rā
	x-ray imaging of the chest to visualize the lungs; directional terms identify the path of the x-ray beam to produce the radiograph:
	    PA (posterior-anterior) = from back to front
	    AP (anterior-posterior) = from front to back
	    lateral = toward the side (e.g., left lateral)

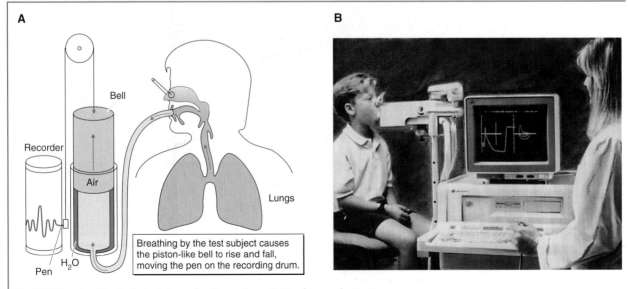

FIGURE 7-11 ■ **A. Principles of spirometry. B. Modern spirometry.**

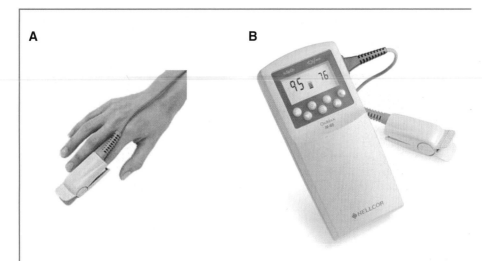

FIGURE 7-12 ■ Pulse oximetry. A. Placement of a sensor on the patient's finger. B. Oxygen saturation reading on a portable monitor.

TEST OR PROCEDURE	EXPLANATION
computed tomography (CT) *kom-pyū'tĕd tō-mog'ră-fē*	CT of the thorax is used to detect lesions in the lung; CT of the head is used to visualize the structures of the nose and sinuses
pulmonary angiography (Fig. 7-13) *pul'mō-năr-ē an-jē-og'ră-fē*	x-ray imaging of the blood vessels of the lungs after the injection of contrast material

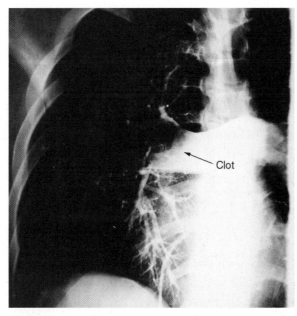

FIGURE 7-13 ■ Pulmonary angiogram showing an embolus obstructing pulmonary circulation (*arrow*).

Programmed Review: Diagnostic Tests and Procedures

ANSWERS	REVIEW
-scopy endoscopy bronchoscopy nasopharyngoscopy	**7.60** Recall that the suffix meaning a process of examination (with an instrument) is _____. Because *endo-* is the prefix for within, the general term for examination within a body cavity using a scope is _____. Use of a special endoscope to examine the airways and bronchi is called _____. Examination of the nasal and throat passages is _____.
chest auscultation	**7.61** A stethoscope is used to listen to _____ sounds. The physical examination procedure for doing this is called _____.
percussion	**7.62** Another physical examination method uses tapping of the body to listen to the resulting sounds and vibrations to make observations about underlying organs and masses. This is called _____.
gases pH PaO_2 $PaCO_2$	**7.63** Laboratory tests analyze arterial blood _____ (ABGs) to determine the adequacy of their function in the lung. The _____ is a measure of blood acidity or alkalinity. The amount of oxygen in the blood is measured as the partial pressure of oxygen and is referred to as _____. The partial pressure of carbon dioxide is referred to as _____.
biopsy	**7.64** Removal of a small sample of lung tissue for pathologic examination is called lung _____. Many different organs and tissues in the body can be biopsied.
many -graphy polysomnography	**7.65** The combining form *somn/o* means sleep, and the prefix *poly-* means _____. The suffix referring to the process of recording is _____. Using these three word parts, the procedure that records many aspects of sleep (respiration, muscle movements, and so on) is called _____.
pulmonary function spirometry	**7.66** Measurement of lung volumes and capacities is called _____ _____ testing (PFT). Formed from the combining term for breathing and the suffix for the process of measuring, the term for the direct measurement of lung volume and capacity is _____. The amount of air exhaled after a

ANSWERS	REVIEW
tidal vital capacity	normal inspiration is called _____ volume. The amount of air exhaled after a maximal inspiration is called _____ _____.
peak expiratory flow	The measure of the fastest flow of exhaled air after a maximal inspiration is called peak flow or _____ _____ _____ rate.
pulse oximetry	**7.67** A noninvasive method of estimating the percentage of oxygen saturation in the blood uses an oximeter attached to the skin at a site of arterial pulsation. This procedure is called _____ _____.
lung scan ventilation, perfusion magnetic resonance imaging	**7.68** Several different imaging modalities are used to visualize the lungs and other respiratory structures. A two-part nuclear scan of the lungs to detect perfusion or ventilation abnormalities is simply called a _____ _____, or a V/Q scan, in which V stands for _____ (breathing) and Q stands for _____ (blood flow). A nonionizing image of the lungs using magnetic fields and radiofrequency waves is produced using a modality called _____ _____ _____ (MRI).
radiology record -graph radiograph chest x-ray posterior-anterior anterior-posterior front, back side angiography computed tomography	**7.69** Using *radi/o*, a combining form meaning x-ray, and the suffix meaning study of, the term for x-ray imaging is _____. A radiogram is an x-ray _____; however, recall that the suffix meaning instrument for recording, _____, is used in the preferred term for an x-ray image: _____. An x-ray of the full thorax to visualize the lungs is a _____ _____ (CXR). The abbreviations PA, for _____-_____, and AP, for _____-_____, indicate the path of the x-ray beam in producing the radiograph. Anterior refers to the _____, and posterior refers to the _____. AP, then, indicates that the x-ray passed from the front of the chest to the back of the chest. A left lateral CXR is taken from the left _____ of the chest. X-ray imaging of the blood vessels of the lungs taken after injection of a contrast medium is called pulmonary _____. The form of x-ray imaging in which a computer creates cross-sectional images of structures such as the lungs is called _____ _____ (CT).

(handwritten note: V/Q scan)

Self-Instruction: Operative Terms

Study the following:

TERM	MEANING
adenoidectomy *ad'ĕ-noy-dek' tŏ-mē*	excision of the adenoids
lobectomy *lō-bek' tŏ-mē*	removal of a lobe of a lung
nasal polypectomy *nā'zăl pol'ip-ek' tŏ-mē*	removal of a nasal polyp
pneumonectomy *nū' mō-nek' tŏ-mē*	removal of an entire lung
thoracentesis (Fig. 7-14) *thōr'ă-sen-tē'sis*	puncture for aspiration of the chest (pleural cavity)
thoracoplasty *thōr'ă-kō-plas-tē*	repair of the chest involving fixation of the ribs
thoracoscopy *thōr-ă-kos' kŏ-pē*	endoscopic examination of the pleural cavity using a thoracoscope
thoracostomy (*see* Fig. 7-14) *thōr-ă-kos' tŏ-mē*	creation of an opening in the chest, usually to insert a tube
thoracotomy *thōr-ă-kot'ŏ-mē*	incision into the chest

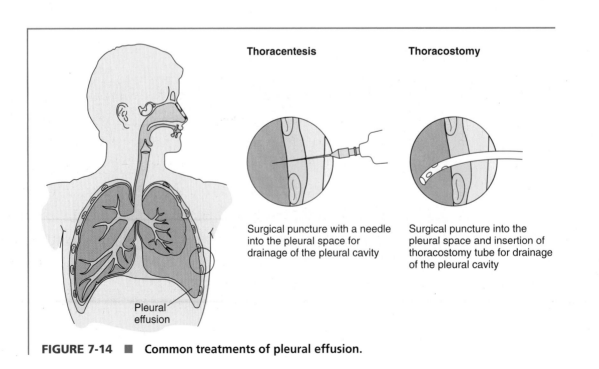

FIGURE 7-14 ■ **Common treatments of pleural effusion.**

Tracheotomy
Incision of the trachea for exploration, for removal of a foreign body, or for obtaining a biopsy specimen

Tracheostomy
Incision of the trachea and insertion of a tube to facilitate passage of air or removal of secretions

Sagittal view, with tracheostomy tube in place

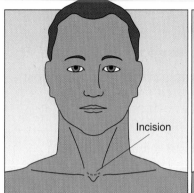
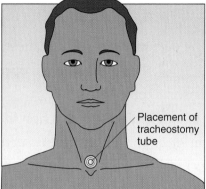
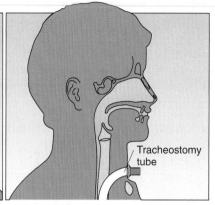

Incision

Placement of tracheostomy tube

Tracheostomy tube

FIGURE 7-15 ■ **Operative procedures related to the trachea.**

Bifurcate ⇒ branches out

TERM	MEANING
tonsillectomy *ton-si-lek'tŏ-mē*	excision of the palatine tonsils
tonsillectomy and adenoidectomy (T&A) *ton-si-lek'tŏ-mē and ad'ĕ-noy-dek'tŏ-mē*	excision of the tonsils and adenoids
tracheostomy (Fig. 7-15) *trā'kē-os'tŏ-mē*	creation of an opening in the trachea, usually to insert a tube
tracheotomy (*see* Fig. 7-15) *trā'kē-ot'ŏ-mē*	incision into the trachea

Programmed Review: Operative Terms

ANSWERS	REVIEW
excision	**7.70** Recall that the suffix *-ectomy* means _____ or removal. The term for the surgical removal of the adenoids is
adenoidectomy	_____. The term for removal of a nasal polyp is
nasal polypectomy	_____ _____. Formed using the combining form that means either air or lung, the term for removal of an entire
pneumonectomy	lung is _____. The removal of the tonsils is called a
tonsillectomy	_____. Sometimes, the tonsils and adenoids are removed
tonsillectomy and	at the same time in a procedure called a _____ _____
adenoidectomy	_____ (T&A). The removal of a lung lobe is called
lobectomy	a _____.

ANSWERS	REVIEW
incision thoracotomy tracheotomy	**7.71** The suffix -*tomy* refers to an _____. An incision into the chest is called a _____. An incision into the trachea is a _____.
opening tracheostomy thoracostomy	**7.72** The operative suffix -*stomy* means surgical creation of an _____. The creation of an opening into the trachea, most often to insert a tube, is called a _____. The surgical creation of an opening into the chest is called _____. (Note that -*tomy* and -*stomy* have related but distinctly different meanings.)
-plasty thoracoplasty	**7.73** The suffix denoting surgical repair or reconstruction is _____. Thus, the surgical repair of the chest that involves fixing the ribs is called a _____.
puncture thoracentesis	**7.74** The suffix -*centesis* means a _____ for aspiration. A puncture that is made surgically for aspiration of fluid or air from the chest (pleural cavity) is called a _____. (Note that thoracocentesis is an acceptable term but is used less often than the shortened form: thoracentesis.)
examination thoracoscopy	**7.75** Recall that the suffix -*scopy* means process of _____. The endoscopic examination of the pleural cavity is called _____. Thoracoscopy is a surgical procedure because an incision must be made for insertion of the endoscope. In contrast, bronchoscopy and nasopharyngoscopy are diagnostic procedures because the scope is inserted through natural body openings.

 ## Self-Instruction: Therapeutic Terms

Study the following:

TERM	MEANING
cardiopulmonary resuscitation (CPR) *kar′dē-ō-pul′mo-nār-ē rē-sŭs-i-tā′shŭn*	method of artificial respiration and chest compressions to move oxygenated blood to vital body organs when breathing and the heart have stopped
continuous positive airway pressure (CPAP) therapy (Fig. 7-16) *kon-tin′yū-ŭs poz′i-tiv ār′wā presh′ŭr thār′ă-pē*	use of a device with a mask that pumps a constant pressurized flow of air through the nasal passages; commonly used during sleep to prevent airway closure in sleep apnea

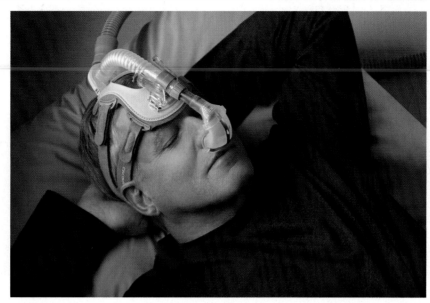

FIGURE 7-16 ■ **Patient wearing a continuous positive airway pressure (CPAP) mask.** (Photo courtesy of Respironics, Inc., Murrysville, PA.)

TERM	MEANING
endotracheal intubation *en'dō-trā'kē-ăl in-tū-bā'shŭn*	passage of a tube into the trachea via the nose or mouth to open the airway for delivering gas mixtures to the lungs (e.g., oxygen, anesthetics, or air)
incentive spirometry (Fig. 7-17) *in-sen'tiv spī-rom'ĕ-trē*	a common postoperative breathing therapy using a specially designed spirometer to encourage the patient to inhale and hold an inspiratory volume to exercise the lungs and prevent pulmonary complications
mechanical ventilation (Fig. 7-18) *mĕ-kan'i-kăl ven-ti-lā'shŭn*	mechanical breathing using a ventilator

COMMON THERAPEUTIC DRUG CLASSIFICATIONS

antibiotic *an'tē-bī-ot'ik*	a drug that kills or inhibits the growth of microorganisms
anticoagulant *an'tē-kō-ag'yū-lant*	a drug that dissolves, or prevents the formation of, thrombi or emboli in the blood vessels (e.g., heparin)
antihistamine *an-tē-his'tă-mēn*	a drug that neutralizes or inhibits the effects of histamine
histamine *his'tă-mēn*	a compound in the body that is released by injured cells during allergic reactions, inflammation, and so on, causing constriction of bronchial smooth muscle and dilation of blood vessels

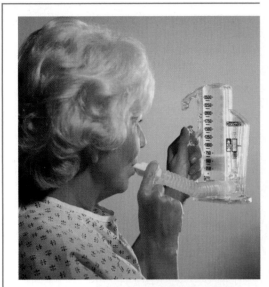

FIGURE 7-17 ■ Incentive spirometer.

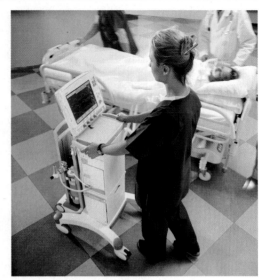

FIGURE 7-18 ■ Mechanical ventilation.

TERM	MEANING
bronchodilator *brong-kō-dī-lā' ter*	a drug that dilates the muscular walls of the bronchi
expectorant *ek-spek' tō-rănt*	a drug that breaks up mucus and promotes coughing

Programmed Review: Therapeutic Terms

ANSWERS	REVIEW
cardiopulmonary resuscitation	**7.76** CPR stands for _____ _____, a method of artificial respiration and chest compressions to move oxygenated blood to vital body organs when breathing and the heart have stopped.
continuous positive airway stopped	**7.77** A patient with sleep apnea may use a device that pumps pressurized air through the nasal passages to prevent airway closure during sleep. This treatment is called _____ _____ _____ pressure (CPAP) therapy. Recall that apnea means _____ breathing.
within endotracheal intubation	**7.78** The prefix *endo-* means _____. The passage of a tube within the trachea via the nose or mouth to deliver oxygen to the lungs is called _____ _____.

ANSWERS	REVIEW
measurement	**7.79** Recall that spirometry is the direct _____ of lung volume and capacity. A similar spirometer is used in postoperative breathing therapy to motivate the patient to inhale and hold a larger inspiratory volume. This therapy is called
incentive spirometry	_____ _____.
mechanical ventilation	**7.80** Mechanical breathing using a ventilator machine is called _____ _____.
against	**7.81** Recall that the prefix *anti-* means _____ or opposed to. Drug classes are commonly named for their actions, such as acting against some thing or process. A drug that acts to prevent the process of coagulation (forming of blood clots) is
anticoagulant	called an _____. The same prefix joined with the combining form for life (*bio*) denotes a drug class that acts to
antibiotic	kill or inhibit bacterial life. This drug is called an _____.
histamine	**7.82** A substance in the body that is released in allergic reactions, and that causes constriction of bronchial muscles, is called a _____. A drug that acts to inhibit the effects
antihistamine	of histamine is called an _____.
bronchodilator	**7.83** A person who has asthma may experience constriction of the bronchi during an attack. A therapeutic drug that counteracts this constriction by dilating the muscular walls of the bronchi is called a _____.
coughing	**7.84** Recall that expectoration means _____ up and spitting out material from the lungs. A type of drug that breaks
expectorant	up mucus to promote coughing is called an _____.

CHAPTER 7 ACRONYMS AND ABBREVIATIONS

ABBREVIATION	EXPANSION
ABG	arterial blood gas
AP	anterior-posterior
Bx	biopsy
COPD	chronic obstructive pulmonary disease
CPAP	continuous positive airway pressure

ABBREVIATION	EXPANSION
CPR	cardiopulmonary resuscitation
CT	computed tomography
CXR	chest x-ray
HIV	human immunodeficiency virus
LTB	laryngotracheobronchitis
MRI	magnetic resonance imaging
PA	posterior-anterior
$PaCO_2$	partial pressure of carbon dioxide
PaO_2	partial pressure of oxygen
PE	pulmonary embolism
PEFR	peak expiratory flow rate
PF	peak flow
PFT	pulmonary function testing
pH	potential of hydrogen
PSG	polysomnography
T&A	tonsillectomy and adenoidectomy
TB	tuberculosis
TV or V_T	tidal volume
URI	upper respiratory infection
VC	vital capacity
V/Q	ventilation-perfusion (scan)

CHAPTER 7 SUMMARY OF TERMS

The terms introduced in chapter 7 are listed below, followed by the page number on which each term can be found and its written pronunciation. For additional practice and reinforcement, write the definition of each term on a separate piece of paper.

adenoid/322
ad'ĕ-noyd

adenoidectomy/344
ad'ĕ-noy-dek'tŏ-mē

alveoli/323
al-vē'ō-lī

antibiotic/347
an'tē-bī-ot'ik

anticoagulant/347
an'tē-kō-ag'yū-lant

antihistamine/347
an-tē-his'tă-mēn

apnea/326
ap'nē-ă

arterial blood gas (ABG)/337
ar-tē'rē-ăl blŭd gas

asthma/330
az'mă

atelectasis/331
at-ĕ-lek'tă-sis

auscultation/338
aws-kŭl-tā'shŭn

bradypnea/325
brad-ip-nē'ă

bronchial tree/323
brong'kē-ăl trē

bronchiectasis/331
brong-kē-ek'tă-sis

bronchioles/323
brong'kē-ōlz

bronchitis/331
brong-kī'tis

bronchodilator/348
brong-kō-dī-lā'ter

bronchogenic carcinoma/331
brong-kō-jen'ik kar-si-nō'mă

bronchoscopy/338
brong-kos'kŏ-pē

bronchospasm/332
brong'kō-spazm

**cardiopulmonary resuscitation
(CPR)**/346
kar'dē-ō-pul'mo-nār-ē rē-sŭs-i-tā'shŭn

caseous necrosis/326
kā'zē-ŭs nĕ-krō'sis

chest x-ray (CXR)/340
chest x-rā

Cheyne-Stokes respiration/326
chān-stōks res-pi-rā'shŭn

**chronic obstructive pulmonary disease
(COPD)**/332
kron'ik ob-strŭk'tiv pūl'mō-nār-ē di-zēz'

cilia/323
sil'ē-ă

computed tomography (CT)/341
kom-pyū'tĕd tō-mog'ră-fē

**continuous positive airway pressure
(CPAP) therapy**/346
*kon-tin'yū-ŭs poz'i-tiv ār'wā presh'ŭr
thār'ă-pē*

crackles/326
krak'ĕlz

croup/332
krūp

cyanosis/327
sī-ă-nō'sis

cystic fibrosis/332
sis'tik fī-brō'sis

diaphragm/323
dī'ă-fram

dysphonia/327
dis-fō'nē-ă

dyspnea/326
disp-nē'ă

emphysema/332
em-fi-sē'mă

empyema/332
em-pī-ē'mă

endoscopy/337
en-dos'kŏ-pē

endotracheal intubation/347
en'dō-trā'kē-ăl in-tū-bā'shŭn

epiglottis/323
ep-i-glot'is

epistaxis/327
ep-i-stak'sis

eupnea/325
yūp-nē'ă

examination methods/338
ek-zam-i-nā'shŭn meth'ŏdz

expectorant/348
ek-spek'tō-rănt

expectoration/327
ek-spek-tō-rā'shŭn

glottis/323
glot'is

hard palate/322
hard pal'ăt

hemoptysis/327
hē-mop'ti-sis

hemothorax/332
hē-mō-thōr'aks

histamine/347
his'tă-mēn

hypercapnia/327
hī-pĕr-kap'nē-ă

hypercarbia/327
hī-pĕr-kar'bē-ă

hyperpnea/326
hī-pĕr-nē'ă

hyperventilation/327
hī'pĕr-ven-ti-lā'shŭn

hypocapnia/327
hī-pō-kap'nē-ă

hypocarbia/327
hī-pō-kar'bē-ă

hypopnea/326
hī-pop'nē-ă

hypoventilation/327
hī'pō-ven-ti-lā'shŭn

hypoxemia/327
hī-pok-sē'mē-ă

hypoxia/327
hī-pok'sē-ă

incentive spirometry/347
in-sen'tiv spī-rom'ĕ-trē

laryngitis/332
lar-in-jī'tis

laryngopharynx/322
lă-ring'gō-fă-ringks

laryngospasm/332
lă-ring'gō-spazm

laryngotracheobronchitis (LTB)/332
lă-ring'gō-trā'kē-o-brong-kī'tis

larynx/323
lar'ingks

lobectomy/344
lō-bek'tŏ-mē

lobes/323
lōbz

lung biopsy (Bx)/338
lŭng bī'op-sē

lung scan/338
lŭng skan

lungs/323
lŭngz

magnetic resonance imaging (MRI)/338
mag-net'ik rez'ō-nănts im'ă-jing

mechanical ventilation/347
mĕ-kan'i-kăl ven-ti-lā'shŭn

mediastinum/323
me'dē-as-tī'nŭm

mucous membranes/323
myū'kus mem'brānz

nasal polypectomy/344
nā'zăl pol'ip-ek'tŏ-mē

nasal polyposis/332
nā'zăl pol'i-pō'sis

nasopharyngoscopy/338
nā'zō-far'ing-gos'kŏ-pē

nasopharynx/322
nā-zō-fă'ringks

nose/322
nōz

obstructive lung disorder/327
ob-strŭk'tiv lŭng dis-ōr'der

oropharynx/322
ŏr'ō-fă-ringks

orthopnea/326
ŏr-thop-nē'ă

palate/322
pal'ăt

parenchyma/323
pă-reng'ki-mă

peak expiratory flow rate (PEFR)/338
pēk ek-spī'ră-tō-rē flō rāt

peak flow (PF)/338
pēk flō

percussion/338
pĕr-kŭsh'ŭn

pharyngitis/332
fă-rin-jī'tis

pharynx/322
fă'ringks

pleura/323
plū'ră

pleural cavity/323
plūr'ăl kav'i-tē

pleural effusion/332
plūr'ăl e-fyū'zhŭn

pleurisy/332
plūr'i-sē

pleuritis/332
plū-rī'tis

pneumoconiosis/332
nū'mō-kō-nē-ō'sis

***Pneumocystis* pneumonia**/333
nū-mō-sis'tis nū-mō'nē-ă

pneumohemothorax/334
nū'mō-hē-mō-thŏr'aks

pneumonectomy/344
nū'mō-nek'tŏ-mē

pneumonia/333
nū-mō'nē-ă

pneumonitis/334
nū-mō-nī'tis

pneumothorax/333
nū-mō-thŏr'aks

polysomnography (PSG)/338
pol'ē-som-nog'ră-fē

pulmonary angiography/341
pŭl'mō-nār-ē an-jē-og'ră-fē

pulmonary edema/327
pŭl'mō-nār-ē e-dē'mă

pulmonary embolism (PE)/334
pŭl'mō-nār-ē em'bō-lizm

pulmonary function testing (PFT)/338
pŭl'mō-nār-ē fŭnk'shŭn test'ing

pulmonary infiltrate/327
pŭl'mō-nār-ē in-fil'trāt

pulmonary tuberculosis (TB)/334
pŭl'mō-nār-ē tū-bĕr-kyū-lō'sis

pulse oximetry/340
pŭls ok-sim'ă-trē

pyothorax/332
pī-ō-thŏr'aks

rales/326
rahlz

restrictive lung disorder/327
rē-strik'tiv lŭng dis-ōr'dĕr

rhinorrhea/327
rī-nō-rē'ă

rhonchi/326
rong'kī

right bronchus and left bronchus/323
rīt brong'kŭs and left brong'kŭs

sinuses/322
sī'nŭs-ĕz

sinusitis/334
sī-nŭ-sī'tis

sleep apnea/334
slēp ap'nē-ă

soft palate/322
soft pal'ăt

spirometry/338
spī-rom'ĕ-trē

sputum/327
spyū'tŭm

stridor/326
strī'dōr

tachypnea/326
tak-ip-nē'ă

thoracentesis/344
thŏr'ă-sen-tē'sis

thoracoplasty/344
thŏr'ă-kō-plas-tē

thoracoscopy/344
thŏr-ă-kos'kŏ-pē

thoracostomy/344
thŏr-ă-kos'tŏ-mē

thoracotomy/344
thŏr-ă-kot'ō-mē

tidal volume (TV or V$_T$)/338
tī'dăl vol'yŭm

tonsillectomy/345
ton'si-lek'tŏ-mē

tonsillectomy and adenoidectomy (T&A)/345
ton'si-lek'tŏ-mē and ad'ĕ-noy-dek'tŏ-mē

tonsillitis/334
ton-si-lī'tis

tonsils/322
ton'silz

trachea/323
trā'kē-ă

tracheostomy/345
trā'kē-os'tŏ-mē

tracheotomy/345
trā'kē-ot'ŏ-mē

upper respiratory infection (URI)/334
up'er rĕs-par'uh-tōr-ē in-fek'shŭn

uvula/322
ū'vyū-lă

ventilation-perfusion (V/Q) scan/338
ven-ti-lā'shŭn-per-fyū'zhŭn skan

vital capacity (VC)/338
vīt-ăl kă-pas'i-tē

wheezes/326
wēz'ez

PRACTICE EXERCISES

For each of the following words, write out the term components (prefixes [P], combining forms [CF], roots [R], and suffixes [S]) on the lines below the word. Then define the term according to the meaning of its components.

EXAMPLE

intranasal

intra / _nas_ / _al_

P   R   S

DEFINITION: within/nose/pertaining to

1. pulmonology

_____ / _____

CF   S

DEFINITION: _____

2. thoracocentesis

_____ / _____

CF   S

DEFINITION: _____

3. nasosinusitis

_____ / _____ / _____

CF   R   S

DEFINITION: _____

4. hypoxemia

_____ / _____ / _____

P   R   S

DEFINITION: _____

5. pleuritis

_____ / _____

R   S

DEFINITION: _____

6. hypercarbia

_____ / _____ / _____

P   R   S

DEFINITION: _____

7. alveolar

_____ / _____

R   S

DEFINITION: _____

8. tracheotomy

_____ / _____

    CF   S

DEFINITION: _____

9. oronasal

_____ / _____ / _____

    CF   R   S

DEFINITION: _____

10. rhinorrhea

_____ / _____

    CF   S

DEFINITION: _____

11. thoracostomy

_____ / _____

    CF   S

DEFINITION: _____

12. tonsillectomy

_____ / _____

    R   S

DEFINITION: _____

13. tracheobronchitis

_____ / _____ / _____

    CF   R   S

DEFINITION: _____

14. bronchospasm

_____ / _____

    CF   S

DEFINITION: _____

15. laryngostenosis

_____ / _____ / _____

    CF   R   S

DEFINITION: _____

16. spirogram

_____ / _____

    CF   S

DEFINITION: _____

Identify the parts of the respiratory system by writing the missing words in the spaces provided:

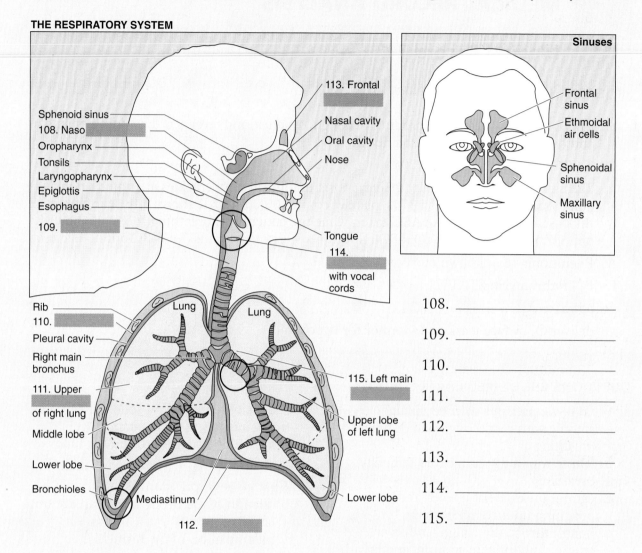

THE RESPIRATORY SYSTEM

Sphenoid sinus
108. Naso
Oropharynx
Tonsils
Laryngopharynx
Epiglottis
Esophagus
109.

113. Frontal
Nasal cavity
Oral cavity
Nose
Tongue
114.
with vocal cords

Sinuses
Frontal sinus
Ethmoidal air cells
Sphenoidal sinus
Maxillary sinus

Rib
110.
Pleural cavity
Right main bronchus
111. Upper
of right lung
Middle lobe
Lower lobe
Bronchioles
Mediastinum
112.

Lung   Lung

115. Left main
Upper lobe of left lung
Lower lobe

108. _____

109. _____

110. _____

111. _____

112. _____

113. _____

114. _____

115. _____

Circle the combining form that corresponds to the meaning given:

116. **nose**	ren/o	rhin/o	nos/o
117. **air or lung**	aden/o	pneum/o	thorac/o
118. **throat**	thorac/o	laryng/o	pharyng/o
119. **chest**	thorac/o	pneum/o	lapar/o
120. **voice box**	laryng/o	trache/o	pharyng/o
121. **breathing**	aer/o	spir/o	crin/o
122. **diaphragm**	phren/o	pleur/o	pneumon/o
123. **mouth**	ox/o	or/o	spir/o

MEDICAL RECORD ANALYSIS

Medical Record 7-1

PROGRESS NOTE

S: This is a 26 y.o. ♀ c/o a nonproductive cough, dyspnea, and fever × 2 d; pt does not smoke and has otherwise been in good health.

O: T 101°F, BP 100/64, R 25, P 104

Tachypnea is accompanied by mild cyanosis, and inspiratory crackles are noted upon auscultation. WBC 31,000, Hct 37%, platelet count 109,000. CXR shows diffuse infiltrates at the bases of both lungs. An ABG taken while the patient was breathing room air showed a pH of 7.54, $PaCO_2$ of 20, PaO_2 of 74. Sputum specimen contains 3+ WBC but no bacteria.

A: Pneumonia of unknown etiology

P: IV erythromycin STAT

admit to ICU

deliver O_2 by face mask and monitor for hypoxemia

QUESTIONS ABOUT MEDICAL RECORD 7-1

1. What is the patient's chief complaint?
   a. afebrile with a dry cough and difficulty breathing
   b. febrile with a dry cough and difficulty breathing
   c. cannot breathe, has a fever, and is coughing up material from the lungs
   d. hoarse throat, dry cough, and fever
   e. febrile, coughing up sputum, and breathing fast

2. What are the findings upon PE?
   a. slow breathing, blue skin, and rhonchi heard in the lungs as the patient exhales
   b. fast breathing, blue skin, and musical sounds heard in the lungs as the patient inhales
   c. slow breathing, blue skin, and rales heard in the lungs as the patient holds her breath
   d. fast heart, blue skin, and rales heard in the lungs as the patient inhales
   e. fast breathing, blue skin, and popping sounds heard in the lungs as the patient inhales

3. What did the chest x-ray show?
   a. tuberculosis
   b. asthma

c. density representing solid material usually indicating inflammation
   d. fluid filling spaces around the lungs
   e. lung cancer

4. What is the impression?
   a. dilation of the bronchi with an accumulation of mucus
   b. inflammation of the bronchi
   c. inflammation of the pleura
   d. inflammation of the lungs because of sensitivity to dust or chemicals
   e. inflammation of the lungs of unknown cause

5. What is an ABG?
   a. analysis of blood to determine the adequacy of lung function in the exchange of gases
   b. measurement of lung volume and capacity
   c. measurement of the flow of air during inspiration
   d. scan to detect breathing abnormalities
   e. image of the lungs used to visualize lung lesions

6. Describe the condition for which the patient was monitored while undergoing oxygen therapy:
   a. blockage of airflow out of the lungs
   b. excessive movement of air into and out of the lungs
   c. deficient amount of oxygen in the blood
   d. deficient amount of oxygen in the tissue cells
   e. excessive level of carbon dioxide in the blood

7. What is the Sig: on the erythromycin?
   a. not mentioned
   b. inject into a vein immediately
   c. take four immediately
   d. insert into the vagina immediately
   e. inject into a muscle immediately

Medical Record 7-2

FOR ADDITIONAL STUDY

Angelica Torrance, a retired painter who for years has boasted to friends that she has the good health of a 30-year-old, suffered a broken ankle when she slipped off a footstool in her basement. The surgical repair of her fracture at Central Medical Center was routine. Soon after surgery, however, Ms. Torrance developed other problems, and a pulmonologist was eventually called in for a consultation. Medical Record 7-2 is the history and physical examination report from Dr. Carl Brownley, the pulmonologist who consulted with Ms. Torrance's doctors after she developed breathing problems.

Read Medical Record 7-2 (pages 366-368), then write your answers to the following questions in the spaces provided.

QUESTIONS ABOUT MEDICAL RECORD 7-2

1. Below are medical terms used in this record that you have not yet encountered in this text. Underline each where it appears in the record, and define the term below.

   morphine _____

   heparin _____

   obese _____

2. In your own words, not using medical terminology, describe what surgery Ms. Torrance had for her broken ankle:

   _____

   _____

   _____

3. Describe in your own words the four symptoms that Ms. Torrance developed postsurgically:

   a. _____

   b. _____

   c. _____

   d. _____

4. Before Ms. Torrance's acute "sense of suffocating," she was being treated with what three pharmacologic treatments?

   a. _____

   b. _____

   c. _____

5. Immediately after her reported "sense of suffocating," Ms. Torrance was given what two treatments?

   a. _____

   b. _____

6. Put the following events that occurred in the hospital in correct order by numbering them from 1 to 8:

    _____ postoperative pulmonary symptoms

    _____ transport to intensive care

    _____ sense of suffocation

    _____ episode of tachycardia

    _____ nuclear lung scan showing high probability of embolus

    _____ evaluation for complications in the lungs

    _____ open reduction, internal fixation

    _____ intravenous drugs first administered

7. In your own words, not using medical terminology, describe the two diagnostic imaging studies performed the morning of 10/24:

    a. _____

    b. _____

8. Name and describe the test that was performed to monitor Ms. Torrance's heparin therapy:

    _____

    _____

    _____

9. Translate into lay language Dr. Brownley's first four assessments from the examination:

    a. _____

    b. _____

    c. _____

    d. _____

10. Dr. Brownley's recommendations include requests for certain tests to be run (or run again) and certain other actions to be taken while Ms. Torrance stays in the hospital. Without using abbreviations, list the tests to be performed and the actions to be taken:

    Tests:

    a. _____

    b. _____

    c. _____

    d. _____

    e. _____

    f. _____

    Actions:

    g. _____

    h. _____

Medical Record 7-2: For Additional Study

CENTRAL MEDICAL CENTER

211 Medical Center Drive • Central City, US 90000-1234 • PHONE: (012) 125-6784 • FAX: (012) 125-9999

HISTORY

DATE OF CONSULTATION:
October 24, 20xx

HISTORY:
The patient is a 75-year-old woman who is admitted to this hospital on October 18, 20xx, after having fractured her right ankle. She underwent an ORIF of this lesion. Upon emerging from surgery, it was noted that she was quite wheezy and was having copious, purulent secretions. She was started on antibiotics; however, fever, cough, and breathlessness persisted. Finally, she was evaluated on October 20, 20xx, for possible pulmonary complications. A V/Q scan at that time showed a high probability for pulmonary emboli, and she was started on IV Heparin along with her antibiotics and bronchodilators. The patient did well with resolution of symptoms and fever and was progressing to the point of discharge.

Late yesterday evening, however, the patient developed the acute onset of "a sense of suffocating." This lasted for about 20-30 minutes and did resolve somewhat with the application of nasal oxygen and morphine sulfate 2 mg. The patient denies any cough, mucus, or actual chest pressure or pain. She denies any wheezing during this episode. Her heart rate went as high as 115-120; however, she was normotensive.

She was transported to ICU for further evaluation and management. An ECG obtained at that time revealed slight ST segment depression and T wave flattening at V4-6 with sinus tachycardia. Arterial blood gases done during the episode on 7 L O_2 showed a PaO_2 of 78, a pH of 7.44, and a $PaCO_2$ of 35. This morning, a chest x-ray revealed continuing resolution of the right upper and right lower lobe infiltrates. A V/Q scan showed evidence of resolving multiple perfusion defects on the right that appeared to actually match the defects noted on the chest x-ray. PTT, which had been continually in control during her Heparin therapy, was as high as 150 on 7 units of Heparin per hour.

PAST MEDICAL HISTORY:
The patient denies a past history of chronic respiratory disease but did have severe pneumonia about 30 years ago. The patient is a nonsmoker who has never smoked, and she has an essentially negative past medical history.

ALLERGIES:
The patient denies any personal allergies, but her family all suffer from chronic post nasal drip.

(continued)

PULMONARY CONSULTATION Page 1	PT. NAME: TORRANCE, ANGELICA W. ID NO: IP-228904 ROOM NO: 663 ATT. PHYS. C. BROWNLEY, M.D.

Medical Record 7-2: For Additional Study (Continued)

CENTRAL MEDICAL CENTER

211 Medical Center Drive • Central City, US 90000-1234 • PHONE: (012) 125-6784 • FAX: (012) 125-9999

PHYSICAL EXAMINATION

GENERAL:
Well-nourished, somewhat overweight woman in no acute distress, having recently come back from x-ray with no undue dyspnea.

VITAL SIGNS:
BP: 110/70. Respirations: 16. Heart Rate: 80 and regular. Temperature: 99°.

CHEST:
LUNGS: Fair expansion bilaterally. Percussion node is normal. There are rare, distant end inspiratory rales at both bases

HEART: No clinical cardiomegaly. There are no murmurs or gallops.

ABDOMEN:
Obese, soft, nontender.

EXTREMITIES:
1+ pretibial edema on the left with a cast on the right.

ASSESSMENT:
1. ACUTE ONSET OF SHORTNESS OF BREATH OF UNCLEAR ETIOLOGY.
2. HYPOXIA.
3. HYPOTHROMBINEMIA (PATIENT ON HEPARIN).
4. STATUS POST PULMONARY EMBOLISM WITH RESOLUTION AND NO EVIDENCE OF RECURRENCE.
5. STATUS POST OPEN REDUCTION INTERNAL FIXATION OF TRIMALLEOLAR FRACTURE ON THE RIGHT.
6. RULE OUT ACUTE MYOCARDIAL INFARCTION VERSUS ISCHEMIA.
7. POSSIBLE MUCOUS PLUG.

(continued)

PULMONARY CONSULTATION Page 2	PT. NAME: TORRANCE, ANGELICA W. ID NO: IP-228904 ROOM NO: 663 ATT. PHYS. C. BROWNLEY, M.D.

Medical Record 7-2: For Additional Study (Continued)

CENTRAL MEDICAL CENTER

211 Medical Center Drive • Central City, US 90000-1234 • PHONE: (012) 125-6784 • FAX: (012) 125-9999

PHYSICAL EXAMINATION

RECOMMENDATIONS:
Cardiac enzymes should be obtained, and the ECG should be repeated as well. Recheck ABGs. Recheck PTT and discontinue Heparin until PTT diminishes to the 60s. Check CBC and comprehensive metabolic panel. Continue to observe in the ICU.

It is somewhat unclear as to what is the etiology of the episode of dyspnea. A possibility might be a mucous plug which has mobilized into the central airway and momentarily caused increased respiratory distress.

Thank you for the opportunity to assist in the management of this patient.

_____
C.Brownley, M.D.
Pulmonologist

CB:im

D: 10/24/20xx
T: 10/25/20xx

PULMONARY CONSULTATION Page 3	PT. NAME:	TORRANCE, ANGELICA W.
	ID NO:	IP-228904
	ROOM NO:	663
	ATT. PHYS.	C. BROWNLEY, M.D.

ANSWERS TO PRACTICE EXERCISES

1. pulmono / logy
   <u>CF</u>   <u>S</u>
   lung/study of

2. thoraco / centesis
   <u>CF</u>   <u>S</u>
   chest/puncture for
   aspiration

3. naso / sinus / itis
   <u>CF</u>   <u>R</u>   <u>S</u>
   nose/sinus/inflammation

4. hyp / ox / emia
   <u>P</u>   <u>R</u>   <u>S</u>
   below or deficient/
   oxygen/blood condition

5. pleur / itis
   <u>R</u>   <u>S</u>
   pleura/inflammation

6. hyper / carb / ia
   <u>P</u>   <u>R</u>   <u>S</u>
   above or excessive/
   carbon dioxide/
   condition of

7. alveol / ar
   <u>R</u>   <u>S</u>
   alveolus (air sac)/
   pertaining to

8. tracheo / tomy
   <u>CF</u>   <u>S</u>
   trachea/incision

9. oro / nas / al
   <u>CF</u> <u>R</u> <u>S</u>
   mouth/nose/
   pertaining to

10. rhino / rrhea
    <u>CF</u>   <u>S</u>
    nose/discharge

11. thoraco / stomy
    <u>CF</u>   <u>S</u>
    chest/creation of an
    opening

12. tonsill / ectomy
    <u>R</u>   <u>S</u>
    tonsil/excision (removal)

13. tracheo / bronch / itis
    <u>CF</u>   <u>R</u>   <u>S</u>
    trachea (windpipe)/
    bronchus/inflammation

14. broncho / spasm
    <u>CF</u>   <u>S</u>
    bronchus (airway)/
    involuntary contraction

15. laryngo / sten / osis
    <u>CF</u>   <u>R</u>   <u>S</u>
    larynx (voice box)/
    narrow/condition or
    increase

16. spiro / gram
    <u>CF</u>   <u>S</u>
    breathing/record

17. lob / ectomy
    <u>R</u>   <u>S</u>
    lobe (a portion)/excision
    (removal)

18. peri / pleur / al
    <u>P</u>   <u>R</u>   <u>S</u>
    around/pleura/
    pertaining to

19. stetho / scope
    <u>CF</u>   <u>S</u>
    chest/instrument for
    examination

20. pneumon / ic
    <u>R</u>   <u>S</u>
    air or lung/pertaining to

21. naso / pharyngo / scopy
    <u>CF</u>   <u>CF</u>   <u>S</u>
    nose/pharynx (throat)/
    process of examination

22. bronchiol / ectasis
    <u>R</u>   <u>S</u>
    bronchiole (little
    airway)/expansion or
    dilation

23. phreno / ptosis
    <u>CF</u>   <u>S</u>
    diaphragm/falling or
    downward displacement

24. pector / al
    <u>R</u>   <u>S</u>
    chest/pertaining to

25. uvulo / palato /pharyngo /
    <u>CF</u>   <u>CF</u>   <u>CF</u>
    plasty
    <u>S</u>
    uvula (grape)/palate/
    throat/surgical repair or
    reconstruction

26. pneumothorax
27. empyema or pyothorax
28. hemothorax
29. auscultation
30. bronchoscope
31. expectoration
32. pleurisy or pleuritis
33. percussion
34. hypoventilation
35. thoracentesis or thora-
    cocentesis
36. nuclear medicine
37. dysphonia
38. laryngitis
39. hypoxia
40. emphysema
41. epistaxis
42. bronchogenic carci-
    noma
43. cystic fibrosis
44. atelectasis
45. sputum
46. stridor
47. pulmonary embolism
48. tracheostomy
49. asthma
50. hyperventilation
51. *Pneumocystis* pneumonia
52. chronic obstructive pul-
    monary disease
53. pneumoconiosis
54. bronchiectasis
55. thoracoplasty
56. pneumonitis
57. spirometry
58. eupnea
59. bradypnea
60. dyspnea
61. orthopnea
62. apnea
63. tachypnea

64. peak expiratory flow rate
65. vital capacity
66. tuberculosis
67. cardiopulmonary resuscitation
68. chronic obstructive pulmonary disease
69. partial pressure of carbon dioxide
70. upper respiratory infection
71. tidal volume
72. pulmonary function testing
73. polysomnography
74. continuous positive airway pressure
75. CXR
76. ABG
77. T&A
78. e
79. h

80. g
81. f
82. i
83. j
84. d
85. c
86. b
87. a
88. auscultation
89. tachypnea
90. eupnea
91. pleurisy
92. hemothorax
93. stethoscope
94. epistaxis
95. rhonchi
96. hemoptysis
97. rhinorrhea
98. emphysema
99. atelectasis
100. orthopnea
101. asthma

102. hypoxia
103. dyspnea
104. pharynx
105. apnea
106. trachea
107. pleurisy
108. pharynx
109. trachea
110. pleura
111. lobe
112. diaphragm
113. sinus
114. larynx
115. bronchus
116. rhin/o
117. pneum/o
118. pharyng/o
119. thorac/o
120. laryng/o
121. spir/o
122. phren/o
123. or/o

ANSWERS TO MEDICAL RECORD ANALYSIS

Medical Record 7-1: Progress Note

1. b   2. e   3. c   4. e   5. a   6. c   7. b

Medical Record 7-2: For Additional Study

See CD-ROM for answers.

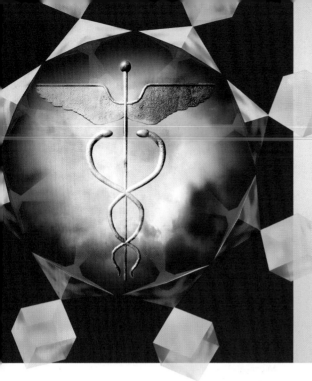

Nervous System and Psychiatry

NERVOUS SYSTEM OVERVIEW

The nervous system is an intricate communication network of neurons and other structures (Fig. 8-1) that activates and controls all functions of the body and receives all input from the environment. The nervous system has three divisions:

🔹 The **central nervous system** consists of the brain and spinal cord.

🔹 The **peripheral nervous system** consists of nerves branching from the central nervous system to all parts of the body.

🔹 The **autonomic nervous system** consists of nerves that carry involuntary impulses to smooth muscle, cardiac muscle, and various glands.

NEURON

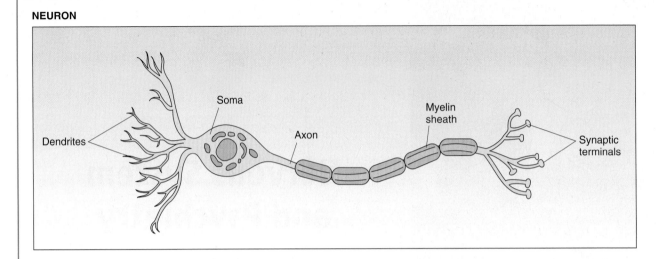

GLIAL CELLS

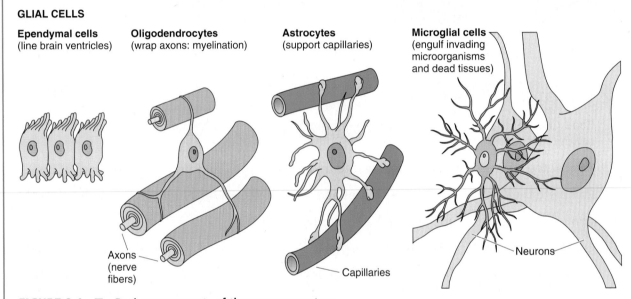

FIGURE 8-1 ■ **Basic components of the nervous system.**

 # Self-Instruction: Term Components

Study the following:

TERM COMPONENT	MEANING
COMBINING FORMS	
cerebr/o	cerebrum (largest part of the brain)
cerebell/o	cerebellum (little brain)
crani/o	skull
encephal/o	entire brain
esthesi/o	sensation
gangli/o	ganglion (knot)

TERM COMPONENT	MEANING
gli/o	glue
gnos/o	knowing
kinesi/o	movement
lex/o	word or phrase
mening/o, meningi/o	meninges (membrane)
myel/o	spinal cord or bone marrow
narc/o	stupor or sleep
neur/o	nerve
phas/o	speech
phob/o	exaggerated fear or sensitivity
phor/o	carry or bear
phren/o, psych/o, thym/o	mind
schiz/o	split
somat/o	body
somn/o, somn/i, hypn/o	sleep
spin/o	spine (thorn)
spondyl/o, vertebr/o	vertebra
stere/o	three-dimensional or solid
tax/o	order or coordination
thalam/o	thalamus (a room)
ton/o	tone or tension
top/o	place
ventricul/o	ventricle (belly or pouch)

PREFIX

cata-	down

SUFFIXES

-asthenia	weakness
-lepsy	seizure
-mania	condition of abnormal impulse toward
-paresis	slight paralysis
-plegia	paralysis

Programmed Review: Term Components

ANSWERS	REVIEW
cerebrum cerebrum spine encephal/o recording	**8.1** The combining form *cerebr/o* means _____ (largest part of the brain). Thus, the adjective cerebrospinal refers to something involving both the _____ and the _____. The combining form referring to the entire brain is _____, as in the term encephalography. Recall that the suffix *-graphy* means the process of _____.
crani/o	**8.2** The brain is housed inside the skull, the combining form for which is _____. The cranium, for example, is the term for the bones of the skull.
cerebell/o adjective cerebellar	**8.3** Another part of the brain is the cerebellum, the combining form for which is _____ (meaning "little brain"). The suffix *-ar* is an _____ ending. A common adjective referring to the cerebellum is _____.
ventricul/o -stomy ventricle	**8.4** Within the brain are interconnected cavities called ventricles. The combining form meaning ventricle is _____. Recall that the surgical suffix for the creation of an opening is _____. Thus, a ventriculostomy is the creation of an opening in a _____.
thalam/o incision	**8.5** The thalamus is a part of the brain. The combining form meaning thalamus is _____. A thalamotomy is an _____ into the thalamus.
meningi/o pouching meninges inflammation	**8.6** The brain and spinal cord are covered with a membrane called the meninges. The two combining forms for meninges are *mening/o* and _____. Recall that the suffix *-cele* means a hernia or _____. Therefore, a meningocele is a pouching of the _____. Meningitis is _____ of the meninges.
spin/o spinal	**8.7** The combining form meaning the spine is _____. The common adjective form is _____.
	8.8 Inside the spine is the spinal cord, a bundle of nerves coming down from the brain and, ultimately, connecting to all areas of the body. The combining form for the spinal cord (and

ANSWERS	REVIEW
myel/o spinal cord	also for bone marrow) is _____, as in the term myelitis, meaning inflammation of the _____ _____.
vertebra spondyl/o vertebral binding or joining vertebra	**8.9** The bones of the spine are vertebrae, the plural form of the term _____. The two combining forms meaning vertebra are *vertebr/o* and _____. A common adjective form made with the first combining form is _____. Spondylosyndesis, meaning spinal fusion, is an example of a term using the second combining form. Syndesis is a surgical technique of _____ together, and *spondyl/o* means _____.
neur/o neurology	**8.10** Nerve cells exist in the brain, spinal cord, and throughout the nervous system. The combining form meaning nerve is _____. The medical specialty studying the nervous system therefore is called _____.
gangli/o ganglia	**8.11** A ganglion is a structure of nerves in the peripheral nervous system. The combining form for ganglion is _____, as in the term ganglioneuroma, a neoplasm affecting ganglions. The other plural form of ganglion is _____.
gli/o glial	**8.12** Glial cells in the nervous system help hold together (glue together) the neurons, which are the primary nervous system cells. The combining term for glue is _____. A common adjective form is _____.
somat/o body	**8.13** Almost all functions in the body are regulated through the nervous system. The combining form meaning body is _____, as in the term psychosomatic, which refers to influences of the mind on the _____.
psych/o, thym/o mind mind faulty	**8.14** The three combining forms meaning mind are *phren/o*, _____, and _____, as in the terms schizophrenia, psychiatry, and dysthymia. Schizophrenia refers to a split _____. Psychiatry is the medical specialty centered on the diagnosis, treatment, and prevention of disorders of the _____. A dysthymia is a psychiatric disorder; the prefix *dys-* means painful, difficult, or _____.

ANSWERS	REVIEW
schiz/o split	**8.15** The combining form meaning split is _____. The thoughts of a patient with schizophrenia are said to be _____ from reality.
gnos/o	**8.16** The combining form that means knowing and is the basis of the term gnosia (meaning the ability to perceive and recognize) is _____.
esthesi/o excessive	**8.17** All physical sensations throughout the body are perceived by the brain. The combining form meaning sensation is _____, as in the term hyperesthesia, an abnormally heightened sensitivity to sensations. The prefix *hyper-* means above or _____.
kinesi/o movement	**8.18** The nervous system also controls body movement. The combining form meaning movement is _____, as in the term kinesiology, which is the study of body _____.
phas/o without adjective	**8.19** The combining form meaning speech is _____. Aphasia is a condition of language loss in which one is often unable to speak. (Recall that the prefix *a-* means _____.) Aphasic is the _____ form of the term.
phrase dyslexia	**8.20** *Lex/o* is a combining form meaning word or _____. A person with a condition of difficulty understanding written or spoken words or phrases is said to have _____.
phob/o	**8.21** Someone with a phobia has an exaggerated fear of or sensitivity to something. The combining form for phobia is _____.
somn/i record sleep many sleep condition	**8.22** Three specific combining forms mean sleep: *somn/o*, _____, and *hypn/o*. Polysomnography, for example, makes a _____ of various physiologic changes that occur during _____. Recall that the prefix *poly-* means _____. Hypnosis is the condition of being in a _____-like state by suggestion. Recall that the suffix *-osis* means increase or _____.
	8.23 Different from the sleep state, a state of stupor can result in various conditions. The combining form meaning stupor is

ANSWERS	REVIEW
narc/o stupor	_____, as in the term narcotic, referring to a class of drugs that induce _____.
carry good	**8.24** The combining form *phor/o* means to bear or _____. Recall that the prefix *eu-* means normal or _____ (well). Thus, the term euphoria, meaning an exaggerated sense of well-being, originates from term components meaning to carry well.
stere/o	**8.25** The combining form meaning three-dimensional or solid is _____, as in the term stereotaxic, referring to an apparatus allowing precise localization in space.
ton/o tone one	**8.26** The combining form meaning tone or tension is _____, as in the term monotone, which refers to speaking in an unchanging single _____. Recall that the prefix *mono-* means _____.
coordination without, condition of ataxia	**8.27** *Tax/o* is a combining form meaning order or _____. Combined with the prefix *a-*, meaning _____, and the suffix *-ia,* meaning _____, the term describing a condition of inability to coordinate muscle movements is _____.
top/o place	**8.28** The combining form for place is _____. For example, the term topesthesia refers to the ability to localize the _____ on which the skin is touched.
down	**8.29** The prefix *cata-* means _____. The term catatonia, for example, which means a state of being unresponsive and unmoving, comes from word roots meaning that all muscle activity is down.
-asthenia weakness	**8.30** The suffix meaning weakness is _____, as in the term myasthenia, which is a condition involving _____ of the muscles (*my/o* = muscle).
sleep -lepsy	**8.31** The term narcolepsy is made from the secondary meaning of the combining form *narc/o*, which is _____, and the suffix _____, meaning seizure. In narcolepsy, sleep comes on unexpectedly and suddenly, as in a seizure.

ANSWERS	REVIEW
impulse or attraction death fear	**8.32** The term mania means a state of abnormal elation and increased activity. The suffix -*mania*, however, refers to an abnormal _____ toward something. For example, necromania is an abnormal attraction to _____. Compare this with necrophobia, which is an abnormal _____ of death.
-paresis half hemi-	**8.33** The suffix meaning a slight paralysis is _____, as in the term hemiparesis, meaning a slight paralysis in _____ of the body (right or left). Recall that the prefix meaning half is _____.
paralysis	**8.34** The suffix -*plegia* means _____, as in the term paraplegia, referring to paralysis of the legs and lower trunk.

◈ Self-Instruction: Anatomic Terms

Study the following:

TERM	MEANING
CENTRAL NERVOUS SYSTEM	
central nervous system (CNS) *sen'trăl nĕr'vŭs sis'tĕm*	brain and spinal cord
brain (Fig. 8-2) *brān*	portion of the central nervous system contained within the cranium
cerebrum *ser'ĕ-brŭm*	largest portion of the brain; divided into right and left halves, known as *cerebral hemispheres,* which are connected by a bridge of nerve fibers called the *corpus callosum*; lobes of the cerebrum are named after the skull bones they underlie
frontal lobe *frŏn'tăl lōb*	anterior section of each cerebral hemisphere; responsible for voluntary muscle movement and personality
parietal lobe *pă-rī'ĕ-tăl lōb*	portion posterior to the frontal lobe; responsible for sensations such as pain, temperature, and touch
temporal lobe *tem'pŏ-răl lōb*	portion that lies below the frontal lobe; responsible for hearing, taste, and smell
occipital lobe *ok-sip'i-tăl lōb*	portion posterior to the parietal and temporal lobes; responsible for vision
cerebral cortex *ser'ĕ-brăl kōr'teks*	outer layer of the cerebrum consisting of gray matter; responsible for higher mental functions (*cortex* = bark)

A

Central sulcus

Frontal lobe

Parietal lobe

Olfactory bulbs

Temporal lobe

Medulla oblongata

Occipital lobe

Cerebellum

Spinal cord

B

Motor area

Speech area, Expression

Somatosensory

Taste

Body awareness

Auditory

Vision

Speech reception

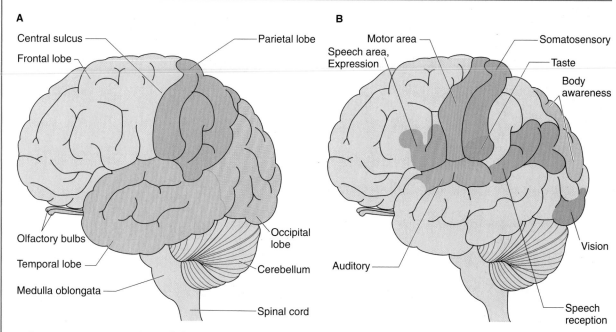

FIGURE 8-2 ■ **A. Lobes of the brain. B. Localized functions of the cerebrum.**

TERM	MEANING
thalamus *thal'ă-mŭs* **diencephalon** *dī-en-sef'ă-lon*	each of two gray matter nuclei deep within the brain; responsible for relaying sensory information to the cortex
gyri *jī'rī*	convolutions (mounds) of the cerebral hemispheres
sulci *sŭl'sī*	shallow grooves that separate gyri
fissures *fish'ŭrz*	deep grooves in the brain
cerebellum (Fig. 8-3) *ser-e-bel'ŭm*	portion of the brain located below the occipital lobes of the cerebrum; responsible for control and coordination of skeletal muscles
brainstem *brān'stem*	region of the brain that serves as a relay between the cerebrum, cerebellum, and spinal cord; responsible for breathing, heart rate, and body temperature; the three levels are the mesencephalon (midbrain), pons, and medulla oblongata
ventricles (Fig. 8-4) *ven'tri-kĕlz*	series of interconnected cavities within the cerebral hemispheres and brainstem filled with cerebrospinal fluid
cerebrospinal fluid (CSF) *ser'ĕ-brō-spī'năl flū'id*	plasma-like clear fluid circulating in and around the brain and spinal cord
spinal cord *spī'năl kōrd*	column of nervous tissue from the brainstem through the vertebrae; responsible for nerve conduction to and from the brain and the body

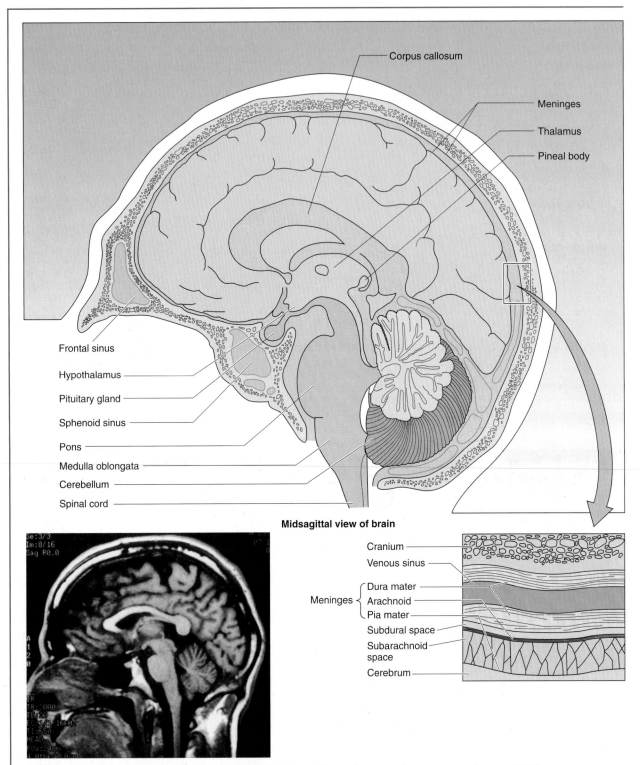

FIGURE 8-3 ■ **Midsagittal view of the brain. Inset: Normal magnetic resonance image (MRI).**

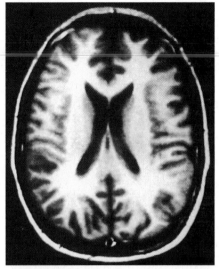

Magnetic resonance image, horizontal view A

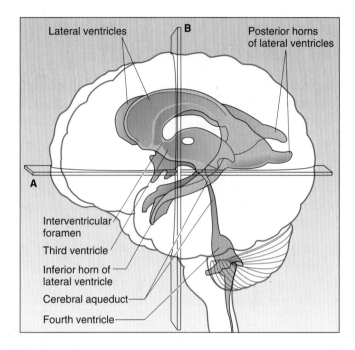

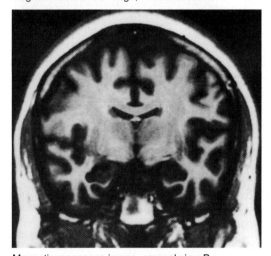

Magnetic resonance image, coronal view B

FIGURE 8-4 ■ **Ventricles of the brain.**

TERM	MEANING
meninges *mĕ-nin'jēz*	three membranes that cover the brain and spinal cord, consisting of the dura mater, pia mater, and arachnoid mater
PERIPHERAL NERVOUS SYSTEM	
peripheral nervous system (PNS) *pĕ-rif'ĕ-răl nĕr'vŭs sis'tĕm*	nerves that branch from the central nervous system including nerves of the brain (cranial nerves) and spinal cord (spinal nerves)
cranial nerves *krā'nē-ăl nĕrvz*	12 pairs of nerves arising from the brain
spinal nerves *spī'năl nĕrvz*	31 pairs of nerves arising from the spinal cord

TERM	MEANING
sensory nerves *sen'sŏ-rē nĕrvz*	nerves that conduct impulses from body parts and carry sensory information to the brain; also called afferent nerves (*ad* = toward; *ferre* = carry)
motor nerves *mō'tŏr nĕrvz*	nerves that conduct motor impulses from the brain to muscles and glands; also called efferent nerves (*e* = out; *ferre* = carry)

AUTONOMIC NERVOUS SYSTEM

autonomic nervous system (ANS) *aw-tō-nom'ik nĕr'vŭs sis'tĕm*	nerves that carry involuntary impulses to smooth muscle, cardiac muscle, and various glands
hypothalamus *hī'pō-thal'ă-mŭs*	control center for the autonomic nervous system located below the thalamus (diencephalon)
sympathetic nervous system *sim-pă-thet'ik nĕr'vŭs sis'tĕm*	division of the autonomic nervous system that is concerned primarily with preparing the body in stressful or emergency situations
parasympathetic nervous system *par-ă-sim-pă-thet'ik nĕr'vŭs sis'tĕm*	division of the autonomic nervous system that is most active in ordinary conditions; it counterbalances the effects of the sympathetic system by restoring the body to a restful state after a stressful experience

🔷 Programmed Review: Anatomic Terms

ANSWERS	REVIEW
central brain	**8.35** The brain and spinal cord comprise the _____ nervous system. The _____ is the part of the central nervous system within the cranium.
cerebrum frontal lobe	**8.36** The largest portion of the brain, the _____, is divided into the two cerebral hemispheres. The lobe at the front of each cerebral hemisphere, called the _____ _____, controls muscle movement and personality. Behind the frontal lobe is the parietal lobe.
parietal	**8.37** The lobe behind the frontal lobe, called the _____ lobe, is responsible for sensations such as pain, temperature, and touch. Below the frontal lobe is the temporal lobe.
temporal	**8.38** The lobe below the frontal lobe, called the _____ lobe, is responsible for hearing, taste, and smell. Posterior to the parietal and temporal lobes is the occipital lobe.

ANSWERS	REVIEW
occipital	**8.39** The lobe posterior to the parietal and temporal lobes, the _____ lobe, is responsible for vision.
cortex	**8.40** The Latin word cortex means bark, referring to an outer layer. The outer layer of the cerebrum is the cerebral _____, which is the gray matter responsible for higher mental functions. Sensory information is relayed to the cortex by the thalamus (diencephalon).
thalamus, diencephalon thalami	**8.41** The two gray matter nuclei deep within the brain that relay sensory information to the cortex are called the _____ or _____. The plural of thalamus is _____.
gyri, gyrus sulci sulcus fissures	**8.42** Gyri, sulci, and fissures are physical characteristics of the cerebral hemispheres. Convolutions (mounds) of the hemispheres are called _____. The singular of gyri is _____. The shallow grooves that separate gyri are called _____. The singular of sulci is _____. The deep grooves in the brain are called _____.
cerebellum	**8.43** Below the occipital lobes is the cerebellum. The _____ is responsible for controlling skeletal muscles. The cerebellum and cerebrum both communicate with the spinal cord through the brainstem.
brainstem	**8.44** The spinal cord communicates with the cerebrum and cerebellum through the _____, which is also responsible for breathing, heart rate, and body temperature. Interconnected cavities within the brainstem and cerebral hemispheres are called ventricles.
ventricles cerebrospinal	**8.45** Cerebrospinal fluid fills the _____, which are the cavities in the cerebral hemispheres and brainstem. The plasma-like fluid circulating in and around the brain and spinal cord is called the _____ fluid.
spinal cord	**8.46** The column of nervous tissue that descends from the brainstem though the vertebrae of the spine is the _____. The spinal cord and brain are covered by membranes called meninges.

ANSWERS	REVIEW
meninges	**8.47** The three membranes covering the brain are called the _____ .
peripheral cranial spinal	**8.48** Nerves branch from the central nervous system to the peripheral nervous system to reach all areas of the body. Cranial nerves, spinal nerves, sensory nerves, and motor nerves are all part of the _____ nervous system. The 12 pairs of nerves arising from the brain are the _____ nerves. The 31 pairs of nerves arising from the spinal cord are the _____ nerves.
sensory motor	**8.49** The nerves in the peripheral nervous system that carry sensory information to the brain are the _____ nerves. The nerves that carry motor impulses from the brain to the muscles and glands are the _____ nerves.
autonomic	**8.50** The autonomic nervous system controls involuntary functions of smooth muscle, cardiac muscle, and various glands. The hypothalamus is the control center for the _____ nervous system.
hypothalamus below	**8.51** The autonomic nervous system is controlled by the _____ , which is located below the thalamus. Recall that the prefix *hypo-* means _____ or deficient.
sympathetic parasympathetic	**8.52** The sympathetic nervous system and the parasympathetic nervous system are divisions of the autonomic nervous system. In stressful or emergency situations, the _____ nervous system prepares the body. In most ordinary conditions, the _____ nervous system is more active, counterbalancing the effects of the sympathetic nervous system.

Self-Instruction: Nervous System Symptomatic Terms

Study the following:

TERM	MEANING
aphasia ă-fā′zē-ă **dysphasia** dis-fā′zē-ă	impairment because of localized brain injury that affects the understanding, retrieving, and formulating of meaningful and sequential elements of language, as demonstrated by an inability to use or comprehend words; occurs as a result of a stroke, head trauma, or disease

Glasgow Coma Scale			A.M.		P.M.				A.M.						
Assessment	Reaction	Score	8	10	12	2	4	6	8	10	12	2	4	6	8
Eye Opening	Spontaneously	4	X							X	X	X	X	X	
Response	To speech	3		X			X								
	To pain	2			X	X	X								
	No response	1													
Motor Response	Obeys verbal command	6	X							X	X	X	X	X	
	Localizes pain	5		X	X										
	Flexion withdrawal	4				X		X							
	Flexion	3					X								
	Extension	2													
	No response	1													
Verbal Response	Oriented x3	5	X							X	X	X	X	X	
	Conversation confused	4		X			X								
	Inappropriate speech	3			X										
	Incomprehensible sounds	2				X	X								
	No response	1													

FIGURE 8-5 ■ Glasgow Coma Scale scoring for a child. A score of 3 to 8 denotes severe trauma; 9 to 12, moderate trauma; and 13 to 15, slight trauma. Note the gradual improvement from coma in this example.

TERM	MEANING
coma (Fig. 8-5) *kō'mă*	a general term referring to levels of decreased consciousness with varying responsiveness; a common method of assessment is the Glasgow Coma Scale
delirium *dē-lir'ē-ŭm*	a state of mental confusion caused by disturbances in cerebral function; the many causes include fever, shock, and drug overdose (*deliro* = to draw the furrow awry when plowing, to go off the rails)
dementia *dē-men'shē-ă*	an impairment of intellectual function characterized by memory loss, disorientation, and confusion (*dementio* = to be mad)
motor deficit *mō'tŏr def'i-sit*	loss or impairment of muscle function
sensory deficit *sen'sŏ-rē def'i-sit*	loss or impairment of sensation
neuralgia *nū-ral'jē-ă*	pain along the course of a nerve
paralysis *pă-ral'i-sis*	temporary or permanent loss of motor control

TERM	MEANING
flaccid paralysis *flak'sid pă-ral'i-sis*	defective (flabby) or absent muscle control caused by a nerve lesion
spastic paralysis *spas'tik pă-ral'i-sis*	stiff and awkward muscle control caused by a central nervous system disorder
hemiparesis *hem'ē-pă-rē'sis*	partial paralysis of the right or left half of the body
sciatica *sī-at'i-kă*	pain that follows the pathway of the sciatic nerve, caused by compression or trauma of the nerve or its roots
seizure *sē'zhŭr*	sudden, transient disturbances in brain function resulting from an abnormal firing of nerve impulses; may or may not be associated with convulsion
convulsion *kon-vŭl'shŭn*	to pull together; type of seizure that causes a series of sudden, involuntary contractions of muscles
syncope *sin'kŏ-pē*	fainting
tactile stimulation *tak'til stim-yū-lā'shŭn*	evoking a response by touching
hyperesthesia *hī'pĕr-es-thē'zē-ă*	increased sensitivity to stimulation such as touch or pain
paresthesia *par-es-thē'zē-ă*	abnormal sensation of numbness and tingling without objective cause

◈ Programmed Review: Nervous System Symptomatic Terms

ANSWERS	REVIEW
speech without condition of aphasia	**8.53** Linking *phas/o* (the combining form meaning _____) with *a-* (the prefix meaning _____) and *–ia* (the suffix meaning _____ _____) forms the term describing one's inability to use or comprehend words due to localized brain injury (such as occurs as the result of a stroke): _____.
faulty dysphasia	**8.54** The prefix *dys-* means painful, difficult, or _____, and is used in the less common synonym for aphasia: _____.
coma	**8.55** A decreased level of consciousness, measured with the Glasgow Coma Scale, is called a _____.
delirium dementia	**8.56** Mental and intellectual function can be disturbed by medical or psychiatric conditions or drugs. A state of mental confusion resulting from disturbed cerebral function is called _____. The impairment of intellectual function characterized by memory loss and disorientation is _____.

ANSWERS	REVIEW
motor sensory	**8.57** A deficit is a loss or impairment related to a nervous system problem. The loss of muscle function is called a _____ deficit. The loss of sensation is called a _____ deficit.
neur/o pain neuralgia	**8.58** The combining form meaning nerve is _____. Recall that the suffix -*algia* means _____. Therefore, the term for pain along the course of a nerve is _____.
paralysis flaccid spastic	**8.59** A temporary or permanent loss of motor control is called _____. A nerve lesion that causes a lack of muscle control, resulting in flabby muscles that do not move, is called _____ paralysis. Stiff, awkward muscle control caused by a central nervous system disorder is called _____ paralysis.
-paresis hemi- hemiparesis	**8.60** The suffix meaning partial paralysis is _____. Recall that the prefix meaning half is _____. The term for partial paralysis of the right or left half of the body is _____.
sciatica	**8.61** The sciatic nerve runs down the leg. Pain along its pathway caused by compression or trauma to this nerve is called _____.
seizure convulsion	**8.62** A sudden, transient disturbance of brain function that results from abnormal firing of nerve impulses is called a _____. A type of seizure that involves sudden, involuntary muscle contractions is termed _____.
syncope	**8.63** The Greek word synkope means cutting short or swoon. From this word, the medical term for fainting is _____.
tactile	**8.64** The process of evoking a response by touching a person's skin is called _____ stimulation.
condition of esthesi/o excessive hyperesthesia	**8.65** Again, the suffix -*ia* means _____ ____. The combining form meaning sensation is _____. The prefix *hyper-* means above or _____. From these three word parts comes the term meaning a condition of increased sensitivity to the sensations of touch and pain: _____.
abnormal paresthesia	**8.66** Recall that the prefix *para-* means alongside of or _____. The term for a condition of an abnormal sensation of numbness and tingling is _____.

Self-Instruction: Nervous System Diagnostic Terms

Study the following:

TERM	MEANING
agnosia *ag-nō′zē-ă*	any of many types of loss of neurologic function involving interpretation of sensory information
astereognosis *ă-stĕr′ē-og-nō′sis*	inability to judge the form of an object by touch (e.g., a coin from a key)
atopognosis *ă-top-og-nō′sis*	inability to locate a sensation properly, such as an inability to locate a point touched on the body
Alzheimer disease *awlz′hī-mĕr di-zēz′*	disease of structural changes in the brain resulting in an irreversible deterioration that progresses from forgetfulness and disorientation to loss of all intellectual functions, total disability, and death
amyotrophic lateral sclerosis (ALS) *ă-mī-ō-trō′fik lat′ĕr-ăl sklĕ-rō′sis*	condition of progressive deterioration of motor nerve cells resulting in total loss of voluntary muscle control; symptoms advance from muscle weakness in the arms and legs, to the muscles of speech, swallowing, and breathing, to total paralysis and death; also known as Lou Gehrig disease
cerebral palsy (CP) *ser′ĕ-brăl pawl′zē*	condition of motor dysfunction caused by damage to the cerebrum during development or injury at birth; characterized by partial paralysis and lack of muscle coordination (*palsy* = paralysis)
cerebrovascular disease *ser′ĕ-brō-vas′kyū-lăr di-zēz′*	disorder resulting from a change within one or more blood vessels of the brain
cerebral arteriosclerosis *ser′ĕ-brăl ar-tēr′ē-ō-skler-ō′sis*	hardening of the arteries of the brain
cerebral atherosclerosis *ser′ĕ-brăl ath′er-ō-skler-ō′sis*	condition of lipid (fat) buildup within the blood vessels of the brain (*ather/o* = fatty [lipid] paste)
cerebral aneurysm *ser′ĕ-brăl an′yū-rizm*	dilation of a blood vessel in the brain (*aneurysm* = dilation or widening)
cerebral thrombosis *ser′ĕ-brăl throm-bō′sis*	presence of a stationary clot in a blood vessel of the brain
cerebral embolism *ser′ĕ-brăl em′bo-lizm*	obstruction of a blood vessel in the brain by an embolus transported through the circulation
cerebrovascular accident (CVA) (Fig. 8-6) *ser′ĕ-brō-vas′kyū-lăr ak′si-dent* **stroke** *strōk*	damage to the brain caused by cerebrovascular disease, such as occlusion of a blood vessel by a thrombus or embolus (ischemic stroke) or intracranial hemorrhage after rupture of an aneurysm (hemorrhagic stroke)
transient ischemic attack (TIA) (Fig. 8-7) *tranz′ē-ent is-kē′mik ă-tak′*	brief episode of loss of blood flow to the brain, usually caused by a partial occlusion that results in temporary neurologic deficit (impairment); often precedes a CVA
encephalitis *en-sef-ă-lī′tis*	inflammation of the brain

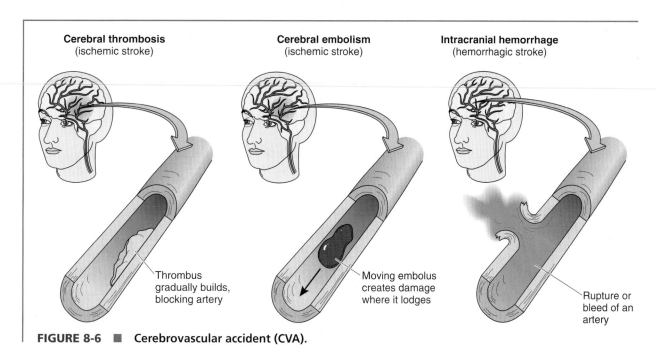

Cerebral thrombosis
(ischemic stroke)

Cerebral embolism
(ischemic stroke)

Intracranial hemorrhage
(hemorrhagic stroke)

Thrombus
gradually builds,
blocking artery

Moving embolus
creates damage
where it lodges

Rupture or
bleed of an
artery

FIGURE 8-6 ■ **Cerebrovascular accident (CVA).**

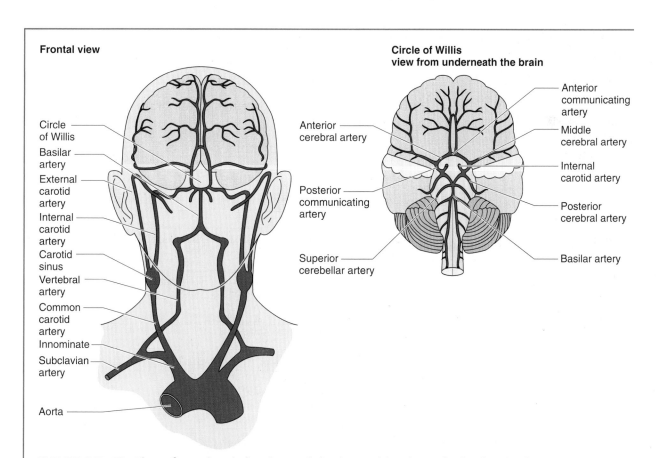

Frontal view

Circle of Willis
view from underneath the brain

Circle
of Willis

Basilar
artery

External
carotid
artery

Internal
carotid
artery

Carotid
sinus

Vertebral
artery

Common
carotid
artery

Innominate

Subclavian
artery

Aorta

Anterior
cerebral artery

Posterior
communicating
artery

Superior
cerebellar artery

Anterior
communicating
artery

Middle
cerebral artery

Internal
carotid artery

Posterior
cerebral artery

Basilar artery

FIGURE 8-7 ■ **Sites of transient ischemic attack (TIA): carotid and vertebrobasilar circulation.**

TERM	MEANING
epilepsy (*see* Fig. 8-12) *ep'i-lep'sē*	disorder affecting the central nervous system; characterized by recurrent seizures
tonic-clonic seizure *ton'ik-klon'ik sē'zhŭr*	stiffening-jerking; a major motor seizure involving all muscle groups; previously termed grand mal (big bad) seizure
absence seizure *ab'sens sē'zhŭr*	seizure involving a brief loss of consciousness without motor involvement; previously termed petit mal (little bad) seizure
partial seizure *par'shăl sē'zhŭr*	seizure involving only limited areas of the brain with localized symptoms
glioma *glī-ō'mă*	tumor of glial cells graded according to degree of malignancy
herniated disk or **disc** (Fig. 8-8) *hĕr'nē-ā-tĕd disk*	protrusion of a degenerated or fragmented intervertebral disk so that the nucleus pulposus protrudes, causing compression on the nerve root
herpes zoster *hĕr'pēz zos'tĕr*	viral disease affecting the peripheral nerves, characterized by painful blisters that spread over the skin following the affected nerves, usually unilateral; also known as shingles
Huntington chorea *hŭn'ting-tŏn kōr-ē'ă* **Huntington disease (HD)** *hŭn'ting-tŏn di-zēz'*	hereditary disease of the central nervous system characterized by bizarre, involuntary body movements and progressive dementia (*choros* = dance)
hydrocephalus (Fig. 8-9) *hī-drŏ-sef'ă-lŭs*	abnormal accumulation of cerebrospinal fluid in the ventricles of the brain as a result of developmental anomalies, infection, injury, or tumor
meningioma *mĕ-nin'jē-ō'mă*	benign tumor of the coverings of the brain (the meninges)
meningitis *men-in-jī'tis*	inflammation of the meninges

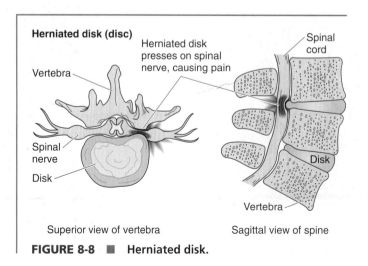

FIGURE 8-8 ▬ Herniated disk.

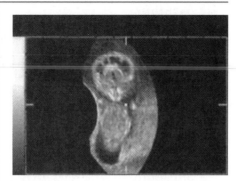

FIGURE 8-9 ■ Sonogram showing hydrocephalus in early pregnancy.

TERM	MEANING
migraine headache *mī'grăn hed'ăk*	paroxysmal (sudden, periodic) attacks of mostly unilateral headache, often accompanied by disordered vision, nausea, or vomiting, lasting hours or days and caused by dilation of arteries
multiple sclerosis (MS) (Fig. 8-10) *mŭl'ti-pul sklĕ-rō'sis*	disease of the central nervous system characterized by the demyelination (deterioration of the myelin sheath) of nerve fibers, with episodes of neurologic dysfunction (exacerbation) followed by recovery (remission)

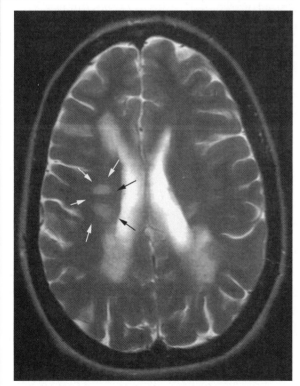

FIGURE 8-10 ■ Magnetic resonance image (MRI) of the brain. Arrows indicate plaque formation in patient with multiple sclerosis.

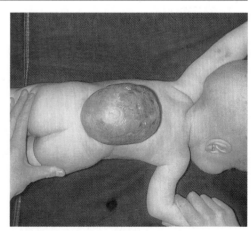

FIGURE 8-11 ■ Spina bifida with myelomeningocele. The infant also has hydrocephaly.

TERM	MEANING
myasthenia gravis *mī-as-thē′nē-ă gra′vis*	autoimmune disorder that affects the neuromuscular junction, causing a progressive decrease in muscle strength; activity resumes and strength returns after a period of rest
myelitis *mī′ĕ-lī′tis*	inflammation of the spinal cord
narcolepsy *nar′kō-lep-sē*	sleep disorder characterized by a sudden, uncontrollable need to sleep, attacks of paralysis (cataplexy), and dreams intruding while awake (hypnagogic hallucinations)
neural tube defects *nūr′ăl tūb dē′fektz*	congenital deformities of the brain and spinal cord caused by incomplete development of the neural tube, the embryonic structure that forms the nervous system
anencephaly *an′en-sef′ă-lē*	defect in closure of the cephalic portion of the neural tube that results in incomplete development of the brain and bones of the skull; the most drastic neural tube defect usually results in a stillbirth
spina bifida (Fig. 8-11) *spī′nă bĭ′fi-dă*	defect in development of the spinal column characterized by the absence of vertebral arches, often resulting in pouching of the meninges (meningocele) or of the meninges and spinal cord (meningomyelocele); considered to be the most common neural tube defect (*spina* = spine; *bifida* = split into two parts)
Parkinson disease *pahr′kin-sĕn di-zēz′*	condition of slowly progressive degeneration in an area of the brainstem (substantia nigra) resulting in a decrease of dopamine (a chemical neurotransmitter necessary for proper movement); characterized by tremor, rigidity of muscles, and slow movements (bradykinesia); usually occurs later in life
plegia *plē′jē-ă*	paralysis
hemiplegia *hem-ē-plē′jē-ă*	paralysis on one side of the body
paraplegia *par-ă-plē′jē-ă*	paralysis from the waist down
quadriplegia *kwah′dri-plĕ′jē-ă*	paralysis of all four limbs
poliomyelitis *po′lē-ō-mī′ĕ-lī′tis*	inflammation of the gray matter of the spinal cord caused by a virus, often resulting in spinal and muscle deformity and paralysis (*polio* = gray)
polyneuritis *pol′ē-nū-rī-tis*	inflammation involving two or more nerves, often caused by a nutritional deficiency, such as lack of thiamine
sleep apnea *slēp ap′nē-ă*	periods of breathing cessation (10 seconds or more) that occur during sleep, often causing snoring

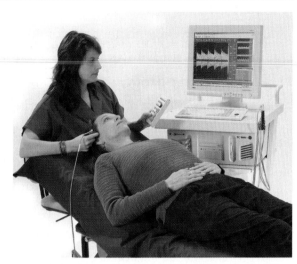

FIGURE 8-18 ■ Transcranial Doppler sonography.

TEST OR PROCEDURE	EXPLANATION
	are either no reflex response or an exaggerated response to stimulus; numbers are often used to record responses Ø = no response (absent reflex) 1+ = diminished response 2+ = normal response 3+ = more brisk than average response 4+ = hyperactive response
Babinski sign (Fig. 8-17) *bă-bin'skē sīn* **Babinski reflex** *bă-bin'skē rē'fleks*	pathologic response to stimulation of the plantar surface of the foot; a positive sign is indicated when the toes dorsiflex (curl upward)
transcranial Doppler sonogram (Fig. 8-18) *trans-krā'nē-ăl dop'lĕr son'ō-gram*	image made by sending ultrasound beams through the skull to assess blood flow in intracranial vessels; used in the diagnosis and management of stroke and head trauma

 ## Programmed Review: Nervous System Diagnostic Tests and Procedures

ANSWERS	REVIEW
	8.93 A wide variety of tests and procedures are used to diagnose conditions of the nervous system, including several electrodiagnostic procedures. The combining form referring to electricity is *electr/o*. The combining form referring to the entire
encephal/o record	brain is _____. Recall that the suffix *-gram* means _____. An EEG is a record of electrical impulses in

ANSWERS	REVIEW
electroencephalogram evoked	the brain; EEG is an abbreviation for _____. Minute electrical waves sorted out of the EEG activity to diagnose specific nerve pathway disorders are called _____ potentials. (Potential is a term referring to electrical charges.)
somn/o poly- recording polysomnography	**8.94** In addition to *hypn/o* and *somn/i*, a combining form meaning sleep is _____. The prefix meaning many is _____. The suffix -*graphy* means process of _____. From these three components comes the term for another electrodiagnostic procedure that measures various physiologic aspects of sleep: _____ (PSG).
lumbar puncture	**8.95** The procedure in which a specialized needle is introduced into the lumbar spine, such as to obtain a sample of cerebrospinal fluid for examination, is called a _____ _____ (LP).
magnetic resonance	**8.96** A nonionizing imaging technique using magnetic fields to visualize structures such as tissues of the brain and spinal cord is called _____ _____ imaging (MRI).
magnetic resonance angiography crani/o, within intracranial outside extracranial	**8.97** An MRI technique for imaging blood vessels (including the combining form *angi/o,* meaning vessel) is termed _____ _____ _____ (MRA). The combining form for skull is _____. The prefix *intra-* means _____. Magnetic resonance imaging of the head to visualize the vessels of the circle of Willis is called _____ MRA. The prefix *extra-* means _____. The term for magnetic resonance imaging of the neck to depict the carotid arteries is called _____ MRA.
medicine photon emission tomography	**8.98** Imaging a structure after administration of a radionuclide is called nuclear _____ imaging. A specialized brain scan that combines nuclear medicine with computed tomography (CT) is called single-_____ _____ computed _____ (SPECT).
emission tomography	**8.99** Another technique that combines nuclear medicine and CT to study brain anatomy and physiology is positron-_____ _____ (PET).

ANSWERS	REVIEW
process recording radiography cerebral angi/o cerebral angiogram	**8.100** Recall that the suffix *-graphy* means the _____ of _____. The process of recording x-ray images is called _____. The adjective form of cerebrum, pertaining to the largest part of the brain, is _____. Again, the combining form for blood vessel is _____. An x-ray of the blood vessels of the cerebrum is called a _____ _____.
computed tomography	**8.101** Cross-sectional x-ray images of the brain produced by _____ _____ are also used to visualize abnormalities, such as brain tumors.
myel/o, record myelogram	**8.102** The combining form meaning spinal cord is _____. Again, the suffix *-gram* means _____. An x-ray record of the spinal cord using an intraspinal contrast medium is called a _____.
Reflex deep tendon	**8.103** A reflex is the body's automatic response to a stimulus. _____ testing is performed to observe such responses. Reflexes that involve involuntary muscle contraction after percussion at a tendon are called _____ _____ reflexes (DTR).
Babinski	**8.104** A response to stimulation of the plantar surface of the foot is a pathologic reflex called the _____ sign, which is named for Babinski, the French neurologist who discovered it.
across transcranial sonogram	**8.105** Ultrasound is also called sonography. The prefix *trans-* means _____ or through. The record of an ultrasound image made by sending ultrasound waves through the skull is called a _____ _____.

 ## Self-Instruction: Nervous System Operative Terms

Study the following:

TERM	MEANING
carotid endarterectomy *ka-rot'id end'ar-tĕr-ek'tŏ-mē*	incision and coring of the lining of the carotid artery to clear a blockage caused by the buildup of atherosclerotic plaque or a clot; an open procedure used to treat patients who are at risk for stroke

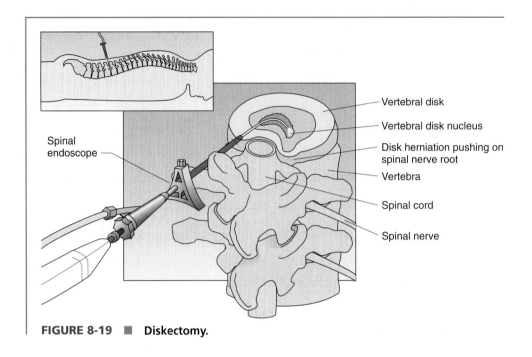

Spinal endoscope

Vertebral disk

Vertebral disk nucleus

Disk herniation pushing on spinal nerve root

Vertebra

Spinal cord

Spinal nerve

FIGURE 8-19 ■ Diskectomy.

TERM	MEANING
craniectomy *krā'nē-ek'tō-mē*	excision of part of the skull to approach the brain
craniotomy *krā-nē-ot'ō-mē*	incision into the skull to approach the brain
diskectomy or **discectomy** (Fig. 8-19) *disk-ek'tŏ-mē*	removal of a herniated disk; often done percutaneously (*per* = through; *cutaneous* = skin)
endovascular neurosurgery *en'dō-vas'kyū-lar nūr'ō-sŭr'jĕr-ē* **interventional neuroradiology** *in'tĕr-ven'shŭn-ăl nū'rō-rā-dē-ol'ŏ-jē*	minimally invasive techniques for diagnosis and treatment of disorders within blood vessels of the neck, brain, and spinal cord using specialized catheters inserted percutaneously (through the skin) into the femoral artery (in the groin) and guided by angiographic imaging to the treatment site; performed in a specialized angiographic laboratory by interventional neuroradiologists; common procedures are: • percutaneous transluminal angioplasty (PTA) with stent (e.g., carotid PTA) • embolization (plugging) of intracranial aneurysms and vascular malformations
laminectomy *lam'i-nek'tŏ-mē*	excision of one or more laminae of the vertebrae to approach the spinal cord
vertebral lamina (*see* Fig. 4-6) *ver'tĕ-brăl lam'i-nă*	flattened posterior portion of the vertebral arch
microsurgery (Fig. 8-20) *mī'krō-sŭr'jĕr-ē*	use of a microscope to dissect minute structures during surgery

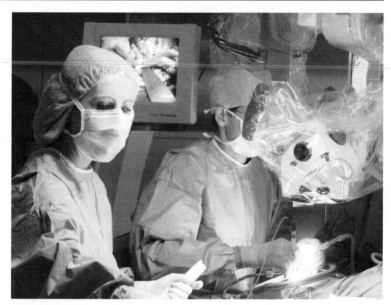

FIGURE 8-20 ■ Microscope for neurologic surgery.

TERM	MEANING
neuroplasty *nū'rō-plas-tē*	surgical repair of a nerve
spondylosyndesis (Fig. 8-21) *spon'di-lō-sin-dē'sis*	spinal fusion

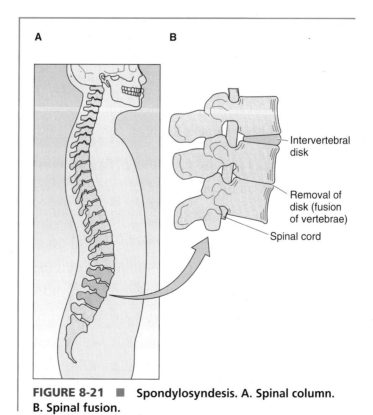

FIGURE 8-21 ■ Spondylosyndesis. A. Spinal column. B. Spinal fusion.

◆ Programmed Review: Nervous System Operative Terms

ANSWERS	REVIEW
within artery removal o endo-	**8.106** Endarterectomy, the open surgical technique that cuts out atherosclerotic blockage from the core lining of the carotid artery, was named by linking *endo-*, the prefix meaning _____, to *arteri/o*, the combining form meaning _____, and the suffix *-ectomy*, meaning excision or _____. Note that occasionally, when a prefix ends in a vowel and the root begins with a vowel, the final vowel is dropped from the prefix. This is why the letter ____ is dropped from the prefix _____ in this term.
-ectomy craniectomy	**8.107** The operative suffix meaning excision is _____. The excision of part of the skull, needed to reach the brain surgically, is termed _____.
diskectomy or discectomy	**8.108** The excision of a herniated spinal disk is termed a _____.
lamina laminectomy	**8.109** The flattened posterior portion of the vertebral arch is called a _____. The excision of one or more laminae is termed a _____.
incision craniotomy	**8.110** The operative suffix *-tomy* means _____. An incision into the skull to approach the brain is a _____.
microsurgery	**8.111** Use of a microscope to dissect minute structures during surgery is called _____.
neur/o -plasty neuroplasty	**8.112** The combining form meaning nerve is _____. Recall that the suffix for surgical repair or reconstruction is _____. The surgical repair of a nerve is called _____.
spondyl/o spondylosyndesis	**8.113** The two combining forms meaning vertebra are *vertebr/o* and _____. Syndesis is a surgical technique of joining bones together. The medical term for spinal fusion, or surgically joining vertebrae together, is _____.

ANSWERS	REVIEW
within	**8.114** Endovascular, a term formed by the combination of *endo-* (meaning _____) with *vascul/o* (meaning
vessel, pertaining to	_____) and *-ar* (meaning _____ _____) is one of the words used to name the minimally invasive techniques for diagnosis and treatment of disorders within blood vessels of the neck, brain, and spinal cord, which are
endovascular neuro	called _____ _____surgery. The synonym for endovascular neurosurgery is interventional
radiology	neuro_____, which is a term that identifies the technology used to guide the endovascular catheters to the treatment sites. The techniques are considered to be minimally invasive, because instruments are guided
skin	percutaneously (through the _____) into blood vessels, as opposed to "open" procedures that cut directly into tissues.

Self-Instruction: Nervous System Therapeutic Terms

Study the following:

TERM	MEANING
chemotherapy *kem-ō-thār'ă-pē*	treatment of malignancies, infections, and other diseases with chemical agents to destroy selected cells or impair their ability to reproduce
radiation therapy (Fig. 8-22) *rā'dē-ā'shŭn thār'ă-pē*	treatment of neoplastic disease using ionizing radiation to impede the proliferation of malignant cells
stereotactic or **stereotaxic radiosurgery** *ster'ē-ō-tak'tik or ster'ē-ō-tak'sik rā'dē-ō-sŭr'jĕr-ē*	radiation treatment to inactivate malignant lesions using multiple, precise external radiation beams focused on a target with the aid of a stereotactic frame and imaging such as CT, MRI, or angiography; used to treat inoperable brain tumors and other lesions
stereotactic or **stereotaxic frame** (Fig. 8-23) *ster'ē-ō-tak'tik or ster'ē-ō-tak'sik frām*	mechanical device used to localize a point in space, targeting a precise site

COMMON THERAPEUTIC DRUG CLASSIFICATIONS

analgesic *an-ăl-jē'zik*	agent that relieves pain

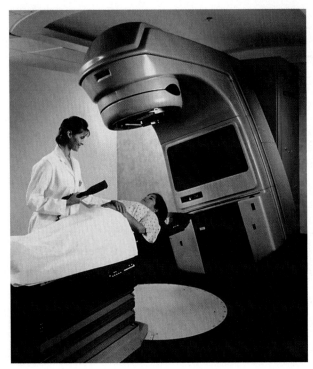

FIGURE 8-22 ■ Radiation therapy linear accelerator.

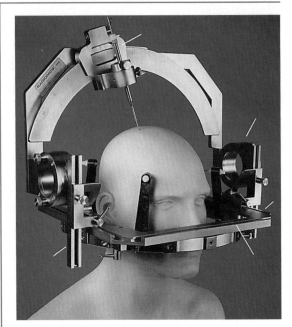

FIGURE 8-23 ■ Stereotactic frame.

TERM	MEANING
anticonvulsant *an'tē-kon-vŭl'sant*	agent that prevents or lessens convulsion
hypnotic *hip-not'ik*	agent that induces sleep

Programmed Review: Nervous System Therapeutic Terms

ANSWERS	REVIEW
chemotherapy	**8.115** The combining form referring to chemical agents is *chem/o*. The treatment of malignancies, infections, and other diseases with chemical agents that destroy targeted cells is called _____.
radiation therapy	**8.116** Some kinds of cancer are treated with radiation, which deters the proliferation of malignant cells. This is called _____ _____.
stere/o	**8.117** The combining form meaning three-dimensional or solid is _____, as in the term stereotactic (or stereotaxic) frame, which is an apparatus allowing precise localization in space.

ANSWERS	REVIEW
stereotactic radiosurgery	Radiation therapy given with precise localization of the radiation beam using a stereotactic frame is called _____ _____.
without analgesic	**8.118** The prefix *an-* means _____. The Greek word algesis means sensation of pain. A drug that relieves pain is called an _____.
against anticonvulsant	**8.119** Many drugs are named according to their action against a condition or symptom. The prefix *anti-* means _____. A drug that works to prevent or lessen convulsion is called an _____.
hypn/o hypnotic	**8.120** The combining forms meaning sleep are *somn/i, somn/o,* and _____. Formed from the last of these, the term for an agent that induces sleep is _____.

Self-Instruction: Psychiatric Symptomatic Terms

Study the following:

TERM	MEANING
affect *af'fekt*	emotional feeling or mood
flat affect *flat af'fekt*	significantly dulled emotional tone or outward reaction
apathy *ap'ă-thē*	a lack of interest or display of emotion
catatonia *kat-ă-tō'nē-ă*	a state of unresponsiveness to one's outside environment, usually including muscle rigidity, staring, and inability to communicate
delusion *dē-lū'zhŭn*	a persistent belief that has no basis in reality
grandiose delusion *grăn-dē-ōs' dē-lū'zhŭn*	a person's false belief that he or she possesses great wealth, intelligence, or power
persecutory delusion *pĕr-se-kyū-tōr'ē dē-lū'zhŭn*	a person's false belief that someone is plotting against him or her with the intent to harm
dysphoria *dis-fōr'ē-ă*	a restless, dissatisfied mood
euphoria *yū-fōr'ē-ă*	an exaggerated, unfounded feeling of well-being

TERM	MEANING
hallucination *ha-lū-si-nā'shŭn*	a false perception of the senses for which there is no reality; most commonly hearing or seeing things (*alucinor* = to wander in mind)
ideation *ī-dē-ā'shŭn*	the formation of thoughts or ideas, such as suicidal ideation (thoughts of suicide)
mania *mā'nē-ă*	state of abnormal elation and increased activity
neurosis *nū-rō'sis*	a psychologic condition in which anxiety is prominent
psychosis *sī-kō'sis*	a mental condition characterized by distortion of reality resulting in the inability to communicate or function within one's environment
thought disorder *thot dis-ōr'dĕr*	thought that lacks clear processing or logical direction

◈ Programmed Review: Psychiatric Symptomatic Terms

ANSWERS	REVIEW
affect emotional	**8.121** An emotional feeling or mood is called an _____. A flat affect is a significantly dulled _____ tone or outward reaction.
apathy	**8.122** A lack of interest or display of emotion is termed _____.
cata- ton/o catatonia	**8.123** Recall that the prefix meaning down is _____, and that the combining term for tone is _____. The original Greek term katatonos means stretching down. The medical term for a state of unresponsiveness that includes muscle rigidity is _____.
false grandiose persecutory delusion	**8.124** A delusion is a persistent _____ belief that has no basis in reality. A delusion that one has great wealth, intelligence, or power is called a _____ delusion. A delusion that one is being persecuted by others plotting against him or her is called a _____ _____.

ANSWERS	REVIEW
carry dysphoria normal euphoria	**8.125** The combining form *phor/o* means to bear or _____. Recall that the prefix *dys-* means painful, difficult, or faulty. Thus, the term dysphoria originated from terms meaning to carry poorly. The medical term for a restless, dissatisfied mood is _____. Incorporating *eu-*, the prefix meaning good or _____, the term for an exaggerated, unfounded feeling of well-being is _____.
hallucination process	**8.126** From the Latin word alucinor, meaning to wander in mind, this medical term means a false perception of the senses: _____. Recall that the suffix *-ation* refers to _____.
ideation	**8.127** The process of forming thoughts or ideas is called _____. For example, thoughts of suicide are called suicidal ideation.
condition of mania	**8.128** Again, the suffix *-ia* means _____ ____. A condition of abnormal elation and increased activity is called _____. The original Greek word mania means frenzy.
increase nerve neurosis	**8.129** The suffix *-osis* means condition or _____. The combining form *neur/o* usually means _____, or, in this case, nervousness. The term for a psychologic condition in which anxiety is prominent is called _____, meaning the condition of nervousness.
psych/o psychosis	**8.130** The combining forms meaning mind are *phren/o*, *thym/o*, and _____. The last of these is used with a suffix that means condition to make the term for a mental condition characterized by a distortion of reality resulting in an inability to function within one's environment: _____.
thought disorder	**8.131** A disorder of thinking in which there is no clear processing or logical direction is called a _____ _____.

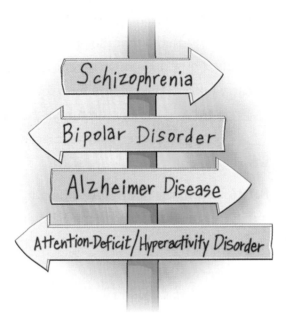

 ## Self-Instruction: Psychiatric Diagnostic Terms

Study the following:

TERM	MEANING
MOOD DISORDERS	
major depression *mā'jor dē-presh'ŭn* **major depressive illness** *mā'jor dē-pres'iv il'nes* **clinical depression** *klin'i-kl dē-presh'ŭn* **major affective disorder** *mā'jor af-fek'tiv dis-ōr'dĕr* **unipolar disorder** *yū'ni-pō'lăr dis-ōr'dĕr*	a disorder causing periodic disturbances in mood that affect concentration, sleep, activity, appetite, and social behavior; characterized by feelings of worthlessness, fatigue, and loss of interest
dysthymia *dis-thī'mē-ă*	a milder affective disorder characterized by chronic depression
manic depression *man'ik dē-presh'ŭn* **bipolar disorder (BD)** *bī-pō'lăr dis-ōr'dĕr*	an affective disorder characterized by mood swings of mania and depression (extreme up and down states)
seasonal affective disorder (SAD) *sē-zŏn'ăl af-fek'tiv dis-ōr'dĕr*	an affective disorder marked by episodes of depression that most often occur during the fall and winter and that remit in the spring

TERM	MEANING
ANXIETY DISORDERS	
generalized anxiety disorder (GAD) *jen'ĕr-ă-līzd ang-zī'ĕ-tē dis-ōr'dĕr*	the most common anxiety disorder; characterized by chronic, excessive, uncontrollable worry about everyday problems; affects the ability to relax or concentrate, but does not usually interfere with social interactions or employment; physical symptoms include muscle tension, trembling, twitching, fatigue, headaches, nausea, and insomnia
panic disorder *pan'ik dis-ōr'dĕr*	a disorder of sudden, recurrent attacks of intense feelings, including physical symptoms that mimic a heart attack (rapid heart rate, chest pain, shortness of breath, chills, sweating, and dizziness) with a general sense of loss of control or feeling that death is imminent; often progresses to agoraphobia
phobia *fō'bē-ă*	exaggerated fear of a specific object or circumstance that causes anxiety and panic; named for the object or circumstance, such as agoraphobia (fear of the marketplace), claustrophobia (fear of confinement), and acrophobia (fear of high places)
posttraumatic stress disorder (PTSD) *pōst-traw'măt-ik strĕs dis-ōr'dĕr*	a condition resulting from an extremely traumatic experience, injury, or illness that leaves the sufferer with persistent thoughts and memories of the ordeal; may occur after a war, violent personal assault, physical or sexual abuse, serious accident, or natural disaster; symptoms include feelings of fear, detachment, exaggerated startle response, restlessness, nightmares, and avoidance of anything or anyone who triggers the painful recollections
obsessive-compulsive disorder (OCD) *ob-ses'iv-kom-pŭl'siv dis-ōr'dĕr*	an anxiety disorder featuring unwanted, senseless obsessions accompanied by repeated compulsions; can interfere with all aspects of a person's daily life; for example, the thought that a door is not locked causing repetitive checking to make sure it is locked, or thoughts that one's body has been contaminated causing repetitive washing
hypochondriasis *hī'pō-kon-drī'ă-sis*	a preoccupation with thoughts of disease and concern that one is suffering from a serious condition that persists despite medical reassurance to the contrary

DISORDERS USUALLY DIAGNOSED IN CHILDHOOD

autism *aw'tizm*	a developmental disability, commonly appearing during the first three years of life, resulting from a neurologic disorder affecting brain function, as evidenced by difficulties with verbal and nonverbal communication and an inability to relate to anything beyond oneself (*auto* = self) in social interactions; persons with autism often exhibit body movements such as rocking and repetitive hand movements; persons commonly become preoccupied with observing

TERM	MEANING
	parts of small objects or moving parts or with performing meaningless rituals
dyslexia *dis-lek'sē-ă*	a developmental disability characterized by difficulty understanding written or spoken words, sentences, or paragraphs that affects reading, spelling, and self-expression
attention-deficit/ hyperactivity disorder (ADHD) *ă-ten'shŭn-def'i-sit/hī-pĕr-ak-tiv'i-tē dis-ōr'dĕr*	a dysfunction characterized by consistent hyperactivity, distractibility, and lack of control over impulses, which interferes with ability to function normally at school, home, or work
mental retardation *men'tăl rē-tar-dā'shŭn*	a condition of subaverage intelligence characterized by an IQ of 70 or less, resulting in the inability to adapt to normal social activities

EATING DISORDERS

anorexia nervosa *an-ō-rek'sē-ă nĕr-vō'să*	a severe disturbance in eating behavior caused by abnormal perceptions about one's body weight, as evidenced by an overwhelming fear of becoming fat that results in a refusal to eat and body weight well below normal
bulimia nervosa *bū-lē'mē-ă nĕr-vō'să*	an eating disorder characterized by binge eating followed by efforts to limit digestion though induced vomiting, use of laxatives, or excessive exercise

SUBSTANCE ABUSE DISORDERS

substance abuse disorders *sŭb'stans ă-byūs' dis-ōr'dĕrz*	mental disorders resulting from abuse of substances such as drugs, alcohol, or other toxins, causing personal and social dysfunction; identified by the abused substance, such as alcohol abuse, amphetamine abuse, opioid (narcotic) abuse, and polysubstance abuse

PSYCHOTIC DISORDERS

schizophrenia *skiz-ō-frē'nē-ă*	a disease of brain chemistry causing a distorted cognitive and emotional perception of one's environment; symptoms include distortions of normal function (such as disorganized thought, delusions, hallucinations, and catatonic behavior), flat affect, apathy, and withdrawal from reality

🔷 Programmed Review: Psychiatric Diagnostic Terms

ANSWERS	REVIEW
	8.132 Psychiatrists use a number of terms referring to major depression, which is a disorder causing mood disturbances that affects concentration, sleep, and activity and is characterized

ANSWERS	REVIEW
clinical affective, disorder	by feelings of worthlessness and apathy. Other terms include major depressive illness, _____ depression, major _____ disorder, and unipolar _____.
manic bipolar one, bipolar	**8.133** The disorder in which a person experiences mood swings between depression and mania is called _____ depression or _____ disorder (BD). Note how unipolar refers to _____ mood, whereas _____ refers to two moods.
thym/o faulty dysthymia	**8.134** Recall that the three combining forms meaning mind are *phren/o*, *psych/o*, and _____. The prefix *dys-* means painful, difficult, or _____. Another mood disorder, _____, uses the third combining form and is a milder affective disorder that is characterized by chronic depression.
seasonal affective disorder	**8.135** An affective disorder in which episodes of depression occur in seasonal cycles is called _____ _____ _____ (SAD).
generalized anxiety	**8.136** There are several anxiety disorders. The most common anxiety disorder occurs generally, not from a specific anxiety-producing situation. It causes excessive and uncontrollable worrying, and it may produce physical symptoms. This disorder is called _____ _____ disorder (GAD).
panic disorder	**8.137** Another anxiety disorder produces sudden attacks of intense feelings of anxiety and panic, with often dramatic physical symptoms. This disorder is called _____ _____.
phob/o condition of phobia	**8.138** Recall that the combining form that means an exaggerated fear or sensitivity is _____. The suffix *-ia* means _____ ____. The psychiatric condition in which one experiences an exaggerated fear of something is called a _____.
post-	**8.139** After a traumatic experience, a person may develop a stressful condition involving persistent thoughts of the ordeal, fear, and other symptoms. Recall that a common prefix meaning after or behind is _____. This condition

ANSWERS	REVIEW
posttraumatic stress disorder	is termed _____ _____ _____ (PTSD).
obsessive-compulsive disorder	**8.140** An obsession is a persistent, uncontrollable thought. A compulsion is a persistent, uncontrollable behavior. An anxiety disorder characterized by obsession and compulsions that often interfere with all aspects of an individual's life is called _____-_____ _____ (OCD).
below presence hypochondriasis	**8.141** The combining form *chondr/o* refers to cartilage of the ribs. The prefix *hypo-* means deficient or _____. Thus, the term hypochondrium refers to the abdomen (beneath the ribs)— once thought to be the place where sensations of a distressing nature were experienced, such as the concern that one is suffering from a serious condition despite medical reassurance to the contrary. Recall that the suffix *-iasis* means formation of or the _____ of. The term for the condition when this concern is present is _____.
condition of autism	**8.142** The prefix *auto-* means self. Recall that the suffix *-ism* means _____ ____. A developmental condition in which the person is unable to relate to anyone other than himself or herself is called _____.
lex/o difficult dyslexia, condition of	**8.143** The combining form meaning word or phrase is _____. The prefix *dys-* means painful, faulty, or _____. The term for the developmental disability of difficulty understanding written words or phrases is _____. The suffix *-ia* means _____ ____.
attention-deficit hyperactivity disorder excessive	**8.144** Typically, ADHD is diagnosed in childhood, when the child has difficulty paying attention to things, is easily distracted, and is generally hyperactive. ADHD is the abbreviation for _____-_____ / _____ _____. Recall that the prefix *hyper-* means above or _____.

ANSWERS	REVIEW
mental retardation	**8.145** The Latin word mens refers to the mind, and the Latin verb retardo means to hinder. The condition of limited intelligence is called _____ _____.
without condition of anorexia nervosa	**8.146** The Greek word orexis means appetite. Recall that the prefix *an-* means _____, and that the suffix *-ia* means _____ _____. Thus, the term for the condition of being without an appetite is _____. When this condition is caused by a psychological disturbance ("nervous" condition) and fear of being fat, it is called anorexia _____.
bulimia	**8.147** An eating disorder characterized by binge eating followed by efforts to limit the digestion of food is called _____ nervosa. Bulimia comes from two Greek words meaning hungry as an ox.
abuse	**8.148** Substance abuse disorders are mental disorders resulting from an _____ of substances, such as drugs or alcohol, that leads to dysfunction.
split mind schizophrenia split	**8.149** The combining form *schiz/o* means _____, and the combining form *phren/o* means _____. Thus, the term for a disease of brain chemistry that causes disorganized thinking, delusions, hallucinations, and other symptoms is _____. Some people mistakenly believe that schizophrenia means a mind that is split in two personalities (multiple personality disorder), but the term actually refers to a mind that is _____ from reality.

Self-Instruction: Psychiatric Therapeutic Terms

Study the following:

TERM	MEANING
electroconvulsive therapy (ECT) *ē-lek'trō-kon-vŭl'siv thār'ă-pē*	electrical shock applied to the brain to induce convulsions; used to treat patients with severe depression
light therapy *līt thār'ă-pē*	use of specialized illuminating light boxes and visors to treat seasonal affective disorder

TERM	MEANING
psychotherapy *sī-kō-thār′ă-pē*	treatment of psychiatric disorders using verbal and nonverbal interaction with patients, individually or in a group, employing specific actions and techniques
behavioral therapy *bē-hāv′yōr-ăl thār′ă-pē*	treatment to decrease or stop unwanted behavior
cognitive therapy *kog′ni-tiv thār′ă-pē*	treatment to change unwanted patterns of thinking

COMMON THERAPEUTIC DRUG CLASSIFICATIONS

psychotropic drugs *sī′kō-trop′ik drŭgz*	medications used to treat mental illnesses (*trop/o* = a turning)
antianxiety agents *an-tī-ang-zī′ĕ-tē ā′jentz* **anxiolytic agents** *ang′zē-ō-lit′ik ā′jentz*	drugs used to reduce anxiety
antidepressant *an′tē-dē-pres′ănt*	agent that counteracts depression
neuroleptic agents *nū-rō-lep′tik ā′jentz*	drugs used to treat psychosis, especially schizophrenia
sedative *sed′ă-tiv*	agent that has a calming effect and quiets nervousness

 # Programmed Review: Psychiatric Therapeutic Terms

ANSWERS	REVIEW
electroconvulsive	**8.150** The combining form *electr/o* refers to electricity. Therapy for patients with severe depression that uses a shock to the brain that induces convulsions is called _____ therapy (ECT).
light	**8.151** One theory for the depression of seasonal affective disorder is that the person suffers from reduced amounts of sunlight in the fall and winter. A treatment for this is therefore _____ therapy.
psych/o psychotherapy	**8.152** The treatment modality for psychiatric patients using verbal and nonverbal interactions was originally named to mean therapy of the mind. Three combining forms meaning mind are *phren/o*, *thym/o*, and _____. Made with the third form, this therapy is termed _____.
behavioral	**8.153** Treatment emphasizing behavioral changes is called _____ therapy.

ANSWERS	REVIEW
cognitive	**8.154** Treatment directed to change unwanted patterns of thinking is called _____ therapy. The term cognitive refers to thought processes.
psychotropic	**8.155** The suffix -*tropic* pertains to turning. The term for the class of drugs used in treating mental illnesses literally means turning of the mind: _____ drugs.
anti- antianxiety anxiolytic	**8.156** Drug classes are frequently named for their actions to cause something or their actions to prevent something. A common prefix meaning against or opposed to is _____. Drugs that work against anxiety, therefore, are termed _____ agents. Another term for these drugs uses the suffix -*lytic*, pertaining to breaking down something. Thus, the term for these drugs literally means breaking down anxiety: _____ agents.
antidepressant	**8.157** A drug that counteracts (works against) depression is called an _____.
neur/o neuroleptic	**8.158** The combining form meaning nerve is _____. Drugs used to treat psychosis, especially schizophrenia, are called _____ agents.
sedative	**8.159** A patient can be sedated to calm his or her anxious state. A drug that quiets nervousness is called a _____.

CHAPTER 8 ACRONYMS AND ABBREVIATIONS

ABBREVIATION	EXPANSION
ALS	amyotrophic lateral sclerosis
ADHD	attention-deficit/hyperactivity disorder
ANS	autonomic nervous system
BD	bipolar disorder
CNS	central nervous system
CP	cerebral palsy
CSF	cerebrospinal fluid
CT	computed tomography
CVA	cerebrovascular accident
DTR	deep tendon reflexes

ABBREVIATION	EXPANSION
ECT	electroconvulsive therapy
EEG	electroencephalogram
GAD	generalized anxiety disorder
HD	Huntington disease
LP	lumbar puncture
MRA	magnetic resonance angiography
MRI	magnetic resonance imaging
MS	multiple sclerosis
NCV	nerve conduction velocity
OCD	obsessive-compulsive disorder
PET	positron-emission tomography
PNS	peripheral nervous system
PSG	polysomnography
PTSD	posttraumatic stress disorder
SAD	seasonal affective disorder
SPECT	single-photon emission computed tomography
TIA	transient ischemic attack

CHAPTER 8 SUMMARY OF TERMS

The terms introduced in chapter 8 are listed below, followed by the page number on which each term can be found and its written pronunciation. For additional practice and reinforcement, write the definition of each term on a separate piece of paper.

absence seizure/390
ab'sens sē'zhŭr

affect/409
af'fekt

agnosia/388
ag-nō'zē-ă

Alzheimer disease/388
awlz'hī-měr di-zēz'

amyotrophic lateral sclerosis (ALS)/388
ă-mī-ō-trō'fik lat'ěr-ăl sklě-rō'sis

analgesic/407
an-ăl-jē'zik

anencephaly/392
an'en-sef'ă-lē

anorexia nervosa/414
an-ō-rek'sē-ă ner-vō'să

antianxiety agents/418
an-tī-ang-zī'e-tē ā'jentz

anticonvulsant/408
an'tē-kon-vŭl'sant

antidepressant/418
an'tē-dē-pres'ănt

anxiolytic agents/418
ang'zē-ō-lit'ik ā'jentz

apathy/409
ap'ă-thē

aphasia/384
ă-fā'zē-ă

PRACTICE EXERCISES

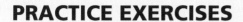

For each of the following words, write out the term components (prefixes [P], combining forms [CF], roots [R], and suffixes [S]) on the lines below the word. Then define the term according to the meaning of its components.

EXAMPLE

anencephaly

<u>an</u> / <u>encephal</u> / <u>y</u>

   P   R   S

DEFINITION: without/brain/condition or process of

1. ganglioma

_____ / _____

   R   S

DEFINITION: _____

2. atopognosia

_____ / _____ / _____ / _____

   P   CF   R   S

DEFINITION: _____

3. catatonic

_____ / _____ / _____

   P   R   S

DEFINITION: _____

4. dystaxia

_____ / _____ / _____

   P   R   S

DEFINITION: _____

5. bradykinesia

_____ / _____ / _____

   P   R   S

DEFINITION: _____

6. meningocele

_____ / _____

   CF   S

DEFINITION: _____

7. dysthymia

_____ / _____ / _____

   P   R   S

DEFINITION: _____

8. polysomnogram

_____ / _____ / _____
    P   CF   S

DEFINITION: _____

9. spondylosyndesis

_____ / _____/_____
   CF   P   S

DEFINITION: _____

10. hemiplegia

_____ / _____
    P   S

DEFINITION: _____

11. craniotomy

_____ / _____
   CF   S

DEFINITION: _____

12. thalamic

_____ / _____
    R   S

DEFINITION: _____

13. neuroglial

_____ / _____ / _____
   CF   R   S

DEFINITION: _____

14. dyslexia

_____ / _____ / _____
    P   R   S

DEFINITION: _____

15. somnipathy

_____ / _____ / _____
   CF   R   S

DEFINITION: _____

16. hydrocephalic

_____ / _____ / _____
   CF   R   S

DEFINITION: _____

17. necromania

_____ / _____
   CF   S

DEFINITION: _____

18. acrophobia

_____ / _____ / _____
    CF   R   S

DEFINITION: _____

19. hypnotic

_____ / _____
    CF   S

DEFINITION: _____

20. euphoria

_____ / _____ / _____
    P   R   S

DEFINITION: _____

21. parasomnia

_____ / _____ / _____
    P   R   S

DEFINITION: _____

22. narcolepsy

_____ / _____
    CF   S

DEFINITION: _____

23. stereotaxy

_____ / _____ / _____
    CF   R   S

DEFINITION: _____

24. hemiparesis

_____ / _____
    P   S

DEFINITION: _____

25. neurasthenia

_____ / _____
    R   S

DEFINITION: _____

26. myelopathy

_____ / _____ / _____
    CF   R   S

DEFINITION: _____

27. intracranial

_____ / _____ / _____
    P   R   S

DEFINITION: _____

28. aphasia

_____ / _____ / _____
     P   R   S

DEFINITION: _____

29. schizophrenia

_____ / _____ / _____
    CF   R   S

DEFINITION: _____

30. cerebrospinal

_____ / _____ / _____
    CF   R   S

DEFINITION: _____

Write the correct medical term for each of the following definitions:

31. _____ inflammation of the meninges

32. _____ excision of a herniated disk

33. _____ inability to locate a sensation properly, such as to locate a point touched on the body

34. _____ a slowly progressive degeneration of nerves in the brain characterized by tremor, rigidity of muscles, and slow movements

35. _____ a pathologic response to stimulation of the plantar surface of the foot indicated by dorsiflexion of the toes

36. _____ numbness and tingling

37. _____ state of unconsciousness

38. _____ a type of seizure that causes a series of sudden, involuntary contractions of muscles

39. _____ congenital neural tube defect of the spinal column characterized by the absence of vertebral arches

40. _____ a type of agnosia indicating an inability to judge the form of an object by touch, for example, not being able to distinguish a coin from a key

Complete each medical term by writing the missing word part:

41. electro_____gram = record of electrical brain impulses

42. _____syndesis = spinal fusion

43. crani_____ = excision of part of the skull

44. cerebral _____sclerosis = fat buildup in blood vessel of brain

45. hyper_____ = increased sensations

46. dys_____ = difficulty speaking

47. _____algesia = loss of sense of pain

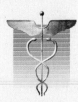

MEDICAL RECORD ANALYSIS

Medical Record 8-1

OUTPATIENT HISTORY AND PHYSICAL, NEUROLOGIC SERVICES

CC: numbness and tingling in feet and hands

HPI: This 44 y.o. right-handed female c/o numbness in her feet for the past two weeks with "pockets" of numbness in the abdomen. Her legs feel heavy and numb. Her hands started tingling a week ago, and she is feeling very nervous. She has had similar episodes over the past 3 years, lasting about a week at a time, often after stressful events or during hot weather.

PMH: Operations: none. No serious illness/accidents

FH: Father, age 71, L&W; Mother, age 66, is bipolar; her only sibling, a sister, age 28, has cerebral palsy.

SH: Denies smoking or use of street drugs, but drinks socially

OH: certified public accountant. Martial Status: single

ROS: noncontributory

VS: T 98.2°F., P 82, R 16, BP 110/68, Ht 5'2", Wt 138#

PE: HEENT: WNL. Neck: negative. Heart/Lungs: normal.

Cranial nerves intact. Reflexes: DTRs are increased, greater on the left than the right, without spasticity.

Toes upgoing bilaterally.

There is numbness to tactile pin stimulation over both extremities. She has no finger-to-nose ataxia. Her gait is steady.

A: R/O MS

P: Schedule MRI of the brain with and without gadolinium (contrast)

RTO for report and further evaluation x 1 wk

QUESTIONS ABOUT MEDICAL RECORD 8-1

1. Which medical term best describes the patient's symptom?
   a. hyperesthesia
   b. paresthesia
   c. ataxia
   d. hemiparesis
   e. neuralgia

2. What is noted in the history about the patient's mother?
   a. she is alive and well
   b. she suffers from depression
   c. she has mood swings of mania and depression
   d. she suffers from generalized anxiety
   e. she is a hypochondriac

3. Describe the sister's condition:
   a. disorder affecting the central nervous system characterized by seizures
   b. hereditary disease of the central nervous system characterized by bizarre involuntary body movements and progressive dementia
   c. abnormal accumulation of cerebrospinal fluid in the ventricles of the brain as a result of developmental abnormality
   d. condition of motor dysfunction caused by damage to the cerebrum during development or injury at birth
   e. slowly progressive degeneration of nerves in the brain characterized by tremor, rigidity, and slow movements

4. Which medical term describes the positive finding of the "toes upgoing" bilaterally?
   a. Babinski sign
   b. neuralgia
   c. hemiparesis
   d. spastic paralysis
   e. flaccid paralysis

5. What is the doctor's impression?
   a. the patient has multiple sclerosis
   b. the patient does not have multiple sclerosis
   c. the patient may have multiple sclerosis
   d. the patient may have hardening of the arteries in the brain
   e. the patient does not have hardening of the arteries in the brain

6. Describe the test noted in the Plan:
   a. x-ray
   b. nuclear image
   c. ultrasound scan
   d. tomographic radiograph
   e. scan produced by magnetic fields and radiofrequency waves

Medical Record 8-2

FOR ADDITIONAL STUDY

Anne Cross has been fairly healthy until she had a stroke about 2 months ago. She was treated by Dr. Paul Jiang, her personal physician, at that time and was discharged from the hospital on medication. At the request of Ms. Cross, Dr. Jiang called for a consultation from a neurologist, Dr. Melvin Classen. Medical Record 8-2 is a consultation report written by Dr. Classen as a letter back to Ms. Cross's physician, Dr. Jiang, after his consultation.

Read Medical Record 8-2 (pages 437-438), then write your answers to the following questions in the spaces provided.

QUESTIONS ABOUT MEDICAL RECORD 8-2

1. Below are medical terms used in this record that you have not yet encountered. Underline each where it appears in the record, and define the term below.

   homonymous hemianopsia _____

   finger-to-nose test _____

   apraxia _____

   clonus _____

2. In your own words, not using medical terminology, briefly describe Ms. Cross's symptoms in April, before she was admitted to the hospital:

   _____

   _____

   _____

3. Complete this table summarizing the diagnostic tests performed in April by writing in the missing parts:

Test	Definition of Test	Findings
CT		
	sound waves through heart	
carotid ultrasound		
		slowed electrical pulse on right side

4. What family member had a problem perhaps similar to that of Ms. Cross?

   _____

5. For each of the following medications given Ms. Cross, translate the dosage instructions:

   Plavix _____

   aspirin _____

Proventil _____

Procardia _____

6. Dr. Classen recommends two diagnostic studies. Describe both in your own words:

   a. _____

   b. _____

7. In one sentence, describe Dr. Classen's rationale for recommending the combination of these two tests:

   _____

   _____

8. Name the preventive surgical procedure Dr. Classen suggests that may be appropriate if changes are found in the carotid blood vessels:

   _____

   Now describe this procedure in your own words:

   _____

   _____

Medical Record 8-2: For Additional Study

CENTRAL MEDICAL GROUP, INC.
Department of Neurology
201 Medical Center Drive • Central City, US 90000-1234 • PHONE: (012) 125-8888 • FAX: (012) 125-3434

June 9, 20xx

Paul Jiang, M.D.
1409 West Ninth Street
Central City, US 90000-1233

Dear Dr. Jiang:

RE: Anne Cross

I had the pleasure of meeting Mrs. Cross today. As you know, she is a 65-year-old right-handed female who began to have difficulties on or about April 17, 20xx. She experienced dizziness that she described as occurring in the midday; there was also some associated slurring of speech. By the next morning, she seemed to have some disorientation with putting on her clothes, and she had some difficulties using the left side of her body. She had no headache or other problems. Prior to that time, she denied having any symptomatology. She was admitted to the hospital, as you are aware, and underwent a series of studies. A CT scan was reviewed and showed evidence of a right ischemic occipital infarct. In addition, she underwent an echocardiogram that was normal and an electroencephalogram that showed some right-sided slowing. A carotid ultrasound study suggested 60-70% stenosis of the bifurcation and/or internal carotids.

The patient was discharged on a combination of Plavix 75 mg daily, and enteric-coated aspirin 81 mg daily for ischemic stroke prophylaxis, Proventil 1 q 12 h p.r.n. for chronic obstructive pulmonary disease, and Procardia XL 1 daily for hypertension. The patient also has stopped smoking.

The patient reports that in the past, she has been essentially well except for some eye surgery. Additionally, after her discharge, she underwent visual field studies which confirmed the presence of an incomplete left-sided homonymous hemianopsia.

By way of family background, her brother died from complications of a stroke at age 78. Her mother died from liver cancer, and her father died from a myocardial infarction.

The patient has no specific allergy to drugs.

The patient's risk factors have been otherwise unremarkable.

On examination today, the patient is a slender female in no acute distress.

Blood pressure from the left arm in a sitting position is 130/95 and from the right arm in the sitting position is 145/95. Her pulse rate is 76 and regular.

No bruits are present over the carotid distributions. The temporal arteries are not enlarged or tender.

On examination of the eyes, the patient showed some mild arteriolar narrowing without hemorrhage or exudate. Gross visual confrontation suggests a neglect of left hemianopsia. The extraocular movements are full. The pupils are symmetrical. There is no ptosis. Facial movements are normal, and speech is normal.

Medical Record 8-2: For Additional Study (Continued)

CENTRAL MEDICAL GROUP, INC.

Department of Neurology

201 Medical Center Drive • Central City, US 90000-1234 • PHONE: (012) 125-8888 • FAX: (012) 125-3434

There is no drift to the outstretched hands. Finger-to-nose test is performed symmetrically.

The patient does not have any asymmetrical topagnosis. She has no evidence of apraxia.

The patient's reflexes are physiologic: they are 2+ at the biceps, triceps, and brachioradialis. The knee and ankle jerks are 2+. No clonus is elicited.

Gait and stance are normal.

OVERALL ASSESSMENT:

Without prior warning, this woman had a new onset of a cerebral infarct. By her description, it is likely that she had a posterior circulatory infarct in the area of the occipital lobe. There may have been an association zone in the parietal area as well. Since that time, she has had some residual hemianopsia as described.

PLAN:

At this time, it is suggested that the most prudent approach would be to do an MRA and an MRI. This should include the great vessels of the neck and the vertebrobasilar system. The MRI would allow us to see the nature of residuals of the stroke, the distribution of the stroke, and would allow us to determine if there are any asymptomatic lesions, including microvascular infarcts which would not be seen on the CAT scan. The MRA would allow us to determine the overall anatomy of the vasculature--including the neck, the bifurcations, and the posterior circulation--in a noninvasive way. Depending on the results of both of these studies, we would have to consider if she needs a full angiogram done with selective views. If, in fact, she has had an infarct of the posterior occipital lobe, then the current treatment with Plavix and aspirin would be adequate. If, by the nature of the MRA, it is determined that there are significant changes or irregularity of the contour of the intima of the vessels at the bifurcations, then there may be an indication for prophylaxis for an endarterectomy despite not having a stroke in that distribution of the vessels. This, of course, would all be determined by the results of this study. The advantage of the MRA-MRI combined would allow us to visualize adequately the vessels combined with the detailed evaluation of her brain.

I think this would be the patient's best and most prudent approach to the patient's health and would help to prevent recurrence of this problem.

Please do not hesitate to call me if there are any questions regarding this patient's evaluation.

Sincerely,

Melvin Classen, M.D.
Department of Neurology
(012) 125-6899

MC:mar
DOT:6/10/20xx

cc: Mrs. Anne Cross

ANSWERS TO PRACTICE EXERCISES

1. gangli/oma
   R   S
   ganglion (knot)/tumor
2. a/topo/gnos/ia
   P CF R S
   without/place/
   knowing/condition of
3. cata/ton/ic
   P R S
   down/tone or
   tension/pertaining to
4. dys/tax/ia
   P R S
   painful, difficult, or
   faulty/order or coordi-
   nation/condition of
5. brady/kines/ia
   P   R   S
   slow/movement/
   condition of
6. meningo/cele
   CF   S
   meninges
   (membrane)/pouching
   or hernia
7. dys/thym/ia
   P R S
   painful, difficult, or
   faulty/mind/condition of
8. poly/somno/gram
   P   CF   S
   many/sleep/record
9. spondylo/syn/desis
   CF   P   S
   vertebra/together or
   with/binding
10. hemi/plegia
    P   S
    half/paralysis
11. cranio/tomy
    CF   S
    skull/incision
12. thalam/ic
    R   S
    thalamus (a room)/
    pertaining to

13. neuro/gli/al
    CF R S
    nerve/glue/
    pertaining to
14. dys/lex/ia
    P R S
    painful, difficult, or
    faulty/speech/
    condition of
15. somni/path/y
    CF   R S
    sleep/disease/condition
    or process of
16. hydro/cephal/ic
    CF   R   S
    water/head/
    pertaining to
17. necro/mania
    CF   S
    death/condition of
    abnormal impulse
    toward
18. acro/phob/ia
    CF   R S
    topmost/exaggerated
    fear/condition of
19. hypno/tic
    CF   S
    sleep/pertaining to
20. eu/phor/ia
    P   R S
    good or normal/carry or
    bear/condition of
21. para/somn/ia
    P   R   S
    abnormal/sleep/
    condition of
22. narco/lepsy
    CF   S
    stupor (sleep)/seizure
23. stereo/tax/y
    CF R S
    three dimensional or
    solid/order or
    coordination/condition
    or process of

24. hemi/paresis
    P   S
    half/slight paralysis
25. neur/asthenia
    R   S
    nerve/weakness
26. myelo/path/y
    CF   R S
    spinal cord/disease/
    condition or process of
27. intra/crani/al
    P   R   S
    within/skull/pertaining
    to
28. a/phas/ia
    P R S
    without/speech/
    condition of
29. schizo/phren/ia
    CF   R   S
    split/mind/condition of
30. cerebro/spin/al
    CF   R   S
    cerebrum/spine/
    pertaining to
31. meningitis
32. diskectomy or
    discectomy
33. atopognosis
34. Parkinson disease
35. Babinski sign or reflex
36. paresthesia
37. coma
38. convulsion
39. spina bifida
40. astereognosis
41. electroencephalogram
42. spondylosyndesis
43. craniectomy
44. cerebral atherosclerosis
45. hyperesthesia
46. dysphasia
47. analgesia
48. i
49. h
50. j
51. a

52. f
53. g
54. e
55. b
56. c
57. d
58. computed tomography
59. magnetic resonance imaging
60. positron-emission tomography
61. multiple sclerosis
62. central nervous system
63. cerebral palsy
64. transient ischemic attack
65. electroencephalogram
66. deep tendon reflexes
67. single-photon emission computed tomography
68. polysomnography
69. amyotrophic lateral sclerosis
70. peripheral nervous system
71. cerebrospinal fluid
72. magnetic resonance angiography
73. cerebrovascular accident
74. encephal/o
75. kinesi/o
76. phas/o
77. somat/o
78. myel/o
79. thym/o
80. esthesi/o
81. top/o
82. hypn/o

83. gnos/o
84. pons
85. cerebellum
86. spinal
87. callosum
88. thalamus
89. cranium
90. meninges
91. cerebrum
92. Alzheimer
93. schizophrenia
94. polysomnography
95. paranoia
96. quadriplegia
97. atopognosis
98. dementia
99. epilepsy
100. catatonia
101. delusion
102. hallucination
103. poliomyelitis
104. epilepsy
105. euphoria
106. cerebellum
107. delusion
108. syncope
109. autism
110. psychosis
111. cerebrum
112. paranoia
113. j
114. d
115. h
116. f
117. a
118. e
119. b
120. i

121. g
122. c
123. generalized anxiety disorder
124. attention-deficit/hyperactivity disorder
125. obsessive-compulsive disorder
126. electroconvulsive therapy
127. bipolar disorder
128. posttraumatic stress disorder
129. c
130. a
131. f
132. e
133. g
134. b
135. d
136. neurosis
137. seasonal affective disorder
138. phobia
139. dysthymia
140. neuroleptic agents
141. psychosis
142. generalized anxiety disorder (GAD)
143. manic depression or bipolar disorder (BD)
144. panic disorder (PD)
145. psychotropic drugs
146. c
147. e
148. b
149. d
150. a

ANSWERS TO MEDICAL RECORD ANALYSIS

Medical Record 8-1: Outpatient History and Physical, Neurologic Services

1. b   2. c   3. d   4. a   5. c   6. e

Medical Record 8-2: For Additional Study

See CD-ROM for answers.

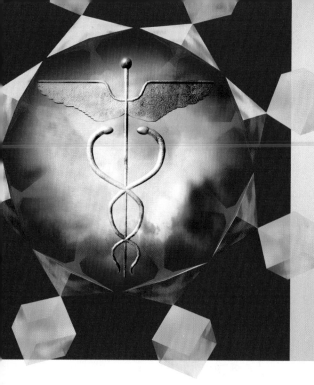

Endocrine System

ENDOCRINE SYSTEM OVERVIEW

The endocrine system secretes hormones and other substances from ductless glands and other structures (Fig. 9-1). Figure 9-2 describes these functions.

Self-Instruction: Combining Forms

Study the following:

COMBINING FORM	MEANING
aden/o	gland
adren/o, adrenal/o	adrenal gland
andr/o	male
crin/o	to secrete

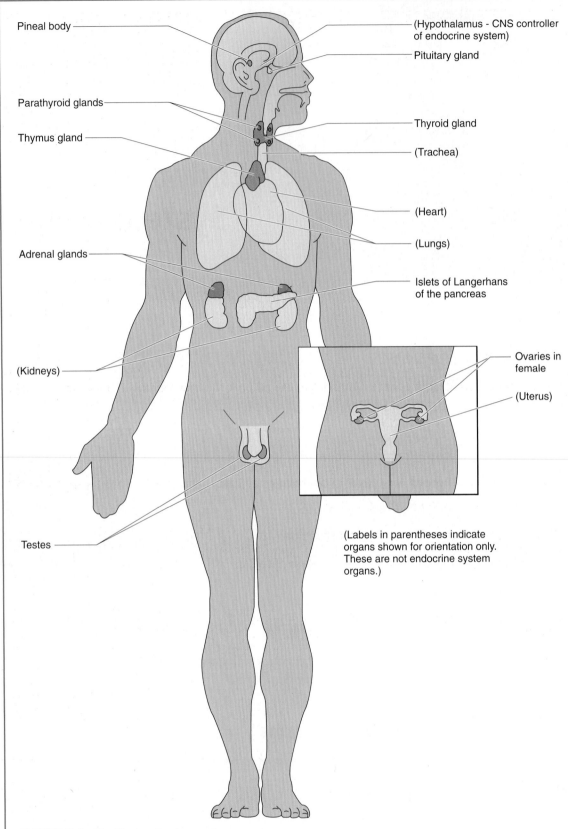

Pineal body

(Hypothalamus - CNS controller of endocrine system)

Pituitary gland

Parathyroid glands

Thyroid gland

Thymus gland

(Trachea)

(Heart)

(Lungs)

Adrenal glands

Islets of Langerhans of the pancreas

(Kidneys)

Ovaries in female

(Uterus)

Testes

(Labels in parentheses indicate organs shown for orientation only. These are not endocrine system organs.)

FIGURE 9-1 ■ **The endocrine system.**

Endocrine gland	Secretions	Function
*Anterior pituitary (adenohypophysis) 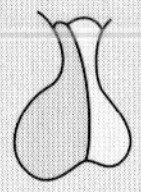	Thyroid-stimulating hormone (TSH)	Stimulates secretion from thyroid gland
	Adrenocorticotrophic hormone (ACTH)	Stimulates secretion from adrenal cortex
	Follicle-stimulating hormone (FSH)	Initiates growth of ovarian follicle; stimulates secretion of estrogen in females and sperm production in males
	Luteinizing hormone (LH)	Causes ovulation; stimulates secretion of progesterone by corpus luteum; causes secretion of testosterone in testes
	Melanocyte-stimulating hormone (MSH)	Affects skin pigmentation
	Growth hormone (GH)	Influences growth
	Prolactin (lactogenic hormone)	Stimulates breast development and milk production during pregnancy
*Posterior pituitary (neurohypophysis) 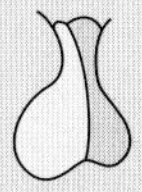	Antidiuretic hormone (ADH)	Influences the absorption of water by kidney tubules
	Oxytocin	Influences uterine contraction
Pineal body	Melatonin	Exact function unknown; effects onset of puberty
	Serotonin	Serves as a precursor to melatonin
Thyroid gland 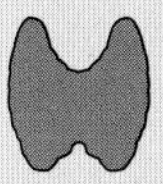	Triiodothyronine (T_3), thyroxine (T_4)	Regulate metabolism
	Calcitonin	Regulates calcium and phosphorus metabolism
Parathyroid glands 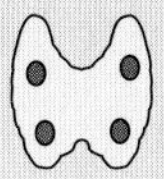	Parathyroid hormone (PTH)	Regulates calcium and phosphorus metabolism
Pancreas (islets of Langerhans) 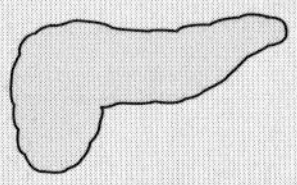	Insulin, glucagon	Regulates carbohydrate/sugar metabolism
Thymus gland 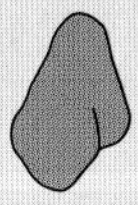	Thymosin	Regulates immune response
Adrenal glands (suprarenal glands) 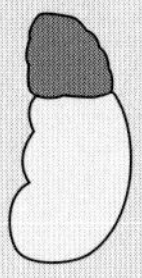	Steroid hormones: glucocorticoids, mineral corticosteroids, androgens	Regulate carbohydrate metabolism and salt and water balance; some effect on sexual characteristics.
	Epinephrine, norepinephrine	Affect sympathetic nervous system in stress response
Ovaries 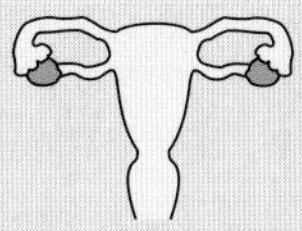	Estrogen, progesterone	Responsible for the development of female secondary sex characteristics and the regulation of reproduction
Testes 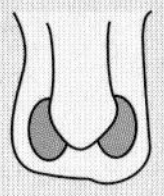	Testosterone	Affects masculinization and reproduction

*Release of hormones in pituitary is controlled by hypothalamus

FIGURE 9-2 ■ Functions of the endocrine glands.

COMBINING FORM	MEANING
dips/o	thirst
gluc/o, glucos/o, glyc/o	glucose (sugar)
hormon/o	hormone (an urging on)
ket/o, keton/o	ketone bodies
pancreat/o	pancreas
thym/o	thymus gland
thyr/o, thyroid/o	thyroid gland (shield)

Programmed Review: Combining Forms

ANSWERS	REVIEW
aden/o -oma adenoma	**9.1** The combining form meaning gland is _____. Put this together with the suffix referring to a tumor, _____, to create the term for a tumor of glandular tissue: _____.
adrenal near enlargement adrenomegaly inflammation adrenalitis	**9.2** The combining forms *adren/o* and *adrenal/o* mean _____ gland. The prefix *ad-* used in these combining forms gives a clue that the gland is to, toward, or _____ the kidney. Using *adren/o* and the suffix *-megaly,* meaning _____, the term describing an enlargement of the adrenal gland is _____. Using the combining form *adrenal/o* and the suffix *-itis,* meaning _____, the term describing an inflammation of the adrenal gland is _____.
andr/o form pertaining to andromorphous	**9.3** The combining form meaning male is _____. Linked to *morph/o,* the combining form meaning _____, and *-ous,* the suffix meaning _____ ____, the term pertaining to male form or appearance is _____.
secrete within endocrine	**9.4** The combining form *crin/o* means to _____. Recall that the prefix *endo-* means _____. Thus, the medical term for the _____ system refers to secreting within. The endocrine system secretes hormones and other substances from ductless glands.
dips/o many condition of polydipsia	**9.5** The combining form meaning thirst is _____. Recall that the prefix *poly-* means _____ or excessive, and that the suffix *-ia* means a _____ ____. Thus, the term for a condition of excessive thirst is _____.

ANSWERS	REVIEW
	9.6 The three combining terms for sugar are *glyc/o, gluc/o,* and
glucos/o	_____. Glucose is a form of sugar that is found in the blood and used for energy. The suffix *-genic* pertains to origin or
production	_____. Combined with *gluc/o,* the term for something
glucogenic	giving rise to or producing glucose is therefore _____.
hyper-	From the combining form *glyc/o* and the prefix _____, meaning too much or excessive, and the suffix *-emia*, referring to a
blood	_____ condition, comes the term hyperglycemia, a condition
glucose or sugar	of too much _____ in the blood.
hormon/o	**9.7** The combining form for hormone is _____, from a Greek word meaning "an urging on." (A hormone is a substance that urges an action to occur.) Hormonal is the _____ form.
adjective	
	9.8 The two combining forms meaning ketone bodies are *ket/o* and
keton/o	_____. Ketone bodies are chemical substances resulting from
ur/o	metabolism. Recall that the combining form for urine is _____, and
condition of	that the suffix *-ia* means a _____ ____. Therefore, the term
ketonuria	for a condition of ketone bodies in the urine is _____.
pancreat/o	**9.9** The combining form meaning the pancreas is _____.
-itis	Recall that the suffix for inflammation is _____. The term for
pancreatitis	inflammation of the pancreas is therefore _____.
pancreatectomy	Excision of the pancreas is termed _____.
thymus	**9.10** The combining form *thym/o* means the _____ gland.
thymoma	A tumor of thymic tissue is called a _____.
	9.11 The two combining forms meaning thyroid gland are
thyr/o, thyroid/o	_____ and _____. The Greek term at the origin of these combining forms means *shield*, and the thyroid
shield	gland is so named because it is resembles a _____. The
pertaining to	suffix *-ic* means _____ _____. Combined with *tox/o,*
poison	a combining form meaning _____, and *thyr/o,* meaning
thyroid gland	_____ _____, the term pertaining to poison
thyrotoxic	of the thyroid gland is _____. Thyroiditis
inflammation, thyroid	describes an _____ of the _____ gland.

Self-Instruction: Anatomic Terms

Study the following:

GLAND OR HORMONE	LOCATION OR FUNCTION
adrenal glands *ă-drē'năl glanz* **suprarenal glands** *sū'pră-rē'năl glanz*	located on the superior surface of each kidney; the adrenal cortex secretes steroid hormones, and the adrenal medulla secretes epinephrine and norepinephrine
steroid hormones *stēr'oyd hōr'mōnz*	hormones secreted by the adrenal cortex
glucocorticoids *glū-kō-kōr'ti-koydz*	regulate carbohydrate metabolism and have antiinflammatory effects; cortisol is the most significant glucocorticoid
mineral corticosteroids *min'ĕr-ăl kōr'ti-kō-stēr'oydz*	maintain salt and water balance
androgens *an'drŏ-jenz*	influence development and maintenance of male sex characteristics, for example, facial hair, deep voice
catecholamines *kat-ĕ-kol'ă-mēnz*	hormones secreted by the adrenal medulla that affect the sympathetic nervous system in stress response
epinephrine *ep-i-nef'rin* **adrenaline** *ă-dren'ă-lin*	secreted in response to fear or physical injury
norepinephrine *nōr'ep-i-nef'rin*	secreted in response to hypotension and physical stress
ovaries *ō'vă-rēz*	located on both sides of the uterus in the female pelvis; secrete estrogen and progesterone
estrogen *es'trō-jen*	responsible for the development of female secondary sex characteristics
progesterone *prō-jes'tĕr-ōn*	regulates uterine conditions during pregnancy
islets of Langerhans of the pancreas *ī'lets of lahng'ĕr-hahnz of the pan'krē-as*	endocrine tissue within the pancreas (the organ located behind the stomach, in front of the 1st and 2nd lumbar vertebrae); secretes insulin and glucagon
insulin *in'sŭ-lin*	a hormone secreted by the beta cells of the islets of Langerhans that is responsible for regulating the metabolism of glucose (*insulin* = island)
glucagon *glū'kă-gon*	a hormone secreted by the alpha cells of the islets of Langerhans that serves to regulate carbohydrate metabolism by raising blood sugar
parathyroid glands *par-ă-thī'royd glanz*	two paired glands located on the posterior aspect of the thyroid gland in the neck; secrete parathyroid hormone
parathyroid hormone (PTH) *par-ă-thī'royd hōr'mōn*	regulates calcium and phosphorus metabolism

GLAND OR HORMONE	LOCATION OR FUNCTION
pineal gland *pin'ē-ăl gland*	located in the center of the brain; secretes melatonin and serotonin
melatonin *mel-ă-tōn'in*	exact function unknown; affects the onset of puberty
serotonin *sĕr-ō-tō'nin*	a neurotransmitter that serves as the precursor to melatonin
pituitary gland *pi-tū'i-tār-ē gland* **hypophysis** *hī-pof'i-sis*	located at the base of the brain; considered the master gland as it secretes hormones that regulate the function of other glands, such as the thyroid gland, adrenal glands, ovaries, and testicles; the anterior pituitary secretes thyroid-stimulating hormone, adrenocorticotropic hormone, follicle-stimulating hormone, luteinizing hormone, melanocyte-stimulating hormone, growth hormone, and prolactin; the posterior pituitary releases antidiuretic hormone and oxytocin
anterior pituitary *an-tēr'ē-ōr pi-tū'i-tār-ē* **adenohypophysis** *ad'ĕ-nō-hī-pof'i-sis*	anterior lobe of the pituitary gland
thyroid-stimulating hormone (TSH) *thī'royd-stim-yū'lā-ting hōr'mōn*	stimulates secretion from thyroid gland
adrenocorticotropic hormone (ACTH) *ă-drē'nō-kōr'ti-kō-trō'pik hōr'mōn*	stimulates secretion from adrenal cortex
follicle-stimulating hormone (FSH) *fol'i-kĕl-stim-yū'lā-ting hōr'mōn*	initiates the growth of ovarian follicle; stimulates the secretion of estrogen in females and the production of sperm in males
luteinizing hormone (LH) *lū-tē-nī'zing hōr'mōn*	causes ovulation; stimulates the secretion of progesterone by the corpus luteum; causes the secretion of testosterone in the testes
melanocyte-stimulating hormone (MSH) *mel'ă-nō-sīt-stim-yū'lā-ting hōr'mōn*	affects skin pigmentation
growth hormone (GH) *grōth hōr'mōn*	influences growth
prolactin *prō-lak'tin* **lactogenic hormone** *lak-tō-jen'ik hōr'mōn*	stimulates breast development and milk production during pregnancy
posterior pituitary *pos-tēr'ē-ōr pi-tū'i-tār-ē* **neurohypophysis** *nūr'ō-hī-pof'i-sis*	posterior lobe of the pituitary gland

GLAND OR HORMONE	LOCATION OR FUNCTION
antidiuretic hormone (ADH) *an'tē-dī-yū-ret'ik hōr'mōn*	influences the absorption of water by kidney tubules
oxytocin *ok-sē-tō'sin*	influences uterine contraction
testes *tes'tēz*	located on both sides within the scrotum in the male; secrete testosterone
testosterone *tes-tos'tĕ-rōn*	affects masculinization and reproduction
thymus gland *thī'mŭs gland*	located in the mediastinal cavity anterior to and above the heart; secretes thymosin
thymosin *thī'mō-sin*	regulates immune response
thyroid gland *thī'royd gland*	located in front of the neck; secretes triiodothyronine (T₃), thyroxine (T₄), and calcitonin
triiodothyronine (T₃) *trī-ī'ō-dō-thī'rō-nēn* **thyroxine (T₄)** *thī-rok'sēn*	known as the thyroid hormones; regulate metabolism
calcitonin *kal-si-tō'nin*	regulates calcium and phosphorus metabolism

 ## Programmed Review: Anatomic Terms

ANSWERS	REVIEW
adrenal above	**9.12** The suprarenal, or _____, glands are located above the kidneys. The term renal refers to the kidneys, and the prefix *supra-* means _____. These glands secrete steroid hormones and other hormones.
corticoids steroids male	**9.13** Steroid hormones have several functions, including an effect on sex characteristics. They include gluco_____ and mineral cortico_____. Androgens are steroids that stimulate the development of _____ sex characteristics.
suprarenal norepinephrine nervous	**9.14** Also secreted by the adrenal, or _____, glands are epinephrine and _____, which are hormones that affect the _____ system in a stress response of the body. For example, epinephrine, also called adrenaline, stimulates the heart and breathing rates.

ANSWERS	REVIEW
	9.15 The ovaries in women are both reproductive and
endocrine	_____ organs, because they produce eggs for reproduction
secrete	and also _____ hormones. The hormones secreted by the
progesterone	two ovaries are estrogen and _____, which stimulate
female	the development of _____ sex characteristics and help to
	regulate reproduction.
	9.16 The islets of Langerhans are groups of cells in the
pancreas	_____, an organ that is located behind the stomach. The
glucagon	pancreas secretes insulin and _____, which help to regulate
	carbohydrate and sugar metabolism. The condition diabetes mellitus
	involves abnormal utilization of insulin. The term glucagon is made
gluc/o	from the combining form for sugar: _____.
alongside	**9.17** Recall that the prefix *para-* means _____
of	____. Located alongside of the thyroid glands in the neck
parathyroid	are the _____ glands. They secrete
parathyroid	_____ hormone (PTH), which regulates calcium
	and phosphorus metabolism.
pineal	**9.18** Located in the center of the brain is the _____ gland,
serotonin	which secretes the neurotransmitter _____. Also secreted
melatonin	by the pineal is the substance _____. The exact function
	of melatonin is unknown, but it affects the onset of puberty.
	9.19 The pituitary gland, located at the base of the brain, secretes a
hypophysis	long list of hormones. It is also called the _____, a term
below	using the prefix *hypo-*, meaning _____ (or deficient), because it
	hangs below the hypothalamus part of the brain. The front subdivision
anterior	of the pituitary gland is called the _____ pituitary, or the
posterior	adenohypophysis. The rear subdivision is called the _____
	pituitary, or the neurohypophysis.
	9.20 The anterior pituitary secretes seven hormones that are often
thyroid	identified by their abbreviations. TSH is _____-stimulating
corticotropic	hormone. ACTH is adreno_____ hormone. FSH is
follicle	_____-stimulating hormone. LH is luteinizing
hormone	_____.

ANSWERS	REVIEW
growth stimulating before, prolactin	**9.21** Also secreted by the anterior pituitary are _____ hormone (GH) and melanocyte-_____ hormone (MSH). The hormone that stimulates breast development and milk during pregnancy (from the combining form *lact/o* meaning milk and the prefix *pro-* meaning _____) is called _____.
neurohypophysis antidiuretic promotes	**9.22** The posterior pituitary, also called the _____, secretes two hormones. ADH, or _____ hormone, influences the absorption of water in the kidney. (Note that diuretic drugs stimulate the body to excrete water; thus, the term antidiuretic would involve an action that _____ the retention of water).
oxytocin	**9.23** The other hormone secreted by the posterior pituitary is _____, which stimulates uterine contractions during labor (childbirth).
testes testosterone testis	**9.24** In males, located within the scrotum are the _____, which are two glands that secrete a hormone affecting masculinization and reproduction: _____. The singular of testes is _____. The testes are also called the testicles.
thymus	**9.25** Located in the mediastinal cavity above and anterior to the heart is the _____ gland. This gland secretes thymosin, which regulates the immune response.
thyroid thyroxine calcitonin	**9.26** From the combining form *thyr/o*, the _____ gland is located in front of the neck and secretes three hormones. Triiodothyronine (T_3) and _____ (T_4) regulate metabolism. The third hormone, called _____, regulates calcium metabolism and is from the same combining form as calcium.

Self-Instruction: Symptomatic Terms

Study the following:

TERM	MEANING
exophthalmos or **exophthalmus** (*see* Fig. 9-6, B) *ek-sof-thal'mos or ek-sof-thal'mŭs*	protrusion of one or both eyeballs, often because of thyroid dysfunction or a tumor behind the eyeball
glucosuria *glŭ-kō-syū'rē-ă* **glycosuria** *glī'kō-sū'rē-ă*	glucose (sugar) in the urine

TERM	MEANING
hirsutism *hĭr′sū-tĭzm*	shaggy; an excessive growth of hair, especially in unusual places (e.g., a woman with a beard)
hypercalcemia *hī′pĕr-kal-sē′mē-ă*	an abnormally high level of calcium in the blood
hypocalcemia *hī′pō-kal-sē′mē-ă*	an abnormally low level of calcium in the blood
hyperglycemia *hī′pĕr-glī-sē′mē-ă*	high blood sugar
hypoglycemia *hī′pō-glī-sē′mē-ă*	low blood sugar
hyperkalemia *hī′pĕr-kă-lē′mē-ă*	an abnormally high level of potassium in the blood (*kalium* = potassium)
hypokalemia *hī′pō-kă-lē′mē-ă*	deficient level of potassium in the blood
hypersecretion *hī′pĕr-se-krē′shŭn*	abnormally increased secretion
hyposecretion *hī′pō-se-krē′shŭn*	abnormally decreased secretion
ketosis *kē-tō′sis* **ketoacidosis** *kē′tō-as-ĭ-dō′sis* **diabetic ketoacidosis (DKA)** *dī-ă-bĕt′ĭk kē′tō-as-ĭ-dō′sĭs*	presence of an abnormal amount of ketone bodies (acetone, beta-hydroxybutyric acid, and acetoacetic acid) in the blood and urine indicating an abnormal use of carbohydrates, such as in uncontrolled diabetes and starvation (*keto* = alter)
metabolism *mĕ-tab′ō-lizm*	all chemical processes in the body that result in growth, generation of energy, elimination of waste, and other body functions
polydipsia *pol-ē-dip′sē-ă*	excessive thirst
polyuria *pol-ē-yū′rē-ă*	excessive urination

Programmed Review: Symptomatic Terms

ANSWERS	REVIEW
away	**9.27** One of the combining forms for eye is *ophthalm/o*. Recall that the prefix *ex-* means _____ or out. The term for the condition in which one or both eyeballs protrude, usually because of a thyroid dysfunction, is
exophthalmos or exophthalmus	_____.

ANSWERS	REVIEW
hirsutism condition of	**9.28** From the Latin word meaning shaggy (hirsutus), the term for an excessive growth of hair in an unusual place is _____. The suffix -ism means _____ _____.
metabolism after	**9.29** Using the same suffix (-ism), though not in reference to a medical condition in this case, the term for all chemical processes in the body involving growth and energy is _____. The prefix meta- means beyond, _____, or change. In this instance, metabolism refers to changes occurring in those chemical processes.
urine, condition of glucosuria	**9.30** Recall that the combining form ur/o means _____, and that the suffix -ia means _____ _____. The condition of glucose (sugar) in the urine is called _____ or glycosuria.
many polyuria	**9.31** The prefix poly- means _____. The condition in which one urinates excessively many times is called _____.
polydipsia	**9.32** Using the same prefix (-poly) and suffix (-ia) as seen earlier, the term for the condition of excessive thirst is _____.
hyper- hypo- hypersecretion hyposecretion	**9.33** The most common prefix meaning above or excessive is _____. The opposite prefix, meaning below or deficient, is _____. These prefixes are used in many symptomatic terms related to levels of secretions and substances in the blood that are influenced by endocrine functions. Abnormally increased secretion is called _____, whereas abnormally decreased secretion is called _____.
-emia hypercalcemia hypocalcemia	**9.34** Recall that the suffix for a blood condition is _____. An abnormally high blood level of calcium is called _____, and an abnormally low blood level of calcium is called _____.

ANSWERS	REVIEW
hypoglycemia hyperglycemia	**9.35** An abnormally low level of blood sugar is called _____, whereas an abnormally high blood sugar level is called _____.
hypokalemia hyperkalemia	**9.36** From the Latin root *kalium* for potassium, the term for an abnormally low level of potassium in the blood is _____, whereas an abnormally high level of potassium in the blood is _____.
increase ketosis keto ketoacidosis	**9.37** The suffix *-osis* means condition or _____. The condition of an increased presence of ketone bodies is called _____, or _____acidosis. The abbreviation DKA refers to diabetic _____.

Self-Instruction: Diagnostic Terms

Study the following:

TERM	MEANING
ADRENAL GLANDS	
Cushing syndrome (Fig. 9-3) *kush'ing sin'drōm*	a collection of signs and symptoms caused by an excessive level of cortisol hormone; may be due to excessive production by the adrenal gland (often because of a tumor), or, more commonly, occurs as a side effect of treatment with glucocorticoid (steroid) hormones, such as prednisone for asthma, rheumatoid arthritis, lupus, or other inflammatory diseases; symptoms include upper body obesity, facial puffiness (moon-shaped appearance), hyperglycemia, weakness, thin and easily bruised skin with stria (stretch marks), hypertension, and osteoporosis

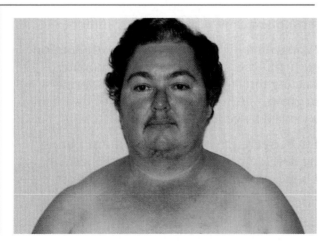

FIGURE 9-3 ■ **Cushing syndrome. A patient with the characteristic upper body obesity and facial puffiness with a moon-shaped appearance is shown.**

TERM	MEANING
adrenal virilism *ă-drē'năl vir'i-lizm*	excessive output of the adrenal secretion of androgen (male sex hormone) in adult women caused by a tumor or hyperplasia; evidenced by amenorrhea (absence of menstruation), acne, hirsutism, and deepening of the voice (*virilis* = masculine)

PANCREAS

TERM	MEANING
diabetes mellitus (DM) *dī-ă-bē'tēz mel'i-tŭs*	metabolic disorder caused by the absence or insufficient production of insulin secreted by the pancreas, resulting in hyperglycemia and glucosuria (*diabetes* = passing through; *mellitus* = sugar)
type 1 diabetes mellitus *tīp 1 dī-ă-bē'tēz mel'i-tŭs*	diabetes in which no beta-cell production of insulin occurs and the patient is dependent on insulin for survival
type 2 diabetes mellitus *tīp 2 dī-ă-bē'tēz mel'i-tŭs*	diabetes in which either the body produces insufficient insulin or insulin resistance (a defective use of the insulin that is produced) occurs; the patient usually is not dependent on insulin for survival
hyperinsulinism *hī'pĕr-in'sū-lin-izm*	a condition resulting from an excessive amount of insulin in the blood that draws sugar out of the bloodstream, resulting in hypoglycemia, fainting, and convulsions; often caused by an overdose of insulin or by a tumor of the pancreas
pancreatitis *pan'krē-ă-tī'tis*	inflammation of the pancreas

PARATHYROID GLANDS

TERM	MEANING
hyperparathyroidism *hī'pĕr-par-ă-thī'royd-izm*	hypersecretion of the parathyroid glands, usually caused by a tumor
hypoparathyroidism *hī'pō-par-ă-thī'royd-izm*	hyposecretion of the parathyroid glands

PITUITARY GLAND (HYPOPHYSIS)

TERM	MEANING
acromegaly (Fig. 9-4) *ak-rō-meg'ă-lē*	disease characterized by enlarged features, especially of the face and hands, caused by hypersecretion of the pituitary growth hormone after puberty, when normal bone growth has stopped; most often caused by a pituitary tumor
pituitary dwarfism (Fig. 9-5) *pi-tū'i-tār-ē dwōrf'izm*	a condition of congenital hyposecretion of growth hormone that slows growth and causes short, yet proportionate, stature (not affecting intelligence); often treated during childhood with growth hormone; other forms of dwarfism are most often caused by genetic defects
pituitary gigantism *pi-tū'i-tār-ē jī'gan-tizm*	a condition of hypersecretion of growth hormone during childhood bone development that leads to an abnormal overgrowth of bone, especially of the long bones; most often caused by a pituitary tumor

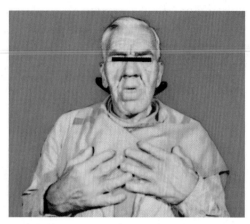

FIGURE 9-4 ■ Enlarged hands and facial features in patient with acromegaly.

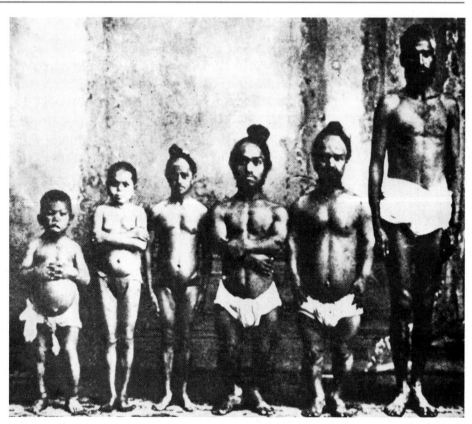

FIGURE 9-5 ■ Normal male (extreme right) and three types of dwarfism. On the extreme left is a child who has failed to grow because of congenital absence of the thyroid gland (cretinism). The next pair of dwarfs have entirely normal proportions but are half-normal in size (pituitary dwarfism). The next pair to the right show disproportionately short extremities but normal-sized trunk and head (disproportionate dwarfism because of gene defect).

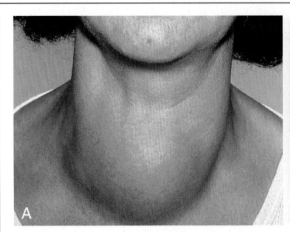 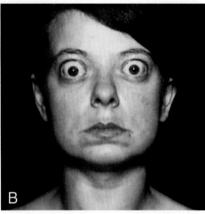

FIGURE 9-6 ■ Hyperthyroidism. A. Patient with goiter. B. Patient with exophthalmos.

TERM	MEANING
THYROID GLAND	
goiter (Fig. 9-6) *goy'tĕr*	enlargement of the thyroid gland caused by thyroid dysfunction, tumor, lack of iodine in the diet, or inflammation (*goiter* = throat)
hyperthyroidism (*see* Fig. 9-6) *hī-pĕr-thī'royd-izm*	a condition of hypersecretion of the thyroid gland characterized by nervousness, weight loss, rapid pulse, protrusion of the eyeball (exophthalmos), goiter, etc.; see Comparison of Symptoms in table on page 457
Graves disease *grāvz diz'ēz*	the most common form of hyperthyroidism; caused by an autoimmune defect that creates antibodies that stimulate the overproduction of thyroid hormones; exophthalmos is a featured characteristic
hypothyroidism *hī'pō-thī'royd-izm*	a condition of hyposecretion of the thyroid gland causing low thyroid levels in the blood that result in sluggishness, slow pulse, and, often, obesity; see Comparison of Symptoms in table on page 457
myxedema *mik-sĕ-dē'mă*	advanced hypothyroidism in adults characterized by sluggishness, slow pulse, puffiness in the hands and face, and dry skin (*myx* = mucus)
cretinism (*see* Fig. 9-5) *krē'tin-izm*	condition of congenital hypothyroidism in children that results in a lack of mental development and dwarfed physical stature; the thyroid gland is either congenitally absent or imperfectly developed

COMPARISON OF SYMPTOMS: HYPERTHYROIDISM VERSUS HYPOTHYROIDISM

HYPERTHYROIDISM	HYPOTHYROIDISM
Restless, nervous, irritable, fine tremor, insomnia	Lethargic, poor memory, slow, expressionless
Fine, silky hair with hair loss	Dry, brittle hair with hair loss
Warm, moist skin	Pale, cold, dry, and scaling skin
Increased perspiration	Decreased perspiration
Fast heart rate (tachycardia)	Slow heart rate (bradycardia)
Weight loss	Weight gain
Protrusion of the eyeball (exophthalmos)	Edema of the face and eyelids
Absence of menses (amenorrhea)	Heavy menses (menorrhagia)
Diffuse goiter	Thick tongue, slow speech

◈ Programmed Review: Diagnostic Terms

ANSWERS	REVIEW
inflammation pancreatitis	**9.38** Recall that the suffix *-itis* means _____. Inflammation of the pancreas is called _____.
high sugar diabetes mellitus 1, no insulin 2 resistance	**9.39** Most endocrine problems involve excessive or deficient secretion of hormones or the body's use of those hormones. The condition caused by the absence or insufficient production of insulin secreted by the pancreas resulting in hyperglycemia (_____ blood sugar) and glycosuria (_____ in the urine) is called _____ _____ (DM). Patients with type ____ diabetes mellitus produce ____ insulin and thereby are dependent on _____ for survival. Patients with type ____ diabetes mellitus produce insulin, but not enough, or have insulin _____ (a defective use of the insulin that is produced).
hyper- condition of hyperinsulinism hypoglycemia	**9.40** Recall that the prefix for excessive is _____, and that the suffix *-ism* refers to a _____ ____. The condition of having excessive insulin is called _____. This condition results in low blood sugar, which is called _____.

ANSWERS	REVIEW
hypoparathyroidism hyperparathyroidism	**9.41** The terms for diagnostic conditions are formed from the combining form for the gland's name with the prefixes for deficient or excessive, referring to the gland's secretion. The condition of hyposecretion of the parathyroid glands is called _____, and hypersecretion of these glands is called _____.
hypothyroidism hyperthyroidism Graves exophthalmos or exophthalmus	**9.42** Similarly, hyposecretion of the thyroid gland is called _____, and hypersecretion of the thyroid gland is called _____. The most common form of hyperthyroidism is called _____ disease. A featured characteristic of Graves disease is the protrusion of the eyeballs, known as _____.
cretinism	**9.43** Congenital hypothyroidism in children, characterized by reduced stature and poor mental development, is called _____.
myxedema	**9.44** The term edema refers to a swollen body area caused by fluid retention. This root is used in the term for a form of advanced hypothyroidism in adults that involves swollen hands and face along with other symptoms: _____.
goiter	**9.45** The Latin word guttur means throat. The condition of an enlarged thyroid gland caused by thyroid dysfunction, tumor, or other causes, and characterized by the appearance of a swollen throat is _____.
Cushing	**9.46** Cortisol is a glucocorticoid hormone that is secreted by the adrenal gland. Excessive levels of cortisol, either caused by tumor or as a side effect of treatment with steroid hormones, result in a collection of signs and symptoms known as _____ syndrome.
andr/o, androgen	**9.47** The adrenal glands also secrete a male sex hormone that is named using the combining form for male: _____. This hormone is called _____.

ANSWERS	REVIEW
adrenal virilism	Hypersecretion of androgen in adult women causes a condition that is named, in part, from the Latin word for masculine (virilis). This condition is called _____ _____.
dwarfism	**9.48** Recall that the pituitary gland produces a number of hormones, including growth hormone. The condition of congenital hyposecretion of growth hormone, marked by small, but proportionate, stature, is called pituitary _____.
enlargement acromegaly pituitary gigantism childhood hyper tumor	**9.49** The combining form *acr/o* refers to the extremities. Recall that the suffix *-megaly* means _____. The condition characterized by enlarged hands and face resulting from pituitary hypersecretion of growth hormone after puberty, when normal bone growth has stopped, is termed _____. The condition of hypersecretion of pituitary growth hormone during childhood bone development that leads to an abnormal overgrowth of bone, especially of the long bones, is called _____ _____. Acromegaly occurs in adulthood, and gigantism occurs in _____. Each is a result of _____secretion of pituitary growth hormone, most often caused by a _____.

◆ Self-Instruction: Diagnostic Tests and Procedures

Study the following:

TEST OR PROCEDURE	EXPLANATION
LABORATORY TESTING	
blood sugar (BS) *blŭd shu-găr* **blood glucose** *blŭd glu′kōs*	measurement of the level of sugar (glucose) in the blood
fasting blood sugar (FBS) *fast-ing blŭd shu-găr*	measurement of blood sugar level after fasting (not eating) for 12 hours

TEST OR PROCEDURE	EXPLANATION
postprandial blood sugar (PPBS) *pōst-pran'dē-ăl blŭd shu-găr*	measurement of blood sugar level after a meal (commonly 2 hours later)
glucose tolerance test (GTT) *glū'kōs tol'ĕr-ănts test*	measurement of the body's ability to metabolize carbohydrates by administering a prescribed amount of glucose after a fasting period, then measuring blood and urine for glucose levels every hour thereafter for 4 to 6 hours
glycohemoglobin *glī'kō-hē-mō-glō'bin* **glycosylated hemoglobin (HbAlc)** *glī'kō-si-lāt-ĕd hē-mō-glō'bin*	a molecule (fraction) in hemoglobin, the level of which rises in the blood as a result of an increased level of blood sugar; a common blood test used in diagnosing and treating diabetes
electrolyte panel *ē-lek'trō-līt păn'l*	measurement of the level of specific ions (sodium, potassium, and chloride) along with carbon dioxide (CO_2) (for indirect measure of bicarbonate ion) in the blood; electrolytes are essential for maintaining water balance (hydration) as well as nerve, muscle, and heart activity
thyroid function study *thi'royd fŭnk'shŭn stŭd'ē*	measurement of thyroid hormone levels in blood plasma to determine the efficiency of glandular secretions, including T_3, T_4, and TSH
urine sugar and ketone studies *yūr'in shu-gar and kē'tōn stŭd'ēz*	chemical tests to determine the presence of sugar or ketone bodies in urine; used as a screen for diabetes (Note: production of a urine specimen for these tests requires one to urinate or void [empty the bladder])

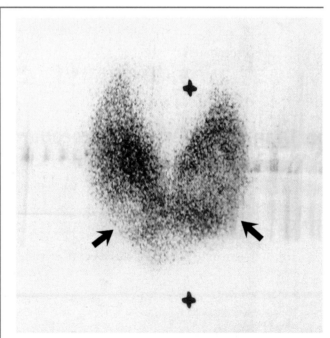

FIGURE 9-7 ■ Thyroid uptake and image detecting the presence of multiple nodules *(arrows)*.

TERM	MEANING
hormone replacement therapy (HRT) *hōr'mōn rē-plās'ment thār'ă-pē*	treatment with a hormone to correct a hormonal deficiency (e.g., estrogen, testosterone, and thyroid)
hypoglycemic *hī'pō-glī-sē'mik* **antihyperglycemic** *an'tē-hī'per-glī-sē'mik*	a drug that lowers the blood glucose level (e.g., insulin)

🔷 Programmed Review: Therapeutic Terms

ANSWERS	REVIEW
continuous subcutaneous insulin infusion 1 diabetes mellitus	**9.68** An insulin pump is a device that subcutaneously infuses programmed doses of insulin through the skin. This therapy, which is called _____ _____ _____ _____ (CSII), is used in the treatment of type ___ _____ _____ (DM).
radioiodine nuclear	**9.69** Because the thyroid gland absorbs iodine, radioactive iodine that is administered into the body becomes localized in the thyroid, where it can kill thyroid tumor cells. This is called _____ therapy, and it is administered in a _____ medicine facility.
anti- antidiabetic -emia hyperglycemia antihyperglycemic hypoglycemic	**9.70** Drug classifications are often named by their action against some process or condition in the body. The prefix meaning against is _____. Any agent that works against the ill effects of diabetes mellitus by controlling blood sugar levels in called an _____ drug. The suffix for a blood condition is _____. Recall that the condition of high blood sugar is called _____. A drug that works against this condition by lowering the blood glucose level is an _____ drug. Another term for this is a _____ drug.
antithyroid	**9.71** An agent that blocks the production of thyroid hormones is called an _____ drug.
hormone replacement therapy	**9.72** A patient with a deficiency of a particular hormone may be treated by administration of that hormone to replace what is missing. This treatment is referred to as _____ _____ _____ (HRT).

CHAPTER 9 ACRONYMS AND ABBREVIATIONS

ABBREVIATION	EXPANSION
ACTH	adrenocorticotropic hormone
ADH	antidiuretic hormone
BS	blood sugar
CO_2	carbon dioxide
CSII	continuous subcutaneous insulin infusion
CT	computed tomography
DKA	diabetic ketoacidosis
DM	diabetes mellitus
FBS	fasting blood sugar
FSH	follicle-stimulating hormone
GH	growth hormone
GTT	glucose tolerance test
HbAlc	glycosylated hemoglobin
HRT	hormone replacement therapy
LH	luteinizing hormone
MRI	magnetic resonance imaging
MSH	melanocyte-stimulating hormone
PPBS	postprandial blood sugar
PTH	parathyroid hormone
T_3	triiodothyronine
T_4	thyroxine
TSH	thyroid-stimulating hormone

CHAPTER 9 SUMMARY OF TERMS

The terms introduced in chapter 9 are listed below, followed by the page number on which each term can be found and its written pronunciation. For additional practice and reinforcement, write the definition of each term on a separate piece of paper.

acromegaly/454
ak-rō-meg′ă-lē

adenohypophysis/447
ad′ĕ-nō-hī-pof′i-sis

adrenal glands/446
ă-drē′năl glanz

adrenal virilism/454
ă-drē′năl vir′i-lizm

adrenalectomy/463
ă-drē-năl-ek′tŏ-mē

adrenaline/446
ă-dren′ă-lin

adrenocorticotropic hormone (ACTH)/447
ă-drē′nō-kōr′ti-kō-trō′pik hōr′mōn

androgens/446
an′drō-jenz

anterior pituitary/447
an-tēr'ē-ōr pi-tū'i-tār-ē

antidiabetic drug/464
an-tē-dī-ă-bet'ik drŭg

**antidiuretic hormone
  (ADH)**/448
an'tē-dī-yū-ret'ik hōr'mōn

antihyperglycemic/465
an'tē-hī'per-glī-sē'mik

antithyroid drug/464
an-tē-thī'royd drŭg

blood glucose/459
blŭd glū'kōs

blood sugar (BS)/459
blŭd shu-găr

calcitonin/448
kal-si-tō'nin

catecholamines/446
kat-ě-kol'ă-mēnz

**computed tomography
  (CT)**/461
kom-pyū'tĕd tō-mog'ră-fē

**continuous subcutaneous insulin
  infusion (CSII)**/464
*kon-tin'yū-ŭs sŭb-kyū-tā'nē-ŭs in'sŭ-lin
  in-fyū'zhŭn*

cretinism/456
krē'tin-izm

Cushing syndrome/453
kush'ing sin'drōm

diabetes mellitus (DM)/454
dī-ă-bē'tēz mel'i-tŭs

diabetic ketoacidosis (DKA)/451
dī-ă-bĕt'ik kē'tō-as-ĭ-dō'sis

electrolyte panel/460
ē-lek'trō-līt păn'l

epinephrine/446
ep-i-nef'rin

estrogen/446
es'trō-jen

exophthalmos or **exophthalmus**/450
ek-sof-thal'mos or ek-sof-thal'mŭs

fasting blood sugar (FBS)/459
fast-ing blŭd shu-găr

**follicle-stimulating hormone
  (FSH)**/447
fol'i-kĕl-stim-yū'lā-ting hōr'mōn

glucagons/446
glū'kă-gon

glucocorticoids/446
glū'kō-kōr'ti-koydz

glucose tolerance test (GTT)/460
glū'kōs tol'ĕr-ănts test

glucosuria/450
glū'kō-syū'rē-ă

glycohemoglobin/460
glī'kō-hē-mō-glō'bin

glycosuria/450
glī-kō-sū'rē-ă

glycosylated hemoglobin (HbAlc)/460
glī'kō-si-lāt-ĕd hē-mō-glō'bin

goiter/456
goy'tĕr

Graves disease/456
grāvz di-zēz'

growth hormone (GH)/447
grōth hōr'mōn

hirsutism/450
hĭr'sū-tizm

**hormone replacement therapy
  (HRT)**/465
hōr'mōn rē-plās'ment thār'ă-pē

hypercalcemia/450
hī'pĕr-kal-sē'mē-ă

hyperglycemia/450
hī'pĕr-glī-sē'mē-ă

hyperinsulinism/454
hī'pĕr-in'sū-lin-izm

hyperkalemia/450
hī'pĕr-kă-lē'mē-ă

hyperparathyroidism/454
hī'pĕr-par-ă-thī'royd-izm

hypersecretion/450
hī'pĕr-se-krē'shŭn

hyperthyroidism/456
hī-pĕr-thī'royd-izm

hypocalcemia/450
hī'pō-kal-sē'mē-ă

hypoglycemia/450
hī'pō-glī-sē'mē-ă

hypoglycemic/465
hī'pō-glī-sē'mik

hypokalemia/450
hī'pō-kă-lē'mē-ă

hypoparathyroidism/454
hī'pō-par-ă-thī'royd-izm

hypophysectomy/463
hī'pof-i-sek'tŏ-mē

hypophysis/447
hī-pof'i-sis

hyposecretion/451
hī'pō-se-krē'shŭn

hypothyroidism/456
hī'pō-thī'royd-izm

insulin/446
in'sŭ-lin

insulin pump therapy/464
in'sŭ-lin pŭmp thār'ă-pē

islets of Langerhans of the pancreas/446
ī'lets of lahng'ĕr-hahnz of the pan'krē-as

ketoacidosis/451
kē'tō-as-i-dō'sis

ketosis/451
kē-tō'sis

lactogenic hormone/447
lak-tō-jen'ik hōr'mōn

luteinizing hormone (LH)/447
lū-tē-nī'zing hōr'mōn

magnetic resonance imaging (MRI)/461
măg-net'ik rez'ō-nănts im'ă-jing

melanocyte-stimulating hormone (MSH)/447
mel'ă-nō-sīt-stim-yū'lā-ting hōr'mōn

melatonin/447
mel-ă-tōn'in

metabolism/451
mĕ-tab'ō-lizm

mineral corticosteroids/446
min'ĕr-ăl kōr'ti-kō-stēr'oydz

myxedema/456
mik-sĕ-dē'mă

neurohypophysis/447
nūr'ō-hī-pof'i-sis

norepinephrine/446
nōr'ep-i-nef'rin

ovaries/446
ō'vă-rēz

oxytocin/448
ok'sē-tō'sin

pancreatectomy/463
pan'krē-ă-tek'tŏ-mē

pancreatitis/454
pan'krē-ă-tī'tis

parathyroid glands/446
par-ă-thī'royd glanz

parathyroid hormone (PTH)/446
par-ă-thī'royd hōr'mōn

parathyroidectomy/463
pa'ră-thī-roy-dek'tŏ-mē

pineal gland/447
pin'ē-ăl gland

pituitary dwarfism/454
pi-tū'i-tār-ē dwōrf'izm

pituitary gigantism/454
pi-tū'i-tār-ē jī'gan-tizm

pituitary gland/447
pi-tū'i-tār-ē gland

polydipsia/451
pol-ē-dip'sē-ă

polyuria/451
pol-ē-yū'rē-ă

posterior pituitary/447
pos-tēr'ē-ŏr pi-tū'i-tār-ē

postprandial blood sugar (PPBS)/460
pōst-pran'dē-ăl blŭd shu-găr

progesterone/446
prō-jes'tĕr-ōn

prolactin/447
prō-lak'tin

radioiodine therapy/464
rā'dē-ō-ī'ō-dīn thār'ă-pē

serotonin/447
sĕr-ō-tō'nin

sonography/461
sŏ-nog'ră-fē

steroid hormones/446
stēr'oyd hor'mōnz

suprarenal glands/446
sū'pră-rē'năl glanz

testes/448
tes'tēz

testosterone/448
tes-tos'tĕ-rōn

thymectomy/463
thī-mek'tō-mē

thymosin/448
thī'mō-sin

thymus gland/448
thī'mŭs gland

thyroid function study/460
thī'royd fŭnk'shŭn stŭd'ē

thyroid gland/448
thī'royd gland

thyroid uptake and image/461
thī'royd ŭp'tāk and im'ăj

thyroidectomy/463
thī-roy-dek'tŏ-mē

**thyroid-stimulating hormone
   (TSH)**/447
thī'royd-stim-yū'lā-ting hōr'mōn

thyroxine (T₄)/448
thī-rok'sēn

triiodothyronine (T₃)/448
trī-ī'ō-dō-thī'rō-nēn

type 1 diabetes mellitus/454
tīp 1 dī-ă-bē'tēz mel'i-tŭs

type 2 diabetes mellitus/454
tīp 2 dī-ă-bē'tēz mel'i-tŭs

**urine sugar and ketone
   studies**/460
yŭr'in shu-găr and kē'tōn stŭd'ēz

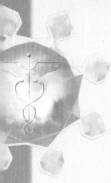

PRACTICE EXERCISES

For each of the following words, write out the term components (prefixes [P], combining forms [CF], roots [R], and suffixes [S]) on the lines below the word. Then define the term according to the meaning of its components.

EXAMPLE

parathyroid

para / _thyr_ / _oid_

P   R   S

DEFINITION: alongside of/thyroid gland/resembling

1. adenitis

_____ / _____

R   S

DEFINITION: _____

2. hyperglycemia

_____ / _____ / _____

P   R   S

DEFINITION: _____

3. thyrotoxicosis

_____ / _____ / _____

CF   R   S

DEFINITION: _____

4. polydipsia

_____ / _____ / _____

P   R   S

DEFINITION: _____

5. hormonal

_____ / _____

R   S

DEFINITION: _____

6. ketosis

_____ / _____

R   S

DEFINITION: _____

7. polyuria

_____ / _____ / _____

P   R   S

DEFINITION: _____

8. endocrine

_____ / _____ / _____

  P   R   S

DEFINITION: _____

9. thyroptosis

_____ / _____

  CF   S

DEFINITION: _____

10. thymoma

_____ / _____

  R   S

DEFINITION: _____

11. acromegaly

_____ / _____

  CF   S

DEFINITION: _____

12. android

_____ / _____

  R   S

DEFINITION: _____

13. adrenotropic

_____ / _____ / _____

  CF   R   S

DEFINITION: _____

14. pancreatogenic

_____ / _____ / _____

  CF   R   S

DEFINITION: _____

15. glycosuria

_____ / _____ / _____

  R   R   S

DEFINITION: _____

Write the correct medical term for each of the following definitions:

16. _____ advanced hypothyroidism in adults

17. _____ congenital hypothyroidism

18. _____ most common form of hyperthyroidism

19. _____ condition resulting from an excessive level of cortisol hormone characterized by obesity, hyperglycemia, and weakness

20. _____ disease characterized by enlarged features, caused by hyper-secretion of the pituitary growth hormone after puberty

21. _____ enlargement of the thyroid gland

22. _____ protrusion of the eyeball

23. _____ condition of hyposecretion of pituitary growth hormone during childhood bone development

24. _____ deficient level of potassium in the blood

25. _____ nuclear image of the thyroid

26. _____ condition of hypersecretion of the pituitary growth hormone during childhood bone development

Write the letter of the matching term in the space after the meaning:

27. congenital hypothyroidism _____   a. gigantism
28. polydipsia _____   b. hirsutism
29. hyperthyroidism _____   c. enlarged thyroid
30. hypophysis _____   d. depends on insulin
31. goiter _____   e. cretinism
32. adult hypothyroidism _____   f. pituitary
33. adrenal virilism _____   g. does not usually depend on insulin
34. type 2 diabetes _____   h. excessive thirst
35. pituitary hypersecretion _____   i. myxedema
36. type 1 diabetes _____   j. Graves disease

Complete each medical term by writing the missing part:

37. poly_____ia = excessive thirst

38. _____secretion = abnormally increased secretion

39. _____glycemia = low blood sugar

40. glucos_____ = sugar in the urine

41. _____secretion = decreased secretion

42. _____glycemia = high blood sugar

43. _____graphy = ultrasound imaging

Write out the expanded term for each abbreviation:

44. CSII _____

45. HRT _____

46. FBS _____

47. DM _____

48. PPBS _____

49. GTT _____

50. DKA _____

Identify the structures of the endocrine system by writing the missing words in the spaces provided:

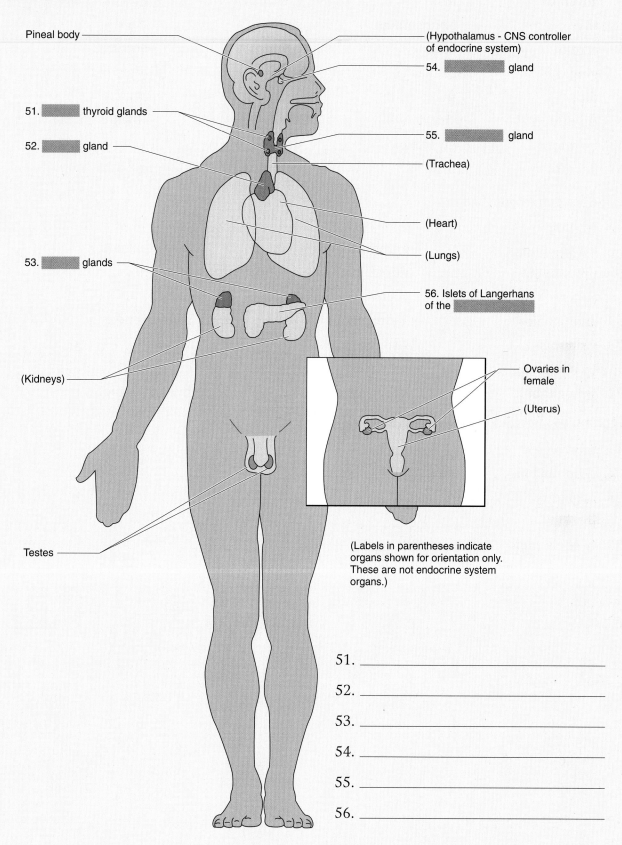

Pineal body

(Hypothalamus - CNS controller of endocrine system)

54. _____ gland

51. _____ thyroid glands

52. _____ gland

55. _____ gland

(Trachea)

(Heart)

(Lungs)

53. _____ glands

56. Islets of Langerhans of the _____

(Kidneys)

Ovaries in female

(Uterus)

Testes

(Labels in parentheses indicate organs shown for orientation only. These are not endocrine system organs.)

51. _____

52. _____

53. _____

54. _____

55. _____

56. _____

Circle the meaning that corresponds to the combining form given:

57. **adren/o**	male	extremity	adrenal gland
58. **thyr/o**	nourishment	shield	chest
59. **crin/o**	blue	cell	secrete
60. **gluc/o**	stomach	sugar	pancreas
61. **dips/o**	thirst	ketones	secrete
62. **thym/o**	shield	hormone	thymus gland
63. **hormon/o**	development	urging on	ketones
64. **aden/o**	male	extremity	gland

Circle the correct spelling:

65.	hirsutism	hirsuitism	hirsitism
66.	exopthalmos	exopthamamos	exophthalmos
67.	myexedema	mixedema	myxedema
68.	goiter	goyter	goitir
69.	androgenius	androgenous	andreogenous
70.	virillism	virilism	viralism
71.	epinephrine	epinefrine	epineprine
72.	hypoglicemic	hypoglicemic	hypoglycemic

Give the noun that is used to form each adjective:

73. acromegalic   _____

74. exophthalmic   _____

75. metabolic   _____

76. diabetic   _____

77. hypoglycemic   _____

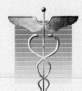

MEDICAL RECORD ANALYSIS

Medical Record 9-1

PROGRESS NOTE

S: This is a 27 y.o. ♀ c̄ a known Hx of diabetes seen in the ER with nausea and vomiting for the past three hours. She has skipped two doses of her insulin because BS levels monitored at home have been low. She is now experiencing a cephalalgia similar to what she has had in the past before coma.

O: T 35.5° C, P 90, R 20, BP 126/68

Lab blood studies: sodium 130, potassium 4.1, CO_2 9, chloride 102, glucose 296

A: Diabetic ketoacidosis

P: Admit to ICU: give 10 units insulin IV; measure BS 1° p̄ insulin given, then q 4 h; check urine for sugar and ketosis q void; repeat electrolytes in a.m.

QUESTIONS ABOUT MEDICAL RECORD 9-1

1. What is the CC?
   a. nausea, vomiting, and headache
   b. nausea, vomiting, and dizziness
   c. nausea, vomiting, and high blood pressure
   d. nausea, vomiting, and ringing in the ears
   e. nausea, vomiting, and unconsciousness

2. What is the diagnosis?
   a. hyperglycemia
   b. hypoglycemia
   c. type 1 DM with ketone bodies in the blood
   d. type 2 DM without ketone bodies in the blood
   e. combination of hyperglycemia and glucosuria

3. As an inpatient, where was treatment provided?
   a. neuropsychiatric facility
   b. coronary care facility
   c. emergency room
   d. recovery room
   e. critical care facility

4. Which of the following are electrolytes?
   1. sodium   2. potassium   3. chloride   4. glucose
   a. only 1, 2, and 3 are electrolytes
   b. only 1 and 3 are electrolytes
   c. only 2 and 4 are electrolytes
   d. only 4 is an electrolyte
   e. all are electrolytes

5. Why were the blood electrolyte studies performed?
   a. to examine the electrical impulses of the brain
   b. to measure the level of ions in the blood in evaluation of metabolism
   c. to measure hormone levels and determine glandular efficiency
   d. to visualize the accumulation of radioactive isotopes to eliminate the presence of tumor
   e. to measure the level of glucose in the blood

6. How should the insulin be administered?
   a. within the skin
   b. absorption through unbroken skin
   c. within the muscle
   d. within the vein
   e. under the skin

7. How often should the blood glucose be measured?
   a. one hour after insulin administration, then every four hours thereafter
   b. once each morning
   c. each time the patient urinates
   d. one hour before insulin administration, then four times a day thereafter
   e. one hour before insulin administration, then every four hours thereafter

Medical Record 9-2

FOR ADDITIONAL STUDY

Tara Nguyen had a long history of hyperthyroidism that was managed by pharmacologic treatment for more than 5 years. She was often unhappy with how she felt, however, and decided on her own to stop taking the drug. Two months ago, the symptoms of hyperthyroidism recurred, and she sought medical attention. Medical Record 9-2 is the report by Dr. Rincon, the physician who analyzed Ms. Nguyen's thyroid uptake and imaging study.

Read Medical Record 9-2 (page 477), then write your answers to the following questions in the spaces provided.

QUESTIONS ABOUT MEDICAL RECORD 9-2

1. Below are medical terms used in this record that you have not yet encountered in this text. Underline each where it appears in the record, and define the term below.

   propylthiouracil (PTU) _____

   uptake _____

   baseline (nonmedical term) _____

2. In your own words, not using medical terminology, briefly describe what seems to have been missing in Ms. Nguyen's past medical management:

   _____

   _____

3. In nonmedical terms, explain how the sodium iodide was administered:

   _____

4. In your own words, not using medical terminology, briefly describe Dr. Rincon's diagnosis:

   _____

   _____

   _____

5. What additional test did Dr. Rincon order on his own authority?

   a. thyroid function study

   b. fasting blood sugar (FBS)

   c. thyroid MRI

   d. thyroid ultrasound

6. Which of the following tests is recommended to be performed in 6 months?

   a. thyroid function study

   b. fasting blood sugar (FBS)

   c. thyroid MRI

   d. thyroid ultrasound

Medical Record 9-2: For Additional Study

CENTRAL MEDICAL CENTER

211 Medical Center Drive • Central City, US 90000-1234 • PHONE: (012) 125-6784 • FAX: (012) 125-9999

THYROID UPTAKE AND IMAGING STUDY

Date of Exam: 5/29/20xx

CLINICAL HISTORY: The patient has more than a six year history of hyperthyroidism which was treated until approximately one year ago with propylthiouracil (PTU). The patient relates some instability in symptomatology during the treatment. She had no previous uptake and imaging study, and radioiodine therapy was never discussed with the patient. She spontaneously discontinued taking the PTU approximately one year ago and has had recurrent symptoms of hyperthyroidism in the last two months.

TECHNIQUE: The patient ingested a capsule containing 200 μCi ^{123}I sodium iodide. Uptakes in the neck were measured at 6 and 24 hours. Images of the thyroid were obtained in multiple projections at 6 hours.

FINDINGS: Radioiodine uptake at 6 hours was 37% (normal: 0-15%), and at 24 hours, uptake was 57% (normal: 5-35%). Thyroid images reveal the gland to be diffusely modestly enlarged. Multiple areas of reduced function correlating with palpable nodules are present in both thyroid lobes with the largest nodule being present in the lower poles of both lobes but with the right lobe being somewhat more severely overall affected than the left lobe. No dominant functioning thyroid nodule is evident.

CONCLUSION:

TOXIC MULTINODULAR GOITER

NOTE: Because of the presence of the multiple nodules which are likely on a benign basis, I took the liberty of ordering a thyroid ultrasound as a baseline. This will be separately reported, and it is suggested that the thyroid ultrasound be repeated in six months to one year.

C. Rincon, M.D.

CR:se

D: 5/29/20xx   T: 5/31/20xx

THYROID UPTAKE AND IMAGING STUDY	PT. NAME: NGUYEN, TARA T. ID NO: NM-384023 Sex: F Age: 58 Y DOB: 02/18/xx ATT. PHYS. T. Hutton

ANSWERS TO PRACTICE EXERCISES

1. aden/itis
   R   S
   gland/inflammation
2. hyper/glyc/emia
   P   R   S
   above or
   excessive/sugar/blood
   condition
3. thyro/toxic/osis
   CF   R   S
   thyroid gland
   (shield)/poison/condition
   or increase
4. poly/dips/ia
   P   R   S
   many/thirst/condition of
5. hormon/al
   R   S
   hormone (an urging
   on)/pertaining to
6. ket/osis
   R   S
   ketone bodies/condition
   or increase
7. poly/ur/ia
   P   R   S
   many/urine/condition of
8. endo/crin/e
   P   R   S
   within/to secrete/noun
   marker
9. thyro/ptosis
   CF   S
   thyroid gland
   (shield)/falling or downward displacement
10. thym/oma
    R   S
    thymus gland/tumor
11. acro/megaly
    CF   S
    extremity/enlargement

12. andr/oid
    R   S
    male/resembling
13. adreno/trop/ic
    CF   R   S
    adrenal gland/
    nourishment or
    development/
    pertaining to
14. pancreato/gen/ic
    CF   R   S
    pancreas/origin or
    production/pertaining to
15. glycos/ur/ia
    R   R   S
    sugar/urine/condition of
16. myxedema
17. cretinism
18. Graves disease
19. Cushing syndrome
20. acromegaly
21. goiter
22. exophthalmos or
    exophthalmus
23. pituitary dwarfism
24. hypokalemia
25. thyroid uptake
    and image
26. gigantism or pituitary
    gigantism
27. e
28. h
29. j
30. f
31. c
32. i
33. b
34. g
35. a
36. d
37. polydipsia
38. hypersecretion
39. hypoglycemia
40. glucosuria

41. hyposecretion
42. hyperglycemia
43. sonography or ultra-
    sonography
44. continuous subcuta-
    neous insulin infusion
45. hormone replacement
    therapy
46. fasting blood sugar
47. diabetes mellitus
48. postprandial blood
    sugar
49. glucose tolerance test
50. diabetic ketoacidosis
51. para
52. thymus
53. adrenal
54. pituitary
55. thyroid
56. pancreas
57. adrenal gland
58. shield
59. secrete
60. sugar
61. thirst
62. thymus gland
63. urging on
64. gland
65. hirsutism
66. exophthalmos
67. myxedema
68. goiter
69. androgenous
70. virilism
71. epinephrine
72. hypoglycemic
73. acromegaly
74. exophthalmos or
    exophthalmus
75. metabolism
76. diabetes
77. hypoglycemia

ANSWERS TO MEDICAL RECORD ANALYSIS

Medical Record 9-1: Progress Note

1. a   2. c   3. e   4. a   5. b   6. d   7. a

Medical Record 9-2: For Additional Study

See CD-ROM for answers.

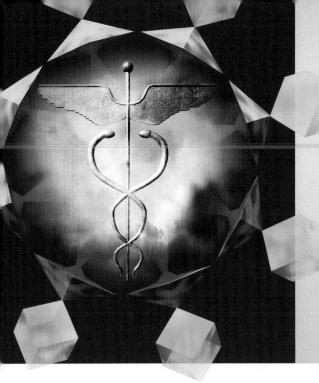

10

The Eye

✓ Chapter 10 Checklist	LOCATION
☐ Read Chapter 10: The Eye and complete all programmed review segments.	pages 481-508
☐ Review the starter set of flash cards and term components related to Chapter 10.	back of book
☐ Complete the Chapter 10 Practice Exercises and Medical Record Analysis 10-1.	pages 511-517
☐ Complete Medical Record Analysis 10-2 For Additional Study.	pages 518-521
☐ Complete the Chapter 10 Exercises by Chapter.	CD-ROM
☐ Complete the Chapter 10 Review and Test Modes.	CD-ROM
☐ Review the Pronunciation Drill for the Chapter 10 terms.	CD-ROM

OVERVIEW OF THE EYE

The eyes are the organs of sight that provide three-dimensional vision (Fig. 10-1):

❀ Light enters the eye through the pupil, the size of which is regulated by the muscles of the iris.

❀ The lens focuses light rays on the retina, the nerve tissue in the inner posterior part of the eye.

❀ Rods and cones, the visual receptor neurons in the retina, respond to the light waves.

❀ Nerve fibers from the rods and cones join in the optic disk, from which the optic nerve carries transmissions to the brain.

❀ Other functions of the eye are performed by protective and lubricating structures.

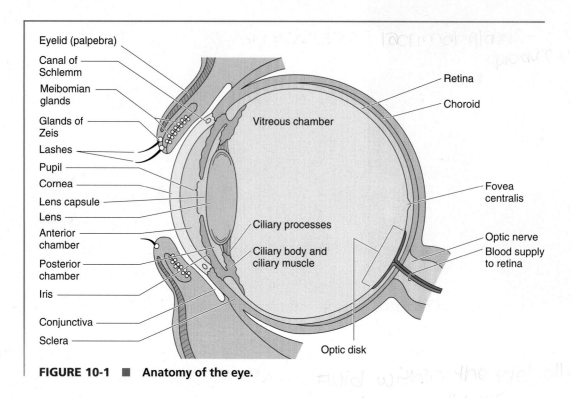

FIGURE 10-1 ▪ Anatomy of the eye.

 ## Self-Instruction: Combining Forms

Study the following:

COMBINING FORM	MEANING
aque/o	water
blephar/o	eyelid
conjunctiv/o	conjunctiva (to join together)
corne/o, kerat/o	cornea
cycl/o	circle, ciliary body
ir/o, irid/o	colored circle, iris
lacrim/o, dacry/o	tear
ocul/o, ophthalm/o, opt/o	eye
phac/o, phak/o	lens (lentil)
phot/o	light
presby/o	old age
retin/o	retina
scler/o	hard or sclera
vitre/o	glassy
-opia (suffix)	condition of vision

TERM	MEANING
trabecular meshwork *tră-bek'yū-lăr mesh'wĕrk*	mesh-like structure in the anterior chamber that filters the aqueous humor as it flows into the canal of Schlemm
vitreous *vit'rē-ŭs*	jelly-like mass filling the inner chamber between the lens and retina that gives bulk to the eye

◆ Programmed Review: Anatomic Terms

ANSWERS	REVIEW
cornea	**10.14** Let's look at the anatomy of the eye in the approximate order of structures involved as light waves enter the eye and result in nerve transmissions to the brain. Light first passes through a transparent outer covering over the iris, pupil, and anterior chamber called the _____.
anterior front aqueous water canal trabecular	**10.15** The _____ chamber is a fluid-filled space between the cornea and iris. It is called anterior because it is the _____ fluid chamber in the eye. The fluid within the anterior chamber is called _____ humor. Recall that the combining form *aque/o* means _____. This watery fluid is carried to the veins through the _____ of Schlemm. As the aqueous humor flows into this canal, it is filtered by a mesh-like structure called the _____ meshwork.
pupil iris light	**10.16** The light waves then pass through the black, circular opening in the center of the iris called the _____. The _____ surrounding the pupil is the colored part of the eye that contracts and dilates to regulate the amount of _____ that passes through the pupil.
posterior humor chamber behind or in back of	**10.17** Between the back of the iris and the upper and lower sections of the lens and vitreous chamber is the _____ chamber, which is also filled with aqueous _____. It is called the posterior _____ because it is _____ the anterior chamber.
lens capsule	**10.18** Light waves passing through the pupil and anterior chamber reach the _____, a transparent structure that focuses the light rays on the retina. The lens is enclosed in a structure called the lens _____.

ANSWERS	REVIEW
ciliary ciliary muscle	**10.19** Tiny muscles control the shape of the lens, allowing it to change its focus for near and far vision. The ring of muscle around the lens, behind the iris, is called the _____ body, and its smooth muscle portion is called the _____ _____.
processes posterior Schlemm	**10.20** Tissue folds on the inner surface of the ciliary body, called ciliary _____, secrete aqueous humor, which fills the anterior and _____ chambers and drains through the canal of _____.
vitreous glassy	**10.21** Light waves focused by the lens now pass through the _____ chamber on the way to the retina. The vitreous is a jelly-like mass that fills this inner chamber and gives bulk to the eye. Recall that the combining form *vitre/o* means _____, referring to the vitreous of the eye.
retina rods bright, rods	**10.22** The light waves passing through the vitreous chamber then strike the _____, the innermost layer at the back of the eye that contains visual receptor neurons that respond to light. These special cells are the _____ and cones. The cones respond to _____ light, and the _____ respond to dim light. These neuron reactions are transmitted to the optic nerve and then to the brain.
macula lutea fovea centralis	**10.23** The central region of the retina, which has a yellow color (*lutea* = yellow), is called the _____ _____. At the center of the macula lutea is a pinpoint depression, which is the site of sharpest vision, called the _____ _____ (*fovea* = pit).
fundus choroid	**10.24** The entire interior surface of the eyeball, including the retina, optic disk, and macula, is termed the _____. The layer behind the retina that provides nourishment to the retina is called the _____.
disk, optic	**10.25** Nerve fibers from the retina come together at the optic _____, the site where the nerves exit the eye. The _____ nerve then carries the nerve impulses to the brain to create the sense of sight.

ANSWERS	REVIEW
sclera	**10.26** The tough outer layer of the eye extending from the cornea around the retina to the optic nerve is called the _____.
palpebra palpebrae	**10.27** Additional eye structures help to protect the eye from the environment. The medical term for eyelid is _____. The plural of this term is _____. The palpebrae can close over the eye.
meibomian Zeis	**10.28** The oil glands located along the rim of the eyelids are called the _____ glands. Other oil glands surrounding the eyelashes are called the glands of _____.
conjunctiva conjunctivitis	**10.29** The mucous membrane that lines the eyelids and outer surface of the eyeball is called the _____, from the combining form *conjunctiv/o*. Because this is the outermost structure of the eye, it is easily irritated by foreign substances, causing an inflammation called _____.
lacrim/o lacrimal glands	**10.30** There are two combining forms meaning tear or tears: *dacry/o*, which is Greek, and _____, which is Latin. Note that the Latin form is used to name the anatomy related to tears. For example, the glands that secrete tears, located in the upper outer region above the eyeball, are called the _____ _____.
ducts sac	**10.31** The tiny tubes that carry tears away from the eye are the lacrimal _____. These ducts carry tears to the lacrimal _____, which collects tears before emptying into the nasolacrimal duct.
nasolacrimal nose	**10.32** Tears from the lacrimal sac reach the nose through the _____ duct. The combining form *nas/o* means _____.

Self-Instruction: Symptomatic Terms

Study the following:

TERM	MEANING
asthenopia *as-thĕ-nō′pē-ă*	eyestrain (*asthenia* = weak condition)
blepharospasm *blef′ă-rō-spazm*	involuntary contraction of the muscles surrounding the eye causing uncontrolled blinking and lid squeezing

TERM	MEANING
diplopia *di-plō'pē-ă*	double vision
exophthalmos or **exophthalmus** *ek-sof-thal'mos* or *ek-sof-thal'mŭs*	abnormal protrusion of one or both eyeballs
lacrimation *lak-ri-mā'shŭn*	secretion of tears
nystagmus *nis-tag'mŭs*	involuntary, rapid, oscillating movement of the eyeball (*nystagmos* = a nodding)
photophobia *fō-tō-fō'bē-ă*	extreme sensitivity to, and discomfort from, light
scotoma *skō-tō'mă*	blind spot in vision (*skotos* = darkness)

Programmed Review: Symptomatic Terms

ANSWERS	REVIEW
vision diplopia	**10.33** Recall that the suffix *-opia* means a condition of _____. The combining form *dipl/o* means double. The condition of having double vision is termed _____.
asthenopia	**10.34** Based on the Greek word asthenia, which means weakness, the condition of eyestrain (weak vision) is called _____.
phot/o photophobia	**10.35** Recall that the combining form meaning light is _____. Extreme sensitivity to, and discomfort from, light is termed _____.
blephar/o blepharospasm	**10.36** Again, the combining form for eyelid is _____. The term for a sudden involuntary contraction of the muscles around the eyelid is _____.
ophthalm/o, out exophthalmos exophthalmus	**10.37** The three combining forms for eye are *ocul/o*, *opt/o*, and _____. The prefix *ex-* means _____ or away. Using the last combining form and this prefix, the term for the condition in which the eyeballs protrude out is termed _____ or _____ (alternate spellings).

ANSWERS	REVIEW
tear process lacrimation	**10.38** *Lacrim/o* is a combining form meaning _____. The suffix *-ation* refers to a _____. The term for the process of secreting tears is _____.
nystagmus	**10.39** The Greek word nystagmos means a nodding, such as the movement of the head up and down or sideways. The condition of rapid oscillation of the eyeballs is called _____.
scotoma	**10.40** The medical term for a visual blind (dark) spot comes from the Greek word that means darkness. The blind spot is called a _____.

Self-Instruction: Diagnostic Terms

Study the following:

TERM	MEANING
refractive errors *rē-frak'tiv er'ōrz*	defects in the bending of light as it enters the eye, causing an improper focus on the retina
astigmatism *ă-stig'mă-tizm*	distorted vision caused by an oblong or cylindrical curvature of the lens or cornea that prevents light rays from coming to a single focus on the retina (*stigma* = point)
hyperopia (Fig. 10-3, B) *hī-pĕr-ō'pē-ă*	farsightedness; difficulty seeing close objects when light rays are focused on a point behind the retina
myopia (Fig. 10-3, C) *mī-ō'pē-ă*	nearsightedness; difficulty seeing distant objects when light rays are focused on a point in front of the retina
presbyopia *prez-bē-ō'pē-ă*	impaired vision caused by old age or loss of accommodation
accommodation *ă-kom'ŏ-dā'shŭn*	ability of the eye to adjust focus on near objects

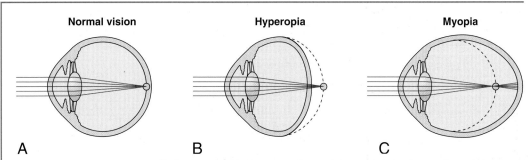

FIGURE 10-3 ■ **A. Proper focus of light rays on the retina. B. Light rays are focused on a point behind the retina in hyperopia. C. Light rays are focused at a point in front of the retina in myopia.**

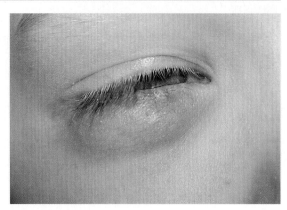

FIGURE 10-4 ▆ Chalazion.

TERM	MEANING
amblyopia *am-blē-ō'pē-ă*	decreased vision in early life because of a functional defect that can occur as a result of strabismus, refractive errors (when one eye is more nearsighted, farsighted, or astigmatic than the other), or trauma; usually occurs in one eye; also known as lazy eye (*ambly/o* = dim)
aphakia *ă-fā'kē-ă*	absence of the lens, usually after cataract extraction
blepharitis *blef'ă-rī'tis*	inflammation of the eyelid
blepharochalasis *blef'ă-rō-kal'ă-sis* **dermatochalasis** *der'mă-tō-kă-lā'sis*	baggy eyelid; overabundance and loss of skin elasticity on the upper eyelid causing a fold of skin to hang down over the edge of the eyelid when the eyes are open (*chalasis* = a slackening)
blepharoptosis *blef'ă-rop'tō-sis* **ptosis** *tō'sis*	drooping of the eyelid; usually caused by paralysis
chalazion (Fig. 10-4) *ka-lā'zē-on*	chronic nodular inflammation of a meibomian gland, usually the result of a blocked duct; commonly presents as a swelling on the upper or lower eyelid (*chalaza* = hailstone)
cataract (Figs. 10-5 and 10-6, B) *kat'ă-rakt*	opaque clouding of the lens causing decreased vision
conjunctivitis *kon-jŭnk-ti-vī'tis*	pinkeye; inflammation of the conjunctiva
dacryoadenitis *dak'rē-ō-ad-ě-nī'tis*	inflammation of the lacrimal gland
dacryocystitis *dak'rē-ō-sis-tī'tis*	inflammation of the tear sac

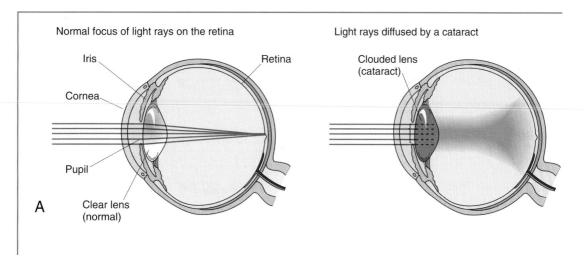

Normal focus of light rays on the retina

Light rays diffused by a cataract

Iris

Retina

Cornea

Clouded lens
(cataract)

Pupil

Clear lens
(normal)

A

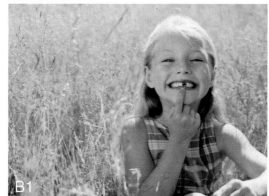

Normal vision

B1

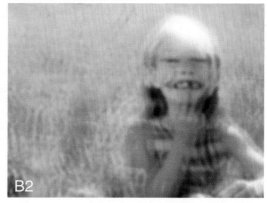

Simulation of cataract vision

B2

FIGURE 10-5 ■ Cataract. A. Normal light focus compared with light focus interference caused by a cataract. B. Simulation of cataract vision.

TERM	MEANING
diabetic retinopathy (Fig. 10-6, C; *see* Fig. 10-13, C) *dī-ă-bet'ik ret-i-nop'ă-thē*	disease of the retina in diabetics characterized by capillary leakage, bleeding, and new vessel formation (neovascularization) leading to scarring and loss of vision
ectropion (Fig. 10-7, A) *ek-trō'pē-on*	outward turning of the rim of the eyelid (*tropo* = turning)
entropion (Fig. 10-7, B) *en-trō'pē-on*	inward turning of the rim of the eyelid
epiphora *ē-pif'ō-ră*	abnormal overflow of tears caused by blockage of the lacrimal duct (*epi* = upon; *phero* = to bear)
glaucoma (Fig. 10-6, D) *glaw-kō'mă*	group of diseases of the eye characterized by increased intraocular pressure that results in damage to the optic nerve, producing defects in vision
hordeolum (Fig. 10-8) *hŏr-dē'ō-lŭm*	sty; an acute infection of a sebaceous gland of the eyelid (*hordeum* = barley)

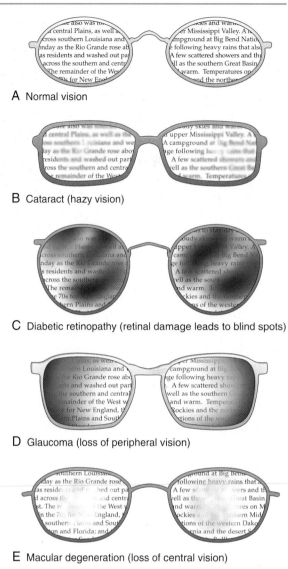

A Normal vision

B Cataract (hazy vision)

C Diabetic retinopathy (retinal damage leads to blind spots)

D Glaucoma (loss of peripheral vision)

E Macular degeneration (loss of central vision)

FIGURE 10-6 ▬ **Simulations of vision loss.**

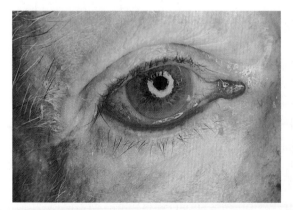
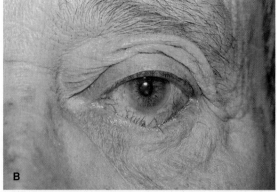

FIGURE 10-7 ▬ **Eyelid abnormalities. A. Severe bilateral lower-lid ectropion. B. Lower-lid entropion causing the lashes to rub on the cornea.**

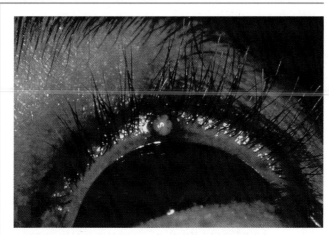

FIGURE 10-8 ■ Upper-lid hordeolum.

TERM	MEANING
iritis ī-rī'tis	inflammation of the iris
keratitis ker-ă-tī'tis	inflammation of the cornea
macular degeneration (Fig. 10-6, E) mak'yū-lăr dē-jen-ĕr-ā'shŭn	breakdown or thinning of the tissues in the macula, resulting in partial or complete loss of central vision
pseudophakia sū-dō-fak'ē-ă	an eye in which the natural lens is replaced with an artificial lens implant (*pseudo* = false)
pterygium (Fig. 10-9) tĕ-rij'ē-ŭm	fibrous, wing-shaped growth of conjunctival tissue that extends onto the cornea, developing most commonly from prolonged exposure to ultraviolet light
retinal detachment ret'i-năl dē-tach'ment	separation of the retina from the underlying epithelium, disrupting vision and resulting in blindness if not repaired surgically

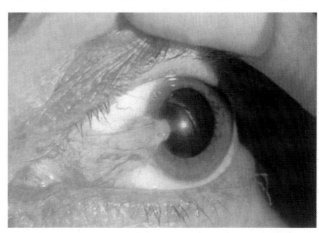

FIGURE 10-9 ■ Pterygium caused by ultraviolet exposure and drying.

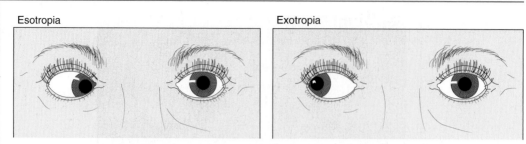

FIGURE 10-10 ■ Strabismus. = lazy eye

TERM	MEANING
retinitis *ret-i-nī'tis*	inflammation of the retina
strabismus (Fig. 10-10) *stra-biz'mŭs* **heterotropia** *het'ĕr-ō-trō'pē-ă*	a condition of eye misalignment caused by intraocular muscle imbalance (*strabismus* = a squinting; *hetero* = other)
esotropia *es-ō-trō'pē-ă*	right or left eye deviates inward, toward nose (*eso* = inward; *tropo* = turning)
exotropia *ek-sō-trō'pē-ă*	right or left eye deviates outward, away from nose (*exo* = out; *tropo* = turning)
scleritis *sklĕ-rī'tis*	inflammation of the sclera
trichiasis *trĭ-kī'ă-sis*	misdirected eyelashes that rub on the conjunctiva or cornea

🔷 Programmed Review: Diagnostic Terms

ANSWERS	REVIEW
inflammation blepharitis conjunctivitis	**10.41** Recall that the suffix -*itis* means _____. Inflammation of the eyelid is therefore termed _____. Inflammation of the conjunctiva is called _____ (or pinkeye).
kerat/o keratitis	**10.42** In addition to *corne/o*, a combining form that means cornea is _____. The term for inflammation of the cornea uses this second form: _____.
ir/o iritis	**10.43** The two combining forms for the iris of the eye are *irid/o* and _____. The latter is used to make the term for inflammation of the iris: _____.

ANSWERS	REVIEW
retinitis scleritis	**10.44** Inflammation of the retina is termed _____. Inflammation of the sclera is _____.
dacry/o dacryocyst dacryocystitis	**10.45** The two combining forms for tears are *lacrim/o* and _____. The combining form *cyst/o* means a sac. Using the latter form for tears, the tear sac is termed the _____. Inflammation of the tear sac is called _____.
inflammation lacrimal or tear	**10.46** The combining form *aden/o* means gland. Thus, the term dacryoadenitis means _____ of the _____ gland.
refractive vision beyond hyperopia myopia	**10.47** Conditions in which the eye incorrectly focuses light on the retina are called _____ errors. Recall that the suffix *-opia* means a condition of _____. The prefix *hyper-* means excessive or _____. The condition of farsightedness occurs when the light rays from near objects focus beyond the retina. This is called _____. The opposite condition of nearsightedness is called _____.
presby/o presbyopia accommodation	**10.48** The combining form meaning old age is _____. The visual condition of impaired vision caused by old age is called _____. This happens because of a loss of accommodation. The ability of the eye to adjust focus on near objects is called _____.
blepharochalasis dermatochalasis	**10.49** The Greek word chalasis means a slackening, such as with baggy skin. The term for a baggy eyelid (using the combining form for eyelid) is _____. The combining form *dermat/o* means skin. Another term for baggy eyelid uses that combining form: _____.
downward blepharoptosis	**10.50** Recall that the suffix *-ptosis* means a falling or _____ displacement. The term for a drooping of the eyelid is _____. This is usually caused by paralysis.
chalazion chalazia	**10.51** From the Greek word for a small hailstone (chalazion), which it may resemble in appearance, comes the term for a chronic nodular inflammation of a meibomian gland: _____. The plural of chalazion is _____.

ANSWERS	REVIEW
cataract	**10.52** The clouding of the lens that causes decreased vision is called a _____.
condition of disease retinopathy	**10.53** The combining form *path/o* means disease, and the suffix *-y* means process of or _____ _____. Thus, *-pathy* refers to a condition of _____. A retinal disease condition in diabetics caused by problems with the capillaries is called diabetic _____.
out ectropion, within entropion	**10.54** The Greek word tropo means turning. The prefix *ec-* means away or _____. The condition of the eyelid rim turning outward is called _____. The prefix *en-*, however, means _____ or inward. The condition of the rim of the eyelid turning in is called _____.
upon epiphora	**10.55** If the lacrimal duct becomes blocked, tears that might otherwise flow to the lacrimal sac overflow. The term for this condition begins with the prefix *epi-*, which means _____. The tears flow upon and out of the outer surface of the eye. This condition is called _____.
glaucoma	**10.56** The group of diseases characterized by increased intraocular pressure, resulting in damage to the ocular nerve and causing visual defects, is called _____.
phak/o condition of pseudophakia	**10.57** Recall that the combining forms for lens are *phac/o* and _____. The latter spelling along with the prefix *pseudo-* (false) and the suffix *-ia,* meaning _____ _____, forms the term for an implanted artificial lens: _____.
strabismus condition of heterotropia esotropia exotropia	**10.58** From the Greek work strabismos, meaning a squinting, comes this term for a condition of eye misalignment: _____. Recall that the word root *tropo* means a turning, and that the suffix *-ia* means a _____ _____. The combining form *heter/o* means the other. Another term for strabismus is named for the appearance of one eye turning toward the other: _____. If the eye turns inward (*eso* = inward) toward the nose, this is called _____. If the eye turns outward (*exo* = outward), this is called _____.

ANSWERS	REVIEW
macular degeneration	**10.59** A breakdown of tissues in the macula that causes a loss of central vision is called _____ _____.
detachment	**10.60** Separation of the retina from the underlying tissue, usually requiring surgical repair, is called retinal _____.
hordeolum	**10.61** The Latin word hordeolus means a little barley grain, which is similar in appearance to a sty, an acute infection of a sebaceous gland of the eyelid. The medical term for a sty is _____.
pterygium ultraviolet	**10.62** The combining form *pteryg/o* means wing-shaped. A triangular, or wing-shaped, fibrous growth of conjunctival tissue extending onto the cornea is called _____. Pterygia are most commonly caused by prolonged exposure to _____ light.
presence trichiasis	**10.63** Recall that the suffix *-iasis* means formation or _____ of. The combining form *trich/o* means hair. The presence of misdirected eyelashes that rub on the conjunctiva or cornea is called _____.
amblyopia	**10.64** *Ambly/o*, a combining form meaning dim, is the foundation of the term _____, commonly called lazy eye, that describes the condition of decreased vision in early life because of a functional defect (e.g., strabismus and refractive error).

◈ Self-Instruction: Diagnostic Tests and Procedures

Study the following:

TEST OR PROCEDURE	EXPLANATION
distance visual acuity (Fig. 10-11) *dis′tănts vizh′yū-ăl ă-kyū′i-tē*	measure of the ability to see the details and shape of identifiable objects from a specified distance, usually from 20 feet (6 meters); normal distance visual acuity is 20/20 (6/6)
fluorescein angiography (Fig. 10-12) *flōr-es′ē-in an-jē-og′ră-fē*	visualization and photography of retinal and choroidal vessels made as fluorescein dye, which is injected into a vein, circulates through the eye

E

T B

D L N

P T E R

F Z B D E

O E L Z T G

L P O R F D Z

FIGURE 10-11 ■ Snellen eye chart for testing distance visual acuity.

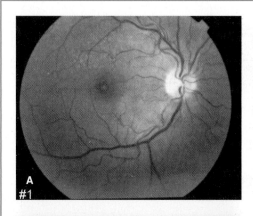

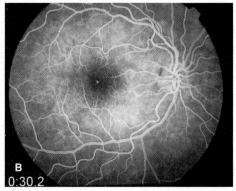

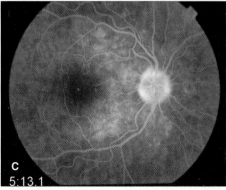

FIGURE 10-12 ■ Fluorescein angiography photographs. A. Right eye before injection of fluorescein. B. Maximal levels of fluorescein circulating through the retinal blood vessels 30 seconds after injection. C. Elimination after 5 minutes.

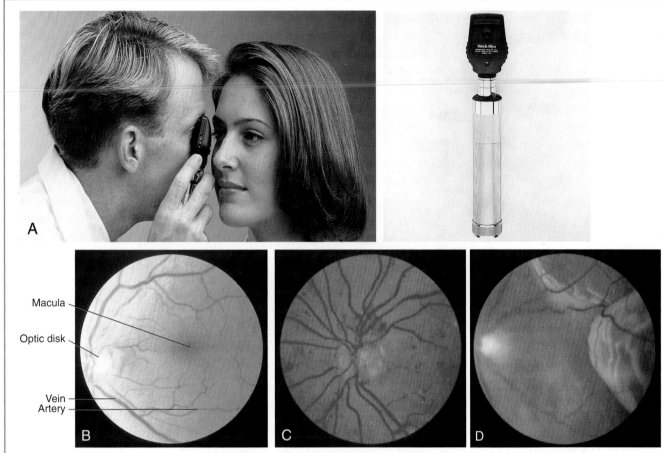

FIGURE 10-13 ■ **A. Doctor performing ophthalmoscopy using an ophthalmoscope. B. Normal retina. C. Aneurysms seen in diabetic retinopathy. D. Retinal detachment.**

TEST OR PROCEDURE	EXPLANATION
ophthalmoscopy (Fig. 10-13) *of-thăl-mos'kŏ-pē*	use of an ophthalmoscope to view the interior of the eye
slit lamp biomicroscopy (Fig. 10-14) *slit lamp bī'ō-mī-kros'kŏ-pē*	use of a tabletop microscope used to examine the eye, especially the cornea, lens, fluids, and membranes
sonography *sŏ-nog'ră-fē*	use of high-frequency sound waves to detect pathology within the eye (e.g., foreign bodies and detached retina)
tonometry (Fig. 10-15) *tō-nom'ĕ-trē*	use of a tonometer to measure intraocular pressure, which is elevated in glaucoma

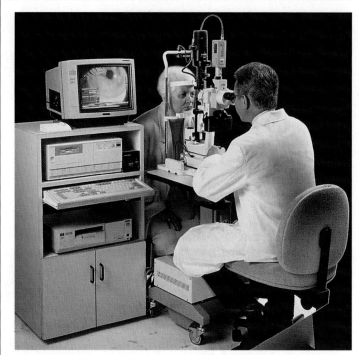

FIGURE 10-14 ■ Slit lamp biomicroscope.

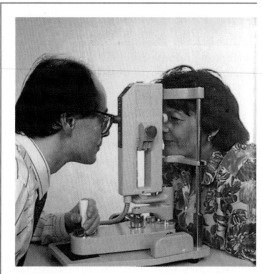

FIGURE 10-15 ■ Tonometer/tonometry.

◈ Programmed Review: Diagnostic Tests and Procedures

ANSWERS	REVIEW
ophthalm/o	**10.65** Again, the three combining forms meaning eye are *ocul/o*, *opt/o*, and _____. The last one is used with the suffix that means the process of examination to make the term for use of an
ophthalmoscopy	ophthalmoscope to view the interior of the eye: _____.

ANSWERS	REVIEW
visual acuity normal	**10.66** The diagnostic test that measures the ability to see objects at a specified distance, usually from 20 feet (6 meters), is called distance _____ _____. A result of 20/20 (6/6) represents _____ distance visual acuity.
fluorescein	**10.67** Angiography, which is radiography of blood vessels after injection of a contrast medium, is used in many body areas. The procedure used with the eye is called _____ angiography, which is named for the fluorescein dye that is injected into a vein to circulate through the eye.
sonography recording	**10.68** The use of high-frequency sound waves to make an image for detecting pathology in the eye is called _____, or ultrasound. The suffix *-graphy* means a process of _____.
tonometry process	**10.69** A tonometer measures intraocular pressure as a test for glaucoma. This procedure is called _____. The suffix *-metry* means a _____ of measuring.
biomicroscopy	**10.70** A special microscope is used to examine eye structures. This procedure is called slit lamp _____.

 ## Self-Instruction: Operative Terms

Study the following:

TERM	MEANING
blepharoplasty *blef'ă-rō-plast-tē*	surgical repair of an eyelid
cataract extraction *kat'ă-rakt ek-strak'shŭn*	excision of a cloudy lens from the eye
cryoretinopexy *krī-ō-ret'i-nō-pek-sē* **cryopexy** *krī'ō-pek-sē*	use of intense cold to seal a hole or tear in the retina; used to treat retinal detachment
dacryocystectomy *dak'rē-ō-sis-tek'tŏ-mē*	excision of a lacrimal sac
enucleation *ē-nū-klē-ā'shŭn*	excision of an eyeball
iridectomy *ir-i-dek'tŏ-mē*	excision of a portion of iris tissue

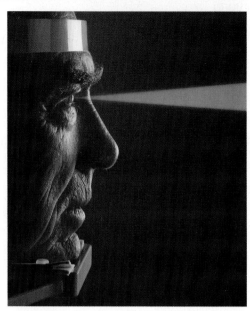

FIGURE 10-16 ■ **Simulation of laser application.**

TERM	MEANING
iridotomy *ir-i-dot'ŏ-mē*	incision into the iris (usually with a laser) to allow drainage of aqueous humor from the posterior to anterior chamber; used to treat a type of glaucoma
keratoplasty *ker'ă-tō-plas-tē*	corneal transplantation; replacement of a diseased or scarred cornea with a healthy one from a matched donor
laser surgery (Fig. 10-16) *lā'zĕr sŭr'jĕr-ē*	use of a laser to make incisions or destroy tissues; used to create fluid passages or obliterate tumors, aneurysms, etc.
laser-assisted in situ keratomileusis (LASIK) *lā'zĕr-ă-sis'tĕd in sī'tū ker'ă-tō-mī-lū'sis (lā'sik)*	a technique using the excimer laser to reshape the surface of the cornea to correct refractive error (e.g., myopia, hyperopia, and astigmatism) (*smileusis* = carving)
intraocular lens (IOL) implant (Fig. 10-17) *in'tră-ok'yū-lăr lenz im'plant*	implantation of an artificial lens to replace a defective natural lens (e.g., after cataract extraction)
phacoemulsification *fak'ō-ē-mŭl-si-fi-kā'shŭn*	use of ultrasound to shatter and break up a cataract, with aspiration and removal
scleral buckling *sklēr'ăl bŭk'ling*	surgery to treat retinal detachment by placing a band of silicone around the sclera to cinch it toward the middle of the eye and relieve pull on the retina; often combined with other techniques to seal retinal tears (e.g., cryoretinopexy)

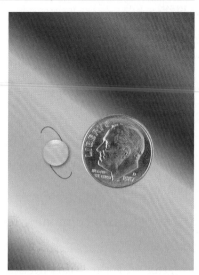

FIGURE 10-17 ▮ Size comparison of an intraocular lens to a dime.

🔷 Programmed Review: Operative Terms

ANSWERS	REVIEW
-plasty blepharoplasty	**10.71** Recall that the suffix for surgical repair or reconstruction is _____. The surgical repair of an eyelid is termed _____.
-pexy cryoretinopexy	**10.72** The combining form *cry/o* means cold. Recall that the operative suffix meaning suspension or fixation is _____. The operative procedure using intense cold to seal a hole in the retina is called _____, or simply cryopexy.
cataract intraocular lens implant within	**10.73** The excision of a cloudy lens from the eye is called a _____ extraction. After the lens has been excised, an artificial lens may be implanted in a procedure called an _____ _____ (IOL) _____. The prefix *intra-* means _____.
lacrimal -ectomy dacryocystectomy	**10.74** Recall that dacryocyst means _____ sac, and that the surgical suffix for excision is _____. Therefore, the term for excision of a lacrimal sac is _____.
iridectomy	**10.75** The excision of a portion of iris tissue is _____.

ANSWERS	REVIEW
-tomy iridotomy	**10.76** The surgical suffix meaning incision is _____. An incision into the iris to allow drainage from the posterior chamber is called an _____.
enucleation	**10.77** The Latin word enucleo means to remove the kernel, such as the kernel of a nut. The medical term for removing an entire structure, such as the eyeball (or a tumor), without rupturing it is _____.
kerat/o keratoplasty	**10.78** The two combining forms referring to the cornea are *corne/o* and _____, which also can mean hard. Combining the latter with the suffix for surgical repair or reconstruction yields this term for a corneal transplant: _____.
laser surgery in situ keratomileusis	**10.79** Lasers are used in many operative techniques to make incisions or destroy tissues. This is generally called _____ _____. A special technique using a laser to reshape the surface of the cornea is termed laser-assisted ____ _____ _____ (LASIK).
phacoemulsification	**10.80** The term emulsification refers to breaking up a substance and distributing it through another substance, generally a liquid. A surgical procedure uses ultrasound to shatter and break up a cataract such that after emulsification, it can be removed by aspiration. This procedure is called _____.
buckling	**10.81** A surgical procedure to treat retinal detachment by placing a "buckle-like" band of silicone around the sclera to cinch it toward the middle of the eye and relieve pull on the retina is simply called scleral _____.

 ## Self-Instruction: Therapeutic Terms

Study the following:

TERM	MEANING
contact lens *kon'takt lenz*	small, plastic, curved disk with optical correction that fits over the cornea; used to correct refractive errors
eye instillation *ī in-sti-lā'shŭn*	introduction of a medicated solution in the eye, usually administered by a drop (gt) or drops (gtt) in the affected eye or eyes

TERM	MEANING
eye irrigation ī ir'i-gā'shŭn	washing of the eye with water or other fluid (e.g., saline)

COMMON THERAPEUTIC DRUG CLASSIFICATIONS

antibiotic ophthalmic solution an'tē-bī-ot'ik of-thal'mik sŏ-lū'shŭn	antimicrobial agent in solution; used to treat bacterial infections (e.g., conjunctivitis and corneal ulcers)
cycloplegic sī-klō-plē'jik	agent that paralyzes the ciliary muscle and the powers of accommodation; commonly used in pediatric eye examinations
mydriatic mi-drē-at'ik	agent that causes dilation of the pupil; used for certain eye examinations
miotic mī-ot'ik	agent that causes the pupil to contract (*mio* = less)

Programmed Review: Therapeutic Terms

ANSWERS	REVIEW
contact lens	**10.82** The plastic lens that the user fits over the cornea to correct refractive errors is called a _____ _____.
instillation, drop gtt irrigation	**10.83** Introduction of a medicated solution in the eye is called an eye _____, usually administered by a _____ (gt) or drops (____) in the affected eye or eyes. Washing the eye with water or other fluid is called eye _____.
antibiotic ophthalmic	**10.84** A solution composed of an antimicrobial agent in a fluid for treatment of bacterial eye infections is called an _____ _____ solution.
mydriatic	**10.85** The term mydriasis means dilation of the pupil. A therapeutic drug that causes dilation of the pupil for an eye examination is called a _____ agent.
miotic	**10.86** In contrast, miosis means contraction of the pupil. A therapeutic drug that causes the pupil to contract is called a _____ agent.
circle ciliary	**10.87** *Cyclo* is a combining form referring either to a _____ or the _____ body, a ring-like structure in the eye that contains

ANSWERS	REVIEW
paralysis	ciliary muscles. Recall from Chapter 8 that *-plegia* is a suffix meaning _____. The term pertaining to an agent that paralyzes the ciliary muscle and powers of accommodation during some eye
cycloplegic	examinations, using the adjective form of *-plegia*, is _____.

CHAPTER 10 ACRONYMS AND ABBREVIATIONS

ABBREVIATION	EXPANSION
IOL	intraocular lens
LASIK	laser-assisted in situ keratomileusis

CHAPTER 10 SUMMARY OF TERMS

The terms introduced in chapter 10 are listed below, followed by the page number on which each term can be found and its written pronunciation. For additional practice and reinforcement, write the definition of each term on a separate piece of paper.

accommodation/491
ă-kom'ŏ-dā'shŭn

amblyopia/492
am-blē-ō'pē-ă

anterior chamber/484
an-tēr'ē-ŏr chām'bĕr

antibiotic ophthalmic solution/507
an'tē-bī-ot'ik of-thal'mik sŏ-lū'shŭn

aphakia/492
ă-fā'kē-ă

aqueous humor/485
ak'wē-ŭs hyū'mŏr

asthenopia/489
as-thĕ-nō'pē-ă

astigmatism/491
ă-stig'mă-tizm

blepharitis/492
blef'ă-rī'tis

blepharochalasis/492
blef'ă-rō-kal'ă-sis

blepharoplasty/503
blef'ă-rō-plast-tē

blepharoptosis/492
blef'ă-rop'tō-sis

blepharospasm/489
blef'ă-rō-spazm

canal of Schlemm/485
kă-nal' of shlem

cataract/492
kat'ă-rakt

cataract extraction/503
kat'ă-rakt ek-strak'shŭn

chalazion/492
ka-lā'zē-on

choroid/485
kō'royd

ciliary body/485
sil'ē-ar-ē bod'ē

ciliary muscle/485
sil'ē-ar-ē mŭs'ĕl

ciliary processes/485
sil'ē-ar-ē pros'es-ēz

cones/486
kōnz

conjunctiva/485
kon-jŭnk-tī'vă

conjunctivitis/492
kon-jŭnk-ti-vī'tis

contact lens/506
kon'takt lenz

cornea/485
kŏr'nē-ă

cryopexy/503
krī'ō-pek-sē

cryoretinopexy/503
krī-ō-ret'i-nō-pek-sē

cycloplegic/507
sī-klō-plē'jik

dacryoadenitis/492
dak'rē-ō-ad-ĕ-nī'tis

dacryocystectomy/503
dak'rē-ō-sis-tek'tō-mē

dacryocystitis/492
dak'rē-ō-sis-tī'tis

dermatochalasis/492
der'mă-tō-kă-lā'sis

diabetic retinopathy/493
dī-ă-bet'ik ret-i-nop'ă-thē

diplopia/490
di-plō'pē-ă

distance visual acuity/499
dis'tănts vĭzh'yū-ăl ă-kyū'i-tē

ectropion/493
ek-trō'pē-on

entropion/493
en-trō'pē-on

enucleation/503
ē-nū-klē-ā'shŭn

epiphora/493
ē-pif'ō-ră

esotropia/496
es-ō-trō'pē-ă

exophthalmos or **exophthalmus**/490
ek-sof-thal'mos or ek-sof-thal'mŭs

exotropia/496
ek-sō-trō'pē-ă

eye instillation/506
ī in-sti-lā'shŭn

eye irrigation/507
ī ir'i-gā'shŭn

eyelid/485
ī'lid

fluorescein angiography/499
flŏr-es'ē-in an-jē-og'ră-fē

fovea centralis/485
fō'vē-ă sen-trā'lis

fundus/485
fŭn'dŭs

glands of Zeis/485
glanz of tsīs

glaucoma/493
glaw-kō'mă

heterotropia/496
het'ĕr-ō-trō'pē-ă

hordeolum/493
hŏr-dē'ō-lŭm

hyperopia/491
hī-pĕr-ō'pē-ă

intraocular lens (IOL) implant/504
in'tră-ok'yū-lăr lenz im'plant

iridectomy/503
ir'i-dek'tŏ-mē

iridotomy/504
ir-i-dot'ŏ-mē

iris/485
ī'ris

iritis/495
ī-rī'tis

keratitis/495
ker-ă-tī'tis

keratoplasty/504
ker'ă-tō-plas-tē

lacrimal ducts/485
lak'ri-măl dŭkts

lacrimal gland/485
lak'ri-măl gland

lacrimal sac/485
lak'ri-măl sak

lacrimation/490
lak-ri-mā'shŭn

laser surgery/504
lā'zĕr sŭr'jĕr-ē

laser-assisted in situ keratomileusis (LASIK)/504
lā'zĕr-ă-sis'tĕd in sī'tū ker'ă-tō-mī-lū'sis (lā'sik)

lens/485
lenz

lens capsule/486
lenz kap'sūl

macula/486
mak'yū-lă

macula lutea/486
mak'yū-lă lū'tĕ-ā

macular degeneration/495
mak'yū-lăr dē-jen-ĕr-ā'shŭn

meibomian glands/485
mī-bō'mē-ăn glanz

miotic/507
mī-ot'ik

mydriatic/507
mi-drē-at'ik

myopia/491
mī-ō'pē-ă

nasolacrimal duct/486
nā-zō-lak'ri-măl dŭkt

nystagmus/490
nis-tag'mŭs

ophthalmoscopy/501
of-thăl-mos'kŏ-pē

optic disk/486
op'tik disk

optic nerve/486
op'tik nĕrv

palpebra/485
pal-pē'bră

phacoemulsification/504
fak'ō-ē-mŭl-si-fi-kā'shŭn

photophobia/490
fō-tō-fō'bē-ă

posterior chamber/486
pos-tēr'ē-ōr chăm'bĕr

presbyopia/491
prez-bē-ō'pē-ă

pseudophakia/495
sū-dō-fak'ē-ă

pterygium/495
tĕ-rij'ē-ŭm

ptosis/492
tō-sis

pupil/486
pyū'pĭl

refractive errors/491
rē-frak'tiv er'ŏrz

retina/486
ret'i-nă

retinal detachment/495
ret'i-năl dē-tach'ment

retinitis/496
ret-i-nī'tis

rods/486
rodz

sclera/486
sklēr'ă

scleral buckling/504
sklēr'ăl bŭk'ling

scleritis/496
sklĕ-rī'tis

scotoma/490
skō-tō'mă

slit lamp biomicroscopy/501
slit lamp bi'ō-mī-kros'kŏ-pē

sonography/501
sŏ-nog'ră-fē

strabismus/496
stra-biz'mŭs

tonometry/501
tō-nom'ĕ-trē

trabecular meshwork/486
tră-bek'yū-lăr mesh'wĕrk

trichiasis/496
tri-kī'ă-sis

vitreous/486
vit'rē-ŭs

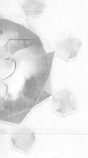

PRACTICE EXERCISES

For each of the following words, write out the term components (prefixes [P], combining forms [CF], roots [R], and suffixes [S]) on the lines below the word. Then define the term according to the meaning of its components.

EXAMPLE

epikeratophakia

epi / kerato / phak/ ia

P   CF   R   S

DEFINITION: upon/cornea/lens/condition of

1. blepharoptosis

_____ / _____
    CF   S

DEFINITION: _____

2. iridotomy

_____ / _____
    CF   S

DEFINITION: _____

3. ophthalmology

_____ / _____
    CF   S

DEFINITION: _____

4. vitrectomy

_____ / _____
    R   S

DEFINITION: _____

5. dacryolithiasis

_____ / _____ / _____
    CF   R   S

DEFINITION: _____

6. lacrimal

_____ / _____
    R   S

DEFINITION: _____

7. photophobia

_____ / _____ / _____
    CF   R   S

DEFINITION: _____

8. keratoplasty

_____ / _____

    CF   S

DEFINITION: _____

9. aqueous

_____ / _____

    R   S

DEFINITION: _____

10. iritis

_____ / _____

    R   S

DEFINITION: _____

11. corneal

_____ / _____

    R   S

DEFINITION: _____

12. phacolysis

_____ / _____

    CF   S

DEFINITION: _____

13. retinopathy

_____ / _____ / _____

    CF   R   S

DEFINITION: _____

14. ocular

_____ / _____

    R   S

DEFINITION: _____

15. conjunctivitis

_____ / _____

    R   S

DEFINITION: _____

16. presbyopia

_____ / _____

    R   S

DEFINITION: _____

6. What caused the pterygium?
   a. misdirected eyelashes that rub on the conjunctiva or cornea
   b. intraocular muscle imbalance
   c. separation of the retina from the underlying epithelium
   d. abnormal overflow of tears
   e. ultraviolet exposure and drying

7. What was the patient told about the pterygium?
   a. it is cancerous
   b. it is not cancerous
   c. it must be removed
   d. both a and c
   e. none of the above

Medical Record 10-2

FOR ADDITIONAL STUDY

Not long ago, Cassandre Aquero had cataract surgery for her left eye and is now losing vision in her right eye because of another cataract. She is consulting an ophthalmologist, Dr. Oanh Tran, about surgery on the right eye. Medical Record 10-2 is the history and physical examination written by Dr. Tran in planning for her surgery.

Read Medical Record 10-2 (pages 520-521), then write your answers to the following questions in the spaces provided.

QUESTIONS ABOUT MEDICAL RECORD 10-2

1. The following are medical terms used in this record that you have not yet encountered in this text. Underline each where it appears in the record, and define each term below.

   appendectomy _____

   irides _____

2. In your own words, briefly describe Ms. Aquero's current complaint and diagnosis as noted under "History of Present Illness:"

   _____

   _____

   _____

3. Describe, in lay language, the two medical conditions that Ms. Aquero has in addition to her current problem and past surgeries:

   _____

   _____

   _____

4. Which of the following findings on physical examination is related to Ms. Aquero's general medical condition in addition to her eye problems?

   a. rales on auscultation

   b. disoriented consciousness

   c. BP 180/100

   d. weight 135 lb.

5. The planned operation involves several risks that the patient has accepted in the hopes of regaining good eyesight. Which of the following was *not* mentioned by Dr. Tran as a risk?

   a. hypertensive crisis

   b. retinal detachment

   c. edema of the macula

   d. bleeding

6. The preoperative nursing staff will ensure that Ms. Aquero receives five medications before surgery. Translate the instructions for these:

   a. _____

   b. _____

   c. _____

   d. _____

   e. _____

7. In your own words, not using medical terminology, briefly describe what will occur in the surgery:

   _____

   _____

   _____

Medical Record 10-2: For Additional Study

CENTRAL MEDICAL GROUP, INC.
Department of Ophthalmology
201 Medical Center Drive • Central City, US 90000-1234 • PHONE: (012) 125-8888 • FAX: (012) 125-3434

HISTORY

HISTORY OF PRESENT ILLNESS:
This 57-year-old female complains of progressive loss of vision in the right eye over the last two years which has been diagnosed as a cataract. The patient recently underwent cataract surgery in the left eye and is currently scheduled for surgery in the right eye due to her decreased vision.

PAST MEDICAL HISTORY:
The patient has had the normal childhood diseases and has essential hypertension and hypothyroidism.

SURGERIES:
Appendectomy 40 years ago. Tonsillectomy and adenoidectomy as a child. Cataract surgery in the left eye with a posterior chamber lens implant in 199x.

ALLERGIES:
None.

MEDICATIONS:
Propranolol 80 mg b.i.d. Hydrochlorothiazide 50 mg b.i.d. Clonidine, 0.1 mg, 2 tablets p.o. t.i.d. Synthroid 0.1 mg q.d. Slow-K 2 tablets p.o. q.d.

PHYSICAL EXAMINATION

VITAL SIGNS:
WEIGHT: 135 lb. BLOOD PRESSURE: 180/100.

HEENT:
HEAD, EARS, EYES, NOSE, THROAT: Normal.

EYES: Best corrected visual acuity in the right eye is counting fingers at two feet and 20/50 in the left eye. Pinhole vision in the left eye is 20/30. Slit lamp examination reveals normal lids, conjunctivae, and sclerae. Corneas are clear. Anterior chambers are clear and deep. Irides are within normal limits in the right eye. Evaluation of the lens reveals a 4+ posterior subcapsular plaquing with 3-4+ nuclear sclerosis, and in the left eye, there is a posterior chamber lens that is in place with posterior lens capsular plaquing. Intraocular pressure: OD: 18. OS: 17. Fundus examination in the right eye was severely hindered due to the dense cataract. However, evaluation of the posterior pole in the right eye was within normal limits.

(continued)

HISTORY AND PHYSICAL Page 1	PT. NAME: AQUERO,CASSANDRE D. ID NO: 008654 ATT PHYS: O. TRAN, M.D.

Medical Record 10-2: For Additional Study (Continued)

CENTRAL MEDICAL GROUP, INC.
Department of Ophthalmology
201 Medical Center Drive • Central City, US 90000-1234 • PHONE: (012) 125-8888 • FAX: (012) 125-3434

PHYSICAL EXAMINATION

CHEST:
Clear to percussion and auscultation. The breasts were normal, and the lungs were clear.

PELVIC/RECTAL:
Within normal limits.

EXTREMITIES:
Within normal limits.

NEUROLOGICAL:
Within normal limits.

IMPRESSION:
1) Cataract, right eye.
2) Pseudophakia, left eye.
3) Essential hypertension.
4) Hypothyroidism.

RISKS/BENEFITS:
The patient is aware of the alternatives, risks, benefits, and possible complications of the procedure that include hemorrhage, infection, loss of vision, reoperation, retinal detachment, macular edema; and the patient still desires to undergo the procedure.

PLAN:
Extracapsular cataract extraction with posterior chamber lens implant under local anesthesia using a +21 diopter posterior chamber lens with the ultraviolet filter. Preoperative medication will consist of the patient's morning dose of Propranolol, 80 mg; Hydrochlorothiazide, 50 mg; Clonidine, 0.2 mg; and Diamox, 250 mg with ¼ glass of water at approximately 10 a.m. on the day of surgery. The patient was also instructed to take Maxitrol, 1 gt OD, q 3 h starting 24 hours prior to the procedure, while awake.

O. Tran, M.D.

OT:mk
D: 10/19/20xx   T: 10/20/20xx

HISTORY AND PHYSICAL Page 2	PT. NAME: AQUERO, CASSANDRE D. ID NO: 008654 ATT PHYS: O. TRAN, M.D.

ANSWERS TO PRACTICE EXERCISES

1. blepharo/ptosis
   CF   S
   eyelid/falling or downward displacement
2. irido/tomy
   CF S
   iris/incision
3. ophthalmo/logy
   CF   S
   eye/study of
4. vitr/ectomy
   R   S
   glassy/excision or
   removal
5. dacryo/lith/iasis
   CF   R S
   tear/stone/formation or
   presence of
6. lacrim/al
   R S
   tear/pertaining to
7. photo/phob/ia
   CF   R S
   light/sensitivity/
   condition of
8. kerato/plasty
   CF   S
   cornea/surgical repair or
   reconstruction
9. aque/ous
   R S
   water/pertaining to
10. ir/itis
    R S
    iris/inflammation
11. corne/al
    R S
    cornea/pertaining to
12. phaco/lysis
    CF   S
    lens (lentil)/breaking
    down or dissolution
13. retino/path/y
    CF   R S
    retina/disease/condition
    or process of

14. ocul/ar
    R S
    eye/pertaining to
15. conjunctiv/itis
    R   S
    conjunctiva (to join
    together)/inflammation
16. presby/opia
    R   S
    old age/condition of
    vision
17. opto/metry
    CF   S
    eye/process of measuring
18. a/phak/ia
    P R S
    without/lens (lentil)/
    condition or process of
19. hyper/opia
    P   S
    above or excessive/
    condition of vision
20. sclero/malacia
    CF   S
    sclera/softening
21. f
22. d
23. a
24. e
25. c
26. b
27. keratitis
28. photophobia
29. dacryocystectomy
30. exophthalmos
31. blepharochalasis or
    dermatochalasis
32. inward turning of the
    rim of the eyelid
33. double vision
34. instrument to measure
    intraocular pressure
35. outward turning of the
    rim of the eyelid
36. blind spot in vision
37. conjunctivitis
38. blepharitis

39. asthenopia
40. mydriatic
41. aphakia
42. hordeolum
43. cataract
44. macular degeneration
45. blepharospasm
46. nystagmus
47. scleral buckling
48. opt/o
49. presby/o
50. vitre/o
51. phot/o
52. scler/o
53. phac/o
54. irid/o
55. dacry/o
56. blephar/o
57. aque/o
58. eyelid
59. cornea
60. lens
61. sclera
62. vitreous
63. ciliary
64. retina
65. optic
66. asthenopia
67. pterygium
68. hordeolum
69. nystagmus
70. chalazion
71. mydriatic
72. scotoma
73. epiphora
74. dacryocyst
75. ophthalmoscope
76. conjunctiva
77. myopia
78. sclera
79. macula
80. exophthalmos or
    exophthalmus

ANSWERS TO MEDICAL RECORD ANALYSIS

Medical Record 10-1: Progress Note

1. d   2. d   3. c   4. a   5. d   6. e   7. b

Medical Record 10-2: For Additional Study

See CD-ROM for answers.

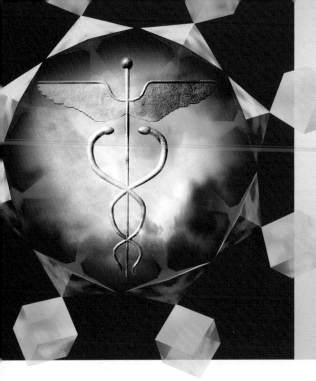

The Ear

OVERVIEW OF THE EAR

The three divisions of the ear function to provide the sense of hearing (Fig. 11-1):

❁ The **external ear**, from the pinna (or auricle), gathers sounds, which funnel through the external auditory canal.

❁ Sounds reach the tympanum, or eardrum, in the **middle ear**. The tympanum transmits sound vibrations to the auditory ossicles (the malleus, incus, and stapes) and to the oval window, which stimulates the auditory fluids in the inner ear. Also in the middle ear, the eustachian tube connects with the throat to maintain equal air pressure.

❁ The **inner ear**, also known as the labyrinth, receives sound vibrations and passes them through intricate, intercommunicating tubes and chambers to the organ of Corti, where nerve impulses are generated and transmitted to the brain for processing.

The inner ear (labyrinth) also helps to maintain the body's equilibrium by stimulating nerve impulses resulting from movement or changes in position.

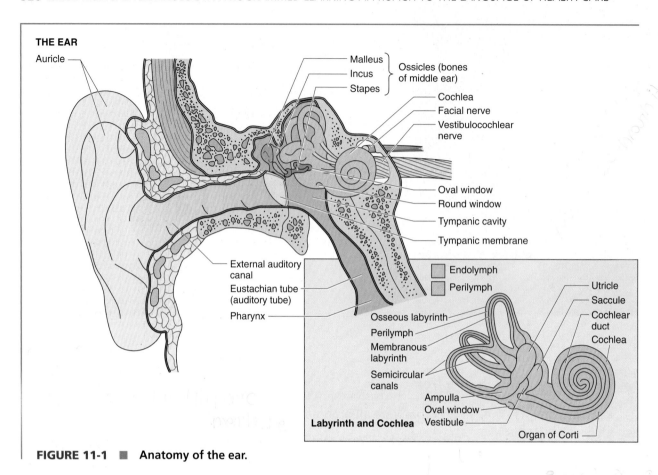

FIGURE 11-1 ■ Anatomy of the ear.

Self-Instruction: Combining Forms

Study the following:

COMBINING FORM	MEANING
acous/o, audi/o	hearing
aer/o	air or gas
aur/i, ot/o	ear
cerumin/o	wax
salping/o	eustachian tube or uterine tube
tympan/o, myring/o	eardrum
-acusis (suffix)	hearing condition

Programmed Review: Combining Forms

ANSWERS	REVIEW
	11.1 The two combining forms for hearing are used in many everyday words in addition to medical terms. People speak of the acoustics of a room, for example, and of audible noises. These two

ANSWERS	REVIEW
acous/o, audi/o	combining forms are _____ and _____. Related to the combining form *acous/o* is the suffix for a hearing condition:
-acusis	_____. The term presbyacusis, for example, means hearing loss because of old age. Recall that the suffix meaning process of
-metry	measuring is _____. The medical process of measuring a person's hearing, using the other combining form, is
audiometry	_____.
aer/o	**11.2** The combining form for air or gas is _____. This combining form is used in many medical terms. An aerobe, for example, is a microbe that lives in the presence of air, whereas a microbe that lives without air (formed with the prefix meaning
anaerobe	without) is an _____.
ot/o	**11.3** The two combining forms for ear are *aur/i* and _____. The medical study of the ear is called otology. The physician who
otologist	specializes in the study and treatment of the ear is an _____. Otology is a subspecialty of otorhinolaryngology (otolaryngology),
ear	involving the study and treatment of the _____, nose, and throat (more commonly known as ENT).
aur/i	**11.4** The other combining form meaning ear is _____. The auricle, for example, is the outer, visible part of the ear.
	11.5 The combining form referring to ear wax comes from the Latin word cera, meaning wax. That combining form is
cerumin/o	_____. Recall that the suffix meaning condition or
-osis	increase is _____; therefore, the term for a condition of
ceruminosis	excessive ear wax is _____.
	11.6 The combining form for the eustachian tube (or uterine tube) comes from the Greek word salpinx, meaning trumpet. That
salping/o	combining form is _____. Using the common suffix for inflammation, the medical term for inflammation of the eustachian
salpingitis	tube in the ear or uterine tube is _____. The context in which the term is used is key to knowing which meaning is appropriate.
	11.7 A kind of drum used in symphony orchestras is called a tympany, from the Greek word for drum. The combining form for

ANSWERS	REVIEW
tympan/o -tomy tympanotomy	the eardrum is _____. Recall that the suffix for surgical incision is _____. An incision into the eardrum is therefore called a _____.
myring/o -ectomy myringectomy	**11.8** A second combining form for eardrum comes from the Latin word for drum membrane: myringa. That combining form is _____. Recall that the suffix for surgical excision is _____. Combine these term components to create the medical term for the excision of the eardrum: _____.

◆ Self-Instruction: Anatomic Terms

Study the following:

TERM	MEANING
external ear *eks-tĕr'năl ēr*	outer structures of the ear that collect sound
pinna *pin'ă*	auricle (little ear); projected part of the external ear (*pinna* = feather)
external auditory meatus or **canal** *eks-tĕr'năl aw'di-tōr-ē mē-ā'tŭs or kă-nal'*	external passage for sounds collected from the pinna to the tympanum
cerumen *sĕ-rū'men*	a waxy substance secreted by glands located throughout the external canal
middle ear *mid'ĕl ēr*	structures in the middle of the ear that vibrate sound from the tympanic membrane to the inner ear
tympanic membrane (TM) (*see* Fig. 11-3, B) *tim-pan'ik mem'brăn*	eardrum; drum-like structure that receives sound collected in the external auditory canal and amplifies it through the middle ear
malleus *mal'ē-ŭs*	hammer; first of the three auditory ossicles of the middle ear
incus *ing'kŭs*	anvil; middle of the three auditory ossicles of the middle ear
stapes *stā'pēz*	stirrup; last of the three auditory ossicles of the middle ear
eustachian tube *yū-stā'shăn tūb* **auditory tube** *aw'di-tōr-ē tūb*	tube connecting the middle ear to the pharynx (throat)

TERM	MEANING
oval window *ō'val win'dō*	membrane that covers the opening between the middle ear and inner ear
inner ear *in'ĕr ēr* **labyrinth** *lab'i-rinth*	intricate, fluid-filled, intercommunicating bony and membranous passages that function in hearing by relaying sound waves to auditory nerve fibers on a path to the brain for interpretation; also sense body movement and position to maintain balance and equilibrium (*labyrinth* = maze)
cochlea *kok'lē-ă*	coiled tubular structure of the inner ear that contains the organ of Corti (*cochlea* = snail)
perilymph *per'i-limf*	fluid that fills the bony labyrinth of the inner ear
endolymph *en'dō-limf*	fluid within the membranous labyrinth of the inner ear
organ of Corti *ōr'gan of kōr'tē*	structure located in the cochlea; contains receptors (hair cells) that receive vibrations and generate nerve impulses for hearing
vestibule *ves'ti-byūl*	middle part of the inner ear, in front of the semicircular canals and behind the cochlea, that contains the utricle and the saccule; functions to provide body balance and equilibrium
utricle *ū'tri-kĕl*	the larger of two sacs within the membranous labyrinth of the vestibule in the inner ear (*uter* = leather bag)
saccule *sak'yūl*	the smaller of two sacs within the membranous labyrinth of the vestibule in the inner ear (*sacculus* = small bag)
semicircular canals *sem'ē-sĕr'kyū-lar kă-nalz'*	three canals within the inner ear that contain specialized receptor cells that generate nerve impulses with body movement

 ## Programmed Review: Anatomic Terms

ANSWERS	REVIEW
pinna pinnae	**11.9** The outer, projecting part of the external ear is called the auricle or _____. The plural form of this term is _____. The adjective form is pinnal.
external auditory cerumen	**11.10** Sound waves travel from the pinna through the _____ _____ canal toward the eardrum. Glands along this canal secrete a waxy substance called _____.
tympanum	**11.11** The tympanic membrane, or _____, is the beginning of the middle ear. Also called the eardrum, this structure amplifies sounds into the middle ear.

ANSWERS	REVIEW
bones malleus incus stapes	**11.12** The middle ear has three ossicles, which are small _____, that are named because of their shapes. The first, named for its hammer shape, is the _____. The malleus receives sound vibrations from the tympanum and transmits them to the anvil-shaped bone, called the _____, which transmits them to the stirrup-shaped bone, called the _____. The stapes transfers the vibrations to the inner ear.
eustachian	**11.13** It is necessary to equalize air pressure outside of the body with that of the middle ear. The tube connecting the middle ear to the throat (pharynx) is the _____ tube (named for the Italian anatomist Eustachio). This is sometimes also called the auditory tube.
oval window inner	**11.14** The opening between the middle ear and the inner ear is covered with a membrane called the _____ _____, which is named for its rounded shape and window-like covering. The stapes transmits sound vibrations to the oval window and, thus, into the _____ ear.
labyrinth	**11.15** The inner ear is a network of interconnecting tubes and chambers that looks like a maze and is also called the _____.
within perilymph endolymph cochlea	**11.16** The combining form *lymph/o* refers to clear liquid. The prefix *peri-* means around, and the prefix *endo-* means _____. The fluid that fills the bony labyrinth in the inner ear is called _____, and the fluid within the membranous labyrinth is called _____. The coiled, snail-shaped structure containing the organ of Corti is the _____.
organ of Corti	**11.17** Nerve receptors are located inside the _____ _____ _____. This organ generates nervous impulses for hearing.
vestibule small utricle, saccule	**11.18** The middle part of the inner ear that contains the utricle and saccule is the _____. Recall that the suffix *-ule* means _____. The larger of the two sacs in the vestibule is the _____, and the smaller of the two sacs is the _____.
semicircular canals	**11.19** The labyrinth structures with partially circular shapes that generate nerve impulses with body movement are called _____ _____. These nerve receptors help to maintain the body's balance and equilibrium.

Self-Instruction: Symptomatic Terms

Study the following:

TERM	MEANING
otalgia ō-tal′jē-ă **otodynia** ō-tō-din′ē-ă	earache
otorrhagia ō-tō-rā′jē-ă	bleeding from the ear
otorrhea ō-tō-rē′ă	purulent drainage from the ear
tinnitus tin′i-tŭs	a jingling; a ringing or buzzing in the ear
vertigo vĕr′ti-gō	a turning round; dizziness

 ## Programmed Review: Symptomatic Terms

ANSWERS	REVIEW
ear pain otalgia	**11.20** The combining form *ot/o* means _____. Recall that the suffix *-algia* means _____. Thus, the term for ear pain, or an earache, is _____.
bleeding or to burst forth otorrhagia	**11.21** The suffix *-rrhagia* means _____. The term for bleeding from the ear is _____.
-rrhea otorrhea	**11.22** Recall that the symptomatic suffix meaning discharge is _____. The term for a purulent drainage (discharge) from the ear is _____.
tinnitus	**11.23** The Latin word tinnitus means to jingle. The symptom of hearing a jingling, ringing, or buzzing sound in the ear is _____.
vertigo	**11.24** The Latin word vertigo means dizziness or turning around. The symptom of feeling that one is turning around, or feeling dizzy, is called _____.

Self-Instruction: Diagnostic Terms

Study the following:

TERM	MEANING
EXTERNAL EAR	
otitis externa (Fig. 11-2, B) *ō-tī'tis eks-tĕr'nă*	inflammation of the external auditory meatus (canal)
cerumen impaction *sĕ-rū'men im-pak'shŭn*	excessive buildup of wax in the ear that often reduces hearing acuity, especially in elderly persons
MIDDLE EAR	
myringitis *mir-in-jī'tis* **tympanitis** *tim-pă-nī'tis*	inflammation of the eardrum
otitis media (Fig. 11-3, C) *ō-tī'tis mē'dē-ă*	inflammation of the middle ear
aerotitis media *ār-o-tī'tis mē'dē-ă*	inflammation of the middle ear from changes in atmospheric pressure; often occurs with frequent air travel
eustachian obstruction *yū-stā'shăn ob-strŭk'shŭn*	blockage of the eustachian tube, usually as a result of infection, as in otitis media
otosclerosis *ō'tō-sklĕ-rō'sis*	hardening of the bony tissue in the ear

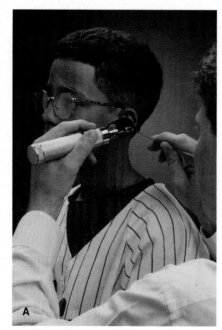

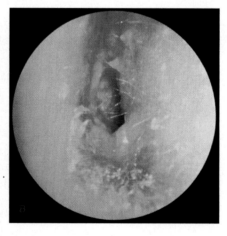

FIGURE 11-2 ■ A. Otoscopic examination of the external auditory meatus (canal). B. Otitis externa.

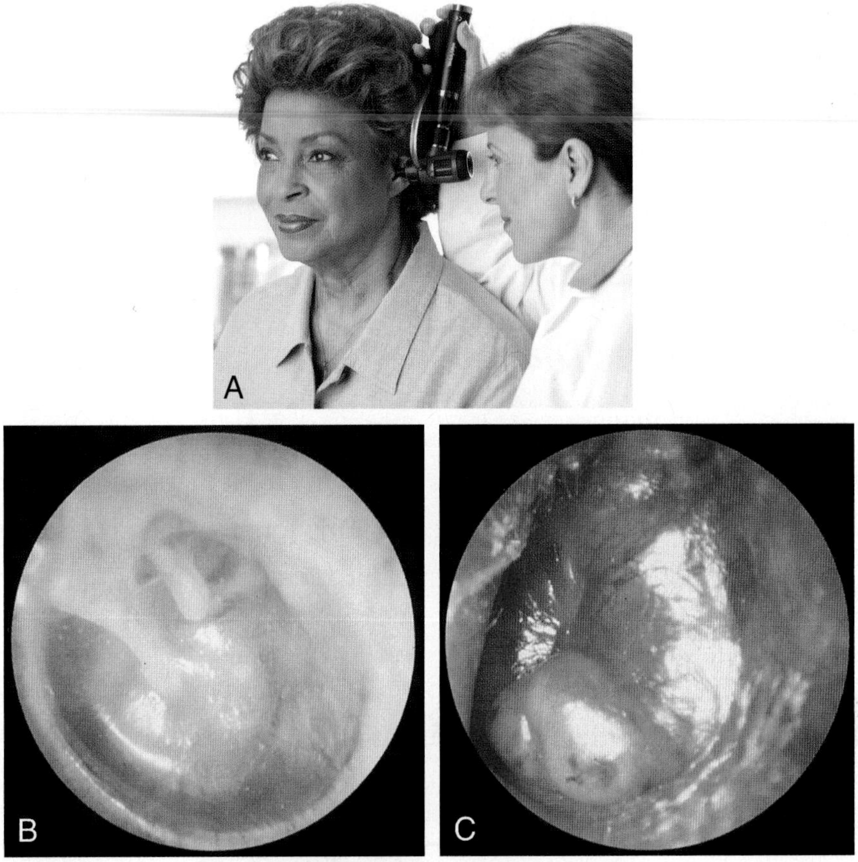

FIGURE 11-3 ■ A. Doctor performing pneumatic otoscopy. B. Normal tympanic membrane. C. Otitis media.

TERM	MEANING
INNER EAR	
acoustic neuroma *ă-kūs'tik nū-rō'mă*	benign tumor on the auditory nerve (8th cranial nerve) that causes vertigo, tinnitus, and hearing loss
labyrinthitis *lab'i-rin-thī'tis*	inflammation of the labyrinth (inner ear)
Ménière disease *měn-yār' di-zēz'*	disorder of the inner ear resulting from an excessive buildup of endolymphatic fluid, causing episodes of vertigo, tinnitus, nausea, vomiting, and hearing loss; one or both ears can be affected, and attacks vary in both frequency and intensity (named after Prosper Ménière, the French physician who first described the condition)
GENERAL	
deafness *def'nes*	general term for partial or complete loss of hearing
conductive hearing loss *kon-dŭk'tiv hēr'ing los*	hearing impairment caused by interference with sound or vibratory energy in the external canal, middle ear, or ossicles

TERM	MEANING
sensorineural hearing loss *sen′sŏr-i-nūr′ăl hēr′ing los*	hearing impairment caused by lesions or dysfunction of the cochlea or auditory nerve
mixed hearing loss *mikst hēr′ing los*	combination of sensorineural and conductive hearing loss
presbyacusis *prez′bē-ă-kū′sis* **presbycusis** *prez-bē-kū′sis*	hearing impairment in old age

◈ Programmed Review: Diagnostic Terms

ANSWERS	REVIEW
-itis myringitis tympanitis	**11.25** Recall that the suffix for inflammation is _____. Using the two different combining forms meaning eardrum, two terms for an inflamed tympanic membrane are _____ and _____.
otitis externa otitis media inflammation labyrinthitis	**11.26** There are three different types of otitis, depending on whether the inflammation is in the external ear, middle ear, or inner ear. Inflammation of the external auditory meatus (canal) is termed _____ _____, and inflammation of the middle ear is termed _____ _____. Otitis interna, or _____ of the inner ear, is more commonly known as inflammation of the labyrinth, or _____.
aerotitis media	**11.27** Using the combining forms for both air and ear, the term for inflammation of the middle ear from changes in atmospheric pressure is _____ _____.
cerumen impaction	**11.28** Ear wax can build up in the external auditory canal and become impacted. This condition of excessive ear wax is called _____ _____.
eustachian obstruction	**11.29** A middle ear infection, such as otitis media, may cause a blockage of the eustachian tube, which is called a _____ _____. This condition is common in young children when the tube is small and easily obstructed.
increase otosclerosis	**11.30** The combining form for *scler/o* means hard. Recall that the suffix *-osis* means condition or _____. The medical term for the hardening (increased hardness) of bony tissue in the ear is therefore called _____.

ANSWERS	REVIEW
hearing pertaining to acoustic neuroma	**11.31** The two-word term describing a benign tumor on the auditory nerve (8th cranial nerve) that causes vertigo, tinnitus, and hearing loss is formed by combining *acous/o*, the combining form meaning _____, and *-ic*, the suffix meaning _____ ____, along with *neur/o*, the combining form meaning nerve and the suffix for tumor: _____ _____.
tinnitus vertigo Ménière	**11.32** Ringing in the ear, or _____, and dizziness, or _____, along with vomiting, nausea, and hearing loss are symptoms of an inner ear disorder resulting from an excessive buildup of endolymphatic fluid called _____ disease (named for the French physician who first described the condition).
deafness conductive sensorineural mixed	**11.33** The general term for partial or complete hearing loss is _____, which is often called hearing impairment or hearing disabled. Hearing loss can be caused by mechanical factors that interfere with the transmission of sound vibrations through the external and middle ears. This is called _____ hearing loss. The term for hearing loss caused by dysfunction of the cochlea or auditory nerve is formed using combining forms referring to the senses and nerves: _____ hearing loss. A combination of sensorineural and conductive hearing loss is known as _____ hearing loss.
hearing condition presbyacusis presbycusis	**11.34** The suffix *-acusis* means _____ _____. Because the combining form *presby/o* means old age, the term for hearing impairment in old age is _____. The shortened form of this term is _____.

◆ Self-Instruction: Diagnostic Tests and Procedures

Study the following:

TEST OR PROCEDURE	EXPLANATION
audiometry (Fig. 11-4) *aw-dē-om'ĕ-trē*	process of measuring hearing
audiometer *aw-dē-om'ĕ-ter*	instrument to measure hearing

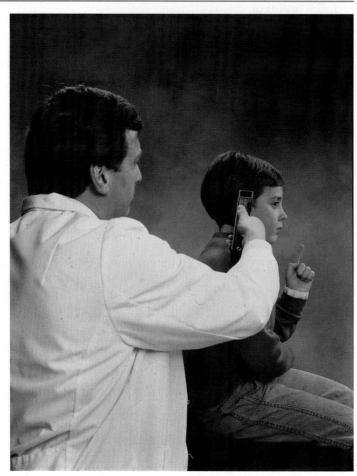

FIGURE 11-4 ■ Audiometry: hearing screening.

TEST OR PROCEDURE	EXPLANATION
audiogram *aw'dē-ō-gram*	record of hearing measurement
audiologist *aw-dē-ol'ō-jist*	health professional who specializes in the study of hearing impairments
auditory acuity testing *aw'di-tōr-ē ă-kyū'i-tē test'ing*	physical assessment of hearing; useful in differentiating between conductive and sensorineural hearing loss
tuning fork (Fig. 11-5) *tū'ning fōrk*	a two-pronged, fork-like instrument that vibrates when struck; used to test hearing, especially bone conduction
brainstem auditory evoked potential (BAEP) (Fig. 11-6) *brān'stem aw'di-tōr-ē ē-vōkt' pō-ten'shăl*	electrodiagnostic testing that uses computerized equipment to measure involuntary responses to sound within the auditory nervous system; commonly used to assess hearing in newborns
brainstem auditory evoked response (BAER) *brān'stem aw'di-tōr-ē ē-vōkt' rē-spons'*	
otoscopy (*see* Fig. 11-2) *ō-tos'kŏ-pē*	use of an otoscope to examine the external auditory canal and tympanic membrane

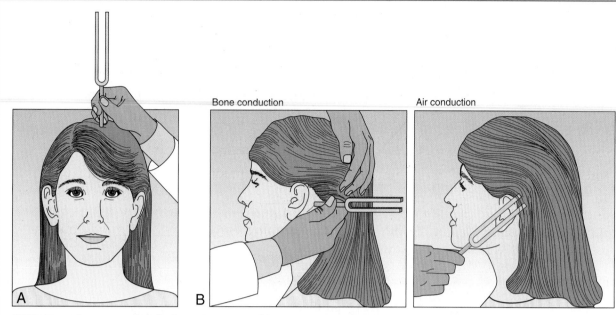

FIGURE 11-5 ■ Tuning fork testing. A. Webber test. B. Rinne test.

TEST OR PROCEDURE	EXPLANATION
pneumatic otoscopy (*see* Fig. 11-3, A) *nū-mat'ik ō-tos'kŏ-pē*	otoscopic observation of the tympanic membrane as air is released into the external auditory meatus; immobility indicates the presence of middle ear effusion (fluid buildup), as occurs as a result of otitis media
tympanometry *tim'pă-nom'ĕ-trē*	measurement of the compliance and mobility (conductibility) of the tympanic membrane and ossicles of the middle ear by monitoring the response to external airflow pressures

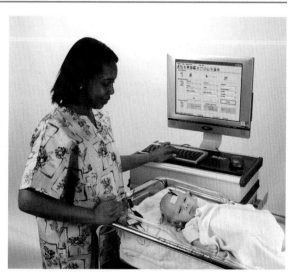

FIGURE 11-6 ■ Brainstem auditory evoked potentials (BAEP) testing of a newborn.

Programmed Review: Diagnostic Tests and Procedures

ANSWERS	REVIEW
-metry audiometry	**11.35** Recall that the suffix referring to the process of measuring is _____. Thus, the term for the process of measuring hearing is _____.
-meter audiometer	**11.36** The suffix for an instrument for measuring is _____. Thus, the term for an instrument that measures hearing is _____.
-gram audiogram	**11.37** The suffix meaning a record is _____. Thus, the term for a record of hearing measurement is _____.
-logist audiologist	**11.38** The suffix for someone who specializes in the study or treatment of a certain subject area is _____. Thus, the term for a health professional who specializes in the study of hearing impairments is an _____.
-metry eardrum tympanometry	**11.39** Again, the suffix for the process of measuring is _____. *Tympan/o* is the combining form for _____ (also called the tympanum). The process of measuring the compliance and mobility (conductibility) of the tympanic membrane is called _____. This test may be used to help diagnose hearing loss.
auditory acuity middle sensorineural	**11.40** A physical assessment of hearing that differentiates between conductive and sensorineural hearing loss is called _____ _____ testing. A conductive hearing loss is usually caused in the external or _____ ear, whereas a _____ hearing loss involves a problem in the cochlea or auditory nerve.
tuning fork bone	**11.41** The vibrating device that is used in acuity testing is a _____ _____. One test uses it to assess the conduction of vibration through _____.
	11.42 The electrodiagnostic test using computerized equipment to measure involuntary responses to sound within the auditory nervous system, such as commonly used to assess

ANSWERS	REVIEW
brainstem auditory evoked potential	hearing in newborns, is called _____ _____ _____ _____ (BAEP).
ot/o	**11.43** The combining forms meaning ear are *aur/i* and _____. The latter is combined with the suffix referring to a process of examination to form this medical term for using an otoscope to examine the external auditory canal and tympanic
otoscopy	membrane: _____. The term describing otoscopic observation of the tympanic membrane as air is released into
pneumatic	the external auditory meatus is called _____ otoscopy (including a combining form meaning lung or air).

◆ Self-Instruction: Operative Terms

Study the following:

TERM	MEANING
microsurgery *mī-krō-sŭr′jĕr-ē*	surgery with the use of a microscope used on delicate tissue, such as the ear
myringotomy *mir-in-got′ŏ-mē* **tympanostomy** (Fig. 11-7) *tim-pan-os′tŏ-mē*	incision into the eardrum, most often for insertion of a small polyethylene (PE) tube to keep the canal open and prevent fluid buildup, such as occurs in otitis media
otoplasty *ō′tō-plas-tē*	surgical repair of the external ear

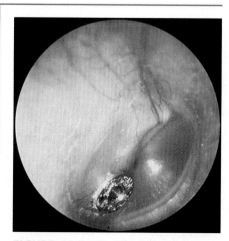

FIGURE 11-7 ■ View through otoscope shows placement of tympanostomy tube.

TERM	MEANING
stapedectomy *stā-pĕ-dek'tō-mē*	excision of the stapes to correct otosclerosis
tympanoplasty *tim'pă-nō-plas-tē*	vein graft of a scarred tympanic membrane to improve sound conduction

Programmed Review: Operative Terms

ANSWERS	REVIEW
-plasty otoplasty	**11.44** Recall that the suffix for surgical repair or reconstruction is _____. A surgeon might repair the external ear after trauma, for example. This is called an _____.
tympanoplasty	**11.45** A surgical repair of the tympanic membrane is a _____. This may include a graft to a scarred membrane to improve sound conduction.
microsurgery	**11.46** Many of the ear's internal structures are small and delicate, and surgery must be performed using a microscope. This type of surgery is called _____.
otitis media tomy stomy	**11.47** Small children often have middle ear infections, which are called _____ _____. To drain fluids from the middle ear, small tubes are often inserted into the eardrum after a surgical incision through the eardrum. There are two terms that describe this procedure. One, using the suffix for incision, is myringo_____. The other, using the suffix describing the creation of an opening, is tympano_____.
-ectomy otosclerosis stapedectomy ossicles or bones middle	**11.48** The suffix meaning excision is _____. For the condition of hardening of the bony tissue of the ear, _____, the stapes may be excised to correct the hearing problem. This procedure is called a _____. The stapes is the last of the three auditory _____ in the _____ ear.

◈ Self-Instruction: Therapeutic Terms

Study the following:

TERM	MEANING
auditory prosthesis *aw'di-tōr-ē pros'thē-sis*	any internal or external device that improves or substitutes for natural hearing
hearing aid *hēr'ing ād*	an external amplifying device designed to improve hearing by more effective collection of sound into the ear
cochlear implant (Fig. 11-8) *kok'lē-ăr im'plant*	an electronic device implanted in the cochlea that provides sound perception to patients with severe or profound sensorineural (nerve) hearing loss in both ears
ear lavage *ēr lă-vahzh'*	irrigation of the external ear canal, often to remove excessive buildup of cerumen
ear instillation *ēr in-sti-lā'shŭn*	introduction of a medicated solution into the external canal, usually administered by drop (gt) or drops (gtt) in the affected ears

COMMON THERAPEUTIC DRUG CLASSIFICATIONS

antibiotic *an'tē-bī-ot'ik*	a drug that inhibits the growth of or destroys microorganisms; used to treat diseases caused by bacteria (e.g., otitis media)
antihistamine *an-tē-his'tă-mēn*	a drug that blocks the effects of histamine
histamine *his'tă-mēn*	a regulatory body substance released in allergic reactions, causing swelling and inflammation of tissues; seen in hay fever and urticaria (hives)

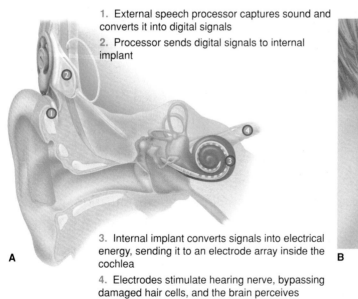

1. External speech processor captures sound and converts it into digital signals
2. Processor sends digital signals to internal implant

3. Internal implant converts signals into electrical energy, sending it to an electrode array inside the cochlea
4. Electrodes stimulate hearing nerve, bypassing damaged hair cells, and the brain perceives signals to hear sound

A

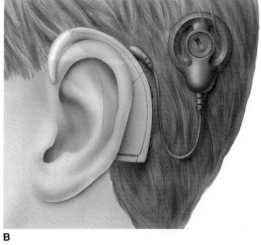

B

FIGURE 11-8 ■ **A. Operation of a cochlear implant. B. Side view showing placement of external speech processor.**

TERM	MEANING
antiinflammatory *an'tē-in-flam'ă-tō-rē*	a drug that reduces inflammation
decongestant *dē-kon-jes'tant*	a drug that reduces congestion and swelling of membranes, such as those of the nose and eustachian tube in an infection

Programmed Review: Therapeutic Terms

ANSWERS	REVIEW
auditory prosthesis hearing aid cochlear	**11.49** Recall from study of Chapter 4 that prosthesis is an artificial replacement for a diseased or missing body part. The term used to refer to any device that is used to improve or substitute for natural hearing is an _____ _____. The external amplifying device designed to improve hearing by more effective collection of sound into the ear is called a _____ _____. The electronic device implanted in the cochlea that provides sound perception to patients with severe or profound sensorineural (nerve) hearing loss in both ears is called a _____ implant.
lavage cerumen impaction	**11.50** The Latin term lavo means to wash. The process by which a cavity or organ is washed out by irrigating it with water or other fluid is called lavage. The external ear canal is often irrigated to remove buildup of cerumen in a process called ear _____. An excessive buildup of earwax is called _____ _____.
instillation drop, gtt	**11.51** The administration of a medicated solution into the ear's external canal is an ear _____, usually introduced by _____ (gt) or drops (____) in the affected ear or ears.
histamine antihistamine against	**11.52** A substance in the body that is released during allergic reactions and that causes swelling and inflammation of tissues is called _____. A drug that acts to inhibit the effects of histamine is an _____. The prefix *anti-* means _____ or opposed to.
antiinflammatory	**11.53** Similarly, a drug that reduces inflammation is an _____.

ANSWERS	REVIEW
antibiotic	**11.54** The same prefix joined with the combining form for life (*bio*) denotes a drug class that kills or inhibits microbial life. This type of drug is called an _____.
not decongestant	**11.55** The prefix *de-* means from, down, or _____. A drug that is given to reduce congestion, such as may occur in the eustachian tube during an infection, is a _____.

CHAPTER 11 ACRONYMS AND ABBREVIATIONS

ABBREVIATION	EXPANSION
BAEP	brainstem auditory evoked potential
BAER	brainstem auditory evoked response
ENT	ear, nose, and throat
PE	polyethylene
TM	tympanic membrane

CHAPTER 11 SUMMARY OF TERMS

The terms introduced in chapter 11 are listed below, followed by the page number on which each term can be found and its written pronunciation. For additional practice and reinforcement, write the definition of each term on a separate piece of paper.

acoustic neuroma/533
ă-kūs'tik nū-rō'mă

aerotitis media/532
ār-ō-tī'tis mē'dē-ă

antibiotic/541
an'tē-bī-ot'ik

antihistamine/541
an-tē-his'tă-mēn

antiinflammatory/542
an'tē-in-flam'ă-tō-rē

audiogram/536
aw'dē-ō-gram

audiologist/536
aw-dē-ol'ō-jist

audiometer/535
aw-dē-om'ĕ-ter

audiometry/535
aw-dē-om'ĕ-trē

auditory acuity testing/536
aw'di-tōr-ē ă-kyū'i-tē test'ing

auditory prosthesis/541
aw'di-tōr-ē pros'thē-sis

auditory tube/528
aw'di-tōr-ē tūb

brainstem auditory evoked potential (BAEP)/536
brān'stem aw'di-tōr-ē ē-vōkt' pō-ten'shăl

brainstem auditory evoked response (BAER)/536
brān'stem aw'di-tōr-ē ē-vōkt' rē-spons'

cerumen/528
sĕ-rū'men

cerumen impaction/532
sĕ-rū'men im-pak'shŭn

cochlea/529
kōk'lē-ă

cochlear implant/541
kōk'lē-ăr im'plant

conductive hearing loss/533
kon-dŭk'tiv hēr'ing los

deafness/533
def'nes

decongestant/542
dē-kon-jes'tant

ear instillation/541
ēr in-sti-lā'shŭn

ear lavage/541
ēr lă-vahzh'

endolymph/529
en'dō-limf

eustachian obstruction/532
yū-stā'shăn ob-strŭk'shŭn

eustachian tube/528
yū-stā'shăn tūb

external auditory meatus or
   canal/528
*eks-tĕr'năl aw'di-tōr-ē mē-ā'tŭs or
   kă-nal'*

external ear/528
eks-tĕr'năl ēr

hearing aid/541
hēr'ing ād

histamine/541
his'tă-mēn

incus/528
ing'kŭs

inner ear/529
in'ĕr ēr

labyrinth/529
lab'i-rinth

labyrinthitis/533
lab'i-rin-thī'tis

malleus/528
mal'ē-ŭs

Ménière disease/533
mĕn-yār' di-zēz'

microsurgery/539
mī-krō-sŭr'jĕr-ē

middle ear/528
mid'ĕl ēr

myringitis/532
mir-in-jī'tis

mixed hearing loss/534
mikst hēr'ing los

myringotomy/539
mir-in-got'ŏ-mē

organ of Corti/529
ōr'gan of kōr'tē

otalgia/531
ō-tal'jē-ă

otitis externa/532
ō-tī'tis eks-tĕr'nă

otitis media/532
ō-tī'tis mē'dē-ă

otodynia/531
ō-tō-din'ē-ă

otoplasty/539
ō'tō-plas-tē

otorrhagia/531
ō-tō-rā'jē-ă

otorrhea/531
ō-tō-rē'ă

otosclerosis/532
ō'tō-sklē-rō'sis

otoscopy/536
ō-tos'kŏ-pē

oval window/529
ō'val win'dō

perilymph/529
per'i-limf

pinna/528
pin'ă

pneumatic otoscopy/537
nū-mat'ik ō-tos'kŏ-pē

presbyacusis/534
prez'bē-ă-kū'sis

presbycusis/534
prez-bē-kū'sis

saccule/529
sak'yūl

semicircular canals/529
sem'ē-sĕr'kyū-lar ka-nălz'

sensorineural hearing loss/534
sen'sōr-i-nūr'ăl hēr'ing los

stapedectomy/540
stā-pĕ-dek'tŏ-mē

stapes/528
stā'pēz

tinnitus/531
tin'i-tŭs

tuning fork/536
tū'ning fōrk

tympanic membrane (TM)/528
tim-pan'ik mem'brān

tympanitis/532
tim-pă-nī'tis

tympanometry/537
tim'pă-nom'ĕ-trē

tympanoplasty/540
tim'pă-nō-plas-tē

tympanostomy/539
tim'pan-os'tŏ-mē

utricle/529
ū'tri-kĕl

vertigo/531
vĕr'ti-gō

vestibule/529
ves'ti-byūl

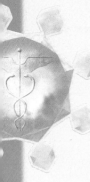

PRACTICE EXERCISES

For each of the following words, write out the term components (prefixes [P], combining forms [CF], roots [R], and suffixes [S]) on the lines below the word. Then define the term according to the meaning of its components.

EXAMPLE

macrotia

<u>macr</u> / <u>ot</u> / <u>ia</u>

P   R   S

DEFINITION: large or long/ear/condition of

1. aerotitis

   _____ / _____ / _____

       R   R   S

   DEFINITION: _____

2. otorrhea

   _____ / _____

       CF   S

   DEFINITION: _____

3. myringoplasty

   _____ / _____

       CF   S

   DEFINITION: _____

4. acoustic

   _____ / _____

       R   S

   DEFINITION: _____

5. ceruminolysis

   _____ / _____

       CF   S

   DEFINITION: _____

6. salpingoscope

   _____ / _____

       CF   S

   DEFINITION: _____

7. audiometry

   _____ / _____

       CF   S

   DEFINITION: _____

8. tympanocentesis

   _____ / _____

      CF   S

   DEFINITION: _____

9. otodynia

   _____ / _____

      CF   S

   DEFINITION: _____

10. auricle

    _____ / _____

       R   S

    DEFINITION: _____

11. myringotomy

    _____ / _____

       CF   S

    DEFINITION: _____

12. ceruminosis

    _____ / _____

       R   S

    DEFINITION: _____

13. audiology

    _____ / _____

       CF   S

    DEFINITION: _____

Complete each medical term by writing the missing part:

14. oto_____osis = condition of hardening of the bony tissue of the ear

15. aero_____ media = inflammation of the middle ear caused by changes in atmospheric pressure

16. _____logist = person who specializes in the study of hearing impairments

17. _____tomy = incision into the eardrum for the insertion of tubes

18. _____scope = instrument used to view the ear canal and tympanum

19. _____ neuroma = benign tumor of the auditory nerve

20. _____ otoscopy = observation of the tympanic membrane as air is released into the external auditory meatus

Write the correct medical term for each of the following definitions:

21. _____ inflammation of the labyrinth

22. _____ dizziness

23. _____ bleeding from the ear

24. _____ electronic device implanted in the cochlea to provide sound perception

25. _____ hearing impairment of old age

26. _____ ringing in the ear

27. _____ excision of stapes to correct otosclerosis

28. _____ excessive buildup of ear wax

29. _____ earache

30. _____ the study of hearing

31. _____ irrigation of the external ear canal

32. _____ disorder of the inner ear characterized by vertigo, tinnitus, nausea, vomiting, and hearing loss, named after the French physician who first described it

Circle the combining form that corresponds to the meaning given:

33. **eardrum**	salping/o	ot/o	myring/o
34. **hearing**	ot/o	audi/o	angi/o
35. **wax**	cerumin/o	crin/o	scler/o
36. **eustachian tube**	tympan/o	myring/o	salping/o
37. **ear**	rhin/o	ot/o	or/o
38. **air**	acr/o	aur/i	aer/o

Identify the parts of the ear by writing the missing words in the spaces provided:

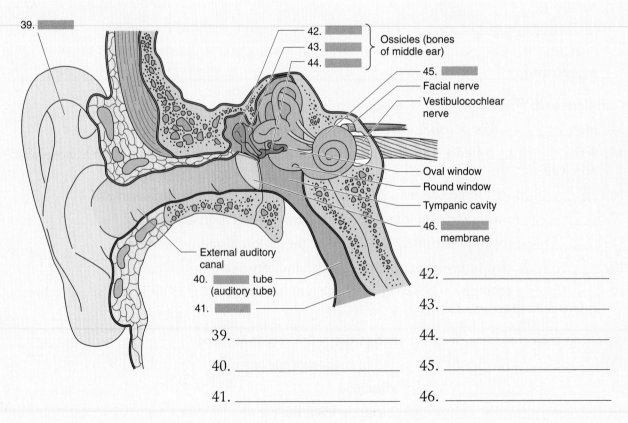

39. ▬▬

42. ▬▬ ⎱ Ossicles (bones
43. ▬▬ ⎰ of middle ear)
44. ▬▬

45. ▬▬
Facial nerve
Vestibulocochlear nerve

Oval window
Round window
Tympanic cavity

46. ▬▬ membrane

External auditory canal

40. ▬▬ tube (auditory tube)

41. ▬▬

39. _____

40. _____

41. _____

42. _____

43. _____

44. _____

45. _____

46. _____

_____ nasopharyngeal examination

_____ polyethylene tube placement in the left tympanum

_____ intubation

10. In your own words, not using medical terminology, briefly describe the condition of Hank's adenoids before adenoidectomy:

_____

_____

_____

Medical Record 11-2A: For Additional Study

CENTRAL MEDICAL CENTER

211 Medical Center Drive • Central City, US 90000-1234 • PHONE: (012) 125-6784 • FAX: (012) 125-9999

HISTORY

DATE OF ADMISSION: August 28, 20xx

HISTORY OF PRESENT ILLNESS: The patient is a 4-year-old white male with recurrent ear infections and ear congestion nonresponsive to antibiotic and decongestant therapy over the past 12 months. The patient also has a history of nasal obstruction and nasal speech. The patient is being admitted for myringotomy, polyethylene tubes, and examination of the nasopharynx and adenoidectomy. The patient has also seen other doctors who have recommended surgery, including Dr. Feldman and Dr. Saunders.

PAST MEDICAL HISTORY: Medications: None. Allergies: None. Hospitalizations: None. Surgeries: None. Childhood Diseases: Normal.

FAMILY HISTORY: No cancer or diabetes, although the patient's grandparents have a history of adult-onset diabetes.

SOCIAL HISTORY: Normal development except for speech.

REVIEW OF SYSTEMS: CARDIOVASCULAR: No hypertension and no heart murmurs. PULMONARY: No croup or asthma. GASTROINTESTINAL: No hepatitis. RENAL: Negative. ENDOCRINE: No diabetes. MUSCULOSKELETAL: No joint disease. HEMATOLOGIC: `No anemia or bleeding tendencies.

(continued)

R. Baird, M.D.

RB:nn

D: 8/28/20xx
T: 8/29/20xx

HISTORY AND PHYSICAL Page 1	PT. NAME: BALL, HANK F. ID NO: OP-372201 ROOM: OPS ADM. DATE: August 28, 20xx ATT. PHYS: R. BAIRD, M.D.

Medical Record 11-2A: For Additional Study (continued)

CENTRAL MEDICAL CENTER

211 Medical Center Drive • Central City, US 90000-1234 • PHONE: (012) 125-6784 • FAX: (012) 125-9999

PHYSICAL EXAMINATION

GENERAL: The patient is alert and afebrile.

HEENT: TMs are dull and slightly retracted; there is decreased mobility. There is dull light reflex bilaterally. No sinus tenderness on percussion of the maxillary or frontal sinuses; there are swollen turbinates on nasal examination. The oropharynx shows hypertrophic tonsils, and there are hypertrophic adenoids on examination of the nasopharynx.

CHEST: LUNGS: Clear to percussion and auscultation. HEART: Pulse: 88 and regular. There are no murmurs, gallops, or rubs. ABDOMEN: There are no masses or tenderness. No hepatosplenomegaly was noted. There was no costovertebral angle (CVA) tenderness.

BACK: Supple. There are no masses or tenderness. There is mild anterior cervical adenopathy.

RECTAL/GENITALIA: Deferred.

EXTREMITIES: There was no peripheral edema, and there were no ecchymoses.

IMPRESSION: CHRONIC OTITIS MEDIA WITH EFFUSION, NASAL SPEECH, AND NASAL OBSTRUCTION SECONDARY TO ADENOID HYPERTROPHY.

PLAN: The patient is to be admitted as an outpatient for adenoidectomy, myringotomy, and polyethylene (PE) tubes as noted above. The surgery and potential risks and complications have been discussed with the grandfather and mother as well as the possible need for further repeat myringotomy and PE tubes.

R. Baird, M.D.

RB:nn

D: 8/28/20xx
T: 8/29/20xx

HISTORY AND PHYSICAL Page 2	PT. NAME: BALL, HANK F. ID NO: OP-372201 ROOM NO: OPS ADM. DATE: August 28, 20xx ATT. PHYS: R. BAIRD, M.D.

Medical Record 11-2B: For Additional Study (continued)

CENTRAL MEDICAL CENTER

211 Medical Center Drive • Central City, US 90000-1234 • PHONE: (012) 125-6784 • FAX: (012) 125-9999

OPERATIVE REPORT

DATE OF OPERATION: August 28, 20xx

PREOPERATIVE DIAGNOSIS: Chronic otitis media with effusion bilaterally and nasal obstruction with chronic adenoiditis and adenoid hypertrophy.

POSTOPERATIVE DIAGNOSIS: Chronic otitis media with effusion bilaterally and adenoid hypertrophy and chronic adenoiditis.

OPERATION PERFORMED: Bilateral myringotomy and tubes with adenoidectomy.

SURGEON: R. Baird, M.D.

ANESTHESIOLOGIST: F. Kodama, M.D.

PROCEDURE AND FINDINGS: After general anesthesia induction and oral intubation, the patient's ears were prepped and draped in the usual manner for microscopic myringotomy surgery. A myringotomy in the right ear was carried out following debridement of cerumen. Incision of the circumferential inferior anterior quadrant was carried out. Mucoid material was aspirated from the middle ear. A Shepard polyethylene tube was placed in position without difficulty. Cotton dressing was applied to the ear. The left ear was examined. A similar dull, nonmobile TM was noted. An inferior anterior myringotomy was carried out again, and thick mucoid material was aspirated. A Shepard polyethylene tube was inserted again in the left ear. Cotton dressing was applied to the ear canal. The patient was repositioned in the Rose's position for examination of the nasopharynx which was carried out with a palate retractor, McIvor mouth gag, tongue retractor, and was stabilized with the Mayo stand. The marked adenoid hypertrophy was noted, and the adenoidectomy was carried out with curette technique. The patient tolerated the procedure well, and following extubation, he was sent back to the recovery room in satisfactory postoperative condition.

FINAL DIAGNOSIS: Chronic otitis media with effusion bilaterally, with chronic adenoiditis, adenoid hypertrophy, and nasal obstruction.

R. Baird, M.D.
R. Baird, M.D.

RB:as
D: 8/28/20xx   T: 8/29/20xx

OPERATIVE REPORT Page 1	PT. NAME: BALL, HANK F. ID NO: OP-372201 ROOM NO: OPS ATT. PHYS: R. BAIRD, M.D.

ANSWERS TO PRACTICE EXERCISES

1. aer/ot/itis
   R R S
   air or gas/ear/
   inflammation
2. oto/rrhea
   CF S
   ear/discharge
3. myringo/plasty
   CF S
   eardrum/surgical repair
   or reconstruction
4. acous/tic
   R S
   hearing/pertaining to
5. cerumino/lysis
   CF S
   wax/breaking down or
   dissolution
6. salpingo/scope
   CF S
   eustachian tube/
   instrument for
   examination
7. audio/metry
   CF S
   hearing/process of
   measuring
8. tympano/centesis
   CF S
   eardrum/puncture for
   aspiration

9. oto/dynia
   CF S
   ear/pain
10. aur/icle
    R S
    ear/small
11. myringo/tomy
    CF S
    eardrum/incision
12. cerumin/osis
    R S
    wax/condition or
    increase
13. audio/logy
    CF S
    hearing/study of
14. otosclerosis
15. aerotitis media
16. audiologist
17. myringotomy
18. otoscope
19. acoustic neuroma
20. pneumatic otoscopy
21. labyrinthitis
22. vertigo
23. otorrhagia
24. cochlear implant
25. presbycusis
26. tinnitus
27. stapedectomy
28. cerumen impaction
29. otalgia

30. audiology
31. ear lavage
32. Ménière disease
33. myring/o
34. audi/o
35. cerumin/o
36. salping/o
37. ot/o
38. aer/o
39. auricle
40. eustachian
41. pharynx
42. malleus
43. incus
44. stapes
45. cochlea
46. tympanic
47. aerotitis
48. cerumen
49. myringotomy
50. vertigo
51. antihistamine
52. tinnitus
53. stapedectomy
54. deafness
55. eustachian

ANSWERS TO MEDICAL RECORD ANALYSIS

Medical Record 11-1: Progress Note

1. d   2. b   3. d   4. c

Medical Record 11-2 and 11-3: For Additional Study

See CD-ROM for answers.

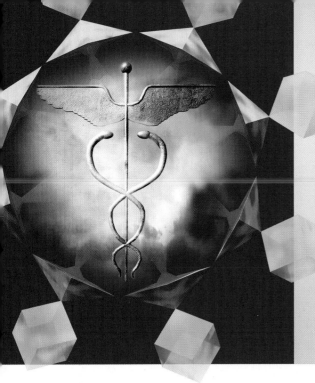

Gastrointestinal System

GASTROINTESTINAL SYSTEM OVERVIEW

The gastrointestinal (GI) system has three functions:

❊ **Digestion**, which is the process of breaking down food by chewing, swallowing, and mixing in digestive juices to convert some of the food into absorbable molecules.

❊ **Absorption**, which is the passage of digested food molecules through the walls of the intestines and into the bloodstream to be carried to cells of the body.

❊ **Excretion**, which is the elimination of nonabsorbable nutrients and waste products from the body.

Self-Instruction: Combining Forms

Study the following:

COMBINING FORM	MEANING
abdomin/o, celi/o, lapar/o	abdomen
an/o	anus
appendic/o	appendix
bil/i, chol/e	bile
bucc/o	cheek
cheil/o	lip
col/o, colon/o	colon
cyst/o	bladder or sac
dent/i	teeth
doch/o	duct
duoden/o	duodenum
enter/o	small intestine
esophag/o	esophagus
gastr/o	stomach
gingiv/o	gum
gloss/o, lingu/o	tongue
hepat/o, hepatic/o	liver
herni/o	hernia
ile/o	ileum
inguin/o	groin
jejun/o	jejunum (empty)
lith/o	stone
or/o, stomat/o	mouth
pancreat/o	pancreas
peritone/o	peritoneum
phag/o	eat or swallow
proct/o	anus and rectum
pylor/o	pylorus (gatekeeper)
rect/o	rectum
sial/o	saliva
sigmoid/o	sigmoid colon (resembles)
steat/o	fat
~emesis (suffix)	vomiting

Programmed Review: Combining Forms

ANSWERS	REVIEW
gastr/o enter/o GI	**12.1** A gastroenterologist specializes in the gastrointestinal tract. The term is built from the combining forms for stomach and intestine. The combining form meaning stomach is _____. The combining form meaning small intestine is _____. The abbreviation for gastrointestinal is _____.
pertaining to adjective duodenal	**12.2** Many combining forms related to the gastrointestinal system are similar to the English words for their meaning. For example, the combining form for duodenum is *duoden/o*. Recall that the suffix *-al*, meaning _____ _____, makes an _____ ending. The adjective form of duodenum is _____.
herni/o hernia	**12.3** There are many other combining forms that are also similar to their meaning. The combining form meaning hernia is _____. For example, a herniorrhaphy is the suturing of a repaired _____.
ile/o ileostomy	**12.4** The combining form for ileum is _____. For example, the surgical creation of an opening for the ileum is _____.
jejun/o inflammation jejunitis	**12.5** The combining form for the jejunum is _____. Recall that the suffix *-itis* means _____. Inflammation of the jejunum is called _____.
pancreat/o pancreatitis	**12.6** The combining form for pancreas is _____. Inflammation of the pancreas is called _____.
an/o anal rectum rectal proct/o anus rectum	**12.7** The combining form for anus is _____. The common adjective form is _____. *Rect/o*, the combining form for _____, is derived from the Latin word rectus, meaning straight. The rectum is so named for its straight passage from the lower bowel to the anus. The common adjective form is _____. The combining form referring to the anus and rectum is _____. A proctological examination involves the study of the _____ and the _____.
appendic/o appendicitis	**12.8** The combining form for appendix is _____. Inflammation of the appendix is called _____.

ANSWERS	REVIEW
peritone/o examination peritoneoscopy	**12.9** The combining form for peritoneum is _____. Link this combining form with *-scopy,* the suffix meaning process of _____, to build the term describing the endoscopic examination of the peritoneum: _____.
pylor/o adjective pertaining to pyloric	**12.10** The combining form for pylorus is _____. Recall that the suffix *-ic* is an _____ ending that means _____ _____. The adjective form of pylorus is _____.
sigmoid/o sigmoidoscopy	**12.11** The combining form for sigmoid colon is _____. The process of examining the sigmoid colon with a sigmoidoscope is called _____.
esophag/o pertaining to adjective esophageal	**12.12** The combining form for esophagus is _____. Recall that the suffix *-eal,* meaning _____ _____, makes an _____ ending. The adjective form of esophagus is _____.
puncture abdominocentesis celi/o, lapar/o	**12.13** In many cases, two or more combining forms have the same meaning. One combining form meaning abdomen is *abdomin/o.* Recall that the suffix *-centesis* means a _____ for aspiration. A puncture of the abdomen for aspiration of an abdominal fluid is called _____. Two other combining forms for abdomen are _____ and _____, as in the terms celiocentesis and laparoscopy.
col/o colon colon/o	**12.14** There are two combining forms for colon. An inflammation of the colon is termed colitis, which is made with the combining form _____. The second form is used in the term colonoscopy, which means examination of the _____. That combining form is _____.
bil/i presence stone	**12.15** There are two combining forms for bile. The term referring to the production of bile is biligenic, which is made from the combining form _____. The second combining form is used to make the term cholelithiasis. Recall that the suffix *-iasis* means formation of or _____ of, and the combining form *lith/o* means _____. Therefore, the term cholelithiasis refers to the

ANSWERS	REVIEW
bile chol/e	presence of a stone in the gallbladder or _____ ducts. The combining form for bile used in this term is _____.
gloss/o under lingu/o	**12.16** There are two combining forms for tongue. An inflammation of the tongue is called glossitis. The combining form used to create this term is _____. The other combining form is used in the term sublingual, which means _____ the tongue. This second combining form is _____.
or/o pain, mouth stomat/o	**12.17** There are two combining forms for mouth. One is used in the common adjective form oral. That combining form is _____. The other is used, for example, in the term stomalgia, which refers to a condition of _____ in the _____. The combining form meaning mouth in this term is _____.
enlargement hepat/o incision hepatic/o	**12.18** There are two similar combining forms meaning liver. The term hepatomegaly, which means an _____ of the liver, is made from the combining form _____. The other is used to make the term hepaticotomy, which refers to an _____ into the liver. That combining form is _____.
bucc/o	**12.19** The adjective buccal pertains to the cheek. The combining form for cheek is _____.
repair cheil/o	**12.20** Recall that the suffix *-plasty* refers to surgical _____ or reconstruction. The term cheiloplasty means repair of the lip. The combining form for lip is _____.
chol/e doch/o	**12.21** A choledochotomy is an incision into a bile duct. The combining form for bile used here is _____. The combining form meaning duct is _____.
dent/i	**12.22** The adjective dental refers to the teeth. The combining form used to make this term is _____.
bile, bladder	**12.23** A cholecystectomy is the excision of the gallbladder. Chol/e means _____, and *cyst/o* means _____ or sac. Put together, these two combining forms refer to the gallbladder, which holds bile.
gums gingiv/o	**12.24** Gingivitis is inflammation of the _____. The combining form meaning gum is _____.

ANSWERS	REVIEW
sial/o	**12.25** A sialolith is a stone of the salivary gland or duct. The combining form for saliva is _____.
inguin/o	**12.26** The adjective inguinal pertains to the groin. The combining form meaning groin is _____.
condition of without phag/o	**12.27** The term aphagia means the condition of being unable to eat. Recall that the suffix -*ia* means _____ _____, and the prefix *a*- means _____. The combining form meaning to eat or to swallow is _____.
dissolution steat/o	**12.28** Recall that the suffix -*lysis* means breaking down or _____. The term steatolysis refers to the breaking down of fat in digestion. The combining form for fat is _____.
blood -emesis	**12.29** The term hematemesis refers to the vomiting of blood. (*Hemat/o* is the combining form for _____.) The suffix meaning vomiting is _____.

Self-Instruction: Anatomic Terms (Fig. 12-1)

Study the following:

TERM	MEANING
oral cavity ōr'ăl kav'i-tē **mouth** mowth	cavity that receives food for digestion
salivary glands sal'i-vār-ē glanz	three pairs of exocrine glands in the mouth that secrete saliva: the parotid, the submandibular (submaxillary), and the sublingual glands
cheeks chēks	lateral walls of the mouth
lips lipz	fleshy structures surrounding the mouth
palate pal'ăt	structure that forms the roof of the mouth; divided into the hard palate and the soft palate
uvula ū'vyū-lă	small projection hanging from the back middle edge of the soft palate
tongue tŭng	muscular structure of the floor of the mouth covered by mucous membrane and secured by a band-like membrane known as the frenulum

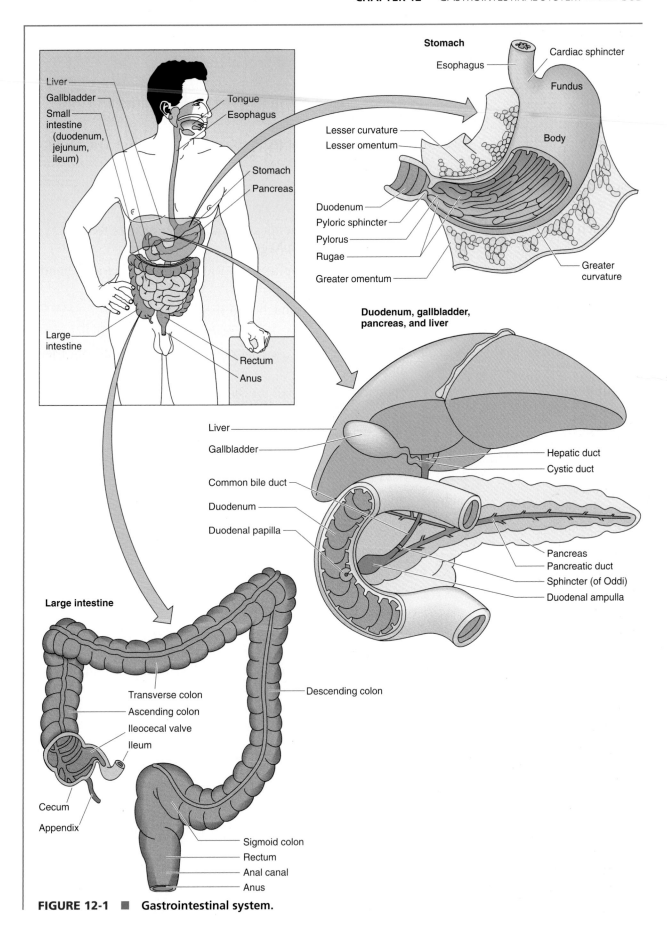

FIGURE 12-1 ■ **Gastrointestinal system.**

TERM	MEANING
gums *gŭmz*	tissue covering the processes of the jaws
teeth *tēth*	hard bony projections in the jaws for masticating (chewing) food
pharynx *fă'ringks*	throat; passageway for food traveling to the esophagus and for air traveling to the larynx
esophagus *ē-sof'ă-gŭs*	muscular tube that moves food from the pharynx to the stomach
stomach *stŏm'ăk*	sac-like organ that chemically mixes and prepares food received from the esophagus
cardiac sphincter *kar'dē-ak sfingk'tĕr*	opening from the esophagus to the stomach (*sphincter* = band)
pyloric sphincter *pī-lōr'ik sfingk'tĕr*	opening from the stomach into the duodenum
small intestine *smawl in-tes'tin*	smaller tubular structure that digests food received from the stomach
duodenum *dū-ō-dē'nŭm*	first portion of the small intestine
jejunum *jĕ-jū'nŭm*	second portion of the small intestine
ileum *il'ē-ŭm*	third portion of the small intestine
large intestine *larj in-tes'tin*	larger tubular structure that receives the liquid waste products of digestion, reabsorbs water and minerals, and forms and stores feces for defecation
cecum *sē'kŭm*	first part of the large intestine
vermiform appendix *vĕr'mi-fōrm ă-pen'diks*	worm-like projection of lymphatic tissue hanging off the cecum with no digestive function; may help to resist infection (*vermi* = worm)
colon *kō'lon*	portions of the large intestine extending from the cecum to the rectum; identified by direction or shape
ascending colon *ă-sen'ding kō'lon*	portion of the colon that extends upward from the cecum
transverse colon *trans-vĕrs' kō'lon*	portion of the colon that extends across from the ascending cecum
descending colon *dē-send'ing kō'lon*	portion of the colon that extends downward from the transverse colon
sigmoid colon *sig'moyd kō'lon*	portion of the colon (resembling an "S" in shape) that terminates at the rectum
rectum *rek'tŭm*	distal (end) portion of the large intestine
rectal ampulla *rek'tăl am-pul'lă*	dilated portion of the rectum just above the anal canal

TERM	MEANING
anus *ā'nŭs*	opening of the rectum to the outside of the body
feces *fē'sēz*	waste formed by the absorption of water in the large intestine; usually solid
defecation *def-ĕ-kā'shŭn*	evacuation of feces from the rectum
peritoneum *per'i-tō-nē'ŭm*	membrane surrounding the entire abdominal cavity and consisting of the parietal layer (lining the abdominal wall) and the visceral layer (covering each organ in the abdomen)
peritoneal cavity *per'i-tō-nē'ăl kav'i-tē*	space between the parietal and visceral peritoneum
omentum *ō-men'tŭm*	an extension of the peritoneum attached to the stomach and connecting it with other abdominal organs
liver *liv'ĕr*	organ in the upper right quadrant that produces bile, which is secreted into the duodenum during digestion
gallbladder *gawl'blad-ĕr*	receptacle that stores and concentrates the bile produced in the liver
pancreas *pan'krē-as*	gland that secretes pancreatic juice into the duodenum, where it mixes with bile to digest food
biliary ducts *bil'ē-ār-ē dŭkts*	ducts that convey bile; include the hepatic, cystic, and common bile ducts

Programmed Review: Anatomic Terms

ANSWERS	REVIEW
oral salivary palate uvula	**12.30** Let's trace the anatomy of the gastrointestinal system from beginning to end. Food is taken in at the _____ cavity, or mouth, where the digestive process begins as food is chewed and saliva from the _____ glands is mixed with the food. Structures of the mouth include the cheeks, lips, tongue, teeth, and gums. The roof of the mouth, or the _____, is divided into the hard palate and the soft palate. The small tissue projection hanging from the back edge of the soft palate is called the _____.
pharynx esophagus	**12.31** Chewed food then passes through the throat to the esophagus and then to the stomach. The medical term for the throat is the _____. From the pharynx, the food reaches the _____, which is a muscular tube descending to the stomach. At the bottom of the esophagus is the

ANSWERS	REVIEW
cardiac stomach	_____ sphincter, the opening from the esophagus to the _____.
stomach pyloric	**12.32** The sac-like organ that mixes and prepares food received from the esophagus is called the _____. From the stomach, food moves next to the small intestine through the _____ sphincter.
sphincter, duodenum jejunum ileum	**12.33** The small intestine does most of the digestive work and has three segments. The first, connected to the stomach at the pyloric _____, is called the _____. After the duodenum comes the second portion, the _____. After the jejunum comes the third portion, the _____. From the ileum, the food passes into the large intestine.
liver biliary gallbladder duodenum	**12.34** Other organs produce substances to help the small intestine digest food. Bile is produced in the _____ and is conveyed through the _____ ducts to the gallbladder. The _____ stores and concentrates the bile that is produced in the liver, which is then conveyed to the first portion of the small intestine, the _____.
pancreas	**12.35** Pancreatic juice, which is produced in the _____, is also secreted into the duodenum. This assists in digestion as well.
large cecum appendix	**12.36** After leaving the small intestine, the digested food enters the _____ intestine, where water and minerals are reabsorbed and wastes are formed into feces for defecation. The first part of the large intestine is called the _____. Hanging from the cecum is a projection of tissue with no known digestive function, which is called the vermiform _____.
colon ascending transverse descending sigmoid	**12.37** The next part of the large intestine, the _____, is identified in four sections that are named for their direction or shape. The portion of the colon extending upward from the cecum is called the _____ colon. The portion that extends from the ascending portion across the body is the _____ colon. The portion extending downward from the transverse colon is the _____ colon. The S-shaped portion at the end of the descending colon is the _____ colon.

ANSWERS	REVIEW
rectum	The sigmoid colon terminates at the _____, which is the end of the large intestine.
ampulla anus feces defecation	**12.38** The dilated portion of the rectum just above the anal canal is called the rectal _____. Waste leaves the body through the opening of the rectum, called the _____. The waste formed in the large intestine is called _____. The evacuation of feces from the rectum is called _____.
peritoneum abdominal peritoneal peritoneum	**12.39** Surrounding the entire abdominal cavity is a membrane called the _____. The peritoneum lines not only the _____ cavity (the parietal layer) but also each organ in the abdomen (the visceral layer). The space between the parietal and visceral peritoneum is called the _____ cavity. The omentum is an extension of the _____ that is attached to the stomach, connecting it with other abdominal organs.

ANATOMIC AND CLINICAL DIVISIONS OF THE ABDOMEN

Anatomic and clinical divisions of the abdomen provide reference points to describe abdominal locations. There are nine specific anatomic divisions and four general clinical divisions (Figs. 12-2 to 12-4). All references are based on the patient's right or left.

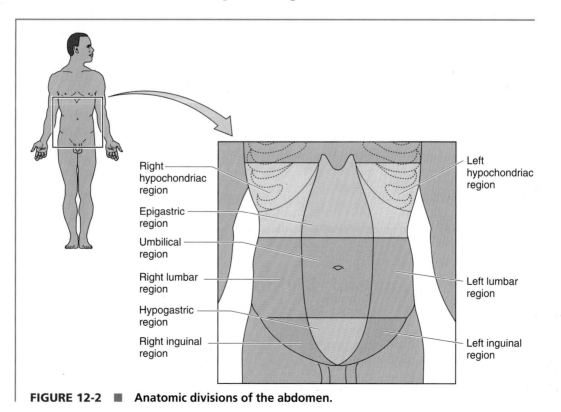

FIGURE 12-2 ■ **Anatomic divisions of the abdomen.**

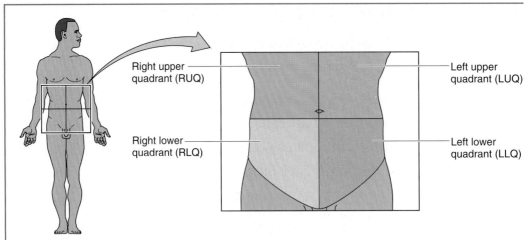

FIGURE 12-3 ■ **Clinical divisions of the abdomen.**

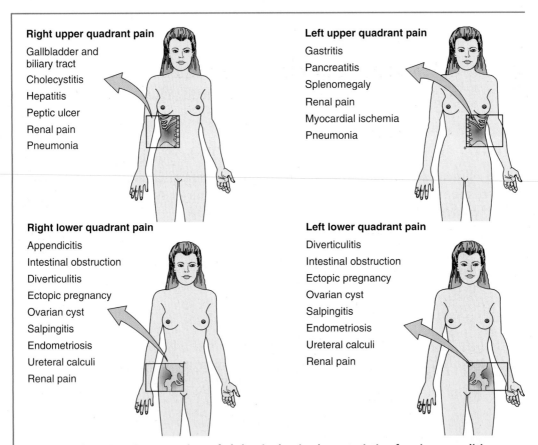

FIGURE 12-4 ■ **Common sites of abdominal pain characteristic of various conditions.**

🔷 **Self-Instruction: Anatomic Divisions** (*see* Fig. 12-2)

Study the following:

REGION	LOCATION
hypochondriac regions *hī-pō-kon'drē-ak rē'jŭnz*	upper lateral regions beneath the ribs

REGION	LOCATION
epigastric region *ep-i-gas'trik rē'jŭn*	upper middle region below the sternum
lumbar regions *lŭm'bar rē'jŭnz*	middle lateral regions
umbilical region *ŭm-bil'i-kăl rē'jŭn*	region of the navel
inguinal regions *ing'gwi-năl rē'jŭnz*	lower lateral groin regions
hypogastric region *hī-pō-gas'trik rē'jŭn*	region below the navel

🔲 Programmed Review: Anatomic Divisions

ANSWERS	REVIEW
below hypochondriac	**12.40** The abdomen is divided into several anatomic regions for reference purposes. Recall that the prefix *hypo-* means _____ or deficient. The upper lateral regions beneath the ribs (*chondro* = cartilaginous) are called the _____ regions.
upon gastr/o epigastric	**12.41** The prefix *epi-* means _____. The combining form meaning stomach is _____. Thus, the name for the upper middle region below the sternum and lying approximately upon the stomach is the _____ region.
lumbar	**12.42** The middle lateral areas of the abdomen, to each side of the lumbar spine, are the _____ regions.
umbilical	**12.43** The medical term for the navel is the umbilicus. The anatomic area in the region of the navel is called the _____ region.
inguin/o inguinal	**12.44** The combining form for groin is _____. The lower lateral groin regions are the _____ regions.
hypo- gastr/o hypogastric	**12.45** The prefix for below is _____, and the combining form for stomach is _____. Thus, the area below the navel, approximately below the stomach, is called the _____ region.

Self-Instruction: Symptomatic Terms

Study the following:

TERM	MEANING
anorexia *an-ō-rek′sē-ă*	loss of appetite (*orexia* = appetite)
aphagia *ă-fā′jē-ă*	inability to swallow
ascites (Fig. 12-5) *ă-sī′tēz*	accumulation of fluid in the peritoneal cavity (*ascos* = bag)
buccal *bŭk′ăl*	in the cheek
diarrhea *dī-ă-rē′ă*	frequent loose or liquid stools
constipation *kon-sti-pā′shŭn*	infrequent or incomplete bowel movements characterized by hardened, dry stool that is difficult to pass (*constipo* = to press together)

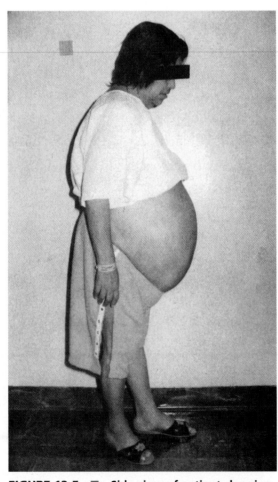

FIGURE 12-5 ■ **Side view of patient showing massive ascites and distention of abdomen.**

TERM	MEANING
dyspepsia *dis-pep'sē-ă*	indigestion (*pepsis* = digestion)
dysphagia *dis-fā'jē-ă*	difficulty in swallowing
eructation *ē-rŭk-tā'shŭn*	belch
flatulence *flat'yū-lents*	gas in the stomach or intestines (*flatus* = a blowing)
halitosis *hal-i-tō'sis*	bad breath (*halitus* = breath)
hematemesis *hē-mă-tem'ě-sis*	vomiting blood
hematochezia *hē'mă-tō-kē'zē-ă*	red blood in stool (*chezo* = defecate)
hepatomegaly *hep'ă-tō-meg'ă-lē*	enlargement of the liver
hyperbilirubinemia *hī'pěr-bil'i-rū-bi-nē'mē-ă*	excessive level of bilirubin (bile pigment) in the blood
icterus *ik'těr-ŭs* **jaundice** (Fig. 12-6) *jawn'dis*	yellow discoloration of the skin, sclera (white of the eye), and other tissues caused by excessive bilirubin in the blood (*jaundice* = yellow)
melena *me-lē'nă*	dark-colored, tarry stool caused by old blood
nausea *naw'zē-ă*	feeling sick in the stomach
steatorrhea *ste'ă-tō-rē'ă*	feces containing fat
sublingual *sŭb-ling'gwăl* **hypoglossal** *hī-pō-glos'ăl*	under the tongue

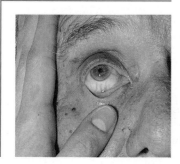

FIGURE 12-6 ■ **The yellow color of jaundice (icterus) is easily seen in the sclera of this patient and in the patient's skin as contrasted with the examiner's hand.**

Programmed Review: Symptomatic Terms

ANSWERS	REVIEW
condition of without phag/o aphagia	**12.46** Recall that the suffix *-ia* means _____ _____. The prefix *a-* means _____. Again, the combining form meaning to eat or swallow is _____. Therefore, the term for the condition of being unable to swallow (without swallowing) is _____.
faulty dysphagia	**12.47** The prefix *dys-* means painful, difficult, or _____. The term for the condition of having difficulty swallowing, then, is _____.
anorexia	**12.48** The condition of loss of (or without) appetite (*orexia* = appetite) is called _____.
dyspepsia	**12.49** The condition of indigestion, or of painful digestion (*pepsis* = digestion), is called _____.
adjective pertaining to bucc/o buccal	**12.50** The suffix *-al* is an _____ ending meaning _____ _____. The combining form meaning cheek is _____. The adjective form meaning pertaining to the cheek is _____.
ascites	**12.51** Formed from the root *ascos* (meaning bag), the term for an accumulation of fluid in the peritoneal cavity is _____.
eructation	**12.52** From the Latin word eructo comes the term for belch: _____.
flatulence	**12.53** From the Latin word flatus (meaning a blowing) comes the term for gas in the stomach or intestines: _____.
condition halitosis	**12.54** The suffix *-osis* means increase or _____. The condition of having bad breath is called _____.
-emesis hematemesis	**12.55** A combining form for blood is *hemat/o*. Again, the suffix meaning vomiting is _____. The term for vomiting blood is _____.
hematochezia	**12.56** Formed from the root word *chezo* (meaning defecate) comes this term for the condition of having red blood in the stool: _____.
hepat/o	**12.57** The two combining forms for liver are *hepatic/o* and _____. Recall that the suffix for enlargement is

ANSWERS	REVIEW
-megaly hepatomegaly	_____. Using the latter combining form for liver, the term for enlargement of the liver is _____.
-emia, excessive hyperbilirubinemia	**12.58** Recall that the suffix meaning blood condition is _____. The prefix *hyper-* means above or _____. The condition of having excessive bilirubin in the blood is _____.
icterus	**12.59** When there is excessive bilirubin in the blood, the skin is discolored yellow. This is called jaundice, or _____.
melena	**12.60** From the Greek word melaina (meaning black) comes this term for dark-colored, tarry stool caused by old blood: _____.
nausea	**12.61** From a Greek word originally referring to seasickness comes the term for feeling sick in the stomach: _____.
steat/o discharge steatorrhea	**12.62** Again, the combining form for fat is _____. Recall that the suffix *-rrhea* means _____. The term for fat in the feces (a discharge of fat) is _____.
lingu/o, below or under sublingual	**12.63** The two combining forms for tongue are *gloss/o* and _____. The prefix *sub-* means _____. Made with the latter combining form, the term for under the tongue is _____.
through, discharge diarrhea constipation	**12.64** Formed from the prefix *dia-*, meaning across or _____, and the suffix *rrhea-*, meaning _____, the term describing frequent loose or liquid stool is _____. In contrast, the term describing hardened, dry stool that is difficult to pass is _____.

 ## Self-Instruction: Diagnostic Terms

Study the following:

TERM	MEANING
RELATED TO THE UPPER GASTROINTESTINAL TRACT	
ankyloglossia *ang′ki-lō-glos′ē-ă*	tongue-tie; a defect of the tongue characterized by a short, thick frenulum (*ankyl/o* = crooked or stiff)

TERM	MEANING
cheilitis *kī-lī′tis*	inflammation of the lip
esophageal varices (*see* Fig. 12-15) *ē-sof′ă-jē′ăl var′i-sēz*	swollen, twisted veins in the esophagus that are especially susceptible to ulceration and hemorrhage
esophagitis *ē-sof-ă-jī′tis*	inflammation of the esophagus
gastritis (*see* Fig. 12-15) *gas-trī′tis*	inflammation of the stomach
gastroesophageal reflux disease (GERD) *gas′trō-ē-sof-ă-jē′ăl rē′flŭks di-zēz′*	backflow of contents of the stomach into the esophagus, often resulting from abnormal function of the lower esophageal sphincter, causing burning pain in the esophagus
gingivitis *jin-ji-vī′tis*	inflammation of the gums
glossitis *glo-sī′tis*	inflammation of the tongue
parotiditis *pă-rot-i-dī′tis* **parotitis** *par-ō-tī′tis*	inflammation of the parotid gland; also called mumps
peptic ulcer disease (PUD) (Fig. 12-7) *pep′tik ŭl′sĕr di-zēz′*	sore on the mucous membrane of the stomach, duodenum, or any other part of the gastrointestinal system exposed to gastric juices; commonly caused by infection with *Helicobacter pylori* bacteria (*pept/o* = to digest)
gastric ulcer *gas′trik ŭl′sĕr*	ulcer located in the stomach
duodenal ulcer *dū′ō-dē′năl ŭl′sĕr*	ulcer located in the duodenum
pyloric stenosis *pī-lōr′ik ste-nō′sis*	narrowed condition of the pylorus
sialoadenitis *sī′ă-lō-ad-ĕ-nī′tis*	inflammation of a salivary gland
stomatitis *stō-mă-tī′tis*	inflammation of the mouth

RELATED TO THE LOWER GASTROINTESTINAL TRACT

anal fistula (Fig. 12-8) *ā′năl fis′tyū-lă*	an abnormal, tube-like passageway from the anus that may connect with the rectum (*fistula* = pipe)
appendicitis *ă-pen-di-sī′tis*	inflammation of the appendix
colitis *kō-lī′tis*	inflammation of the colon (large intestine)

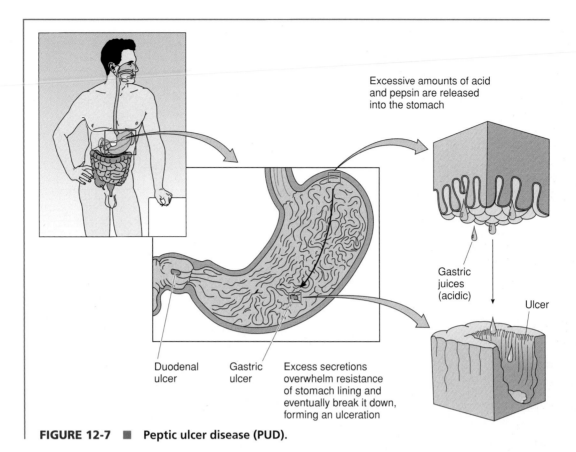

Excessive amounts of acid and pepsin are released into the stomach

Gastric juices (acidic)

Ulcer

Duodenal ulcer

Gastric ulcer

Excess secretions overwhelm resistance of stomach lining and eventually break it down, forming an ulceration

FIGURE 12-7 ■ **Peptic ulcer disease (PUD).**

TERM	MEANING
ulcerative colitis *ŭl'sĕr-ă-tiv kō-lī'tis*	chronic inflammation of the colon with ulcerations
colorectal polyps (*see* Fig. 12-15) *kol'ō-rek'tăl pol'ips*	benign tissue growths on the mucous membrane lining the large intestine and rectum; adenomatous types are precancerous and likely to develop into malignancy
pediculated polyp *pĕ-dik'yū-lā'tĕd pol'ip*	projected on a stalk (*ped/o* = foot)
sessile polyp *ses'il pol'ip*	lying flat on the surface (*sessilis* = low growing)

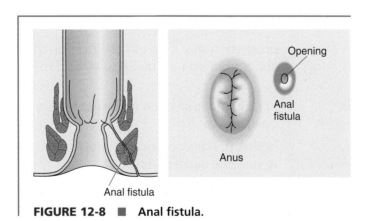

Opening

Anal fistula

Anus

Anal fistula

FIGURE 12-8 ■ **Anal fistula.**

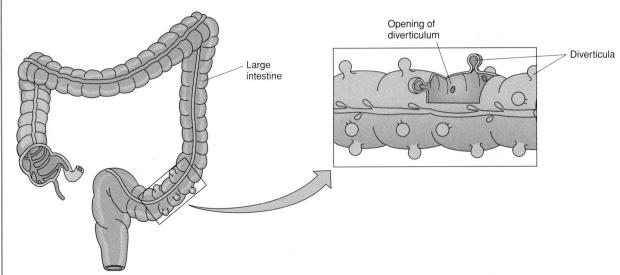

FIGURE 12-9 ■ **Diverticulosis.**

TERM	MEANING
diverticulum *dī-vĕr-tik'yū-lŭm*	an abnormal side pocket in the gastrointestinal tract; usually related to a lack of dietary fiber
diverticulosis (Fig. 12-9; *see* Fig. 12-15) *dī'vĕr-tik-ū-lō'sis*	presence of diverticula in the gastrointestinal tract, especially the colon
diverticulitis *dī'vĕr-tik-yū-lī'tis*	inflammation of diverticula
dysentery *dis'en-ter-ē*	inflammation of the intestine characterized by frequent, bloody stools; most often caused by bacteria or protozoa (e.g., amebic dysentery)
enteritis *en-tĕr-ī'tis*	inflammation of the small intestine
hemorrhoid *hem'ŏ-royd*	swollen, twisted vein (varicosity) in the anal region (*haimorrhois* = a vein likely to bleed)
hernia *hĕr'nē-ă*	protrusion of a part from its normal location
hiatal hernia (Fig. 12-10; *see* Fig. 12-18) *hī-ā'tăl hĕr'nē-ă*	protrusion of a part of the stomach upward through the opening in the diaphragm
inguinal hernia (Fig. 12-10) *ing'gwi-năl hĕr'nē-ă*	protrusion of a loop of the intestine through layers of the abdominal wall in the inguinal region
incarcerated hernia *in-kar'sĕr-ā-tĕd hĕr'nē-ă*	hernia that is swollen and fixed within a sac, causing an obstruction
strangulated hernia *strang'gyū-lā-tĕd hĕr'nē-ă*	hernia that is constricted, cut off from circulation, and likely to become gangrenous
umbilical hernia *ŭm-bil'i-kăl hĕr'nē-ă*	protrusion of the intestine through a weakness in the abdominal wall around the umbilicus (navel)

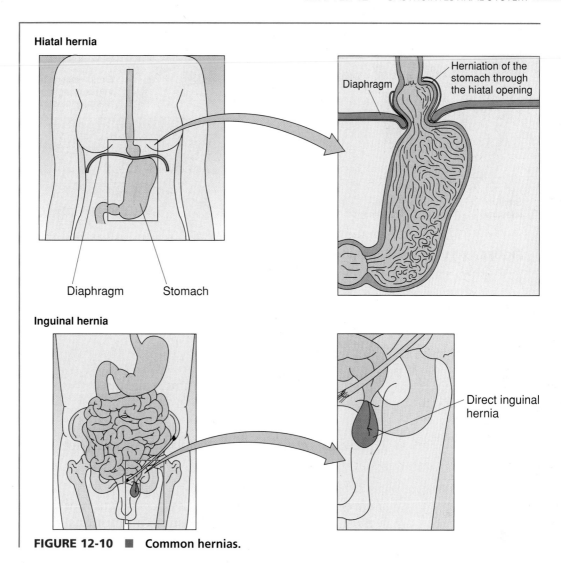

Hiatal hernia

Diaphragm

Herniation of the stomach through the hiatal opening

Diaphragm   Stomach

Inguinal hernia

Direct inguinal hernia

FIGURE 12-10 ■ **Common hernias.**

TERM	MEANING
ileitis *il-ē-ī'tis*	inflammation of the lower portion of the small intestine
intussusception (Fig. 12-11) *in'tŭs-sŭs-sep'shŭn*	prolapse of one part of the intestine into the lumen of the adjoining part (*intus* = within; *suscipiens* = to take up)
peritonitis *per'i-tō-nī'tis*	inflammation of the peritoneum
proctitis *prok-tī'tis*	inflammation of the rectum and the anus
volvulus (Fig. 12-12) *vol'vyū-lŭs*	twisting of the bowel on itself, causing obstruction (*volvo* = to roll)

RELATED TO THE ACCESSORY ORGANS OF THE GASTROINTESTINAL SYSTEM

cholangitis *kō-lan-jī'tis*	inflammation of the bile ducts

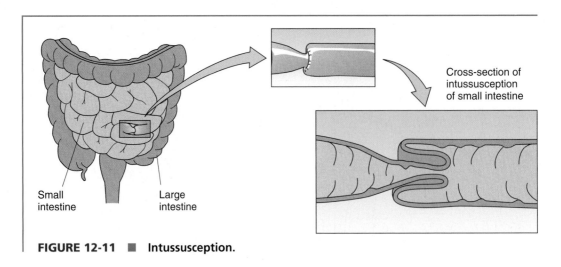

FIGURE 12-11 ■ Intussusception.

TERM	MEANING
cholecystitis *kō'lē-sis-tī'tis*	inflammation of the gallbladder
choledocholithiasis (Fig. 12-13; *see* Fig. 12-15) *kō-led'ō-kō-lith-ī'ă-sis*	presence of stones in the common bile duct
cholelithiasis (*see* Fig. 12-13) *kō'lē-li-thī'ă-sis*	presence of stones in the gallbladder or bile ducts
cirrhosis *sir-rō'sis*	chronic disease characterized by degeneration of liver tissue; most often caused by alcoholism or a nutritional deficiency (*cirrho* = yellow)
hepatitis *hep-ă-tī'tis*	inflammation of the liver
hepatitis A *hep-ă-tī'tis A*	inflammation of the liver caused by the hepatitis A virus (HAV), usually transmitted orally through fecal contamination of food or water

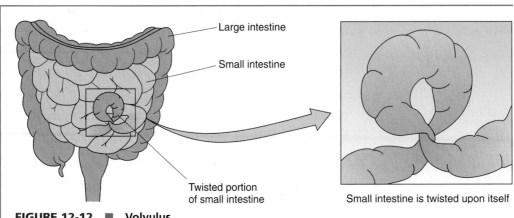

FIGURE 12-12 ■ Volvulus.

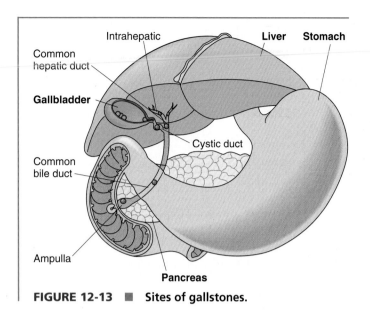

Labels: Intrahepatic · **Liver** · **Stomach** · Common hepatic duct · **Gallbladder** · Cystic duct · Common bile duct · Ampulla · **Pancreas**

FIGURE 12-13 ■ Sites of gallstones.

TERM	MEANING
hepatitis B *hep-ă-tī'tis B*	inflammation of the liver caused by the hepatitis B virus (HBV), which is transmitted sexually or by exposure to contaminated blood or body fluids
hepatitis C *hep-ă-tī'tis C*	inflammation of the liver caused by the hepatitis C virus (HCV), which is transmitted by exposure to infected blood; this strain is rarely contracted sexually
pancreatitis *pan'krē-ă-tī'tis*	inflammation of the pancreas

🔷 Programmed Review: Diagnostic Terms

ANSWERS	REVIEW
-itis stomat/o stomatitis	**12.65** The suffix for inflammation is _____. Many parts of the gastrointestinal system can become inflamed; thus, there are many diagnostic terms for inflammation of different organs. The two combining forms for mouth are *or/o* and _____. Made with the latter, the term for inflammation of the mouth is _____.
sial/o sialoadenitis parotiditis or parotitis	**12.66** The combining form for saliva is _____. Using that combining form along with *aden/o*, meaning gland, the term for inflammation of a salivary gland is _____. Inflammation of the parotid gland is called _____ (also known as mumps).

ANSWERS	REVIEW
cheil/o cheilitis	**12.67** The combining form meaning lip is _____. Inflammation of the lip is called _____.
gloss/o glossitis gingiv/o gingivitis	**12.68** The two combining forms for tongue are *lingu/o* and _____. Using the latter, the term for inflammation of the tongue is _____. The combining form for gums is _____, and the term for inflammation of the gums is _____.
esophag/o esophagitis gastr/o gastritis	**12.69** The combining form for esophagus is _____, and the term for inflammation of the esophagus is _____. The combining form for stomach is _____, and the term for inflammation of the stomach is _____.
enter/o enteritis	**12.70** The combining form for small intestine is _____, and the term for inflammation of the small intestine is _____.
ile/o ileitis col/o colitis ulcerative colitis	**12.71** The combining form for the ileum is _____, and inflammation of the ileum (the lower portion of the small intestine) is called _____. The two combining forms for the colon are *colon/o* and _____. Made from the latter form, the term for inflammation of the colon is _____. When this occurs chronically along with ulcerations, it is called _____ _____.
condition of diverticulosis diverticulitis	**12.72** Recall that the suffix *-osis* means increase or _____ _____. The condition of having diverticula (abnormal little pockets in the gastrointestinal tract) is called _____. If the diverticula are inflamed, this is called _____.
appendic/o appendicitis peritone/o, inflammation peritoneum	**12.73** The combining form for the appendix is _____, and inflammation of the appendix is called _____. The combining form for the peritoneum is _____. Peritonitis describes _____ of the _____.

ANSWERS	REVIEW
proct/o proctitis	**12.74** The combining form referring to the anus and rectum is _____. It is used in the term for inflammation of the rectum and the anus: _____.
gallbladder cholecystitis cholangitis	**12.75** *Cholecyst/o* refers to the _____. Inflammation of the gallbladder is termed _____. Formed from *chol/e* (bile) and *angi/o* (vessels), which, when combined, refer to the bile ducts, the term for inflammation of the bile ducts is _____.
pancreat/o pancreatitis	**12.76** The combining form for pancreas is _____. Inflammation of the pancreas is _____.
hepat/o hepatitis A fecal B sexually blood, C blood	**12.77** The two combining forms for liver are *hepatic/o* and _____. Made from the latter, the term for inflammation of the liver is _____. The different types of hepatitis are named after the viruses that cause them. The hepatitis _____ virus (HAV) is transmitted orally through _____ contamination of food or water. Hepatitis _____ virus (HBV) is transmitted _____ or by exposure to contaminated _____ or body fluids. Hepatitis _____ virus (HCV) is transmitted primarily through exposure to infected _____.
condition of cirrhosis	**12.78** Again, the suffix *-osis* refers to an increase or _____ _____. The chronic liver condition that causes yellowing (*cirrho* = yellow) of tissues is called _____. It is usually caused by alcoholism or a nutritional deficiency.
colon rectum pertaining to colorectal polyps pediculated sessile malignancy or cancer	**12.79** *Col/o* is a combining form referring to the _____. Combined with *rect/o,* meaning _____, and the suffix *-al,* meaning _____ _____, the adjective referring to the colon and the rectum is _____. The mucous membranes lining the colon and the rectum are common sites for the development of benign tissue growths called _____. Those that project from a stalk are called _____ polyps, and those that lie flat on the surface are called _____ polyps. Adenomatous types are likely to develop into a _____.

ANSWERS	REVIEW
pyloric stenosis	**12.80** Stenosis refers to a narrowed condition of an organ. A narrowing of the pylorus is termed _____ _____.
condition of gloss/o ankyloglossia	**12.81** The combining form *ankyl/o* means crooked or stiff. Recall that the suffix *-ia* means a _____ _____. The two combining forms for tongue are *lingu/o* and _____. Made from the latter, the term for a condition of a tongue-tie defect with a stiff, short frenulum is _____.
esophageal varices	**12.82** Varices are swollen, twisted veins. When they occur in the esophagus, this condition is called _____ _____.
gastroesophageal reflux disease	**12.83** Reflux is a backflow. When stomach contents flow back into the esophagus, this is called _____ _____ _____ (GERD).
peptic ulcer disease gastric duodenal	**12.84** An ulcer is a sore on the skin or a mucous membrane. The disease characterized by ulcer formation on the mucous membrane of the stomach, duodenum, or any other part of the GI system exposed to gastric juices is called _____ _____ _____ (PUD). An ulcer located in the stomach is called a _____ ulcer, and an ulcer in the duodenum is called a _____ ulcer.
enter/o condition of or process of dysentery	**12.85** The prefix *dys-* means painful, difficult, or faulty. The combining form for small intestine is _____. The suffix *-y* means _____ _____. The condition of a painful inflammation of the intestine (usually caused by bacteria or protozoa) is called _____.
hernia hiatal inguinal umbilical	**12.86** The protrusion of a part from its normal location is termed a _____. Hernias are often named according to the location of the protrusion. The protrusion of a part of the stomach upward through the opening in the diaphragm (hiatus) is called a _____ hernia. Protrusion of a loop of intestine through the abdominal wall in the inguinal region is an _____ hernia. Protrusion of the intestine through a weakness in the abdominal wall around the umbilicus is called an _____ hernia.

ANSWERS	REVIEW
incarcerated strangulated	**12.87** A hernia that is swollen and becomes fixed within a sac is called an _____ hernia. A hernia that becomes constricted and cut off from circulation is called a _____ hernia.
intussusception volvulus	**12.88** A section of intestine may prolapse into the lumen of an adjoining section, causing an _____. If a section of intestine twists upon itself, an obstruction may result; this condition is called _____ (*volvo* = to roll).
anal fistula	**12.89** A fistula (*fistula* = pipe) is an abnormal connection. A fistula from the anus to the rectum is called an _____ _____.
hemorrhoid	**12.90** *Hem/o* is a combining form referring to blood. A swollen, twisted vein in the anal region that is liable to bleed is called a _____.
bile lith/o -iasis cholelithiasis	**12.91** The combining form *chol/e* means _____. The combining form for stone is _____. The suffix meaning formation of or presence of is _____. Therefore, the term for the presence of stones in the gallbladder or bile ducts is _____.
choledocholithiasis	**12.92** The combining forms *chol/e* and *doch/o* together refer to the common bile duct. The term for the presence of stones in the common bile duct is _____.

 ## Self-Instruction: Diagnostic Tests and Procedures

Study the following:

TEST OR PROCEDURE	EXPLANATION
BIOPSY	
biopsy (Bx) *bī'op-sē*	removal and microscopic study of tissue for pathological examination
incisional biopsy *in-sizh'ŭn-ăl bī'op-sē*	removal of a portion of a lesion
excisional biopsy *ek-sizh'ŭn-ăl bī'op-sē*	removal of an entire lesion

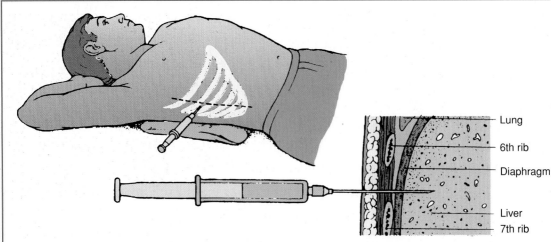

Lung
6th rib
Diaphragm
Liver
7th rib

FIGURE 12-14 ■ **Needle biopsy of the liver.**

TEST OR PROCEDURE	EXPLANATION
needle biopsy (Fig. 12-14) *nē'dĕl bī'op-sē*	percutaneous removal of tissue or fluid using a special, hollow needle (e.g., for liver biopsy)

ENDOSCOPY

endoscopy (Fig. 12-15) *en-dos'kŏ-pē*	examination within a body cavity with a flexible endoscope for diagnosis or treatment; used in the gastrointestinal tract to detect abnormalities and to perform procedures such as biopsy, excision of lesions, and therapeutic interventions

Lower Gastrointestinal Endoscopy

colonoscopy *kō-lon-os'kŏ-pē*	examination of the colon using a flexible colonoscope
proctoscopy *prok-tos'kŏ-pē*	examination of the rectum and anus with a proctoscope
sigmoidoscopy *sig-moy-dos'kŏ-pē*	examination of the sigmoid colon with a rigid or flexible sigmoidoscope

Upper Gastrointestinal Endoscopy

esophagogastroduodenoscopy (EGD) *ē-sof'ă-gō-gas'trō-dū'ō-den-os-kŏ-pē*	examination of the lining of the esophagus, stomach, and duodenum with a flexible endoscope for diagnostic and/or therapeutic purposes, such as biopsy, excision of lesions, removal of swallowed objects, dilation of obstructions, stent placement, measures to control hemorrhage, etc.
capsule endoscopy *kap'sūl en-dos'kŏ-pē*	examination of the small intestine made by a tiny video camera placed in a capsule and then swallowed; images are transmitted to a waist-belt recorder and then downloaded onto a computer for assessment of possible abnormalities; traditional endoscopy cannot completely access the small intestine because of its length and complexity

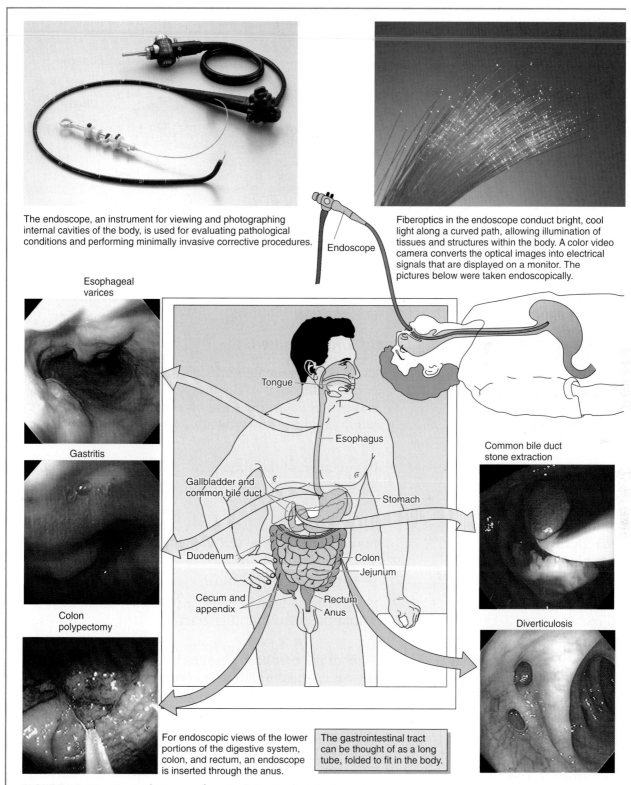

The endoscope, an instrument for viewing and photographing internal cavities of the body, is used for evaluating pathological conditions and performing minimally invasive corrective procedures.

Endoscope

Fiberoptics in the endoscope conduct bright, cool light along a curved path, allowing illumination of tissues and structures within the body. A color video camera converts the optical images into electrical signals that are displayed on a monitor. The pictures below were taken endoscopically.

Esophageal varices

Gastritis

Colon polypectomy

Tongue

Esophagus

Gallbladder and common bile duct

Stomach

Duodenum

Colon

Jejunum

Cecum and appendix

Rectum

Anus

Common bile duct stone extraction

Diverticulosis

For endoscopic views of the lower portions of the digestive system, colon, and rectum, an endoscope is inserted through the anus.

The gastrointestinal tract can be thought of as a long tube, folded to fit in the body.

FIGURE 12-15 ■ **Endoscopy of gastrointestinal system.**

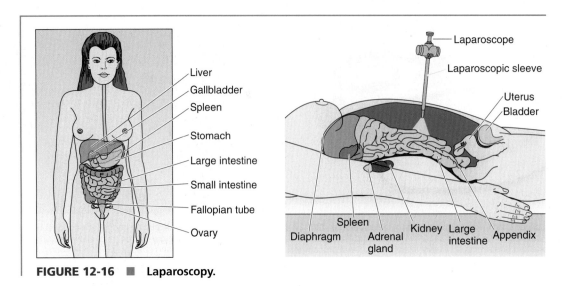

FIGURE 12-16 ■ **Laparoscopy.**

TEST OR PROCEDURE	EXPLANATION
Endoscopy of the Accessory Organs and Abdomen	
endoscopic retrograde cholangiopancreatography (ERCP) *en-dō-skop'ik ret'rō-grād kō-lan'jē-ō-pan-krē-ă-tog'ră-fē*	endoscopic procedure including x-ray fluoroscopy to examine the ducts of the liver, gallbladder, biliary ducts, and pancreas; includes use of instruments to obtain tissue samples, extract biliary stones, relieve obstructions, etc.
laparoscopy (Fig. 12-16) *lap-ă-ros'kŏ-pē*	examination of the abdominal cavity with a laparoscope for diagnostic purposes and/or to perform surgery

IMAGING STUDIES

magnetic resonance imaging (MRI) *mag-net'ik rez'ō-nănts im'ă-jing*	nonionizing imaging technique for visualizing the abdominal cavity to identify disease or deformity in the gastrointestinal tract
radiography (Figs. 12-17 to 12-19) *rā'dē-og'ră-fē*	x-ray imaging used to detect a condition or anomaly within the gastrointestinal tract
upper gastrointestinal (GI) series (*see* Fig. 12-18) *ŭp'ĕr gas'trō-in-tes'ti-năl sēr'ēz*	x-ray of the esophagus, stomach, and duodenum after the patient has swallowed a contrast medium; barium is the most commonly used medium
barium swallow (*see* Fig. 12-19) *ba'rē-ŭm swahl'ō*	x-ray of the esophagus only; often used to locate swallowed objects
fluoroscopy *flōr-os'kŏ-pe*	x-ray imaging with a fluorescent screen to visualize structures in motion (e.g., during a barium swallow)
small bowel series *smawl bow'el sēr'ēz*	x-ray examination of the small intestine; generally done in conjunction with an upper GI series

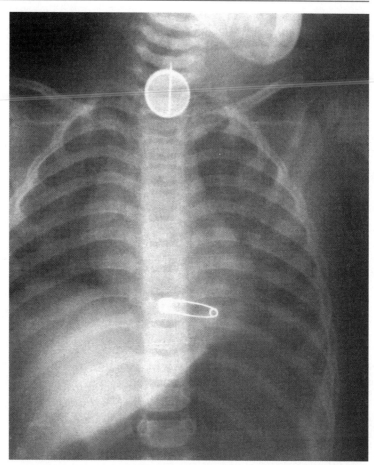

FIGURE 12-17 ■ Plain radiograph (without contrast) showing two impacted foreign bodies in a child 2½ years of age. The child ingested a safety pin and an ornamental pin. Endoscopic removal was required.

TEST OR PROCEDURE	EXPLANATION
lower gastrointestinal (GI) series *lō'ĕr gas'trŏ-in-tes'ti-năl sēr'ēz* **barium enema** *ba'rē-yŭm en'ĕ-mă*	x-ray imaging of the colon after administration of an enema containing a contrast medium
cholangiogram *kō-lan'jē-ō-gram*	x-ray image of the bile ducts; often performed during surgery
cholecystogram *kō-lē-sis'tō-gram*	x-ray image of the gallbladder obtained after oral ingestion of iodine
computed tomography (CT) of the abdomen *kom-pyū'tĕd tō-mog'ră-fē of the ab'dō-men*	cross-sectional x-ray imaging of the abdomen used to identify a condition or anomaly within the gastrointestinal tract
sonography *sŏ-nog'ră-fē*	ultrasound imaging
abdominal sonogram (Fig. 12-20, B) *ab-dom'i-năl son'ō-gram*	ultrasound image of the abdomen to detect disease or deformity in organs and vascular structures (e.g., liver, pancreas, gallbladder, spleen, and aorta)

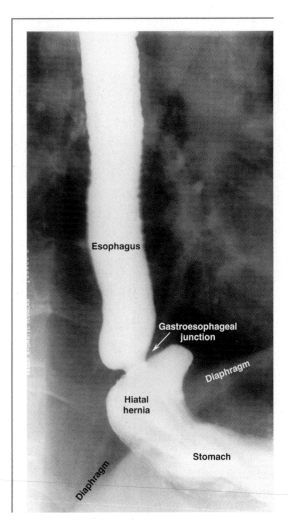

FIGURE 12-18 ■ Upper gastrointestinal (GI) radiograph showing hiatal hernia.

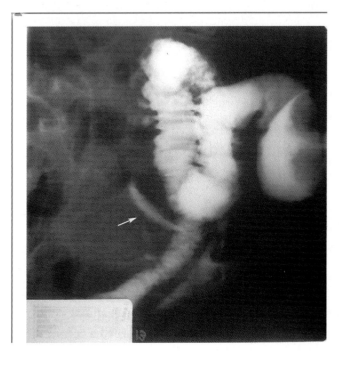

FIGURE 12-19 ■ Barium enema radiograph of colon showing ruptured diverticulum. The elongated appearance is similar to that of a deflated balloon.

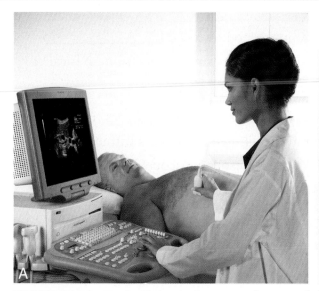
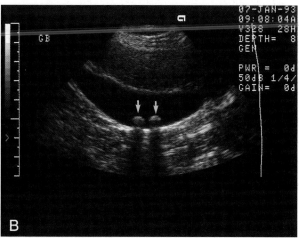

FIGURE 12-20 ■ A. Abdominal sonography procedure. B. Abdominal sonogram of two stones present in the gallbladder (*arrows*).

TEST OR PROCEDURE	EXPLANATION
endoscopic ultrasonography (EUS) *en-dō-skop'ik ŭl'tră-sŏ-nog'ră-fē*	images produced using a sonographic transducer within an endoscope to evaluate abnormalities of the upper and lower gastrointestinal tracts and adjacent structures (e.g., biliary ducts, gallbladder, and pancreas); also used to guide needle biopsy of tissue and in determining the stage of a malignancy

STOOL STUDIES

stool culture and sensitivity (C&S) *stūl kŭl'chŭr and sen-si-tiv'i-tē*	isolation of a stool specimen in a culture medium to identify disease-causing organisms; if organisms are present, the drugs to which they are sensitive are listed
stool occult blood study *stūl ŏ-kŭlt' blŭd stŭd'ē*	chemical test of a stool specimen to detect the presence of blood; positive findings indicate bleeding in the gastrointestinal tract

 Programmed Review: Diagnostic Tests and Procedures

ANSWERS	REVIEW
-scopy, within	**12.93** Recall that the suffix for the process of examination is _____. The prefix *endo-* means _____. The general term for a scope used for conducting an

ANSWERS	REVIEW
endoscope endoscopy	examination within the body is an _____. The process of examination using this instrument is called _____.
esophagoscopy	**12.94** Many specialized kinds of endoscopes have been developed to examine different structures within the gastrointestinal tract. An esophagoscope, for example, is used for examination of the esophagus. This examination is called _____.
colonoscopy sigmoidoscopy	**12.95** Examination of the colon with a special scope is called _____. Examination of the sigmoid colon with a special scope is called _____.
proct/o proctoscopy	**12.96** Recall that the combining form for the anus and the rectum is _____. The term for examination of the rectum and the anus with a special scope is _____.
lapar/o laparoscopy	**12.97** Recall that the three combining forms for abdomen are *abdomin/o*, *celi/o*, and _____. Built from the last of these, the term for examination of the abdominal cavity with a special scope is _____.
esophagogastroduodenoscopy	**12.98** Upper gastrointestinal endoscopy includes examination of the whole upper part of the gastrointestinal tract—the esophagus, stomach, and duodenum—using a flexible endoscope. Using the combining forms for esophagus, stomach, and duodenum, the technical term is _____ (EGD).
endoscopic retrograde cholangiopancreatography	**12.99** Another endoscopic procedure is performed under x-ray fluoroscopy to examine the ducts of the liver, gallbladder, and pancreas. Abbreviated ERCP, this procedure is called _____ _____ _____.
	12.100 Because most of the 20 feet of small intestine lies beyond the reach of either upper or lower endoscopic instruments, a tiny video camera placed in a capsule may

ANSWERS	REVIEW
capsule endoscopy	be swallowed and used for examination. This procedure is called _____ _____.
biopsy excisional portion skin needle	**12.101** The removal and microscopic study of suspicious lesions or tissues is called a _____. Specimens for biopsy are collected in various ways. When a lesion is removed entirely, the procedure is called an _____ biopsy. Incisional biopsy removes a _____ of a lesion for examination. Recall that the term cutaneous pertains to the _____. Another type of biopsy that uses a hollow needle inserted percutaneously (through the skin) to remove tissue for analysis is simply called a _____ biopsy.
magnetic resonance imaging	**12.102** The nonionizing imaging technique used in many body systems is also used in the gastrointestinal system to visualize the abdominal cavity. Abbreviated MRI, this procedure is called _____ _____ _____.
-graphy radiography	**12.103** Recall that the suffix meaning process of recording is _____. The general term for recording an x-ray image is _____.
gastrointestinal swallow	**12.104** Several specialized radiographic procedures are performed to depict the _____ (GI) tract. An x-ray of the esophagus after the patient swallows a barium contrast medium is called a barium _____. A series of x-ray images of the upper part of the gastrointestinal tract, from the esophagus to the duodenum, obtained after the patient swallows barium is called an
upper gastrointestinal series	_____ _____ (GI) _____.
small bowel series	**12.105** Bowel is another term for intestine. Using the term bowel, the x-ray examination of the small intestine is called a _____ _____ _____.
	12.106 Barium contrast can also be introduced into the lower gastrointestinal tract through an enema. An x-ray

ANSWERS	REVIEW
lower gastrointestinal	image of the colon after a barium enema has been administered is called either a barium enema or a _____ _____ (GI) series.
record cholangiogram cholecystogram	**12.107** The suffix *-gram* means _____. Using the combining form referring to bile ducts, an x-ray record of bile ducts is called a _____. Using the combining form referring to the gallbladder, an x-ray image of the gallbladder is called a _____.
fluoroscopy	**12.108** The type of x-ray examination using a fluorescent screen to visualize structures in motion is called _____.
computed tomography	**12.109** The process of obtaining computer cross-sectional x-ray images of the abdomen is called _____ _____ (CT) of the abdomen.
recording sonography abdominal sonogram endoscopic ultrasonography	**12.110** The suffix *-graphy* means process of _____. Another term for ultrasound imaging is _____. An ultrasound image of the abdomen is called an _____ _____. When the sonographic transducer is placed inside an endoscope for examining a body cavity with ultrasound, this is called _____ _____ (EUS).
stool culture, sensitivity	**12.111** Stool specimens can be diagnostically examined to detect pathology. Isolation of a specimen in a culture medium to grow and identify microorganisms and to determine the drugs to which they are sensitive is called a _____ _____ and _____ (C&S).
occult blood	**12.112** The term occult means hidden or not obvious. A chemical test of a stool specimen to detect unseen blood and, thereby, bleeding in the GI tract is called a stool _____ _____ study.

Self-Instruction: Operative Terms

Study the following:

TERM	MEANING
abdominocentesis *ab-dom'i-nō-sen-tē'sis*	puncture of the abdomen for aspiration of fluid
abdominal paracentesis *ab-dom'i-năl par'ă-sen-tē'sis*	puncture of the abdomen for aspiration of fluid in the peritoneal cavity (e.g., fluid accumulated in ascites)
anal fistulectomy *ā'năl fis-tyū-lek'tŏ-mē*	excision of an anal fistula
anastomosis *ă-nas'tŏ-mō'sis*	union of two hollow vessels; a technique used in bowel surgery
appendectomy *ap-pen-dek'tŏ-mē*	excision of a diseased appendix
bariatric surgery *bar-ē-at'rik sūr'jĕr-ē*	treatment of morbid obesity by surgery to the stomach and/or intestines; procedures include restrictive techniques that limit the size of the stomach and malabsorptive techniques that limit the absorption of food (*baros* = weight; *iatric* = pertains to treatment)
cheiloplasty *kī'lō-plas-tē*	repair of the lip
cholecystectomy *kō'lē-sis-tek'tŏ-mē*	excision of the gallbladder; common treatment for symptomatic gallbladder disease (e.g., cholelithiasis, cholecystitis, and cholangitis)
laparoscopic cholecystectomy *lap'ă-rŏ-skop'ik kō'lē-sis-tek'tŏ-mē*	excision of the gallbladder through a laparoscope
colostomy (Fig. 12-21) *kō-los'tŏ-mē*	creation of an opening in the colon through the abdominal wall to create an abdominal anus, allowing stool to bypass a diseased portion of the colon; performed to treat ulcerative colitis, cancer, or obstructions
esophagoplasty *ē-sof'ă-gō-plas-tē*	repair of the esophagus

1. Ascending colostomy   2. Transverse colostomy   3. Descending colostomy   4. Sigmoid colostomy

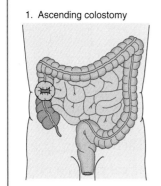 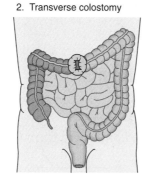 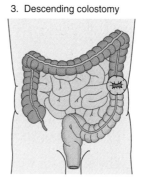 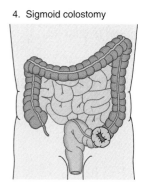

FIGURE 12-21 ■ Common colostomy sites.

TERM	MEANING
gastrectomy *gas-trek'tŏ-mē*	partial or complete removal of the stomach
gastric resection *gas'trik rē-sek'shŭn*	partial removal and repair of the stomach
gastroenterostomy *gas'trō-en-tĕr-os'tŏ-mē*	formation of an artificial opening between the stomach and small intestine; often performed at the time of gastrectomy to route food from the remainder of the stomach to the intestine; also performed to repair a perforated duodenal ulcer
glossectomy *glo-sek'tŏ-mē*	excision of all or part of the tongue
glossorrhaphy *glo-sōr'ă-fē*	suture of the tongue
hemorrhoidectomy *hem'ō-roy-dek'tŏ-mē*	excision of hemorrhoids
hepatic lobectomy *he-pat'ik lō-bek'tŏ-mē*	excision of a lobe of the liver
herniorrhaphy *hĕr'nē-ōr'ă-fē* **hernioplasty** *hĕr'nē-ō-plas-tē*	repair of a hernia
ileostomy *il-ē-os'tŏ-mē*	surgical creation of an opening on the abdomen to which the end of the ileum is attached, providing a passageway for ileal discharges; performed after removal of the colon, such as to treat chronic inflammatory bowel diseases (e.g., ulcerative colitis)
laparoscopic surgery *lap'ă-rō-skop'ik sūr'jĕr-ē*	abdominal surgery using a laparoscope
laparotomy *lap-ă-rot'ō-mē*	incision into the abdomen
pancreatectomy *pan'krē-ă-tek'tō-mē*	excision of the pancreas
polypectomy (*see* Fig. 12-15) *pol'ip-ek'tŏ-mē*	excision of polyps
proctoplasty *prok'tō-plas-tē*	repair of the anus and rectum

🔷 Programmed Review: Operative Terms

ANSWERS	REVIEW
gastr/o	**12.113** Recall that the combining form for stomach is _____.
-ectomy	The suffix for excision is _____. The surgical excision of
gastrectomy	part or all of the stomach is called _____.

ANSWERS	REVIEW
hemorrhoidectomy	**12.114** Excision of hemorrhoids is called _____.
pancreat/o pancreatectomy	**12.115** The combining form for pancreas is _____. Surgical excision of the pancreas is called _____.
gloss/o glossectomy	**12.116** The two combining forms for tongue are *lingu/o* and _____. Made from the latter, the term for surgical excision of all or part of the tongue is _____.
cholecystectomy laparoscopic	**12.117** Excision of the gallblader is called _____. When performed through a laparoscope, it is called _____ cholecystectomy.
lobectomy	**12.118** Excision of a lobe of the liver is called a hepatic _____.
appendic/o appendectomy	**12.119** The combining form for appendix is _____. Surgical excision of the appendix is termed _____. (*Note:* The "ic" in the combining form is removed to prevent the unwieldy "ic-ec" sound.)
polypectomy	**12.120** The procedure of surgical excision of polyps is called _____.
anal fistulectomy	**12.121** Excision of an anal fistula is termed an _____ _____.
-plasty cheiloplasty esophagoplasty hernioplasty proctoplasty	**12.122** Recall that the suffix for surgical repair or reconstruction is _____. Surgical repair of the lip is termed _____. Repair of the esophagus is called _____. Repair of a hernia is called _____. Repair of the anus and rectum is called _____.
-rrhaphy glossorrhaphy herniorrhaphy	**12.123** Recall that the suffix meaning suture is _____. Suture of the tongue is therefore called _____. Surgical repair and suture of a hernia is called _____.
gastric resection	**12.124** Resection typically involves less tissue removal than a full excision. The procedure of partial removal and repair of the stomach is called _____ _____.

ANSWERS	REVIEW
opening colostomy ileostomy	**12.125** Recall that the operative suffix *-stomy* means creation of an _____. The surgical creation of an opening in the colon through the abdominal wall, allowing stool to bypass a diseased portion of the colon, is called a _____. The creation of an opening from the end of the ileum to the abdomen, done when the colon has been removed, is called an _____.
gastroenterostomy	**12.126** The term for the creation of an artificial opening between the stomach and the small intestine is built from the combining forms for both the stomach and the intestine. This procedure is called a _____.
-tomy lapar/o laparotomy	**12.127** The operative suffix meaning incision is _____. Recall that the three combining forms meaning abdomen are *adomin/o, celi/o,* and _____. Formed from the last of these, the term for an incision into the abdomen is _____.
-centesis abdomin/o abdominocentesis paracentesis puncture of aspiration	**12.128** Recall that the suffix meaning puncture for aspiration is _____. The three combining forms meaning abdomen are *celi/o, lapar/o,* and _____. Made from the last of these, the term for puncture of the abdomen for the aspiration of a fluid is _____. Another general term for the aspiration of fluid from any cavity is _____. Abdominal paracentesis describes _____ _____ the abdomen for the _____ of fluid (e.g., the fluid that accumulates in ascites).
anastomosis	**12.129** The term for the operative procedure in which two hollow vessels are joined is _____. This technique is often used in bowel surgery.
laparoscopic	**12.130** A general term for abdominal surgery performed using a laparoscope is _____ surgery.
weight treatment, bariatric	**12.131** The term describing surgery to the stomach and/or intestines to treat morbid obesity is formed by joining *baros*, a combining form meaning _____, with *-iatric*, a suffix meaning _____, creating the term _____ surgery.

Self-Instruction: Therapeutic Terms

Study the following:

TERM	MEANING
gastric lavage *gas'trik lă-vahzh'*	oral insertion of a tube into the stomach for examination and treatment, such as to remove blood clots from the stomach or to monitor bleeding (*lavage* = to wash)
nasogastric (NG) intubation *nā'sō-gas'trik in'tū-bā'shŭn*	insertion of a tube through the nose and into the stomach for various purposes, such as to obtain a gastric fluid specimen for analysis
COMMON THERAPEUTIC DRUG CLASSIFICATIONS	
antacid *ant-as'id*	drug that neutralizes stomach acid
antiemetic *an'tē-ē-met'ik*	drug that prevents or stops vomiting
antispasmodic *an'tē-spaz-mod'ik*	drug that decreases motility in the gastrointestinal tract to arrest spasm or diarrhea
cathartic *kă-thar'tik*	drug that causes movement of the bowels; also called a laxative

Programmed Review: Therapeutic Terms

ANSWERS	REVIEW
gastric lavage	**12.132** The word lavage means to wash. The therapeutic procedure in which a tube is inserted into the stomach from the mouth to remove fluids, such as blood clots, is termed _____ _____.
nasogastric intubation	**12.133** A tube can be inserted through the nose to the stomach for purposes such as obtaining a gastric fluid specimen for analysis. This is called _____ (NG) _____.
anti-	**12.134** Therapeutic drug classifications are often named for their actions against some process or condition. The common prefix meaning against is _____.
pertaining to antiemetic	**12.135** Recall that *-emesis* means vomiting and that the suffix *-ic*, which is often used in names of drug classes, means _____ ____. A drug that prevents or stops vomiting (against vomiting) is called an _____.

ANSWERS	REVIEW
antispasmodic	**12.136** Similarly, a drug used to stop spasms (of the gastrointestinal tract) is called an _____.
antacid	**12.137** A drug that works against excess stomach acid by neutralizing it is called an _____. (*Note:* In this case, the *-ic* ending is not used.)
cathartic	**12.138** The Greek word katharsis means purification by purging. A drug that purges the large intestine by stimulating a bowel movement is called a _____; such a drug is also called a laxative.

CHAPTER 12 ACRONYMS AND ABBREVIATIONS

ABBREVIATION	EXPANSION
Bx	biopsy
C&S	culture and sensitivity
CT	computed tomography
EGD	esophagogastroduodenoscopy
ERCP	endoscopic retrograde cholangiopancreatography
EUS	endoscopic ultrasonography
GERD	gastroesophageal reflux disease
GI	gastrointestinal
HAV	hepatitis A virus
HBV	hepatitis B virus
HCV	hepatitis C virus
LLQ	left lower quadrant
LUQ	left upper quadrant
MRI	magnetic resonance imaging
NG	nasogastric
PUD	peptic ulcer disease
RLQ	right lower quadrant
RUQ	right upper quadrant

CHAPTER 12 SUMMARY OF TERMS

The terms introduced in chapter 12 are listed below, followed by the page number on which each term can be found and its written pronunciation. For additional practice and reinforcement, write the definition of each term on a separate piece of paper.

abdominal paracentesis/595
ab-dom'i-năl par'ă-sen-tē'sis

abdominal sonogram/589
ab-dom'i-năl son'ō-gram

abdominocentesis/595
ab-dom'i-nō-sen-tē'sis

anal fistula/576
ā'năl fis'tyū-lă

anal fistulectomy/595
ā'năl fis-tyū-lek'tŏ-mē

anastomosis/595
ă-nas'tō-mō'sis

ankyloglossia/575
ang'ki-lō-glos'ē-ă

anorexia/572
an-ō-rek'sē-ă

antacid/599
ant-as'id

antiemetic/599
an'tē-ĕ-met'ik

antispasmodic/599
an'tē-spaz-mod'ik

anus/567
ā'nŭs

aphagia/572
ă-fā'jē-ă

appendectomy/595
ap-pen-dek'tō-mē

appendicitis/576
ă-pen-di-sī'tis

ascending colon/566
ă-sen'ding kō'lon

ascites/572
ă-sī'tēz

bariatric surgery/595
bār-ē-at'rik sūr'jĕr-ē

barium enema/589
ba'rē-yŭm en'ĕ-mă

barium swallow/588
ba'rē-ŭm swahl'ō

biliary ducts/567
bil'ē-ār-ē dŭkts

biopsy (Bx)/585
bī'op-sē

buccal/572
bŭk'ăl

capsule endoscopy/586
kap'sūl en-dos'kŏ-pē

cardiac sphincter/566
kar'dē-ak sfingk'tĕr

cathartic/599
kă-thar'tik

cecum/566
sē'kŭm

cheeks/564
chēks

cheilitis/576
kī-lī'tis

cheiloplasty/595
kī'lō-plas-tē

cholangiogram/589
kō-lan'jē-ō-gram

cholangitis/579
kō-lan-jī'tis

cholecystectomy/595
kō'lē-sis-tek'tō-mē

cholecystitis/580
kō'lē-sis-tī'tis

cholecystogram/589
kō-lē-sis'tō-gram

choledocholithiasis/580
kō-led'ō-kō-lith-ī'ă-sis

cholelithiasis/580
kō'lē-li-thī'ă-sis

cirrhosis/580
sir-rō'sis

colitis/576
kō-lī'tis

colon/566
kō'lon

colonoscopy/586
kō-lon-os'kŏ-pē

colorectal polyps/577
kol'ō-rek'tăl pol'ips

colostomy/595
kō-los'tō-mē

computed tomography (CT) of the abdomen/589
kom-pyū'tĕd tō-mog'ră-fē of the ab'dō-men

constipation/572
kon-sti-pā'shŭn

defecation/567
def-ĕ-kā'shŭn

descending colon/566
dē-send'ing kō'lon

diarrhea/572
dī-ă-rē'ă

diverticulitis/578
dī'vĕr-tik-yū-lī'tis

diverticulosis/578
dī'vĕr-tik-yū-lō'sis

diverticulum/578
dī-vĕr-tik'yū-lŭm

duodenal ulcer/576
dū'ō-dē'năl ŭl'sĕr

duodenum/566
dū-ō-dē'nŭm

dysentery/578
dis'en-ter-ē

dyspepsia/573
dis-pep'sē-ă

dysphagia/573
dis-fā'jē-ă

endoscopic retrograde cholangiopancre-atography (ERCP)/588
en-dō-skop'ik ret'rō-grād kō-lan'jē-ō-pan-krē-ă-tog'ră-fē

endoscopic ultrasonography (EUS)/591
en-dō-skop'ik ŭl'tră-sŏ-nog'ră-fē

endoscopy/586
en-dos'kŏ-pē

enteritis/578
en-tĕr-ī'tis

epigastric region/571
ep-i-gas'trik rē'jŭn

eructation/573
ē-rŭk-tā'shŭn

esophageal varices/576
ē-sof'ă-jē'ăl var'i-sēz

esophagitis/576
ē-sof-ă-jī'tis

esophagogastroduodenoscopy (EGD)/586
ē-sof'ă-gō-gas'trō-dū'ō-den-os-kŏ-pē

esophagoplasty/595
ē-sof'ă-gō-plas-tē

esophagus/566
ē-sof'ă-gŭs

excisional biopsy/585
ek-sizh'ŭn-ăl bī'op-sē

feces/567
fē'sēz

flatulence/573
flat'yū-lents

fluoroscopy/588
flōr-os'kŏ-pe

gallbladder/567
gawl'blad-ĕr

gastrectomy/596
gas-trek'tŏ-mē

gastric lavage/599
gas'trik lă-vahzh'

gastric resection/596
gas'trik rē-sek'shŭn

gastric ulcer/576
gas'trik ŭl'sĕr

gastritis/576
gas-trī'tis

gastroenterostomy/596
gas'trō-en-tĕr-os'tŏ-mē

gastroesophageal reflux disease (GERD)/576
gas'trō-ē-sof-ă-jē'ăl rē'flŭks di-zēz'

gingivitis/576
jĭn-jĭ-vī'tis

glossectomy/596
glos-sek'tŏ-mē

glossitis/576
glos-sī'tis

glossorrhaphy/596
glo-sōr'ă-fē

gums/566
gŭmz

halitosis/573
hal-i-tō'sis

hematemesis/573
hē-mă-tem'ĕ-sis

hematochezia/573
hē'mă-tō-kē'zē-ă

hemorrhoid/578
hem'ŏ-royd

hemorrhoidectomy/596
hem'ŏ-roy-dek'tŏ-mē

hepatic lobectomy/596
he-pat'ik lō-bek'tŏ-mē

hepatitis A/580
hep-ă-tī'tis A

hepatitis B/581
hep-ă-tī'tis B

hepatitis C/581
hep-ă-tī'tis C

hepatomegaly/573
hep'ă-tō-meg'ă-lē

hernia/578
hĕr'nē-ă

hernioplasty/596
hĕr'nē-ō-plas-tē

herniorrhaphy/596
hĕr'nē-ōr'ă-fē

hiatal hernia/578
hī-ā'tăl hĕr'nē-ă

hyperbilirubinemia/573
hī'pĕr-bil'i-rū-bi-nē'mē-ă

hypochondriac regions/570
hī-pō-kon'drē-ak rē'jŭnz

hypogastric region/571
hī-pō-gas'trik rē'jŭn

hypoglossal/573
hī-pō-glos'ăl

icterus/573
ik'tĕr-ŭs

ileitis/579
il-ē-ī'tis

ileostomy/596
il-ē-os'tŏ-mē

ileum/566
il'ē-ŭm

incarcerated hernia/578
in-kar'sĕr-ā-tĕd hĕr'nē-ă

incisional biopsy/585
in-sizh'ŭn-ăl bī'op-sē

inguinal hernia/578
ing'gwi-năl hĕr'nē-ă

inguinal regions/571
ing'gwi-năl rē'jŭnz

intussusception/579
in'tŭs-sŭs-sep'shŭn

jaundice/573
jawn'dis

jejunum/566
jĕ-jū'nŭm

laparoscopic cholecystectomy/595
lap'ă-rō-skop'ik kō'l ē-sis-tek'tŏ-mē

laparoscopic surgery/596
lap'ă-rō-skop'ik sŭr'jĕr-ē

laparoscopy/588
lap-ă-ros'kŏ-pē

laparotomy/596
lap-ă-rot'ō-mē

large intestine/566
larj in-tes'tin

lips/564
lipz

liver/567
liv'ĕr

lower gastrointestinal (GI) series/589
lō'ĕr gas'trō-in-tes'ti-năl sēr'ēz

lumbar regions/571
lŭm'bar rē'jŭnz

magnetic resonance imaging (MRI)/588
mag-net'ik rez'ō-nănts im'ă-jing

melena/573
me-lē'nă

mouth/564
mowth

nasogastric (NG) intubation/599
nā'sō-gas'trik in'tū-bā'shŭn

nausea/573
naw'zē-ă

needle biopsy/586
nē'dĕl bī'op-sē

omentum/567
ō-men'tŭm

oral cavity/564
ōr'ăl kav'i-tē

palate/564
pal'ăt

pancreas/567
pan'krē-as

pancreatectomy/596
pan'krē-ă-tek'tō-mē

pancreatitis/581
pan'krē-ă-tī'tis

parotitis/576
par-ō-tī'tis

pediculated polyp/577
pĕ-dik-yū-lā'tĕd pol'ip

peptic ulcer disease (PUD)/576
pep'tik ŭl'sĕr di-zēz'

peritoneal cavity/567
per'i-tō-nē'ăl kav'i-tē

peritoneum/567
per'i-tō-nē'ŭm

peritonitis/579
per'i-tō-nī'tis

pharynx/566
fă'ringks

polypectomy/596
pol'ip-ek'tō-mē

proctitis/579
prok-tī'tis

proctoplasty/596
prok'tō-plas-tē

proctoscopy/586
prok-tos'kŏ-pē

pyloric sphincter/566
pī-lōr'ik sfingk'tĕr

pyloric stenosis/576
pī-lōr'ik ste-nō'sis

radiography/588
rā'dē-og'ră-fē

rectal ampulla/566
rek'tăl am-pul'lă

rectum/566
rek'tŭm

salivary glands/564
sal'i-văr-ē glanz

sessile polyp/577
ses'il pol'ip

sialoadenitis/576
sī'ă-lō-ad-ĕ-nī'tis

sigmoid colon/566
sig'moyd kō'lon

sigmoidoscopy/586
sig-moy-dos'kŏ-pē

small bowel series/588
smawl bow'el sēr'ēz

small intestine/566
smawl in-tes'tin

sonography/589
sŏ-nog'ră-fē

steatorrhea/573
stē'ă-tō-rē'ă

stomach/566
stŏm'ăk

stomatitis/576
stō-mă-tī'tis

stool culture and sensitivity (C&S)/591
stūl kŭl'chŭr and sen-si-tiv'i-tē

stool occult blood study/591
stūl ŏ-kŭlt' blŭd stŭd'ē

strangulated hernia/578
strang'gyū-lā-tĕd hĕr'nē-ă

sublingual/573
sŭb-ling'gwăl

teeth/566
tēth

tongue/564
tŭng

transverse colon/566
trans-vĕrs' kō'lon

ulcerative colitis/577
ŭl'sĕr-ă-tiv kō-lī'tis

umbilical hernia/578
ŭm-bil'i-kăl hĕr'n ē-ă

umbilical region/571
ŭm-bil'i-kăl rē'jŭn

**upper gastrointestinal (GI)
  series**/588
up'ĕr gas'trō-in-tes'ti-năl sĕr'ēz

uvula/564
ū'vyū-lă

vermiform appendix/566
vĕr'mi-fōrm ă-pen'diks

volvulus/579
vol'vyū-lŭs

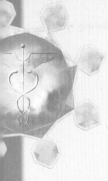

PRACTICE EXERCISES

For each of the following words, write out the term components (prefixes [P], combining forms [CF], roots [R], and suffixes [S]) on the lines below the word. Then define the term according to the meaning of its components.

EXAMPLE

sublingual

$$\frac{sub}{P} / \frac{lingu}{R} / \frac{al}{S}$$

DEFINITION: below or under/tongue/pertaining to

1. transabdominal

_____ / _____ / _____
    P   R   S

DEFINITION: _____

2. proctocolectomy

_____ / _____ / _____
    CF   R   S

DEFINITION: _____

3. sialolithotomy

_____ / _____ / _____
    CF   CF   S

DEFINITION: _____

4. glossorrhaphy

_____ / _____
    CF   S

DEFINITION: _____

5. hematemesis

_____ / _____
    R   S

DEFINITION: _____

6. cheilostomatoplasty

_____ / _____ / _____
    CF   CF   S

DEFINITION: _____

7. appendicitis

_____ / _____
    R   S

DEFINITION: _____

8. celiac

   _____ / _____
       R   S

   DEFINITION: _____

9. cholangiogram

   _____ / _____ / _____
       R   CF   S

   DEFINITION: _____

10. anorectal

    _____ / _____ / _____
        CF   R   S

    DEFINITION: _____

11. enterocolitis

    _____ / _____ / _____
        CF   R   S

    DEFINITION: _____

12. orolingual

    _____ / _____ / _____
        CF   R   S

    DEFINITION: _____

13. dysphagia

    _____ / _____ / _____
         P   R   S

    DEFINITION: _____

14. pancreatoduodenostomy

    _____ / _____ / _____
        CF   CF   S

    DEFINITION: _____

15. hernioplasty

    _____ / _____
        CF   S

    DEFINITION: _____

16. biliary

    _____ / _____
        R   S

    DEFINITION: _____

17. gastroesophageal

_____ / _____ / _____
    CF   R   S

DEFINITION: _____

18. steatorrhea

_____ / _____
    CF   S

DEFINITION: _____

19. dentalgia

_____ / _____
    R   S

DEFINITION: _____

20. pylorospasm

_____ / _____
    CF   S

DEFINITION: _____

21. hepatotoxic

_____ / _____ / _____
    CF   R   S

DEFINITION: _____

22. ileojejunitis

_____ / _____ / _____
    CF   R   S

DEFINITION: _____

23. buccogingival

_____ / _____ / _____
    CF   R   S

DEFINITION: _____

24. cholecystectomy

_____ / _____ / _____
    CF   R   S

DEFINITION: _____

25. perirectal

_____ / _____ / _____
    P   R   S

DEFINITION: _____

Write the correct medical term for each of the following definitions:

26. _____ inflammation of the stomach

27. _____ loss of appetite

28. _____ inability to swallow

29. _____ in the cheek

30. _____ gas in the stomach or intestines

31. _____ protrusion of a part from its normal location

32. _____ black tarry stool

33. _____ belch

34. _____ examination of the small intestine made by a tiny video camera placed in a capsule and swallowed

35. _____ inflammation of the large intestine

36. _____ type of polyp projected on a stalk

37. _____ accumulation of fluid in the peritoneal cavity

38. _____ inflammation of the gallbladder

39. _____ feces containing fat

40. _____ presence of inflamed, abnormal side pockets in the gastrointestinal tract

41. _____ peptic ulcer located in the stomach

42. _____ enlargement of the liver

43. _____ a tongue-tie condition

44. _____ type of hernia that is swollen and fixed within a sac, causing obstruction

45. _____ type of biopsy that involves the removal of an entire growth

Complete each medical term by writing the missing word or word part:

46. hemi_____ectomy = removal of half of the stomach

47. _____itis = inflammation of the appendix

48. pyloric _____ = narrowed condition of the pylorus

49. _____plasty = surgical repair of the mouth

50. chol_____gram = x-ray image of bile ducts (vessels)

51. _____bilirubin_____ = excessive level of bilirubin in the blood

52. gastric _____ = partial removal and repair of the stomach

53. diverticul_____ = presence of diverticula

Name the anatomic divisions of the abdomen:

54. lower lateral groin regions _____

55. upper lateral regions beneath the ribs _____

56. upper middle region below the sternum _____

57. region below the navel _____

58. middle lateral regions _____

59. region of the navel _____

Name the four clinical divisions of the abdomen:

60. _____

61. _____

62. _____

63. _____

Write the letter of the matching term in the space provided:

64. cathartic   _____   a. cholecystectomy

65. herniorrhaphy   _____   b. barium swallow

66. appendicitis   _____   c. bariatric surgery

67. lower gastrointestinal series _____   d. appendectomy

68. icterus   _____   e. colostomy

69. peptic ulcer disease _____   f. hernioplasty

70. abdominocentesis   _____   g. *H. pylori* bacterial infection

71. parotitis   _____   h. barium enema

72. sublingual   _____   i. mumps

73. upper gastrointestinal series _____   j. paracentesis

74. ulcerative colitis _____   k. jaundice

75. cholelithiasis   _____   l. hypoglossal

76. morbid obesity   _____   m. laxative

An endoscope is an instrument used to examine within the body. Name the specific type of endoscope used to examine the body parts listed here:

77. abdomen   _____

78. anus   _____

79. sigmoid colon _____

80. colon   _____

Write out the expanded term for each abbreviation:

81. NG   _____

82. ERCP   _____

83. GERD   _____

84. LUQ   _____

85. GI   _____

86. MRI   _____

87. EGD   _____

Circle the combining form that corresponds to the meaning given:

88. **abdomen**	gastr/o	lapar/o	stomat/o
89. **tongue**	gloss/o	proct/o	gingiv/o
90. **small intestine**	col/o	appendic/o	enter/o
91. **teeth**	dent/i	chol/e	lingu/o
92. **stomach**	lapar/o	stomat/o	gastr/o
93. **cheek**	bucc/o	or/o	proct/o
94. **bile**	col/o	celi/o	chol/e
95. **mouth**	gastr/o	stomat/o	lapar/o
96. **liver**	hepat/o	nephr/o	ren/o
97. **eat**	phas/o	phag/o	gloss/o
98. **rectum**	an/o	proct/o	col/o

Write in the term components related to each of the gastrointestinal organs in the spaces provided:

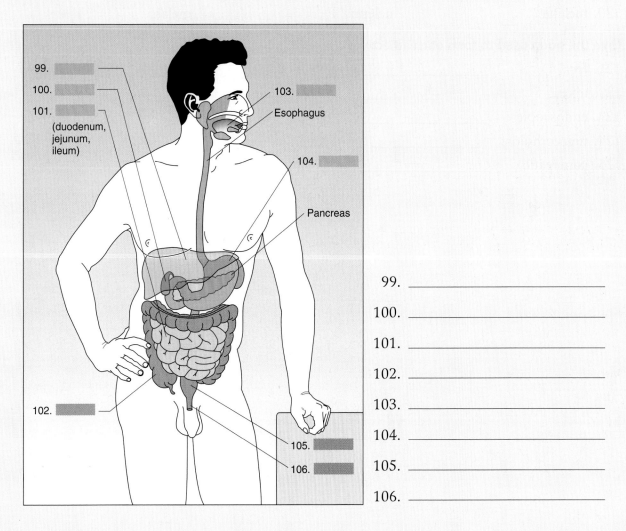

99. _____

100. _____

101. _____

102. _____

103. _____

104. _____

105. _____

106. _____

Circle the correct spelling:

107. anorexia	annorexia	anorrexia
108. asites	ascitis	ascites
109. hematochesia	hemochezia	hematochezia
110. icterus	ickterus	icteris
111. ankleoglossia	ankyloglosia	ankyloglossia
112. volvulis	volvulus	volvolus
113. cirhosis	cirrhosus	cirrhosis
114. glossectomy	glozectomy	glosectomy
115. hernniorhaphy	herniorraphy	herniorrhaphy
116. hemorroidectomy	hemroidectomy	hemorrhoidectomy
117. anteacid	anacid	antacid
118. antiemetic	antemetic	antaemetic
119. cathartik	cathartic	catarthic
120. melena	melenna	melana

Give the noun used to form each adjective:

121. fecal _____

122. icteric _____

123. endoscopic _____

124. hemorrhoidal _____

125. pancreatic _____

MEDICAL RECORD ANALYSIS

Medical Record 12-1

EMERGENCY ROOM REPORT

S: This is a 36 y.o. ♂ with a complaint of abdominal pain. He describes having lifted a 75-lb. beam yesterday at work. He noticed a sharp pain in his navel but continued to work. The pain intensified as the day went on and persisted through last night and today. He claims his navel now bulges forward. He denies fever, chills, dysphagia, anorexia, or vomiting.

PMH: No hospitalizations or surgeries

Meds: none

Allergies: NKDA

O: T 97.5°F, P 87, R 18, BP 128/86

WDWN male in moderate distress secondary to abdominal pain. Upon palpation, the abdomen is soft, with spasm of the muscles in the periumbilical region, and there is an obvious bulge in the umbilicus. The omentum is also palpable. There is no hepatosplenomegaly.

A: Incarcerated umbilical hernia

P: Admit for STAT umbilical hernia repair

QUESTIONS ABOUT MEDICAL RECORD 12-1

1. Which of the following summarizes the subjective information?
   a. pain in stomach
   b. pain in abdomen
   c. pain in the groin area
   d. generalized abdominal pain with chills and fever
   e. stomach pain and has difficulty swallowing

2. What kind of an appetite does the patient have?
   a. normal
   b. increased
   c. decreased

3. What is the condition of the patient's liver?
   a. not stated
   b. enlarged
   c. not enlarged
   d. inflamed
   e. ruptured

4. What were the objective findings?
   a. involuntary contraction of the muscles around the navel
   b. pouching of the muscles under the navel
   c. contraction of abdominal muscles and enlargement of the spleen
   d. protrusion of the navel and enlargement of the liver
   e. pouching of the stomach and omentum

5. Which of the following best describes the diagnosis?
   a. a portion of the bowel has protruded through the abdominal wall and been cut off from circulation
   b. one part of the intestine has prolapsed into the lumen of the adjoining part
   c. a portion of the intestine has protruded through a weakness in the abdominal wall around the navel and is swollen and fixed in a sac
   d. a portion of the bowel has twisted on itself, causing obstruction
   e. the stomach and small intestine are inflamed

6. Which of the following medical terms describes the planned surgery?
   a. laparotomy
   b. gastroenterostomy
   c. hernioplasty
   d. ileostomy
   e. abdominal paracentesis

Medical Record 12-2

FOR ADDITIONAL STUDY

Mr. Antonio Villata undergoes a comprehensive physical examination each year as part of a wellness program promoted by his employer. This year, after a routine sigmoidoscopic exam revealed a polyp in his intestine, he was referred to Dr. Blain, a gastroenterologist at Central Medical Center, for evaluation. Medical Record 12-2 is a procedure dictated by Dr. Blain after his evaluation and treatment of Mr. Villata in the endoscopy suite at Central Medical Center.

   Read Medical Record 12-2 (page 617), then write your answers to the following questions in the spaces provided.

QUESTIONS ABOUT MEDICAL RECORD 12-2

1. Below are medical terms used in this record that you have not yet encountered in this text. Underline each where it appears in the record, and define the term below:

   cannulated _____

   verge _____

   snare _____

2. Describe the screening procedure performed by Dr. Kolima prior to Mr. Villata's referral to Dr. Blain:

   _____

   _____

   _____

3. In your own words, not using medical terminology, briefly describe the procedure performed by Dr. Blain and the indications for which the patient was referred:

   _____

   _____

   _____

4. What position was Mr. Villata in when the procedure was performed?

   a. lying flat, face down

   b. lying flat, face up

   c. lying on his side

   d. sitting

5. Put the following actions in order by numbering them from 1 to 12:

   _____ location of the cecum was confirmed by internal and external landmarks

   _____ video colonoscope was inserted in the rectum and advanced carefully to the cecum

   _____ hemorrhoids were noted

   _____ terminal ileum was cannulated

   _____ scope was straightened, air aspirated, and scope withdrawn

   _____ scattered diverticula were noted in the sigmoid colon

   _____ lining of the colon was thoroughly inspected

____ polyp was removed using a snare and submitted to the pathology lab for biopsy

____ pediculated, 4-mm polyp was seen in the sigmoid colon

____ scope was brought back to the rectum and retroflexed

____ patient was placed in the left lateral decubitus position

____ scope was brought back to the cecum and then gradually withdrawn

6. Translate the statement "a pediculated 4-mm polyp was seen in the sigmoid colon":

_____

_____

_____

7. How many inches from the anal verge was the polyp? _____

8. Copy the sentence from the medical record that indicates how the polypectomy was performed:

_____

_____

_____

9. Name and describe the condition for which a high-fiber diet was indicated in the plan:

_____

_____

_____

10. Describe the third condition Dr. Blain listed in his assessment of Mr. Villata. Include the degree of severity and any treatment planned:

_____

_____

_____

11. In your own words, describe the recommendations outlined in the plan that will be made depending on the results of the biopsy:

_____

_____

_____

Medical Record 12-2: For Additional Study

CENTRAL MEDICAL CENTER

211 Medical Center Drive • Central City, US 90000-1234 • PHONE: (012) 125-6784 • FAX: (012) 125-9999

ENDOSCOPY LABORATORY REPORT

PATIENT: Villata, Antonio   DATE: 4/29/20xx

PROCEDURE PERFORMED: COLONOSCOPY WITH BIOPSY

INDICATIONS: This is a 54-year-old white male referred to me for evaluation of a polyp found during a screening sigmoidoscopy by Dr. Kolima. A complete colonoscopy is being done to remove the polyp and rule out other concurrent lesions.

CONSENT: The procedure and its risks including bleeding, infection, perforation, and sedative reaction have been explained to the patient, and informed consent was obtained.

INSTRUMENT USED: Olympus video colonoscope.

MEDICATIONS GIVEN: Demerol 50 mg and Versed 3 mg in divided doses. The patient had stable vital signs. A Fleets Phospho-Soda prep provided good visualization.

PROCEDURE: The patient was placed in the left lateral decubitus position. After adequate sedation, a rectal examination was performed. No masses were felt. The video colonoscope was inserted in the rectum and advanced carefully to the cecum. The location of the cecum was confirmed by internal and external landmarks, and photographic documentation was obtained. The terminal ileum was then cannulated. This was normal to about 2 cm. The scope was brought back to the cecum and then gradually withdrawn. The lining of the colon was thoroughly inspected. There were scattered diverticula noted in the sigmoid colon. A pediculated 4 mm polyp was seen in the sigmoid colon at 30 cm from the anal verge. This was removed using a snare and submitted to pathology lab for biopsy. The scope was brought back to the rectum and retroflexed. Minimal hemorrhoids were noted. The scope was straightened, air was aspirated, and the scope was withdrawn. The patient tolerated the procedure well.

IMPRESSION:
1. POLYP ON SIGMOID COLON AT 30 CM.
2. SIGMOID DIVERTICULAR DISEASE.
3. HEMORRHOIDS.

PLAN:
1. A high-fiber diet is indicated.
2. Await pathology results. If adenomatous, a full colonoscopy is indicated in 3 years. If hyperplastic or normal, a colonoscopy is indicated in 10 years.

Roger Blain, M.D.

RB:mw
D: 4/29/xx
T: 5/1/xx
cc: R. Kolima, M.D.

ANSWERS TO PRACTICE EXERCISES

1. trans/abdomin/al
   P   R   S
   across or
   through/abdomen/
   pertaining to

2. procto/col/ectomy
   CF   R   S
   anus and
   rectum/colon/excision
   or removal

3. sialo/litho/tomy
   CF   CF   S
   saliva/stone/incision

4. glosso/rrhaphy
   CF   S
   tongue/suture

5. hemat/emesis
   R   S
   blood/vomiting

6. cheilo/stomato/plasty
   CF   CF   S
   lip/mouth/surgical
   repair or reconstruction

7. appendic/itis
   R   S
   appendix/inflammation

8. celi/ac
   R S
   abdomen/pertaining to

9. chol/angio/gram
   R   CF   S
   bile/vessel/record

10. ano/rect/al
    CF R   S
    anus/rectum/pertaining
    to

11. entero/col/itis
    CF   R   S
    small intestine/colon/
    inflammation

12. oro/lingu/al
    CF R   S
    mouth/tongue/
    pertaining to

13. dys/phag/ia
    P   R   S
    painful, difficulty, or
    faulty/eat or
    swallow/condition of

14. pancreato/duodeno/stomy
    CF   CF   S
    pancreas/duodenum/
    creation of an opening

15. hernio/plasty
    CF   S
    hernia/surgical repair or
    reconstruction

16. bil/iary
    R   S
    bile/pertaining to

17. gastro/esophag /eal
    CF   R   S
    stomach/esophagus/
    pertaining to

18. steato/rrhea
    CF   S
    fat/discharge

19. dent/algia
    R   S
    teeth/pain

20. pyloro/spasm
    CF   S
    pylorus
    (gatekeeper)/involuntary
    contraction

21. hepato/tox/ic
    CF   R   S
    liver/poison/pertaining
    to

22. ileo/jejun/itis
    CF   R   S
    ileum/jejunum/
    inflammation

23. bucco/gingiv/al
    CF   R   S
    cheek/gum/pertaining to

24. chole/cyst/ectomy
    CF   R   S
    bile/bladder or sac/
    excision (removal)

25. peri/rect/al
    P   R   S
    around/rectum/
    pertaining to

26. gastritis
27. anorexia
28. aphagia
29. buccal
30. flatulence
31. hernia
32. melena
33. eructation
34. capsule endoscopy
35. colitis
36. pediculated polyp
37. ascites
38. cholecystitis
39. steatorrhea
40. diverticulitis
41. gastric ulcer
42. hepatomegaly
43. ankyloglossia
44. incarcerated
45. excisional
46. hemigastrectomy
47. appendicitis
48. pyloric stenosis
49. stomatoplasty
50. cholangiogram
51. hyperbilirubinemia
52. gastric resection
53. diverticulosis
54. inguinal regions
55. hypochondriac regions
56. epigastric region
57. hypogastric region
58. lumbar regions
59. umbilical region
60. right upper quadrant
    (RUQ)
61. left upper quadrant
    (LUQ)
62. right lower quadrant
    (RLQ)
63. left lower quadrant
    (LLQ)
64. m
65. f

66. d
67. h
68. k
69. g
70. j
71. i
72. l
73. b
74. e
75. a
76. c
77. laparoscope
78. anoscope or procto-scope
79. sigmoidoscope
80. colonoscope
81. nasogastric
82. endoscopic retrograde cholangiopancreatography
83. gastroesophageal reflux disease
84. left upper quadrant
85. gastrointestinal
86. magnetic resonance imaging
87. esophagogastroduo-denoscopy
88. lapar/o
89. gloss/o
90. enter/o
91. dent/i
92. gastr/o
93. bucc/o
94. chol/e
95. stomat/o
96. hepat/o
97. phag/o
98. proct/o
99. hepat/o or hepatic/o
100. cholecyst
101. enter/o
102. col/o or colon/o
103. gloss/o or lingu/o
104. gastr/o
105. proct/o or rect/o
106. an/o
107. anorexia
108. ascites
109. hematochezia
110. icterus
111. ankyloglossia
112. volvulus
113. cirrhosis
114. glossectomy
115. herniorrhaphy
116. hemorrhoidectomy
117. antacid
118. antiemetic
119. cathartic
120. melena
121. feces
122. icterus
123. endoscopy
124. hemorrhoid
125. pancreas

ANSWERS TO MEDICAL RECORD ANALYSIS

Medical Record 12-1: Emergency Room Report

1. b   2. a   3. c   4. a   5. c   6. c

Medical Record 12-2: For Additional Study

See CD-ROM for answers.

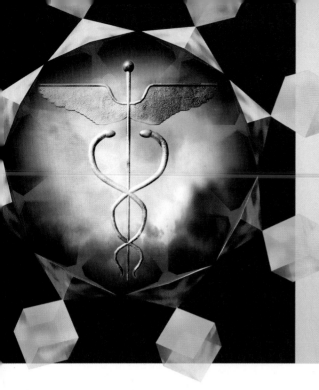

CHAPTER

13

Urinary System

URINARY SYSTEM OVERVIEW

The urinary system includes the organs and structures involved in the secretion and elimination of urine (Fig. 13-1):

✱ The kidneys filter the blood and secrete water and nitrogenous wastes in urine.

✱ The kidneys regulate the levels of critical elements, such as water, sodium, and potassium, in the blood.

✱ The ureters carry urine from the kidney.

✱ The urinary bladder holds urine until it is expelled.

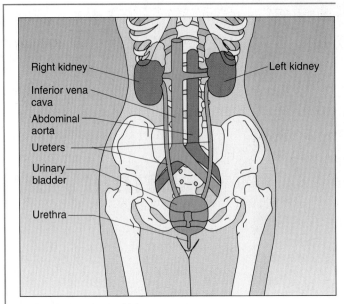

FIGURE 13-1 ■ Urinary system.

 ## Self-Instruction: Combining Forms

Study the following:

COMBINING FORM	MEANING
albumin/o	protein
bacteri/o	bacteria
cyst/o, vesic/o	bladder or sac
dips/o	thirst
glomerul/o	glomerulus (small ball)
gluc/o, glucos/o, glyc/o	glucose (sugar)
ket/o, keton/o	ketone bodies
lith/o	stone
meat/o	meatus (opening)
nephr/o, ren/o	kidney
pyel/o	renal pelvis (basin)
py/o	pus
ureter/o	ureter
urethr/o	urethra
ur/o, urin/o	urine

Programmed Review: Combining Forms

ANSWERS	REVIEW
albumin/o resembling, albuminoid	**13.1** The combining form meaning protein comes from the Latin term for egg white: albumen. That combining form is _____. Recall that the suffix *-oid* means _____. Therefore, the term _____ means resembling albumin (referring to any protein).
bacteri/o against pertaining to antibacterial	**13.2** The combining form meaning bacteria is _____. Using the prefix *anti-*, meaning _____, and the suffix *-al*, meaning _____ ____, an agent such as a soap that kills bacteria is called an _____.
bladder -scope cystoscope	**13.3** The combining form *cyst/o* means sac or _____. Using the suffix referring to an instrument for examination, _____, the term for the special kind of endoscope that is used to examine the bladder is _____.
vesic/o -tomy vesicotomy or cystotomy	**13.4** Another combining form meaning bladder or sac is _____ (from the Latin word vesica, meaning bladder). Using the operative suffix for incision, _____, the term for an incision into the bladder is _____.
dips/o many, condition of polydipsia	**13.5** The combining form meaning thirst (from the Greek word dipsa) is _____. Recall that the suffix *poly-* means _____. The suffix *-ia* refers to a _____ ____. Thus, the term for excessive thirst (the need to drink many times) is _____.
urine -logist urologist urin/o	**13.6** *Ur/o* is a combining form meaning _____. Recall that the suffix for a specialist in the study of a particular area is _____. The physician who specializes in conditions of the urinary system is therefore called a _____. Used to form the adjective urinary, a second combining form for urine is _____.
glucos/o urine	**13.7** The three combining terms for sugar are *glyc/o, gluc/o,* and _____. Glucose is a form of sugar that is found in the blood and used for energy. Because the combining form *ur/o* means _____ and the suffix *-ia* means a

ANSWERS	REVIEW
condition of sugar	_____ _____, the term glucosuria therefore refers to a condition of _____ in the urine.
glomerul/o, glomeruli	**13.8** The combining form that means glomerulus (a small, ball-shaped cluster of capillaries in the kidney) is _____. The plural of glomerulus is _____. Because each nephron in the kidney has a glomerulus, each kidney has as many as 1,000,000 glomeruli.
keton/o urine condition of ketonuria	**13.9** The two combining forms meaning ketone bodies are *ket/o* and _____. Ketone bodies are chemical substances resulting from metabolism. Recall that *ur/o* is a combining form meaning _____. Combined with *-ia,* the suffix meaning _____ _____, the term for a condition of ketone bodies in the urine is _____.
increase ketosis	**13.10** Recall that the suffix *-osis* means condition or _____. Therefore, the term for the condition of increased ketone bodies in the body is _____.
lith/o lithiasis	**13.11** The combining form meaning stone is _____ (from the Greek word for stone, lithos). The suffix meaning formation of, or presence of, is *-iasis.* Therefore, the term for the formation of any stone is _____.
ureter/o ureterolithiasis	**13.12** Two similar words refer to different urinary system structures that carry urine. The ureters carry urine from the kidneys to the bladder. The urethra carries urine from the bladder to the outside of the body. The combining form for ureter is _____. The condition of having a stone form in the ureter is _____.
urethr/o -algia -dynia urethralgia urethrodynia	**13.13** The combining form for urethra is _____. Recall that there are two suffixes meaning pain: _____ and _____. Each suffix is used to form synonyms meaning pain in the urethra: _____ or _____.
meat/o urine	**13.14** The combining form that means opening is _____ (from the Latin word meatus). The urethral meatus is the structure through which _____ leaves the body.

ANSWERS	REVIEW
ren/o	**13.15** Two different combining forms refer to the kidneys: *nephr/o* and _____. As often happens, these two forms come from Greek and Latin roots, both of which mean the kidneys. Recall that the suffix *-osis* refers to an increase or a
condition of nephrosis	_____ _____; it is combined with the first combining form to make this term for a kidney condition: _____. The second form combines with the common suffix *-al* to create
renal	this common adjective referring to the kidney: _____.
py/o	**13.16** The Greek word pyon is the origin of the combining form referring to pus: _____. This form is combined with *nephr/o* and the suffix for inflammation to create the term for suppurative (forming pus) inflammation of the kidney:
pyonephritis	_____.
pyel/o	**13.17** The combining form meaning basin is _____. This combining form also can refer to the pelvis, although it usually refers to the renal pelvis, a basin-like portion of the ureter within the kidney. Recall that the suffix for surgical repair or
-plasty pyeloplasty	reconstruction is _____. Thus, a surgical repair of the renal pelvis is called a _____.

Self-Instruction: Anatomic Terms

Study the following:

TERM	MEANING
kidneys (Fig. 13-2) *kid'nēz*	two structures located on each side of the lumbar region that filter blood and secrete impurities, forming urine
cortex *kōr'teks*	outer part of the kidney (*cortex* = bark)
hilum *hī'lŭm*	indented opening in the kidney where vessels enter and leave
medulla *me-dūl'ă*	inner part of the kidney
calices or **calyces** *kal'i-sēz*	ducts that carry urine from the nephrons to the renal pelvis (*kalyx* = cup of a flower)
nephron *nef'ron*	microscopic functional units of the kidney, comprised of kidney cells and capillaries, each of which is capable of forming urine

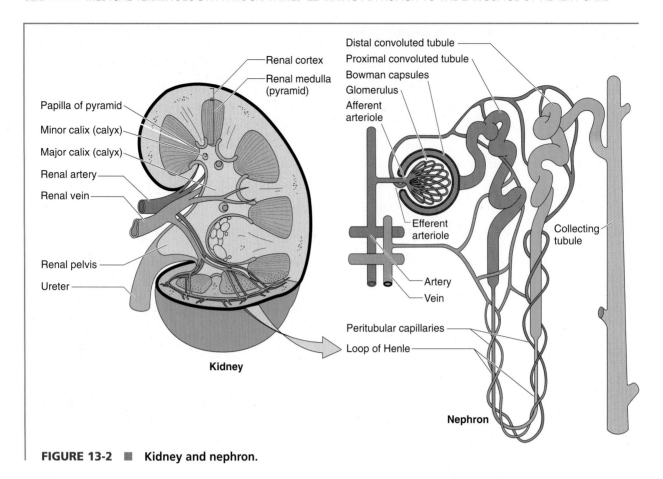

FIGURE 13-2 ■ Kidney and nephron.

TERM	MEANING
glomerulus *glō-mer′yū-lŭs*	small, ball-shaped cluster of capillaries located at the top of each nephron
Bowman capsule *bō′măn kap′sŭl*	top part of the nephron that encloses the glomerulus
renal tubule *rē′năl tū′byūl*	stem portion of the nephron
ureter *yū-rē′tĕr*	tube that carries urine from the kidney to the bladder
renal pelvis *rē′năl pel′vis*	basin-like portion of the ureter within the kidney
ureteropelvic junction *yū-rē′tĕr-ō-pel′vĭk jŭngk′shŭn*	point of connection between the renal pelvis and the ureter
urinary bladder *yūr′i-nār-ē blad′ĕr*	sac that holds the urine
urethra *yū-rē′thră*	single canal that carries urine to the outside of the body
urethral meatus *yū-rē′thrăl mē-ā′tŭs*	opening in the urethra to the outside of the body

TERM	MEANING
urine *yūr′in*	fluid produced by the kidneys, containing water and waste products
urea *yū-rē′ă*	waste product formed in the liver, filtered out of the blood by the kidneys, and excreted in urine
creatinine *krē-at′i-nēn*	waste product of muscle metabolism, filtered out of the blood by the kidneys, and excreted in urine

◈ Programmed Review: Anatomic Terms

ANSWERS	REVIEW
kidneys cortex medulla medullae	**13.18** The two structures to the sides of the lumbar region that filter blood to remove wastes are the _____. The outer part of the kidney is called the _____ (from a word originally meaning bark, as tree bark is the outer part of a tree trunk). The inner part, where the urine is collected, is called the _____. (This same term, meaning middle, is used to refer to the middle part of a number of body structures.) The plural of medulla is _____.
hilum	**13.19** The indented opening in the kidney where vessels enter and leave is called the _____.
nephrons glomerulus capsule renal tubule kidney	**13.20** Inside the cortex of the kidneys are the microscopic functional units that form urine; these units are called _____. At the top of each nephron is a ball-shaped cluster of capillaries, called a _____, that carries blood to and away from each nephron. Enclosing each glomerulus is a structure called the Bowman _____. From the Bowman capsule, the urine flows through the _____ _____. Recall that the adjective renal refers generally to the _____.
urine urea creatinine	**13.21** The fluid secreted by the nephrons that contains water and waste products is called _____. The waste product formed in the liver but filtered from the blood in the kidneys is called _____. A second waste product filtered from the blood in the kidneys is a product of muscle metabolism: _____.
calices or calyces calix or calyx	**13.22** Urine flows through the renal tubules from each nephron through a system of ducts called _____. The singular form of this term is _____. The calices (also spelled calyces)

ANSWERS	REVIEW
	carry the urine to the renal pelvis, the basin-like portion of the ureter within the kidney.
renal pelvis ureteropelvic	**13.23** The basin-like portion of the ureter collecting urine from the calyces is called the _____ _____. The point of connection between the renal pelvis and the ureter is called the _____ junction.
ureter hilum	**13.24** From the renal pelvis, urine moves through the _____ to the bladder, a sac that holds the urine before its excretion. Each kidney has one ureter, which exits the kidney at the same point where the arteries and veins enter it, at the _____ of the kidney.
bladder urethra	**13.25** The sac that holds urine is called the urinary _____. From the bladder, the urine exits through a canal called the _____.
urethral meatus	**13.26** Made from the combining forms meaning urethra and opening, the opening from the urethra to the outside of the body, through which urine leaves the body, is called the _____ _____.

 ## Self-Instruction: Symptomatic Terms

Study the following:

TERM	MEANING
albuminuria *al-byū-mi-nyū'rē-ă* **proteinuria** *prō-tē-nū'rē-ă*	presence of albumin in the urine, such as occurs in renal disease or in normal urine after heavy exercise
anuria *an-yū'rē-ă*	absence of urine formation
bacteriuria *bak-tēr-ē-yū'rē-ă*	presence of bacteria in the urine
dysuria *dis-yū'rē-ă*	painful urination
enuresis *en-yū-rē'sis*	involuntary discharge of urine, usually referring to a lack of bladder control
nocturnal enuresis *nok-tūr'năl en-yū-rē'sis*	bed-wetting during sleep

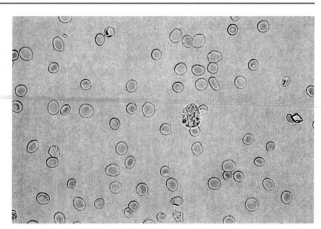

FIGURE 13-3 ■ Hematuria. Microscopic view of urine showing a large number of red blood cells. One lone white blood cell is present in the center of the field.

TERM	MEANING
glucosuria *glū-kō-syū'rē-ă* **glycosuria** *glī'kō-sū'rē-ă*	glucose (sugar) in the urine
hematuria (Fig. 13-3) *hē-mă-tyū'rē-ă*	presence of blood in the urine
incontinence *in-kon'ti-nents*	involuntary discharge of urine or feces
stress urinary incontinence (SUI) *stres yūr'i-nār-ē in-kon'ti-nents*	involuntary discharge of urine with coughing, sneezing, and/or strained exercise
ketonuria *kē-tō-nyū'rē-ă*	presence of ketone bodies in the urine
ketone bodies *kē'tōn bod'ēz* **ketone compounds** *kē'tōn kom'powndz*	acetone, beta-hydroxybutyric acid, and acetoacetic acid; products of metabolism that appear in the urine from the body's abnormal utilization of carbohydrates, such as occurs in uncontrolled diabetes or starvation
nocturia *nok-tū'rē-ă*	urination at night
oliguria *ol-i-gū'rē-ă*	scanty production of urine
polyuria *pol-ē-yū'rē-ă*	condition of excessive urination
pyuria (Fig. 13-4) *pī-yū'rē-ă*	presence of white cells in the urine, usually indicating infection
urinary retention *yūr'i-nār-ē rē-ten'shŭn*	retention of urine resulting from an inability to void (urinate) naturally because of spasm or obstruction

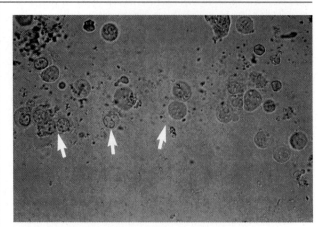

FIGURE 13-4 ■ Pyuria. Microscopic view of urine showing the presence of white blood cells *(arrows).*

🔷 Programmed Review: Symptomatic Terms

ANSWERS	REVIEW
urine condition of bacteriuria	**13.27** *Ur/o* is a combining form for _____. The suffix *-ia* refers to a _____ ____. Many symptomatic terms therefore end in *-uria*, referring to the presence of abnormal amounts of a substance in the urine. For example, the presence of bacteria in the urine is called _____.
 hematuria	**13.28** A combining form meaning blood is *hemat/o*. The presence of blood in the urine is called _____.
py/o pyuria	**13.29** The combining form for pus is _____. Pus consists mostly of white blood cells that fight infection. The presence of white blood cells in the urine is therefore termed _____, which often indicates a urinary tract infection (UTI).
albumin/o albuminuria	**13.30** The combining form meaning protein is _____. The presence of protein in the urine is therefore termed _____. Another term for protein in the blood is proteinuria.
  without anuria	**13.31** The ending *-uria* is also used with other urinary conditions, not just with those indicating the presence of some substance in the urine. The prefix *an-* means _____; therefore, the term for absence of urine formation (being without urine) is _____.

ANSWERS	REVIEW
nocturia	Another term modified by *-uria* describes excessive voluntary urination at night: _____.
within enuresis nocturnal	**13.32**　The term uresis is synonymous with urination. When combined with *en-*, the prefix meaning _____, the term referring to involuntary urinating because of lack of bladder control is _____. An involuntary discharge of urine during sleep is called _____ enuresis (bed-wetting).
glycosuria	**13.33**　The presence of glucose (sugar) in urine is not a normal finding. The two synonyms used to indicate the presence of sugar in urine are glucosuria and _____.
painful dysuria	**13.34**　Recall that the prefix *dys-* means difficult, faulty, or _____. The term for a condition of painful urination is _____.
deficient oliguria	**13.35**　Recall that *oligo-* is a prefix meaning few or _____. Therefore, the term for a condition of scanty (deficient) production of urine is _____. (Recall that the final vowel is occasionally dropped from the prefix when joined with a root that begins with a vowel.)
urine polyuria	**13.36**　Again, *-uria* is a common word ending that refers to a condition of _____. It is linked to the prefix meaning many to describe a condition of excessive urination: _____.
urine incontinence stress	**13.37**　Enuresis is the involuntary discharge of _____; however, the general term for the involuntary discharge of urine or feces is _____. When an involuntary discharge of urine occurs during the stress of coughing, sneezing, or exercise, it is called _____ urinary incontinence (SUI).
urine	**13.38**　Urinary retention is the retention of _____ resulting from an inability to void (urinate) naturally because of spasm, an obstruction, or other factors.
ketone ketonuria	**13.39**　The combining form *ket/o* means _____ bodies or ketone compounds. These are metabolic products that may appear in the urine because of abnormal use of carbohydrates. The condition in which ketone bodies appear in the urine is called _____.

Self-Instruction: Diagnostic Terms

Study the following:

TERM	MEANING
adult polycystic kidney disease (APKD) *ă-dŭlt' pol-ē-sis' tik kid' nē di-zēz'*	inherited condition of multiple cysts that gradually form in the kidney, causing destruction of normal tissue that leads to renal failure; diagnosed in adults presenting with hypertension, kidney enlargement, and recurrent urinary tract infections (UTIs)
glomerulonephritis *glō-mer' yū-lō-nef-rī' tis*	form of nephritis involving the glomerulus
hydronephrosis (Fig. 13-5) *hī' drō-ne-frō' sis*	pooling of urine in dilated areas of the renal pelvis and calices of one or both kidneys caused by an obstructed outflow of urine
nephritis *ne-frī' tis*	inflammation of the kidney
pyelonephritis *pī' ě-lō-ne-frī' tis*	inflammation of the renal pelvis
nephrosis *ne-frō' sis*	degenerative disease of the renal tubules
nephrolithiasis (Fig. 13-6) *nef' rō-li-thī' ă-sis*	presence of a renal stone or stones
cystitis *sis-tī' tis*	inflammation of the bladder

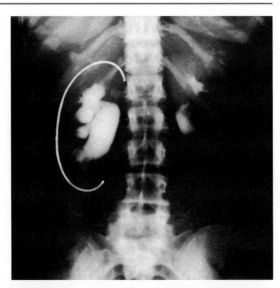

FIGURE 13-5 ■ **Hydronephrosis. Collection of contrast media in the kidney displays an extraordinary amount of material, which indicates right-sided hydronephrosis caused by obstruction of the ureter.**

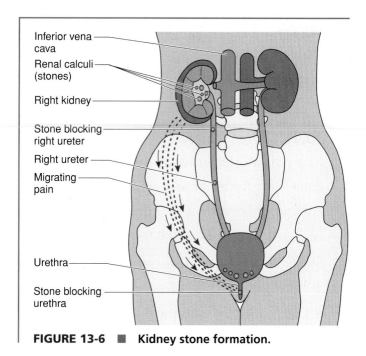

FIGURE 13-6 ■ **Kidney stone formation.**

TERM	MEANING
urethritis *yū-rē-thrī′tis*	inflammation of the urethra
urethrocystitis *yū-rē′thrō-sis-tī′tis*	inflammation of the urethra and bladder
urethral stenosis *yū-rē′thrăl ste-nō′sis*	narrowed condition of the urethra
urinary tract infection (UTI) *yūr′i-nār-ē trakt in-fek′shŭn*	invasion of pathogenic organisms (commonly bacteria) in the urinary tract, especially the urethra and bladder; symptoms include dysuria, urinary frequency, and malaise
uremia *yū-rē′mē-ă* **azotemia** *az-ō-tē′mē-ă*	excess of urea and other nitrogenous waste in the blood caused by kidney failure

◈ Programmed Review: Diagnostic Terms

ANSWERS	REVIEW
 sac many	**13.40** *Cyst/o* is a combining form meaning either bladder or _____. *Cyst*, a root word, describes an abnormal sac. The term polycystic therefore pertains to _____ cysts. This term describes the inherited disease of multiple cysts that gradually form in the kidney, causing destruction of normal tissue and

ANSWERS	REVIEW
adult polycystic kidney disease	renal failure. Most commonly diagnosed in adulthood, this disease is called _____ _____ _____ _____ (APKD).
-itis nephr/o nephritis glomerulonephritis	**13.41** Recall that the suffix meaning inflammation is _____. Many diagnostic terms are formed by adding this suffix to the combining forms for anatomic structures. In addition to the combining form *ren/o*, another combining form meaning kidney is _____. Using that form, the term for inflammation of the kidney is _____. A form of nephritis involving the glomerulus is called _____.
cyst/o cystitis	**13.42** In addition to the combining form *vesic/o*, another combining form for the bladder is _____. Using that form, the term for inflammation of the bladder is _____.
urethritis	**13.43** Inflammation of the urethra is called _____.
urethrocystitis	**13.44** Inflammation of both the urethra and the bladder is called _____.
pyel/o renal pelvis pyelonephritis	**13.45** Recall that the combining form meaning basin is _____. The basin-like portion of the ureter is called the _____ _____. Therefore, the term for inflammation of the renal pelvis area of the kidney is _____.
condition nephrosis	**13.46** Recall that the suffix -*osis* means an increase or _____. That suffix is used to make the term for degenerative disease of the kidney (specifically, the renal tubules): _____.
condition of hydronephrosis	**13.47** A combining form meaning water (or watery fluid) is *hydr/o*. Recall that the suffix -*osis* means _____ ____ or increase. The term referring to a condition of urine pooling in the renal pelvis because of an outflow obstruction is _____.
lith/o -iasis nephrolithiasis	**13.48** Recall that the combining form for stone is _____. The suffix for formation of or presence of is _____. These word parts, along with the combining form *nephr/o*, create the term for the presence of stones in the kidney: _____.

ANSWERS	REVIEW
urethral stenosis	**13.49** A general medical term for the condition of a narrowed structure is stenosis. A narrowed condition of the urethra is called _____ _____.
urinary tract infection	**13.50** The invasion of pathogenic bacteria into urinary structures is called a _____ _____ _____ (UTI).
-emia uremia, azotemia	**13.51** Recall that the suffix for a blood condition is _____. Using the combining form for urine (in this case, referring to urea and waste products normally excreted in urine), the condition of nitrogenous wastes in the blood because of kidney failure is _____. A synonym for uremia is _____, a term that is made with the prefix *azo-,* which refers to a nitrogen molecule.

Self-Instruction: Diagnostic Tests and Procedures

Study the following:

TEST OR PROCEDURE	EXPLANATION
cystoscopy (Fig. 13-7) *sis-tos′kŏ-pē*	examination of the bladder using a rigid or flexible cystoscope

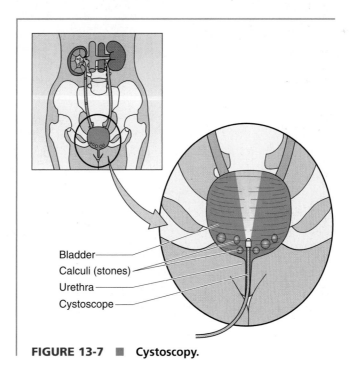

Bladder
Calculi (stones)
Urethra
Cystoscope

FIGURE 13-7 ▉ Cystoscopy.

TEST OR PROCEDURE	EXPLANATION
kidney biopsy (Bx) *kid′ nē bī′ op-sē* **renal biopsy (Bx)** *rē′ năl bī′ op-sē*	removal of kidney tissue for pathologic examination

RADIOGRAPHY

intravenous pyelogram (IVP) (*see* Fig. 13-5) *in′ tră-vē′ nŭs pī′ el-ō-gram* **intravenous urogram (IVU)** *in′ tră-vē′ nŭs yūr′ō-gram*	x-ray image of the urinary tract obtained after an iodine contrast medium has been injected into the bloodstream; the contrast passes through the kidney and may reveal an obstruction, evidence of trauma, etc.
kidneys, ureters, bladder (KUB) (Fig. 13-8) *kid′ nēz, yū-rē′ tĕrz, blad′ĕr*	abdominal x-ray image of the kidneys, ureters, and bladder; typically used as a scout film before obtaining an intravenous pyelogram (IVP)

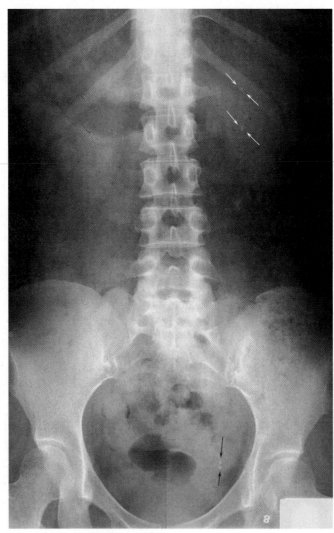

FIGURE 13-8 ▬ KUB radiograph showing kidney stones in ureters and bladder *(arrows).*

TEST OR PROCEDURE	EXPLANATION
scout film *skowt film*	plain-film x-ray image obtained to detect any obvious pathology before further imaging (e.g., a KUB before an IVP)
renal angiogram *rē'năl an'jē-ō-gram* **renal arteriogram** *rē'năl ar-tēr'ē-ō-gram*	x-ray image of the renal artery obtained after injecting contrast material into a catheter in the artery
retrograde pyelogram (RP) *ret'rō-grăd pī'el-ō-gram* **retrograde urogram** *ret'rō-grăd yūr'ō-gram*	x-ray image of the bladder, ureters, and renal pelvis obtained after contrast medium has been injected up to the kidney by way of a small catheter passed through a cystoscope; used to detect the presence of stones, obstruction, etc.
voiding cystourethrogram (VCU or VCUG) *voy'ding sis-tō-yū-rēth'rō-gram*	x-ray image of the bladder and urethra obtained during urination (*voiding* = urinating)
abdominal sonogram *ab-dom'i-năl son'ō-gram*	abdominal ultrasound image of the urinary tract, including the kidney and bladder

LABORATORY TESTING

urinalysis (UA) (Fig. 13-9) *yū-ri-nal'i-sis*	physical, chemical, and microscopic examination of urine
specific gravity (SpGr) *spĕ-sif'ik grav'i-tē*	measure of the concentration or dilution of urine
pH	measure of the acidity or alkalinity of urine
glucose *glū'kōs*	chemical test used to detect sugar in the urine; most often used to screen for diabetes (*glucose* = sugar)
albumin (alb) *al-byū'min* **protein** *prō'tēn*	chemical test used to detect the presence of albumin in the urine
ketones *kē'tōnz*	chemical test used to detect the presence of ketone bodies in the urine; positive test indicates that fats are being used by the body instead of carbohydrates, which occurs during starvation or an uncontrolled diabetic state
urine occult blood *yūr'in ŏ-kŭlt' blŭd*	chemical test for the presence of hidden blood in the urine resulting from red blood cell hemolysis; indicates bleeding in the kidneys (*occult* = hidden)
bilirubin *bil-i-rū'bin*	chemical test used to detect bilirubin in the urine; seen in gallbladder and liver disease
urobilinogen *yūr'ō-bī-lin'ō-jen*	chemical test used to detect bile pigment in the urine; increased amounts are seen in gallbladder and liver disease
nitrite *nī'trīt*	chemical test to determine the presence of bacteria in the urine
microscopic findings (*see* Figs. 13-3 and 13-4) *mī'krō-skop'ik fīnd'ings*	microscopic identification of abnormal constituents in the urine (e.g., red blood cells, white blood cells, and casts); reported per high- or low-power field (hpf or lpf, respectively)

CENTRAL MEDICAL CENTER

211 Medical Center Drive • Central City, US 90000-1234 • PHONE: (012) 125-6784 • FAX: (012) 125-9999

11//02/20xx
13:49

NAME :   TEST, PATIENT   LOC: TEST   DOB: 2/2/XX   AGE: 38Y
MR#   :   TEST-221   SEX: M
ACCT # :   H111111111

M63560 COLL: 11/2/20xx 13:24   REC: 11/2/20xx   13:25

URINE BASIC
   Color   STRAW
   Appearance   CLEAR
   Specific Gravity   1.010   [1.003 - 1.035]
   pH   5.5   [5.0 - 9.0]
   Protein   NEG   [0 - 10]   MG/DL
   Glucose   NEG   [NEG]
   Ketones   NEG   [NEG]
   Bilirubin   NEG   [NEG]
   Urine Occult Blood   NEG   [NEG]
   Nitrites   NEG

URINE MICROSCOPIC
   Epithelial Cells   3 to 4   /HPF
   WBCs   0 to 1   /HPF
   RBCs   0   /HPF
   Bacteria   0
   Mucous Threads   0

TEST, PATIENT   TEST-221   END OF REPORT   PAGE 1
11/02/20xx   13:49   INTERIM REPORT
INTERIM REPORT COMPLETED

FIGURE 13-9 ▬ Sample urinalysis (UA) report.

TEST OR PROCEDURE	EXPLANATION
urine culture and sensitivity (C&S) *yūr'in kŭl'chŭr and sen-si-tiv'i-tē*	isolation of a urine specimen in a culture medium to propagate the growth of microorganisms; organisms that grow in the culture are identified, as are drugs to which they are sensitive
blood urea nitrogen (BUN) *blŭd yū-rē'ă nī'trō-jen*	blood test to determine the level of urea in the blood; a high BUN indicates the inability of one or both kidneys to excrete urea
creatinine, serum *krē-at'i-nēn, sēr'ŭm*	test to determine the level of creatinine in the blood; useful in assessing kidney function
creatinine, urine *krē-at'i-nēn, yūr'in*	test to determine the level of creatinine in the urine
creatinine clearance testing *krē-at'i-nēn klēr'ănts test'ing*	measurements of the level of creatinine in the blood and in a 24-hour urine specimen to determine the rate at which creatinine is "cleared" from the blood by the kidneys

Programmed Review: Diagnostic Tests and Procedures

ANSWERS	REVIEW
vesic/o cystoscopy	**13.52** Recall that the two combining forms for bladder are *cyst/o* and _____. The first of these, combined with the suffix for process of examination with an instrument, forms the term for examination of the bladder with a special scope: _____.
biopsy renal	**13.53** The general term for removal of any body tissue for pathologic examination is _____ (Bx). The removal of kidney tissue is called a kidney biopsy or a _____ biopsy.
recording radiography	**13.54** Recall that the suffix *-graphy* means the process of _____ (e.g., an image). The process of making x-ray studies of internal body structures, such as the urinary tract, is termed _____.
scout KUB	**13.55** A plain-film x-ray image obtained to detect any obvious pathology before further imaging is called a _____ film. An abdominal x-ray image of the kidneys, ureters, and bladder (called a _____) is often obtained as a scout film before additional images are taken using a contrast medium.

ANSWERS	REVIEW
record renal pelvis intravenous pyelogram urogram within	**13.56** Recall that the suffix *-gram* means a _____. The combining form *pyel/o* means basin, referring to the basin-like portion of the ureter in the kidney known as the _____ _____. These components are used to name a type of x-ray image of the urinary tract that is obtained after contrast iodine has been injected into the bloodstream to reveal obstruction, trauma, or other problems in the kidney: _____ _____ (IVP). The other term for this x-ray, using the combining form for urine, is intravenous _____. Recall that the prefix *intra-* means _____, referring in this case to the contrast medium administered within a vein.
vessel renal angiogram arteriogram	**13.57** The term angiogram comes from the combining form *angi/o*, meaning _____; angiograms are x-ray images of blood vessels in many parts of the body. Therefore, the general term describing an x-ray image of the renal artery that is obtained after a contrast medium has been injected into it is _____ _____. The specific term uses the combining for artery: renal _____ .
retrograde pyelogram	**13.58** The type of x-ray image of urinary structures that is obtained after a contrast medium is sent up (backward) through a catheter is called a _____ _____ (RP). The word retrograde refers to the insertion of the medium in a direction against the usual flow (of urine in this case).
urinate voiding cystourethrogram	**13.59** To void means to _____. An x-ray image of the bladder and urethra (using the combining forms for both) that is obtained during urination is called a _____ _____ (VCU or VCUG).
abdominal sonogram	**13.60** Ultrasound is also used with the urinary tract. An ultrasound image of the abdomen showing the kidneys and bladder is called an _____ _____.
urinalysis	**13.61** Many different laboratory tests are conducted on the urine to aid in diagnosing conditions of the urinary system. The term for a full set of physical, chemical, and microscopic examinations of urine is _____ (UA).

ANSWERS	REVIEW
specific gravity	**13.62** The measurement of the concentration of urine, showing the kidney's ability to concentrate or dilute urine, is called _____ _____ (SpGr).
pH	**13.63** The measurement of the acidity or alkalinity of any fluid is called its _____. Urinalysis (UA) includes the urine pH.
glucose	**13.64** Sugar in the blood or urine is called _____. When detected in the urine, glucose may be an indication of diabetes.
albumin/o albumin	**13.65** Recall that the combining form meaning protein is _____. The test in urinalysis (UA) that detects the presence of protein in the urine is called an _____ or protein test.
ketones	**13.66** The test to detect the presence of ketone bodies in the urine is simply called _____.
breaking down urine occult blood	**13.67** Recall that the suffix *-lysis* means dissolution or _____ _____. Hemolysis occurs when the intact membranes of red blood cells break down. The cells, once intact, are now hidden. The presence of free-flowing hemoglobin (the pigment normally contained within red blood cells) is a clue to their hidden state. The chemical test of urine to determine the presence of these once intact and now hidden blood cells is called _____ _____ _____.
bilirubin	**13.68** Bilirubin is a component of bile, which is secreted by the liver and is not normally present in urine. During urinalysis (UA), the chemical test for its presence in urine is simply called _____.
urobilinogen liver	**13.69** The chemical test for the presence of a bile pigment in the urine is called _____. Increased amounts of urobilinogen are seen in gallbladder and _____ disease.
bacteriuria nitrite	**13.70** The presence of bacteria in the urine is termed _____. Nitrite is a waste product that is produced by bacteria. The chemical test to determine the presence of this waste product in urine, thereby indicating bacteriuria, is simply called _____.

ANSWERS	REVIEW
microscopic findings	**13.71** Urine is examined under a microscope to identify abnormal constituents, such as blood cells. The results of this examination are called _____ _____.
urine culture sensitivity	**13.72** The isolation of a urine specimen in a culture medium to grow microorganisms and to identify drugs to which they are sensitive is called a _____ _____ and _____ (C&S).
creatinine urine creatinine	**13.73** Recall that a waste product of muscle metabolism is _____. The test that determines the level of creatinine in the urine is called _____ _____.
serum creatinine creatinine clearance	**13.74** Blood tests (serum tests) also help to diagnose problems in the urinary system. The test to determine the level of creatinine in the blood is called _____ _____. Measurements taken in the blood and in a 24-hour urine specimen are used to determine the rate at which creatinine is cleared by the kidneys; this is called _____ _____ testing.
blood urea nitrogen	**13.75** BUN is the abbreviation for _____ _____ _____, a blood test to determine the level of urea in the blood. The results of this test may indicate a kidney disorder.

Self-Instruction: Operative Terms

Study the following:

TERM	MEANING
urologic endoscopic surgery (Fig. 13-10) *yūr-ō-loj'ik en-dō-skop'ik sŭr'jĕr-ē*	use of specialized endoscopes (e.g., resectoscope) within the urinary tract to perform various surgical procedures, such as resection of a tumor, repair of an obstruction, stone retrieval, placement of a stent, etc.
resectoscope *rē-sek'tŏ-skōp*	urologic endoscope inserted through the urethra to resect (cut and remove) lesions of the bladder, urethra, or prostate
intracorporeal lithotripsy (Fig. 13-11) *in'tră-kōr-pō'rē-ăl lith'ō-trip-sē*	method of destroying stones within the urinary tract using discharges of electrical energy that are transmitted to a probe within a flexible endoscope; most commonly used to pulverize bladder stones

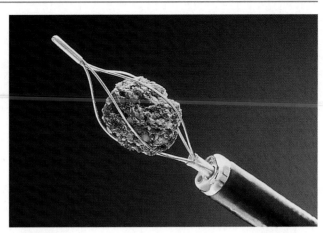

FIGURE 13-10 ■ Stone basket used in kidney stone retrieval.

TERM	MEANING
nephrotomy *ne-frot'ŏ-mē*	incision into the kidney
nephrorrhaphy *nef-rōr'ă-fē*	suture of an injured kidney
nephrolithotomy *nef'rō-li-thot'ŏ-mē*	incision into the kidney for the removal of stones
nephrectomy *ne-frek'tŏ-mē*	excision of a kidney
pyeloplasty *pī'e-lō-plas-tē*	surgical reconstruction of the renal pelvis
stent placement (Fig. 13-12) *stent plās'ment*	use of a device (stent) to hold open vessels or tubes (e.g., an obstructed ureter)

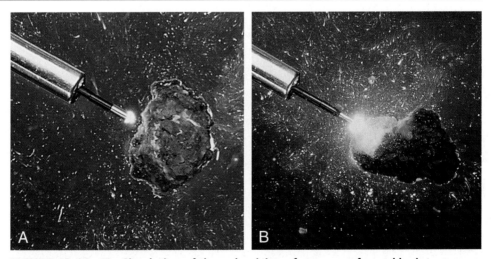

FIGURE 13-11 ■ Simulation of the pulverizing of stones performed by intracorporeal lithotripsy.

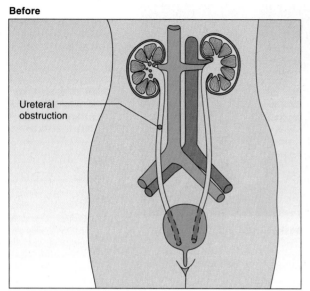
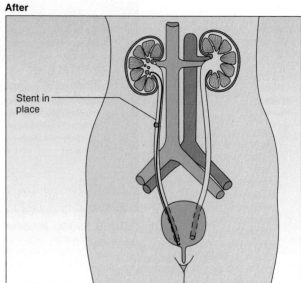

FIGURE 13-12 ■ **Placement of a double-J stent to relieve ureteral obstruction (kidney stone).**

TERM	MEANING
kidney transplantation *kid'nē tranz-plan-tā'shŭn* **renal transplantation** *rē'năl tranz-plan-tā'shŭn*	transfer of a kidney from the body of one person (donor) to another (recipient)
urinary diversion *yūr'i-nār-ē di-vĕr'zhŭn*	creation of a temporary or permanent diversion of the urinary tract to provide a new passage through which urine exits the body; used to treat defects or diseases (e.g., bladder cancer)
noncontinent ileal conduit (Fig. 13-13) *non-kon'ti-nent il'e-ăl kon'dū-it*	removal of a portion of the ileum to use as a conduit to which the ureters are attached at one end; the other end is brought through an opening (stoma) created in the abdomen; urine drains continually into an external appliance (bag);

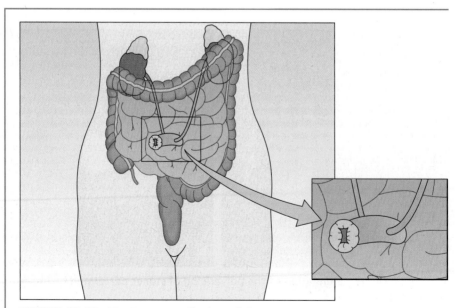

FIGURE 13-13 ■ **Urostomy: ileal conduit.**

TERM	MEANING
	noncontinent indicates that urine cannot be held and drains continually
continent urostomy *kon' ti-nent yū-ros-tō' mē*	an internal reservoir (pouch) constructed from a segment of intestine that diverts urine through an opening (stoma) that is brought through the abdominal wall; a valve is created internally to prevent leakage, and the patient empties the pouch by catheterization; continent refers to the ability to hold or retain urine
orthotopic bladder *ōr-thō-top' ik blad'ĕr* **neobladder** *nē'ō-blad'ĕr*	bladder constructed from portions of intestine connected to the urethra, allowing "natural" voiding

◈ Programmed Review: Operative Terms

ANSWERS	REVIEW
-tomy nephrotomy lith/o nephrolithotomy	**13.76** Recall that the suffix meaning incision is _____. The term for an incision into the kidney is therefore _____. The combining form meaning stone is _____. An incision into the kidney to remove a stone (using the combining forms for both kidney and stone) is therefore _____.
excision or removal nephrectomy	**13.77** The suffix *-ectomy* means _____. Therefore, the excision of a kidney is called _____.
-plasty pyeloplasty	**13.78** The suffix referring to surgical repair or reconstruction is _____. Therefore, the term for surgical reconstruction of the renal pelvis (using the combining form meaning basin, for this basin-like structure) is _____.
-rrhaphy nephrorrhaphy	**13.79** Recall that the suffix for suturing is _____. The procedure of suturing an injured kidney is therefore called _____.
resectoscope stent resecto	**13.80** Urologic endoscopic surgery uses a specialized endoscope, called a _____, to resect tumors or to perform other surgical procedures within the urinary tract. A device that is surgically placed to hold open a vessel or tube is called a _____. Urologic stent placement also may be performed through the _____scope.

ANSWERS	REVIEW
within intracorporeal lithotripsy intracorporeal lithotripsy	**13.81** Stones within the urinary tract may be destroyed by the transmission of electrical energy through an endoscope. The prefix *intra-* means _____, and *corpor/o* combined with the suffix *-eal* pertains to the body. Thus, this process, performed within the body, is described as being _____. The suffix *-tripsy* means crushing; thus, the crushing of a stone is termed _____. Together, these two terms form the name for the procedure of electrically destroying stones within the urinary tract, usually in the bladder: _____ _____.
kidney or renal transplantation	**13.82** In patients with two diseased kidneys, a kidney from a donor may be surgically implanted in the patient. This procedure is called _____ _____.
bladder ileal conduit continent	**13.83** Defects or diseases such as bladder cancer can require the temporary or permanent surgical diversion of the urinary tract. When cystectomy, or removal of the _____, is required, it is necessary to create a new permanent passage for urine to exit the body. One method that uses a portion of the ileum as a conduit, diverting urine from the ureters to the outside of the body is called an _____ _____. The term continent refers to the ability to hold or retain urine. This method is considered to be non_____, because urine cannot be held and drains continually into a bag.
urostomy continent	**13.84** The internal reservoir constructed of intestine that diverts urine to a stoma on the abdomen with a valve attachment to allow catheter draining is called _____. Because the reservoir is capable of retaining urine, the procedure is called _____ urostomy.
neo urination, orthotopic correct pertaining to	**13.85** Construction of a new bladder, or a _____bladder, provides a straight connection to the urethra, allowing a more natural voiding or _____. A neobladder is also called an _____ bladder, a term formed from the combination of *orth/o,* meaning straight, normal, or _____; *top/o,* meaning place; and *-ic,* meaning _____ _____.

Self-Instruction: Therapeutic Terms

Study the following:

TERM	MEANING
extracorporeal shock wave lithotripsy (ESWL) *eks'tră-kōr-pō'rē-ăl shok wăv lith'ō-trip'sē*	procedure using ultrasound outside the body to bombard and disintegrate a stone within; most commonly used to treat urinary stones above the bladder
kidney dialysis *kid'nē dī-al'i-sis*	methods of filtering impurities from the blood, replacing the function of one or both kidneys lost in renal failure
hemodialysis *hē'mō-dī-al'i-sis*	method of removing impurities by pumping the patient's blood through a dialyzer, the specialized filter of the artificial kidney machine (hemodialyzer)
peritoneal dialysis *per'i-tō-nē'ăl dī-al'i-sis*	method of removing impurities using the peritoneum as the filter; a catheter inserted in the peritoneal cavity delivers cleansing fluid (dialysate) that is washed in and out in cycles
urinary catheterization *yūr'i-nār-ē kath'ĕ-ter-ī-zā'shun*	methods of placing a tube into the bladder to drain or collect urine
straight catheter *strāt kath'ĕ-tĕr*	a type of catheter that is inserted through the urethra into the bladder to relieve urinary retention or to collect a sterile specimen of urine for testing; the catheter is removed immediately after the procedure
Foley catheter *fō'lē kath'ĕ-tĕr*	indwelling catheter inserted through the urethra and into the bladder that includes a collection system allowing urine to be drained into a bag; the catheter can remain in place for an extended period
suprapubic catheter *sū'pra-pyū-bĭk kath'ĕ-tĕr*	indwelling catheter inserted directly in the bladder through an abdominal incision above the pubic bone that includes a collection system that allows urine to be drained into a bag; used in patients requiring long-term catheterization

COMMON THERAPEUTIC DRUG CLASSIFICATIONS

analgesic *an-ăl-jē'zik*	drug that relieves pain
antibiotic *an'tē-bī-ot'ik*	drug that kills or inhibits the growth of microorganisms
antispasmodic *an'tē-spaz-mod'ik*	drug that relieves spasm
diuretic *dī-yū-ret'ik*	drug that increases the secretion of urine

Programmed Review: Therapeutic Terms

ANSWERS	REVIEW
body, outside extracorporeal extracorporeal shock wave lithotripsy	**13.86** Recall that the term intracorporeal pertains to within the _____. In contrast, the prefix *extra-* means _____. Therefore, the term for outside the body is _____. The procedure using the shock waves of ultrasound from outside the body to break up urinary stones is termed _____ _____ _____ _____ (ESWL).
kidney dialysis hemodialysis	**13.87** Dialysis is a general medical term that means filtration. This process of filtering impurities from the blood in patients with renal failure is called _____ _____. The combining form for blood is *hem/o,* which is used to create the term for the process of pumping a patient's blood through an artificial kidney machine: _____.
peritoneal dialysis	**13.88** Another method for removing impurities uses the patient's peritoneum (an abdominal cavity) for a filtering bath and is called _____ _____.
urinary catheterization	**13.89** A catheter is a tube that is placed in a body cavity or vessel to allow passage of fluid through it. The process is called catheterization. Catheter placement in the bladder to drain or collect urine is therefore called _____ _____.
straight	**13.90** The type of catheter that is inserted straight through the urethra and into the bladder to relieve urinary retention or to collect a sterile specimen of urine for testing and that is removed immediately after the procedure is simply called a _____ catheter.
Foley catheter	**13.91** An indwelling catheter is one that is left in place. One type is named for its developer, Dr. Frederick Foley, and is inserted through the urethra and into the bladder and includes a collection system that allows urine to be drained into a bag. This type of catheter, called a _____ _____, can remain in place for an extended period.

ANSWERS	REVIEW
above suprapubic	**13.92** Another type of indwelling catheter is used when the patient needs long-term catheterization. It is inserted directly in the bladder through an abdominal incision made above the pubic bone. *Supra-*, a prefix meaning excessive or _____, is used in the name of this catheter in reference to its placement above the pubic bone: _____ catheter.
against antispasmodic antibiotic	**13.93** Recall that the prefix *anti-* means _____ or opposed to. Drug classes are commonly named for their actions, such as acting against some thing or process. A drug that acts to prevent or relieve a spasm is called an _____. The same prefix when joined with the combining form for life (*bio*) denotes a drug class that acts to kill or inhibit microbial life. This drug is called an _____.
without analgesic	**13.94** The Greek word algesis means sensation of pain. Recall that the prefix *an-* means _____. A type of drug that relieves pain is called an _____.
diuretic	**13.95** A drug that increases the secretion of urine is called a _____. Other common substances, such as coffee and alcohol, also have diuretic effects.

CHAPTER 13 ACRONYMS AND ABBREVIATIONS

ABBREVIATION	EXPANSION
alb	albumin
APKD	adult polycystic kidney disease
BUN	blood urea nitrogen
Bx	biopsy
C&S	culture and sensitivity
ESWL	extracorporeal shock wave lithotripsy
hpf	high-power field
IVP	intravenous pyelogram
IVU	intravenous urogram
KUB	kidneys, ureters, bladder
lpf	low-power field
RP	retrograde pyelogram

ABBREVIATION	EXPANSION
SpGr	specific gravity
SUI	stress urinary incontinence
UA	urinalysis
UTI	urinary tract infection
VCU or VCUG	voiding cystourethrogram

CHAPTER 13 SUMMARY OF TERMS

The terms introduced in chapter 13 are listed below, followed by the page number on which each term can be found and its written pronunciation. For additional practice and reinforcement, write the definition of each term on a separate piece of paper.

abdominal sonogram/637
ab-dom'i-năl son'ō-gram

adult polycystic kidney disease (APKD)/632
ă-dŭlt' pol-ē-sis'tik kid'nē di-zēz'

albumin (alb)/637
al-byū'min

albuminuria/628
al-byū-mi-nyū'rē-ă

analgesic/647
an-ăl-jē'zik

antibiotic/647
an'tē-bī-ot'ik

antispasmodic/647
an'tē-spaz-mod'ik

anuria/628
an-yū'rē-ă

azotemia/633
az-ō-tē'mē-ă

bacteriuria/628
bak-tēr-ē-yū'rē-ă

bilirubin/637
bil-i-rū'bin

blood urea nitrogen (BUN)/639
blŭd yū-rē'ă nī'trō-jen

Bowman capsule/626
bō'măn kap'sūl

calices or calyces/625
kal'i-sēz

continent urostomy/645
kon'ti-nent yū-ros-tō'mē

cortex/625
kōr'teks

creatinine/627
krē-at'i-nēn

creatinine clearance testing/639
krē-at'i-nēn klēr'ănts test'ing

creatinine, serum/639
krē-at'i-nēn, sēr'ŭm

creatinine, urine/639
krē-at'i-nēn, yūr'in

cystitis/632
sis-tī'tis

cystoscopy/635
sis-tos'kŏ-pē

diuretic/647
dī-yū-ret'ik

dysuria/628
dis-yū'rē-ă

enuresis/628
en-yū-rē'sis

extracorporeal shock wave lithotripsy (ESWL)/647
eks'tră-kōr-pō'rē-ăl shok wāv lith'ō-trip'sē

Foley catheter/647
fō'lē kath'ĕ-tĕr

glomerulonephritis/632
glō-mer'yū-lō-nef-rī'tis

glomerulus/626
glō-mer'yū-lŭs

glucose/637
glū'kōs

glucosuria/629
glū-kō-syū'rē-ă

glycosuria/629
glī'kō-sū'rē-ă

hematuria/629
hē-mă-tyū'rē-ă

hemodialysis/647
hē'mō-dī-al'i-sis

hilum/625
hī'lŭm

hydronephrosis/632
hī'drō-ne-frō'sis

incontinence/629
in-kon'ti-nents

intracorporeal lithotripsy/642
in'tră-kōr-pō'rē-ăl lith'ō-trip-sē

**intravenous pyelogram
   (IVP)**/636
in'tră-vē'nŭs pī'el-ō-gram

intravenous urogram (IVU)/636
in'tră-vē'nŭs yūr'ō-gram

ketone bodies/629
kē'tōn bod'ēz

ketone compounds/629
kē'tōn kom'powndz

ketones/637
kē'tōnz

ketonuria/629
kē-tō-nyū'rē-ă

kidney biopsy (Bx)/636
kid'nē bī'op-sē

kidney dialysis/647
kid'nē dī-al'i-sis

kidney transplantation/644
kid'nē tranz-plan-tā'shŭn

kidneys/625
kid'nēz

kidneys, ureters, bladder (KUB)/636
kid'nēz, yū-rē'tĕrz, blad'ĕr

medulla/625
me-dūl'ă

microscopic findings/637
mī'krō-skop'ik fīnd'ings

neobladder/645
nē'ō-blad'ĕr

nephrectomy/643
ne-frek'tŏ-mē

nephritis/632
ne-frī'tis

nephrolithiasis/632
nef'rō-li-thī'ă-sis

nephrolithotomy/643
nef'rō-li-thot'ŏ-mē

nephron/625
nef'ron

nephrorrhaphy/643
nef-rōr'ă-fē

nephrosis/632
ne-frō'sis

nephrotomy/643
ne-frot'ŏ-mē

nitrite/637
nī'trīt

nocturia/629
nok-tū'rē-ă

nocturnal enuresis/628
nok-tūr'năl en-yū-rē'sis

noncontinent ileal conduit/644
non-kon'ti-nent il'ē-ăl kon'dū-it

oliguria/629
ol-i-gū'rē-ă

orthotopic bladder/645
ōr-thō-top'ik blad'ĕr

peritoneal dialysis/647
per'i-tō-nē'ăl dī-al'i-sis

pH/637

polyuria/629
pol-ē-yū'rē-ă

protein/637
prō'tēn

proteinuria/628
prō-tē-nū'rē-ă

pyelonephritis/632
pī'ĕ-lō-ne-frī'tis

pyeloplasty/643
pī'e-lō-plas-tē

pyuria/629
pī-yū'rē-ă

renal angiogram/637
rē'năl an'jē-ō-gram

renal arteriogram/637
rē'năl ar-tēr'ē-ō-gram

renal biopsy (Bx)/636
rē'năl bī'op-sē

renal pelvis/626
rē'năl pel'vis

renal transplantation/644
rē'năl tranz-plan-tā'shŭn

renal tubule/626
rē'năl tū'byūl

resectoscope/642
rē-sek'tŏ-skōp

retrograde pyelogram (RP)/637
ret'rō-grād pī'el-ō-gram

retrograde urogram/637
ret'rō-grād yūr'ō-gram

scout film/637
skowt film

specific gravity (SpGr)/637
spĕ-sif'ik grav'i-tē

stent placement/643
stent plās'ment

straight catheter/647
strāt kath'ĕ-tĕr

stress urinary incontinence (SUI)/629
stres yūr'i-nār-ē in-kon'ti-nents

suprapubic catheter/647
sū'pra-pyū-bĭk kath'ĕ-tĕr

urea/627
yū-rē'ă

uremia/633
yū-rē'mē-ă

ureter/626
ū-rē'tĕr

ureteropelvic junction/626
yū-rē'tĕr-ō-pel'vĭk jŭngk'shŭn

urethra/626
yū-rē'thră

urethral meatus /626
yū-rē'thrăl mē-ā'tŭs

urethral stenosis/633
yū-rē'thrăl ste-nō'sis

urethritis/633
yū-rē-thrī'tis

urethrocystitis/633
yū-rē'thrō-sis-tī'tis

urinalysis (UA)/637
yū-ri-nal'i-sis

urinary bladder/626
yūr'i-nār-ē blad'ĕr

urinary catheterization/647
yūr'i-nār-ē kath'ĕ-ter-ī-zā'shun

urinary diversion/644
yūr'i-nār-ē di-vĕr'zhŭn

urinary retention/629
yūr'i-nār-ē rē-ten'shŭn

urinary tract infection (UTI)/633
yūr'i-nār-ē trakt in-fek'shŭn

urine/627
yūr'in

urine culture and sensitivity (C&S)/639
yūr'in kŭl'chŭr and sen-si-tiv'i-tē

urine occult blood/637
yūr'in ŏ-kŭlt' blŭd

urobilinogen/637
yūr'ō-bī-lin'ō-jen

urologic endoscopic surgery/642
yūr-ō-loj'ik en-dō-skop'ik sŭr'jĕr-ē

voiding cystourethrogram (VCU or VCUG)/637
voy'ding sis-tō-yū-rēth'rō-gram

PRACTICE EXERCISES

For each of the following words, write out the term components (prefixes [P], combining forms [CF], roots [R], and suffixes [S]) on the lines below the word. Then define the term according to the meaning of its components.

EXAMPLE

pericystitis

peri / cyst / itis

P   R   S

DEFINITION: around/bladder or sac/inflammation

1. pyuria

   _____ / _____ / _____

       R   R   S

   DEFINITION: _____

2. bacteriosis

   _____ / _____

       R   S

   DEFINITION: _____

3. transurethral

   _____ / _____ / _____

       P   R   S

   DEFINITION: _____

4. urogram

   _____ / _____

       CF   S

   DEFINITION: _____

5. urethrocystitis

   _____ / _____ / _____

       CF   R   S

   DEFINITION: _____

6. nephroptosis

   _____ / _____

       CF   S

   DEFINITION: _____

7. polyuria

   _____ / _____ / _____

       P   R   S

   DEFINITION: _____

8. glomerulosclerosis

_____ / _____ / _____
    CF   R   S

DEFINITION: _____

9. pyonephritis

_____ / _____ / _____
    CF   R   S

DEFINITION: _____

10. urinal

_____ / _____
    R   S

DEFINITION: _____

11. ureterovesicostomy

_____ / _____ / _____
    CF   CF   S

DEFINITION: _____

12. glucosuria

_____ / _____ / _____
    R   R   S

DEFINITION: _____

13. meatorrhaphy

_____ / _____
    CF   S

DEFINITION: _____

14. pyelonephrosis

_____ / _____ / _____
    CF   R   S

DEFINITION: _____

15. cystoscopy

_____ / _____
    CF   S

DEFINITION:_____

16. suprarenal

_____ / _____ / _____
    P   R   S

DEFINITION: _____

17. nephrolithiasis

_____ / _____ / _____
    CF   R   S

DEFINITION: _____

18. urostomy

_____ / _____
    CF   S

DEFINITION: _____

19. albuminuria

_____ / _____ / _____
    R   R   S

DEFINITION: _____

20. ketosis

_____ / _____
    R   S

DEFINITION: _____

Write the correct medical term for each of the following definitions:

21. _____ inflammation of the bladder

22. _____ urinating at night

23. _____ involuntary discharge of urine

24. _____ suture of a torn kidney

25. _____ degenerative disease of the kidney without inflammation

26. _____ protein in urine

27. _____ inherited condition of multiple cysts that gradually form in the kidney in adult life

28. _____ incision into the kidney

29. _____ cytologic study of kidney tissue

30. _____ physical, chemical, and microscopic study of urine

Complete each medical term by writing the missing part or word:

31. _____scopy = examination of the bladder

32. urethral _____osis = a narrowed condition of the urethra

33. extracorporeal shock wave _____ = procedure for disintegration of stones

34. _____scope = specialized endoscope used to cut and remove lesions from the bladder, urethra, or prostate

35. _____uria = scanty urination

36. _____uria = painful or difficult urination

37. _____uria = presence of infection in urine

38. _____uria = blood in the urine

39. _____uria = condition without urine formation

40. _____ catheter = indwelling catheter inserted into the bladder through an incision above the pubic bone

41. _____ _____ incontinence = involuntary discharge of urine when coughing or sneezing

42. _____ blood = hidden blood

Give the appropriate abbreviation for the following:

43. kidney x-ray image obtained after contrast medium is sent "backward" through a cystoscope _____

44. cytologic study of kidney tissue _____

45. physical, chemical, and microscopic study of urine _____

Write the letter of the matching term in the space provided:

46. sugar	_____	a.	cyst/o
47. proteinuria	_____	b.	bacteriuria
48. uremia	_____	c.	renal Bx
49. ren/o	_____	d.	albuminuria
50. vesic/o	_____	e.	neobladder
51. diuretic	_____	f.	Foley
52. kidney biopsy	_____	g.	glyc/o
53. nitrite	_____	h.	nephr/o
54. catheter	_____	i.	azotemia
55. urinary diversion	_____	j.	urobilinogen
56. bile pigment	_____	k.	urination

Write out the expanded term for each abbreviation:

57. C&S _____

58. VCU _____

59. BUN _____

60. IVU _____

61. ESWL _____

62. KUB _____

63. SpGr _____

64. UTI _____

65. RP _____

Circle the combining form that corresponds to the meaning given:

66. **urine**	hydr/o	ur/o	ren/o
67. **thirst**	dips/o	crin/o	hidr/o
68. **pus**	pyel/o	py/o	albumin/o
69. **bladder**	cyt/o	vesic/o	nephr/o
70. **protein**	albumin/o	lip/o	bacteri/o
71. **kidney**	hepat/o	cyst/o	nephr/o
72. **opening**	or/o	meat/o	orth/o
73. **basin**	meat/o	vesic/o	pyel/o
74. **stone**	scler/o	lip/o	lith/o

Identify the parts of the urinary system by writing the missing words in the spaces provided:

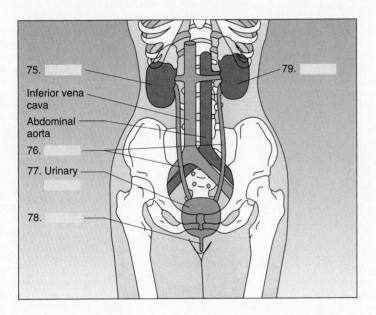

75. _____

76. _____

77. _____

78. _____

79. _____

Circle the correct spelling in each set of words:

80.	cystascope	cystoskope	cystoscope
81.	pyleogram	pyelogram	pielogram
82.	oliguria	oleguria	oligouria
83.	hydronefrosis	hidronephrosis	hydronephrosis
84.	azootemia	azothemia	azotemia
85.	urinalysis	urinelysis	uranalysis
86.	glowmerular	glomerular	glomarular
87.	nefrectomy	nephrecktomy	nephrectomy
88.	diuretic	dyuretic	diuretik
89.	hemadialysis	hemodialysis	hemidialysis

Give the noun used to form each adjective:

90. urinary   _____

91. glomerular   _____

92. meatal   _____

93. uremic   _____

94. urethral   _____

95. nephrotic   _____

MEDICAL RECORD ANALYSIS

Medical Record 13-1

CHART NOTE

S: This 70 y.o. female has had polyuria, nocturia, and dysuria × 2–3 days. She had a similar infection 6 months ago and was treated with Macrobid, 50 mg, q.i.d. × 3 d. She has occasional stress incontinence with hard sneezing.

O: The patient is afebrile. UA shows a trace of leukocytes and blood.

A: R/O recurrent UTI

P: C&S

Cipro 500 mg tab p.o. b.i.d. pending culture

pt instructed to ↑ fluid intake and call for culture results in 48 h

1. What is the patient's CC?
   a. presence of red and white blood cells in her urine
   b. a urinary tract infection
   c. pain when she urinates, with the need to go often, even at night
   d. urinary retention

2. What were the objective findings?
   a. culture showed leukocytes and blood in the urine
   b. urinalysis indicated red and white blood cells present in urine
   c. infection of the bladder and urethra
   d. return of infection of the bladder and urethra

3. What was the doctor's impression?
   a. leukocytes and blood in the patient's urine
   b. patient has pain when she urinates, with the need to go often, even at night
   c. patient has a bladder infection
   d. patient may have another bladder infection

4. Which medical terms describe the UA findings?
   a. pyuria and hematuria
   b. dysuria and enuresis
   c. bacteriuria and hematuria
   d. bacteriuria and nocturia

5. To what does C&S refer?
   a. condition of urinary stress
   b. isolation of microorganisms in the urine
   c. inflammation of the bladder
   d. physical, chemical, and microscopic study of urine

6. How should the Cipro be administered?
   a. two, by mouth every day
   b. one, by mouth two times a day
   c. one, by mouth three times a day
   d. one, by mouth four times a day

7. Was the patient's temperature elevated?
   a. yes
   b. no
   c. nothing is stated about the patient's temperature

Medical Record 13-2 A and B

FOR ADDITIONAL STUDY

Charles Mercier had urination problems and abdominal pain when he saw his doctor, who referred him to Central Medical Center for a possible kidney infection. Dr. Zlatkin performed surgery, and Mr. Mercier was soon doing fine and was discharged. As planned, he later returned for surgical removal of a device that had been temporarily placed during the first surgery. Medical Record 13-2A is the discharge summary from the first surgery, dictated by Dr. Zlatkin. The second document, Medical Record 13-2B, is the operative report for Mr. Mercier's return surgery 6 weeks later, also dictated by Dr. Zlatkin.

   Read Medical Record 13-2 (pages 662–663), then write your answers to the following questions in the spaces provided.

QUESTIONS ABOUT MEDICAL RECORD 13-2

1. Below are medical terms used in this record that you have not yet encountered in this text. Underline each where it appears in the record, and define the term below.

   stent (double-J) _____

   drain (Jackson-Pratt) _____

   lithotomy position _____

   ureteral catheter _____

   patency _____

2. In your own words, not using medical terminology, briefly describe the history of Mr. Mercier's medical problems identified in the "Discharge Summary":

   _____

   _____

   _____

3. Put the following events reported in the "Discharge Summary" in chronological order by numbering them from 1 to 5:

   _____ removal of drain

   _____ reconstruction of renal pelvis

   _____ difficulty with micturition

   _____ urine test for microorganisms

   _____ insertion of stent

4. While at home after the operation, Mr. Mercier is instructed to do two things and to not do three things. List them below:

   Mr. Mercier should _____

   _____

   Mr. Mercier should not _____

   _____

   _____

5. When Mr. Mercier returned 6 weeks later for follow-up surgery, describe in your own words the preoperative diagnosis:

   _____

   _____

   _____

6. During the second surgery, an endoscopic procedure and two different x-ray procedures were used to visualize internal structures. List and define each procedure, and describe the findings:

Procedure	Definition	Finding
_____	_____	_____
_____	_____	_____
_____	_____	_____

7. The first surgery included insertion of a specialized device, which was then removed in the second surgery. What was this device, and what function did it perform during the time between the two surgeries?

   _____

   _____

   _____

8. In the second surgery, did Mr. Mercier experience any complications? Copy the sentence from the report that supports your answer.

   _____

   _____

Medical Record 13-2A For Additional Study

CENTRAL MEDICAL CENTER

211 Medical Center Drive • Central City, US 90000-1234 • PHONE: (012) 125-6784 • FAX: (012) 125-9999

DISCHARGE SUMMARY

DATE OF ADMISSION: 10/25/20xx   DATE OF DISCHARGE: 10/29/20xx

ADMITTING DIAGNOSIS:
Left ureteropelvic junction obstruction.

DISCHARGE DIAGNOSIS:
Left ureteropelvic junction obstruction.

PROCEDURE PERFORMED:
Left dismembered pyeloplasty and placement of stent.

BRIEF SUMMARY:
The patient is a 19-year-old male who was admitted to the hospital a month ago with left pyelonephritis. He was found to have a left ureteropelvic junction obstruction. The patient was brought to the hospital at this time for repair of the moderately to severely obstructed left kidney. A preoperative urine culture was sterile. The patient underwent the procedure without complication. A double-J stent was placed. The Jackson-Pratt drain was removed on the second postoperative day because of minimal drainage. The patient initially had urinary retention, but this resolved by the third postoperative day. He was doing fine at the time of discharge. His condition on discharge is good.

INSTRUCTIONS TO THE PATIENT:
1) Regular diet. 2) No heavy lifting, straining, or driving an automobile for six weeks from the day of surgery. He should also keep the incision relatively dry this week. 3) Follow up in my office in three weeks. 4) It is anticipated the stent will remain indwelling for six weeks and then will be removed cystoscopically at that time. 5) Discharge medication is Tylenol #3, 1-2 q 4 h p.r.n. pain.

L. Zlatkin, M.D.
_____
L. Zlatkin, M.D.

LZ:mr

D: 10/29/20xx
T: 10/30/20xx

DISCHARGE SUMMARY	PT. NAME: MERCIER, CHARLES F.
	ID NO: IP-392689
	ROOM NO: 444
	ATT. PHYS: L.ZLATKIN, M.D.

Medical Record 13-2B For Additional Study

CENTRAL MEDICAL CENTER

211 Medical Center Drive • Central City, US 90000-1234 • PHONE: (012) 125-6784 • FAX: (012) 125-9999

OPERATIVE REPORT

DATE: December 7, 20xx

PREOPERATIVE DIAGNOSIS: Congenital left ureteropelvic junction obstruction status post pyeloplasty. Indwelling left ureteral stent.

POSTOPERATIVE DIAGNOSIS: Congenital left ureteropelvic junction obstruction status post pyeloplasty. Indwelling left ureteral stent, removed

OPERATION: Cystoscopy, removal of left ureteral stent, and left retrograde pyelogram.

PROCEDURE: The patient was identified, was placed on the operating table, and was administered a general anesthetic. He was placed in the lithotomy position, and a KUB was obtained. The genitalia were prepped and draped in a sterile fashion. After reviewing the KUB, it was noted at this time that the position of the stent was normal. Cystoscopy was performed with a #22 French cystoscope. The stent was identified coming from the left ureteral orifice, and the end was grasped with forceps and removed through the cystoscope. A #8 French cone-tipped ureteral catheter was then placed in the left ureteral orifice and passed to 10 cm. Then, 20 cm^3 of contrast was injected into a left collecting system. A film was exposed, and this showed patency without extravasation at the left ureteropelvic junction. There was some filling of calyces and partial filling of the dilated renal pelvis. A drainage film was subsequently obtained showing complete emptying of the pelvis and partial emptying of the mid and distal ureters. Dilated calyces were noted in the kidney. The patient was allowed to awaken and was returned to the recovery room in satisfactory condition. There were no intraoperative complications. He had no bleeding. The patient did receive 1 gm Ancef one-half hour prior to the onset of the procedure.

L. Zlatkin, M.D.

LZ:mr
D: 12/07/20xx
T: 12/08/20xx

OPERATIVE REPORT		
	PT. NAME:	MERCIER, CHARLES F.
	ID NO:	OP-912689
	ROOM NO:	ASC
	ATT. PHYS:	L.ZLATKIN, M.D.

ANSWERS TO PRACTICE EXERCISES

1. py/ur/ia
   R R S
   pus/urine/condition of
2. bacteri/osis
   R   S
   bacteria/condition or
   increase
3. trans/urethr/al
   P   R   S
   across or through/
   urethra/pertaining to
4. uro/gram
   CF   S
   urine/record
5. urethro/cyst/itis
   CF   R   S
   urethra/bladder/
   inflammation
6. nephro/ptosis
   CF   S
   kidney/falling or downward displacement
7. poly/ur/ia
   P   R S
   many/urine/condition of
8. glomerulo/scler/osis
   CF   R   S
   glomerulus (small
   ball)/hard/condition or
   increase
9. pyo/nephr/itis
   CF   R   S
   pus/kidney/inflammation
10. urin/al
    R   S
    urine/pertaining to
11. uretero/vesico/stomy
    CF   CF   S
    ureter/bladder/creation of
    an opening
12. glucos/ur/ia
    R   R S
    sugar/urine/condition of
13. meato/rrhaphy
    CF   S
    meatus (opening)/suture

14. pyelo/nephr/osis
    CF   R   S
    renal pelvis (basin)/
    kidney/condition or
    increase
15. cysto/scopy
    CF   S
    bladder/process of exami-
    nation
16. supra/ren/al
    P   R   S
    above/kidney/pertaining
    to
17. nephro/lith/iasis
    CF   R   S
    kidney/stone/formation
    or presence of
18. uro/stomy
    CF   S
    urine/creation of an
    opening
19. albumin/ur/ia
    R   R S
    protein/urine/condition
    of
20. ket/osis
    R   S
    ketone bodies/condition
    or increase
21. cystitis
22. nocturia
23. enuresis
24. nephrorrhaphy
25. nephrosis
26. albuminuria or
    proteinuria
27. adult polycystic kidney
    disease (APKD)
28. nephrotomy
29. renal or kidney biopsy
30. urinalysis
31. cystoscopy
32. urethral stenosis
33. extracorporeal shock
    wave lithotripsy
34. resectoscope
35. oliguria

36. dysuria
37. pyuria
38. hematuria
39. anuria
40. suprapubic
41. stress urinary inconti-
    nence
42. occult blood
43. RP
44. renal Bx or kidney Bx
45. UA
46. g
47. d
48. i
49. h
50. a
51. k
52. c
53. b
54. f
55. e
56. j
57. culture and sensitivity
58. voiding cystourethro-
    gram
59. blood urea nitrogen
60. intravenous urogram
61. extracorporeal shock
    wave lithotripsy
62. kidneys, ureters, bladder
63. specific gravity
64. urinary tract infection
65. retrograde pyelogram
66. ur/o
67. dips/o
68. py/o
69. vesic/o
70. albumin/o
71. nephr/o
72. meat/o
73. pyel/o
74. lith/o
75. right kidney
76. ureters
77. bladder
78. urethra
79. left kidney
80. cystoscope
81. pyelogram

ANSWERS	REVIEW
perine/o	**14.4** The adjective perineal comes from the combining form _____, referring to the perineum, an anatomic area between the scrotum and the anus in males.
prostat/o, pain prostatalgia	**14.5** The Latin term prostata has its origins in a Greek word that means one who stands before. Perhaps the prostate gland was so named because it stands before the opening for sperm leaving the body to exit through the penis. The combining form for prostate is _____. Recall that the suffix -*algia* means _____. Using this combining form, the term for a painful prostate is _____.
sperm/o, spermat/o sperm/o spermat/o	**14.6** The Greek word sperma means seed; thus, sperm are the reproductive "seed" of males. The two combining forms for sperm are _____ and _____. The combining form used to make the term oligospermia, meaning too few sperm in the semen, is _____. The combining form used to make the adjective form spermatic is _____.
vas/o -rrhaphy vasorrhaphy	**14.7** The Latin word vas refers to vessel, which includes ducts as well as blood vessels. The combining term for vessel is _____. Recall that the surgical suffix meaning suture is _____. Thus, the procedure of suturing a vessel is called a _____.

◆ Self-Instruction: Anatomic Terms (Fig. 14-1)

Study the following:

TERM	MEANING
scrotum *skrō'tŭm*	skin-covered pouch in the groin divided into two sacs, each containing a testis and an epididymis
testis *tes'tis* **testicle** *tes'tĭ-kĕl*	one of the two male reproductive glands, located in the scrotum, that produce sperm and the hormone testosterone
sperm *spĕrm* **spermatozoon** *spĕr' mă-tō-zō'on*	male gamete or sex cell produced in the testes that unites with the ovum in the female to produce offspring

THE MALE REPRODUCTIVE SYSTEM

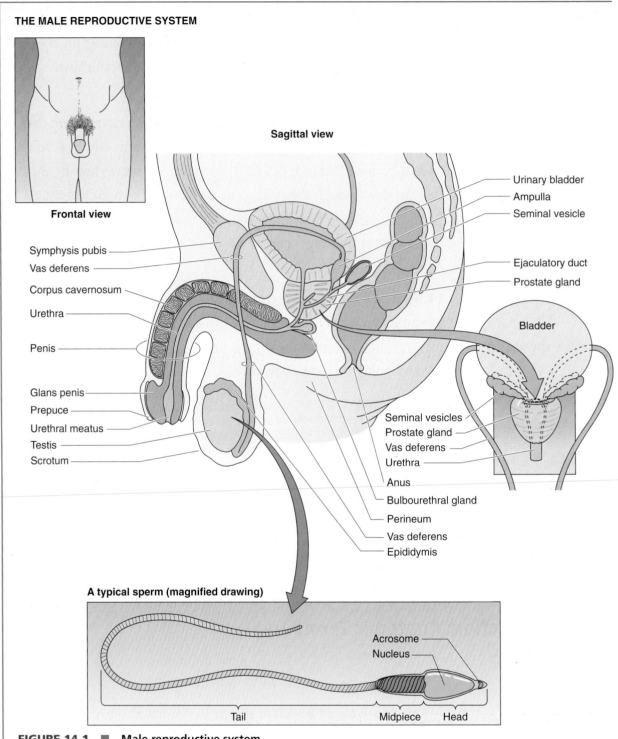

Frontal view

Sagittal view

Symphysis pubis
Vas deferens
Corpus cavernosum
Urethra
Penis
Glans penis
Prepuce
Urethral meatus
Testis
Scrotum

Urinary bladder
Ampulla
Seminal vesicle
Ejaculatory duct
Prostate gland
Bladder

Seminal vesicles
Prostate gland
Vas deferens
Urethra
Anus
Bulbourethral gland
Perineum
Vas deferens
Epididymis

A typical sperm (magnified drawing)

Acrosome
Nucleus

Tail   Midpiece   Head

FIGURE 14-1 ■ Male reproductive system.

TERM	MEANING
epididymis *ep-i-did′i-mis*	coiled duct on the top and at the side of the testis that stores sperm before emission
penis *pē′nis*	erectile tissue covered with skin that contains the urethra for urination and the ducts for secretion of seminal fluid (semen)

TERM	MEANING
glans penis *glanz pē'nis*	bulging structure at the distal end of the penis (*glans* = acorn)
prepuce *prē'pūs*	foreskin; loose casing that covers the glans penis; removed by circumcision
vas deferens *vas def'ĕr-ens*	duct that carries sperm from the epididymis to the ejaculatory duct (*vas* = vessel; *deferens* = carrying away)
seminal vesicle *sem'i-năl ves'i-kĕl*	one of two sac-like structures behind the bladder and connected to the vas deferens on each side; secretes an alkaline substance into the semen to enable the sperm to live longer
semen *sē'mĕn*	a mixture of the secretions of the testes, seminal vesicles, prostate, and bulbourethral glands discharged from the male urethra during orgasm (*semen* = seed)
ejaculatory duct *ē-jak'yū-lă-tōr-ē dŭkt*	duct formed by the union of the vas deferens with the duct of the seminal vesicle; its fluid is carried into the urethra
prostate gland *pros'tāt gland*	trilobular gland that encircles the urethra just below the bladder and secretes an alkaline fluid into the semen (*pro* = before; *stat* = to stand)
bulbourethral glands *bŭl'bō-yū-rē'thrăl glanz* **Cowper glands** *kow'per glanz*	pair of glands below the prostate, with ducts opening into the urethra, that adds a viscid (sticky) fluid to the semen
perineum *per'i-nē'ŭm*	external region between the scrotum and anus in a male and between the vulva and anus in a female

---

> **TERM TIP Prostrate versus Prostate**
>
> **Prostate,** a Greek word that literally means to stand before, describes the gland encircling the male urethra at the base of the bladder. Its spelling is often confused with **prostrate,** which describes helplessness or exhaustion (*pro* = before; *stratus* = to strew).

Programmed Review: Anatomic Terms

ANSWERS	REVIEW
	14.8 The testicles (or testes), which produce sperm and testosterone, are enclosed inside the skin-covered pouch called
scrotum	the _____.
testis testes	**14.9** Sperm are produced by each _____ (testicle). The plural of testis is _____.

ANSWERS	REVIEW
sperm, spermatozoon	**14.10** Produced by the testes, the male gamete (sex cell) is called _____ or _____.
epididymis epididymides	**14.11** On each testis is a coiled duct that stores the sperm before emission and is called an _____. The plural of epididymis is _____.
vas deferens vessel	**14.12** The duct that carries the sperm from the epididymis to the ejaculatory duct is called the _____ _____. Recall that the combining form *vas/o* means _____ (or duct). Deferens means carrying away.
ejaculatory duct	**14.13** From the epididymis, the sperm is carried by the vas deferens to the _____ _____.
semen	**14.14** Various secretions are mixed with the sperm to make the fluid called _____, which is discharged through the male urethra during orgasm. The semen is sometimes called the male seed.
seminal	**14.15** Connected to the vas deferens on each side is another structure that secretes an alkaline substance into the semen. This is called the _____ vesicle. This alkaline substance enables the sperm to live longer.
prostate	**14.16** The trilobular gland encircling the urethra below the bladder, which also secretes an alkaline substance into the semen, is called the _____ gland. Malignancies of this gland, called prostate cancer, are common in men.
bulbourethral Cowper	**14.17** Finally, a pair of glands below the prostate, with ducts opening into the urethra, secrete a viscous fluid into the semen. These are called the _____ glands, or the _____ glands.
penis glans	**14.18** The semen containing sperm and various secretions exits the body through the urethra, which passes through the skin-covered erectile tissue in the male called the _____. The acorn-shaped end of the penis where semen is ejaculated from the urethra is called the _____ penis. The medical term

ANSWERS	REVIEW
prepuce	for foreskin, which covers the glans penis and is removed by circumcision in some men, is the _____.
perineum	**14.19** Between the scrotum and the anus is the external area called the _____.

Self-Instruction: Symptomatic Terms

Study the following:

TERM	MEANING
aspermia ā-spĕr′mē-ă	inability to secrete or ejaculate sperm
azoospermia ā-zō-ō-spĕr′mē-ă	semen without living spermatozoa; a sign of infertility in a male (*zoo* = life)
oligospermia ol′i-gō-spĕr′mē-ă	scanty production and expulsion of sperm
mucopurulent discharge myū-kō-pū′rū-lent dis′charj	drainage of mucus and pus

Programmed Review: Symptomatic Terms

ANSWERS	REVIEW
without condition of aspermia	**14.20** Recall that the prefix *a-* means _____, and that the suffix *-ia* means _____. Use the shorter combining form for sperm to create the term for the condition in which one is unable to produce or ejaculate sperm (without sperm): _____.
sperm or seed condition of azoospermia	**14.21** *Zoo* is a term component meaning life. Join this term component with *sperm/o* (a combining form meaning _____) and then modify it with the prefix meaning without and *–ia* (a suffix meaning _____) to create the term for a condition of semen without living sperm: _____.
few or deficient oligospermia	**14.22** Recall that the prefix *oligo-* means _____. The condition of deficient production and expulsion of sperm is called _____.

ANSWERS	REVIEW
mucopurulent	**14.23** The term purulent refers to pus. The combining form for mucus is *muc/o*. The drainage of mucus and pus is called a _____ discharge.

◆ Self-Instruction: Diagnostic Terms

Study the following:

TERM	MEANING
anorchism *an-ōr′kizm*	absence of one or both testes
balanitis *bal-ă-nī′tis*	inflammation of the glans penis
cryptorchism (Fig. 14-2) *krip-tōr′kizm* **cryptorchidism** *krip-tōr′ki-dizm*	undescended testicle, or failure of a testis to descend into the scrotal sac during fetal development; the testis most often remains lodged in the abdomen or inguinal canal, requiring surgical repair (*crypt* = to hide)
epididymitis *ep′i-did-i-mī′tis*	inflammation of the epididymis
erectile dysfunction (ED) *ē′rek-tīl dis-fŭnk′shŭn*	failure to initiate or maintain an erection until ejaculation because of physical or psychologic dysfunction; formerly termed impotence (*im* = not; *potis* = able)

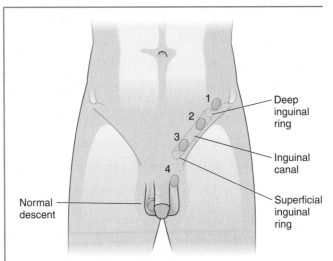

FIGURE 14-2 ▬ Cryptorchism (cryptorchidism). Four degrees of incomplete descent of the testis. 1. In the abdominal cavity close to the deep inguinal ring. 2. In the inguinal canal. 3. At the superficial inguinal ring. 4. In the upper part of the scrotum.

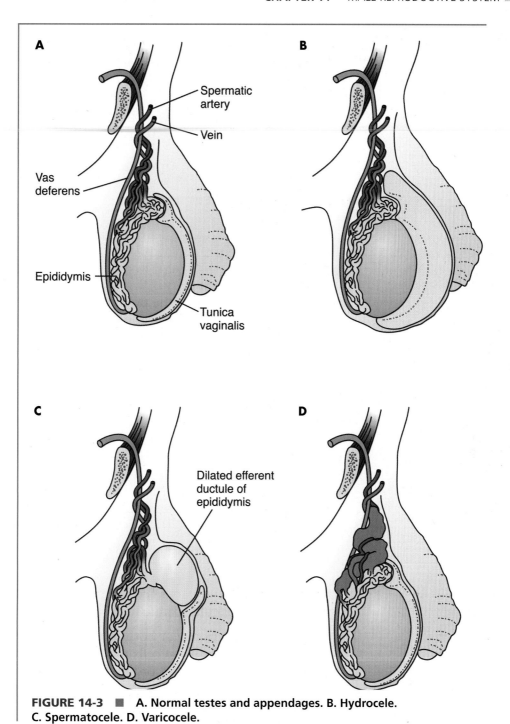

FIGURE 14-3 ■ **A. Normal testes and appendages. B. Hydrocele. C. Spermatocele. D. Varicocele.**

TERM	MEANING
hydrocele (Fig. 14-3, B) *hī'drō-sēl*	hernia of fluid in the testis or in the tubes leading from the testis
hypospadias (Fig. 14-4) *hī'pō-spā'dē-ăs*	congenital opening of the male urethra on the undersurface of the penis (*spadias* = to draw away)
Peyronie disease (Fig. 14-5) *pā-rō-nē' di-zēz'*	disorder characterized by a buildup of hardened fibrous tissue in the corpus cavernosum, causing pain and a defective curvature of the penis, especially during erection

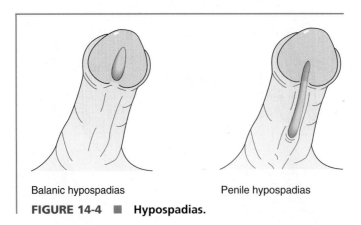

Balanic hypospadias   Penile hypospadias

FIGURE 14-4 ■ **Hypospadias.**

TERM	MEANING
phimosis (Fig. 14-6) *fī-mō′sis*	a narrowed condition of the prepuce (foreskin) resulting in its inability to be drawn over the glans penis, often leading to infection; commonly requires circumcision (*phimo* = muzzle)
benign prostatic hyperplasia (BPH) (Fig. 14-7) *bē-nīn′ pros-tat′ik hī-pěr-plā′zhē-ă* **benign prostatic hypertrophy (BPH)** *bē-nīn′ pros-tat′ik hī-pěr′trō-fē*	enlargement of the prostate gland, common in older men, causing urinary obstruction
prostate cancer *pros′tāt kan′sěr*	malignancy of the prostate gland
prostatitis *pros-tă-tī′tis*	inflammation of the prostate
spermatocele (Fig. 14-3, C) *spěr′mă-tō-sēl*	painless, benign cystic mass containing sperm lying above and posterior to, but separate from, the testicle
testicular cancer *tes-tik′yū-lăr kan′sěr*	malignant tumor in one or both testicles commonly developing from the germ cells that produce sperm; classified in two groups according to growth potential

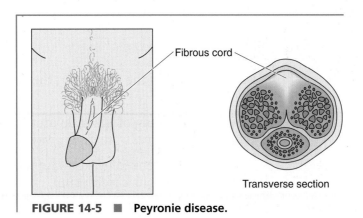

Fibrous cord

Transverse section

FIGURE 14-5 ■ **Peyronie disease.**

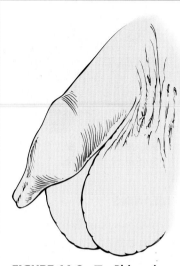

FIGURE 14-6 ■ **Phimosis.**

TERM	MEANING
seminoma *sem-i-nō'mă*	most common type of testicular tumor, composed of immature germ cells; highly treatable with early detection
nonseminoma *non-sem-i-nō'mă*	testicular tumor arising from more mature germ cells; these tumors have a tendency to be more aggressive than seminomas and often develop earlier in life; includes choriocarcinoma, embryonal carcinoma, teratoma, and yolk sac tumors
varicocele (*see* Fig. 14-3, D) *var'i-kō-sēl*	enlarged, swollen, herniated veins near the testis (*varico* = twisted vein)

SEXUALLY TRANSMITTED DISEASE (STD)

Major Bacterial STDs

chlamydia *kla-mid'ē-ă*	most common sexually transmitted bacterial infection in North America; often occurs with no symptoms and is treated only after it has spread

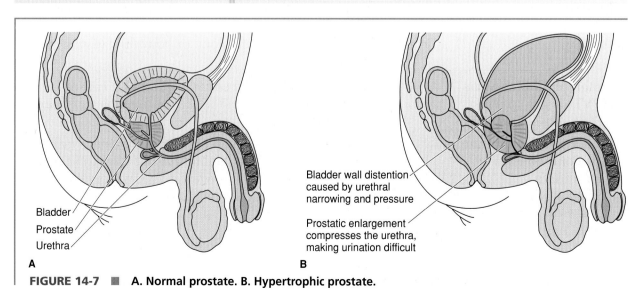

Bladder

Prostate

Urethra

Bladder wall distention caused by urethral narrowing and pressure

Prostatic enlargement compresses the urethra, making urination difficult

A

B

FIGURE 14-7 ■ **A. Normal prostate. B. Hypertrophic prostate.**

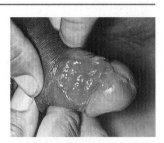

FIGURE 14-8 ▰
Syphilitic chancre.

TERM	MEANING
gonorrhea *gon-ō-rē'ă*	contagious inflammation of the genital mucous membranes caused by invasion of the gonococcus *Neisseria gonorrhea;* the condition was named for the urethral discharge characteristic of the infection, which was first thought to be a leakage of semen (*gono* = seed; *rrhea* = discharge); the genus is named for the Polish dermatologist Albert Neisser
syphilis (Fig. 14-8) *sif'i-lis*	sexually transmitted infection caused by a spirochete and which may involve any organ or tissue over time; usually manifests first on the skin, with the appearance of small, painless, red papules that erode and form bloodless ulcers called chancres

Major Viral STDs

TERM	MEANING
hepatitis B virus (HBV) *hep-ă-tī'tis B vī'rŭs*	virus that causes inflammation of the liver; transmitted through any body fluid, including vaginal secretions, semen, and blood
herpes simplex virus type 2 (HSV-2) (*see* Fig. 15-8) *her'pēz sim'pleks vī'rŭs tīp 2*	virus that causes ulcer-like lesions of the genital and anorectal skin and mucosa; after initial infection, the virus lies dormant in the nerve cell root and may recur at times of stress
human immunodeficiency virus (HIV) *hyū'măn im'yū-nō-dē-fish'en-sē vī'rŭs*	virus that causes acquired immunodeficiency syndrome (AIDS), which permits various opportunistic infections, malignancies, and neurologic diseases; contracted through exposure to contaminated blood or body fluid (e.g., semen or vaginal secretions)
human papilloma virus (HPV) (*see* Fig. 15-9) *hyū'măn pap-i-lō'mă vī'rŭs*	virus transmitted by direct sexual contact that causes an infection that can occur on the skin or mucous membranes of the genitals
condyloma acuminatum (pl. condylomata acuminata) *kon-di-lō'mă ă-kū-mi-nā'tŭm (kon-di-lō-mah'tă ă-kū-mĭ-nā'tă)*	lesion that appears as a result of human papilloma virus; on the skin, lesions appear as cauliflower-like warts, and on mucous membranes, they have a flat appearance; also known as venereal or genital warts

Programmed Review: Diagnostic Terms

ANSWERS	REVIEW
-itis balan/o balanitis	**14.24** Recall that the suffix meaning inflammation is _____. The combining form for glans penis is _____. Inflammation of the glans penis is therefore called _____.
epididymitis	**14.25** Inflammation of the epididymis is called _____.
prostatitis	**14.26** Inflammation of the prostate gland is called _____.
condition of, without testis anorchism	**14.27** Recall that the suffix *-ism* means _____ ____. The prefix *an-* means _____. The combining form *orch/o* means _____. The medical term for the condition in which one or both testes are absent is _____.
condition of cryptorchism or cryptorchidism	**14.28** The combining form *crypt/o* means hidden. Again, the suffix *-ism* means _____ ____. The condition in which a testicle does not descend during development but remains "hidden" in the abdomen is called _____.
hernia hydrocele varicocele sperm spermatocele	**14.29** Recall that the suffix *-cele* means pouching or _____. The combining form *hydr/o* refers to water or fluid. A hernia of fluid in the testis or tubes leading from the testis is called a _____. The combining form *varic/o* means swollen, twisted vein. A condition of swollen, herniated veins near the testis is therefore called _____. *Spermat/o*, a combining from meaning _____, is used in the term describing a painless, benign cystic mass containing sperm and lying near the testicle: _____.
hypospadias	**14.30** The congenital condition in which the urethra opens on the undersurface of the penis is called _____.

ANSWERS	REVIEW
erectile dysfunction	**14.31** Impotence is a term formerly used to describe a failure to have or maintain an erection until ejaculation. This condition is now called _____ _____ (ED).
disease	**14.32** The disorder characterized by a buildup of hardened fibrous tissue in the corpus cavernosum, causing pain and a defective curvature of the penis, is called Peyronie _____.
condition of phimosis	**14.33** Phimos, a word meaning muzzle, combined with *-osis*, the suffix meaning _____ ____, was used to name a narrowed condition of the prepuce that results in its inability to be drawn over the glans penis: _____.
benign above excessive benign prostatic hyperplasia or hypertrophy	**14.34** The opposite of malignant is _____. Recall that the prefix *hyper-* means _____ or _____. Hyperplasia refers to a condition of excessive formation of tissue. Hypertrophy refers to the excessive growth or enlargement of a structure. Using either of these terms, the nonmalignant enlargement of the prostate gland is called _____ _____ _____ (BPH).
prostate cancer	**14.35** Malignancy of the prostate is called _____ _____.
-oma seminoma	**14.36** Recall that the suffix for tumor is _____. The term for a malignant tumor of the testicle uses the root for semen instead of testicle: _____.
chlamydia	**14.37** Most sexually transmitted diseases (STDs) are caused by bacteria or viruses. The most common bacterial STD in North America, which often occurs without symptoms, is _____. Like many bacterial diseases, chlamydia gets its name from the Latin genus name for the bacteria: *Chlamydia*.
	14.38 The name for another bacterial STD, the genus of which was named for the Polish dermatologist Albert

ANSWERS	REVIEW
gonorrhea	Neisser, was coined in ancient times based on the thought that the urethral discharge characteristic of the infection was a leakage of semen: *Neisseria* _____.
syphilis	**14.39** The bacterial STD caused by a spirochete that can, over time, involve any body tissue or organ is _____.
hepatitis B	**14.40** Several viruses also cause STDs. The virus that causes inflammation of the liver, which can be spread through any body fluid, is _____ ____ virus (HBV).
herpes simplex virus	**14.41** HSV-2 is the abbreviation for this sexually transmitted virus, which typically lies dormant after the initial infection but recurs at times of stress: _____ _____ _____ type 2.
human immunodeficiency virus	**14.42** The virus that causes acquired immunodeficiency syndrome (AIDS) is _____ _____ _____ (HIV).
papilloma condylomata acuminata	**14.43** HPV is the abbreviation for human _____ virus, which causes an STD characterized by lesions on the skin or mucous membranes. A condyloma is a warty growth; the plural of this term is _____. Condylomata _____ are warty growths in the genital area caused by HPV.

Self-Instruction: Diagnostic Tests and Procedures

Study the following:

TEST OR PROCEDURE	EXPLANATION
biopsy (Bx) *bī'op-sē*	tissue sampling used to identify neoplasia
biopsy of the prostate *bī'op-sē of the pros'tāt*	needle biopsy of the prostate; often performed using ultrasound guidance (*see* Fig. 14-9)
testicular biopsy *tes-tik'yū-lăr bī'op-sē*	biopsy of a testicle

TEST OR PROCEDURE	EXPLANATION
digital rectal exam (DRE) *dij'i-tăl rek'tăl ek-zam'*	insertion of a finger into the male rectum to palpate the rectum and prostate
prostate-specific antigen (PSA) test *pros'tāt-spĕ-sif'ik an'ti-jen test*	blood test used to screen for prostate cancer; an elevated level of the antigen indicates the possible presence of tumor
urethrogram *yū-rē'thrō-gram*	x-ray of the urethra and prostate
semen analysis *sē'mĕn ă-nal'i-sis*	study of semen, including a sperm count with observation of morphology (form) and motility; usually performed to rule out male infertility
endorectal sonogram of the prostate (Fig. 14-9) *en'dō-rek'tăl son'ō-gram of the pros'tāt* **transrectal sonogram of the prostate** *tranz-rek'tăl son'ō-gram of the pros'tāt*	scan of the prostate made after introducing an ultrasonic transducer into the rectum; also used to guide needle biopsy

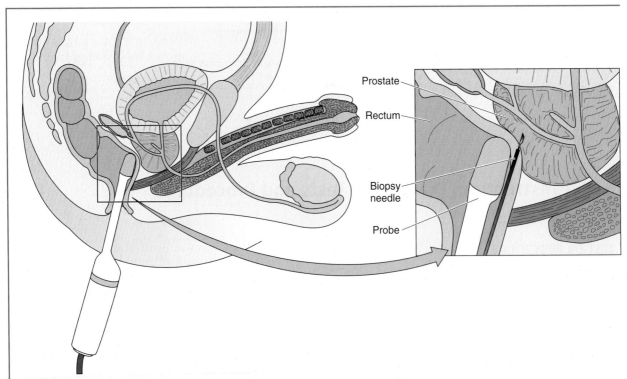

FIGURE 14-9 ■ Ultrasound and biopsy (inset) of prostate.

Programmed Review: Diagnostic Tests and Procedures

ANSWERS	REVIEW
biopsy testicular	**14.44** The general term for removal of any body tissue for pathologic examination is _____, which is abbreviated Bx. The removal of testicular tissue is called a _____ biopsy.
prostate	**14.45** A needle biopsy of the prostate, often performed with ultrasound guidance, is called a _____ biopsy. This may be performed if prostate cancer is suspected.
prostate specific antigen	**14.46** Prostate cancer often causes the blood level of a specific antigen to become elevated. Thus, the _____-_____ _____ (PSA) test may indicate the possible presence of a prostate tumor.
digital rectal	**14.47** The physical examination procedure involving the physician inserting a finger (digit) into the rectum to palpate the rectum and prostate is called a _____ _____ exam (DRE). An enlarged or tender prostate can be detected with this exam.
within endorectal sonogram	**14.48** Recall that the prefix *endo-* means _____. Another type of examination of the prostate involves introducing an ultrasonic transducer within the rectum to produce an _____ (or transrectal) _____ of the prostate, which can also be used to guide a needle biopsy.
record urethrogram	**14.49** Recall that the suffix *-gram* means a _____. An x-ray record of the urethra and prostate is called a _____.
semen analysis	**14.50** A study of semen that includes a sperm count and observations of other characteristics of sperm is called a _____ _____. This analysis is often performed to help determine a man's fertility.

Self-Instruction: Operative Terms

Study the following:

TERM	MEANING
circumcision *ser-kŭm-sizh'ŭn*	removal of the foreskin (prepuce), exposing the glans penis

TERM	MEANING
epididymectomy *ep'i-did-i-mek'tŏ-mē*	removal of an epididymis
orchiectomy *ōr-kē-ek'tŏ-mē* **orchidectomy** *ōr-ki-dek'tŏ-mē*	removal of a testicle
orchioplasty *ōr'kē-ō-plas-tē*	repair of a testicle
orchiopexy *ōr'kē-ō-pek'sē*	fixation of an undescended testis in the scrotum
prostatectomy *pros-tă-tek'tŏ-mē*	excision of the prostate gland
transurethral resection of the prostate (TURP) (Fig. 14-10) *tranz-yū-rē'thral rē-sek'shŭn of the pros'tāt*	removal of prostatic gland tissue through the urethra using a resectoscope, a specialized urologic endoscope; common treatment for benign prostatic hyperplasia/hypertrophy (BPH)
vasectomy (Fig. 14-11) *va-sek'tŏ-mē*	removal of a segment of the vas deferens to produce sterility in the male
vasovasostomy *vā'sō-vă-sos'tŏ-mē*	restoration of the function of the vas deferens to regain fertility after a vasectomy

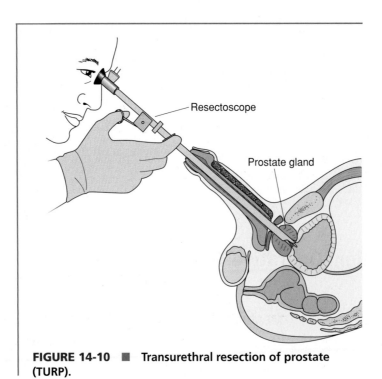

Resectoscope

Prostate gland

FIGURE 14-10 ■ **Transurethral resection of prostate (TURP).**

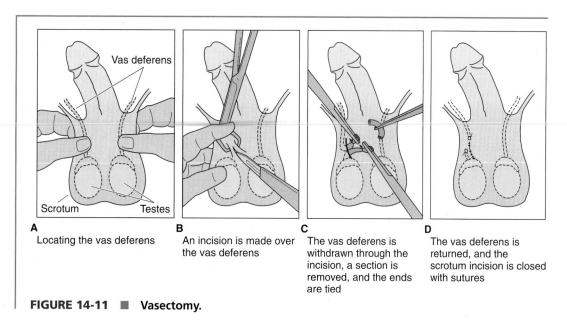

FIGURE 14-11 ■ **Vasectomy.**

A — Locating the vas deferens
B — An incision is made over the vas deferens
C — The vas deferens is withdrawn through the incision, a section is removed, and the ends are tied
D — The vas deferens is returned, and the scrotum incision is closed with sutures

🔷 Programmed Review: Operative Terms

ANSWERS	REVIEW
excision epididymectomy	**14.51** Recall that the operative suffix *-ectomy* means _____ or removal. The excision of an epididymis is termed an _____.
orchiectomy orchidectomy	**14.52** The excision of a testicle is called an _____ or _____.
prostatectomy	**14.53** The surgical removal of the prostate gland is called a _____.
vasectomy	**14.54** Excision of part of the vas deferens is called a _____. This is done to produce male sterility.
opening vasovasostomy	**14.55** In contrast, the operative suffix *-stomy* means to create an _____. The operation performed to restore the function of the vas deferens after a vasectomy (to restore fertility) is called a _____. The combining form *vas/o* is used twice in the term to refer to both free ends of the vas deferens (which had been cut during the vasectomy), as both ends must be reopened so that they can be reattached.
repair orchioplasty	**14.56** Recall that the suffix *-plasty* means surgical reconstruction or _____. The surgical repair of a testicle is called _____.

ANSWERS	REVIEW
-pexy orchiopexy	**14.57** The suffix for surgical fixation or suspension is _____. The fixation of an undescended testis in the scrotum is called an _____.
around circumcision prepuce	**14.58** The Latin word root for *-cision* (e.g., incision) means to cut. Recall that the prefix *circum-* means _____. The surgical procedure that cuts the foreskin from around the penis is called a _____. The medical term for the foreskin is _____.
through transurethral resection	**14.59** Resect is synonymous with excise. A specialized endoscope allows resection using an instrument through the scope; this is called a resectoscope. Recall that the prefix *trans-* means across or _____. The surgical procedure of removing prostatic gland tissue using a resectoscope through the urethra is called a _____ _____ of the prostate (TURP).

 ## Self-Instruction: Therapeutic Terms

Study the following:

TERM	MEANING
chemotherapy *kem'ō-thār-ă-pē*	treatment of malignancies, infections, and other diseases with chemical agents that destroy selected cells or impair their ability to reproduce
radiation therapy *rā'dē-ā'shŭn thār'ă-pē*	treatment of neoplastic disease using radiation, usually from a cobalt source, to stop the proliferation of malignant cells
brachytherapy *brak-ē-thār'ă-pē*	radiation therapy technique involving internal implantation of radioactive isotopes, such as radioactive seeds to treat prostate cancer; *brachy-,* meaning short distance, refers to localized application
hormone replacement therapy (HRT) *hōr'mōn rē-plās'ment thār'ă-pē*	use of a hormone to remedy a deficiency or regulate production (e.g., testosterone)
penile prosthesis *pē'nīl pros'thē-sis*	implantation of a device designed to provide an erection of the penis; used to treat physical impotence
penile self-injection *pē'nīl self-in-jek'shŭn*	intracavernosal injection therapy causing an erection; used in treatment of erectile dysfunction

⬡ Programmed Review: Therapeutic Terms

ANSWERS	REVIEW
chemotherapy	**14.60** The combining form referring to chemical agents is *chem/o*. The treatment of malignancies, infections, and other diseases with chemical agents that destroy targeted cells is called _____.
radiation therapy brachytherapy	**14.61** Some kinds of cancer are also treated with radiation, which deters the proliferation of malignant cells. This is called _____ _____. *Brachy-*, a term component meaning short distance, is used to name the technique involving internal implantation of radioactive isotopes, such as radioactive seeds to treat prostate cancer. Signaling its localized application, this therapy is called _____.
hormone replacement	**14.62** If a patient is deficient in the production of a hormone, such as testosterone, treatment may involve administering a replacement hormone. This is called _____ _____ therapy (HRT).
penile prosthesis	**14.63** A prosthesis is an artificial substitute for a nonfunctioning or missing body part or organ. A device that is implanted in the penis to provide an erection because the penis cannot become erect naturally is called a _____ _____.
penile	**14.64** Another therapy to treat erectile dysfunction involves self-injection of a medication into the corpus cavernosum to cause an erection. This therapy is called _____ self-injection.

CHAPTER 14 ACRONYMS AND ABBREVIATIONS

ABBREVIATION	EXPANSION
BPH	benign prostatic hyperplasia; benign prostatic hypertrophy
Bx	biopsy
DRE	digital rectal exam
ED	erectile dysfunction
HBV	hepatitis B virus
HIV	human immunodeficiency virus
HPV	human papilloma virus

ABBREVIATION	EXPANSION
HRT	hormone replacement therapy
HSV-2	herpes simplex virus type 2
PSA	prostate-specific antigen
STD	sexually transmitted disease
TURP	transurethral resection of the prostate

CHAPTER 14 SUMMARY OF TERMS

The terms introduced in chapter 14 are listed below, followed by the page number on which each term can be found and its written pronunciation. For additional practice and reinforcement, write the definition of each term on a separate piece of paper.

anorchism/674
an-ōr'kizm

aspermia/673
ā-spěr'mē-ă

azoospermia/673
ā-zō-ō-spěr'mē-ă

balanitis/674
bal-ă-nī'tis

benign prostatic hyperplasia (BPH)/676
bē-nīn' pros-tat'ik hī-pěr-plā'zhē-ă

benign prostatic hypertrophy (BPH)/676
bē-nīn' pros-tat'ik hī-pěr'trō-fē

biopsy (Bx)/681
bī'op-sē

biopsy of the prostate/681
bī'op-sē of the pros'tāt

brachytherapy/686
brak-ē-thār'ă-pē

bulbourethral glands/671
bŭl'bō-yū-rē'thrăl glanz

chemotherapy/686
kem'ō-thār-ă-pē

chlamydia/677
kla-mid'ē-ă

circumcision/683
ser-kŭm-sizh'ŭn

condyloma acuminatum/678
kon-di-lō'mă ă-kū-mi-nā'tŭm

condylomata acuminata/678
kon-di-lō-mah'tă ă-kū'mĭ-nā'tă

Cowper glands/671
kow'per glanz

cryptorchism/674
krip-tōr'kizm

cryptorchidism/674
krip-tōr'ki-dizm

digital rectal exam (DRE)/682
dij'i-tăl rek'tăl ek-zam'

ejaculatory duct/670
ē-jak'yū-lă-tōr-ē dŭkt

endorectal sonogram of the prostate/682
en'dō-rek'tăl son'ō-gram of the pros'tāt

epididymectomy/684
ep'i-did-i-mek'tŏ-mē

epididymis/670
ep-i-did'i-mis

epididymitis/674
ep'i-did-i-mī'tis

erectile dysfunction (ED)/674
ē'rek-tīl dis-fŭnk'shŭn

glans penis/671
glanz pē'nis

gonorrhea/678
gon-ō-rē'ă

hepatitis B virus (HBV)/678
hep-ă-tī'tis B vī'rŭs

**herpes simplex virus type 2
   (HSV-2)**/678
her'pēz sim'pleks vī'rŭs tīp 2

**hormone replacement therapy
   (HRT)**/686
hōr'mōn rē-plās'ment thăr'ă-pē

**human immunodeficiency virus
   (HIV)**/678
hyū'măn im'yū-nō-dē-fish'en-sē vī'rŭs

human papilloma virus (HPV)/678
hyū'măn pap-i-lō'mă vī'rŭs

hydrocele/675
hī'drō-sēl

hypospadias/675
hī'pō-spā'dē-ăs

mucopurulent discharge/673
myū-kō-pū'rū-lent dis'charj

nonseminoma/677
non-sem-i-nō'mă

oligospermia/673
ol'i-gō-spĕr'mē-ă

orchidectomy/684
ōr-ki-dek'tŏ-mē

orchiectomy/684
ōr-kē-ek'tŏ-mē

orchiopexy/684
ōr'kē-ō-pek'sē

orchioplasty/684
ōr'kē-ō-plas-tē

penile prosthesis/686
pē'nīl pros'thē-sis

penile self-injection/686
pē'nīl self-in-jek'shŭn

penis/670
pē'nis

perineum/671
per'i-nē'ŭm

Peyronie disease/675
pā-rō-nē' di-zēz'

phimosis/676
fī-mō'sis

prepuce/671
prē'pūs

prostate cancer/676
pros'tāt kan'sĕr

prostate gland/671
pros'tāt gland

prostatectomy/684
pros-tă-tek'tŏ-mē

**prostate-specific antigen (PSA)
   test**/682
pros'tāt-spĕ-sif'ik an'ti-jen test

prostatitis/676
pros-tă-tī'tis

radiation therapy/686
rā'dē-ā'shŭn thăr-ă-pē

scrotum/669
skrō'tŭm

semen/671
sē'měn

semen analysis/682
sē'měn ă-nal'i-sis

seminal vesicle/671
sem'i-năl ves'i-kěl

seminoma/677
sem-i-nō'mă

sperm/669
spěrm

spermatocele/676
spěr'mă-tō-sēl

spermatozoon/669
spěr'mă-tō-zō'on

syphilis/678
sif'i-lis

testicle/669
tes'tĭ-kěl

testicular biopsy/681
tes-tik'yū-lăr bī'op-sē

testicular cancer/676
tes-tik'yū-lăr kan'sĕr

testis/669
tes'tis

transrectal sonogram of the prostate/682
tranz-rek'tăl son'ō-gram of the pros'tāt

transurethral resection of the prostate (TURP)/684
tranz-yū-rē'thral rē-sek'shŭn of the pros'tāt

urethrogram/682
yū-rē'thrō-gram

varicocele/677
var'i-kō-sēl

vas deferens/671
vas def'ĕr-enz

vasectomy/684
va-sek'tŏ-mē

vasovasostomy/684
vā'sō-vă-sos'tŏ-mē

PRACTICE EXERCISES

For each of the following words, write out the term components (prefixes [P], combining forms [CF], roots [R], and suffixes [S]) on the lines below the word. Then define the term according to the meaning of its components.

EXAMPLE

synorchism

syn / *orch* / *ism*

P   R   S

DEFINITION: together/testis or testicle/condition of

1. oligospermia

    _____ / _____ / _____

        P   R   S

    DEFINITION: _____

2. perineoplasty

    _____ / _____

        CF   S

    DEFINITION: _____

3. testalgia

    _____ / _____

        R   S

    DEFINITION: _____

4. balanic

    _____ / _____

        R   S

    DEFINITION: _____

5. prostatomegaly

    _____ / _____

        CF   S

    DEFINITION: _____

6. orchidectomy

    _____ / _____

        R   S

    DEFINITION: _____

7. anorchism

    _____ / _____ / _____

        P   R   S

    DEFINITION: _____

8. vasectomy

_____ / _____

    R   S

DEFINITION: _____

9. aspermia

_____ / _____ / _____

    P   R   S

DEFINITION: _____

10. prostatorrhea

_____ / _____

   CF   S

DEFINITION: _____

11. balanitis

_____ / _____

    R   S

DEFINITION: _____

12. orchioplasty

_____ / _____

   CF   S

DEFINITION: _____

13. spermatocele

_____ / _____

   CF   S

DEFINITION: _____

14. epididymotomy

_____ / _____

   CF   S

DEFINITION: _____

15. vasovasostomy

_____ / _____ / _____

   CF   CF   S

DEFINITION: _____

Write the correct medical term for each of the following definitions:

16. _____ absence of a testicle

17. _____ inflammation of the glans penis

18. _____ failure to maintain an erection

19. _____ enlarged, herniated veins near the testicle

20. _____ most common type of testicular cancer tumor

21. _____ semen without living sperm

22. _____ scanty production of sperm

23. _____ operative treatment for cryptorchism

24. _____ specialized endoscope used to approach the prostate when performing a TURP

25. _____ enlargement of prostate

26. _____ fluid hernia in the testis

27. _____ removal of a portion of the vas deferens to produce male sterility

28. _____ disorder that is caused by a buildup of hardened fibrous tissue in the corpora cavernosa in the penis

29. _____ removal of foreskin to expose the glans penis

Complete each medical term by writing the missing word(s) or word part:

30. _____orchism = undescended testicle

31. _____ _____ exam = insertion of a finger into the male rectum to palpate the rectum and prostate

32. _____ sonogram of the prostate = ultrasound scan of prostate made after introduction of the transducer into the rectum

33. _____ penis = bulging structure at the distal end of the penis

34. _____spermia = inability to secrete or ejaculate semen

Write the letter of the matching term in the space provided:

35. semen analysis _____   a. orchiopexy

36. testis _____   b. foreskin

37. testo _____   c. sperm morphology

38. BPH _____   d. testes

39. cryptorchism _____   e. TURP

40. prepuce _____   f. orchido

Write out the expanded term for each abbreviation:

41. PSA _____

42. BPH _____

43. TURP _____

44. DRE _____

45. Bx _____

Circle the combining form that corresponds to the meaning given:

46. **testis**   prostat/o   epididym/o   orchi/o
47. **perineum**   peritone/o   perine/o   prostat/o
48. **sperm**   test/o   orchi/o   spermat/o
49. **vessel**   aden/o   angin/o   vas/o
50. **glans penis**   prostat/o   orchid/o   balan/o
51. **epididymis**   sperm/o   vas/o   epididym/o

Identify the parts of the male reproductive anatomy by writing the missing words in the spaces provided:

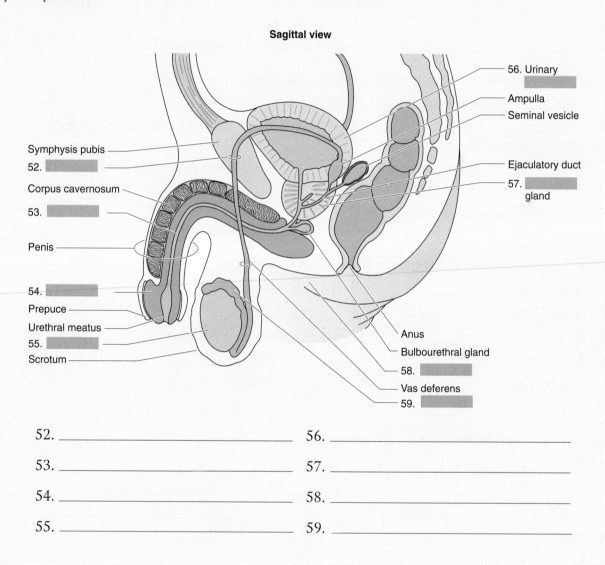

Sagittal view

56. Urinary

Ampulla
Seminal vesicle

Symphysis pubis
52.

Ejaculatory duct
57.   gland

Corpus cavernosum

53.

Penis

54.
Prepuce
Urethral meatus
55.
Scrotum

Anus
Bulbourethral gland
58.
Vas deferens
59.

52. _____   56. _____

53. _____   57. _____

54. _____   58. _____

55. _____   59. _____

Circle the correct spelling in each set of words:

60. fimosis   phemosis   phimosis
61. oligspermia   oligospermia   oligispermia
62. azospermia   asospermia   azoospermia
63. anorchesm   anorchism   anorschizm
64. balanitis   balanitus   balantis
65. creptorchism   criptorchism   cryptorchism
66. hypospadias   hypospadeas   hypespadias
67. clamidyia   chlamidya   chlamydia
68. syphilis   syphillis   syphyllis

Give the noun used to form each adjective:

69. prostatic _____
70. epididymal _____
71. perineal _____
72. penile _____
73. gonorrheal _____

MEDICAL RECORD ANALYSIS

Medical Record 14-1

CHART NOTE

S: Twelve days ago, this 34 y.o. male had a flu-like syndrome that lasted about 2 to 3 hours. For the past two days, he has felt lousy again and is experiencing left testicular pain and swelling s̄ voiding Sx

   Allergies: none

   PH: negative

   Habits: smoking—no alcohol—occasional beer

   ROS: otherwise negative

O: Slightly small testes bilaterally; tender Ⓛ epididymis; normal circumcised penis

   UA: WNL

A: Ⓛ epididymitis

P: Rx: Maxaquin 400 mg #16

   Sig: ii̇ STAT, then i̇ daily × 14 d; return in two weeks for follow-up

QUESTIONS ABOUT MEDICAL RECORD 14-1

1. What was the patient's diagnosis?
   a. testicular pain and swelling
   b. inflammation of the testicle
   c. swollen veins near the testis
   d. inflammation of the coiled duct that stores sperm
   e. fluid hernia in a testicle

2. What was the condition of the patient's penis?
   a. small but normal
   b. prepuce had been excised
   c. inflamed
   d. swollen and tender
   e. not stated

3. What was the Sig: on the prescription?
   a. two every day for 14 days
   b. two immediately, then one a day for 14 days
   c. one immediately, then one a day for 14 days
   d. one as needed every day for 14 days

4. Did the patient have any trouble urinating?
   a. yes
   b. no

5. What was the condition of the right testicle?
   a. inflamed
   b. enlarged
   c. small
   d. normal
   e. had been excised

6. What was the result of the urinalysis?
   a. not stated
   b. normal
   c. not performed, because the patient could not void
   d. hematuria
   e. glucosuria

ANSWERS TO PRACTICE EXERCISES

1. oligo/sperm/ia
   P   R   S
   few or deficient/sperm/
   condition of

2. perineo/plasty
   CF   S
   perineum/surgical repair
   or reconstruction

3. test/algia
   R   S
   testis or testicle/pain

4. balan/ic
   R   S
   glans penis/pertaining to

5. prostato/megaly
   CF   S
   prostate/enlargement

6. orchid/ectomy
   R   S
   testis or testicle/excision
   (removal)

7. an/orch/ism
   P   R   S
   without/testis or
   testicle/condition of

8. vas/ectomy
   R   S
   vessel/excision (removal)

9. a/sperm/ia
   P   R   S
   without/sperm
   (seed)/condition of

10. prostato/rrhea
    CF   S
    prostate/discharge

11. balan/itis
    R   S
    glans penis/inflammation

12. orchio/plasty
    CF   S
    testis or testicle/surgical
    repair or reconstruction

13. spermato/cele
    CF   S
    sperm (seed)/pouching or
    hernia

14. epididymo/tomy
    CF   S
    epididymis/incision

15. vaso/vaso/stomy
    CF CF   S
    vessel/vessel/creation of
    an opening

16. anorchism
17. balanitis
18. erectile dysfunction
19. varicocele
20. seminoma
21. azoospermia
22. oligospermia
23. orchiopexy
24. resectoscope
25. benign prostatic hyper-
    plasia or hypertrophy
26. hydrocele
27. vasectomy
28. Peyronie disease
29. circumcision
30. cryptorchism or cryp-
    torchidism
31. digital rectal exam
32. endorectal or transrectal
    sonogram of prostate
33. glans penis
34. aspermia
35. c
36. d

37. f
38. e
39. a
40. b
41. prostate-specific antigen
42. benign prostatic hyper-
    plasia or hypertrophy
43. transurethral resection of
    the prostate
44. digital rectal exam
45. biopsy
46. orchi/o
47. perine/o
48. spermat/o
49. vas/o
50. balan/o
51. epididym/o
52. vas deferens
53. urethra
54. glans penis
55. testis
56. bladder
57. prostate
58. perineum
59. epididymis
60. phimosis
61. oligospermia
62. azoospermia
63. anorchism
64. balanitis
65. cryptorchism
66. hypospadias
67. chlamydia
68. syphilis
69. prostate
70. epididymis
71. perineum
72. penis
73. gonorrhea

ANSWERS TO MEDICAL RECORD ANALYSIS

Medical Record 14-1: Chart Note

1. d   2. b   3. b   4. b   5. c   6. b

Medical Record 14-2: For Additional Study

See CD-ROM for answers.

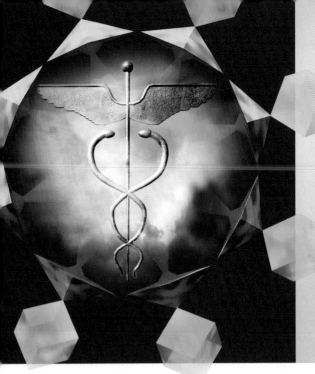

CHAPTER 15

Female Reproductive System

✓ Chapter 15 Checklist	LOCATION
☐ Read Chapter 15: Female Reproductive System and complete all programmed review segments.	pages 703–750
☐ Review the starter set of flash cards and term components related to Chapter 15.	back of book
☐ Complete the Chapter 15 Practice Exercises and Medical Record Analysis 15-1.	pages 758–765
☐ Complete Medical Record Analysis 15-2 For Additional Study.	pages 766–769
☐ Complete the Chapter 15 Exercises by Chapter.	CD-ROM
☐ Complete the Chapter 15 Review and Test Modes.	CD-ROM
☐ Review the Pronunciation Drill for the Chapter 15 terms.	CD-ROM

FEMALE REPRODUCTIVE SYSTEM OVERVIEW

Functions of the female reproductive system:

- Produce and maintain ova
- Provide a place for the implantation and nurturing of the fertilized ovum through the embryonic and fetal stages to birth
- Produce some female sex hormones

Self-Instruction: Combining Forms

Study the following:

COMBINING FORM	MEANING
cervic/o	neck or cervix
colp/o, vagin/o	vagina (sheath)
episi/o, vulv/o	vulva (covering)
gynec/o	woman
hyster/o, metr/o, uter/o	uterus
lact/o	milk
mast/o, mamm/o	breast
men/o	menstruation
obstetr/o	midwife
oophor/o, ovari/o	ovary
ov/i, ov/o	egg
pelv/i	pelvis (basin); hip bone
salping/o	uterine (fallopian) tube; also, eustachian tube
toc/o	labor or birth
-arche (suffix)	beginning

 ## Programmed Review: Combining Forms

ANSWERS	REVIEW
cervic/o	**15.1** The Latin word cervix means neck; the cervix in the female is like a neck between the vagina and the uterus. The combining term for cervix is _____. The common adjective form, for example, is cervical.
vagin/o colp/o -scope colposcope	**15.2** As often happens, there are two combining forms for vagina, one from a Latin word and one from a Greek word. The Latin word vagina means sheath (the vagina sheaths the penis during intercourse); the combining form is _____. The Greek word kolpos means a hollow; the combining form is _____. Using the latter combining form and the suffix for an instrument of examination, _____, forms the term for a special kind of scope designed to examine the vagina: _____.

ANSWERS	REVIEW
episi/o, incision episiotomy	**15.3** The Greek term episeion, meaning pubic region, is the origin for the combining form for the vulva (the external female genitalia): _____. The operative suffix *-tomy* means _____. Using this combining form, an incision made in the perineum to facilitate childbirth is an _____.
vulv/o	**15.4** A second combining form meaning vulva comes from the Latin word vulva: _____. It is used, for example, to create the common adjective form vulvar.
women gynec/o midwife	**15.5** A gynecologist is a physician who specializes in the reproductive system of _____. The combining form meaning women is _____. Obstetrics is the specialty pertaining to the care and treatment of mother and fetus throughout pregnancy, childbirth, and the immediate postpartum period. *Obstetr/o* is a combining form meaning _____. OB-GYN is the abbreviation for the combined field of obstetrics (OB) and gynecology (GYN).
uter/o hyster/o excision or removal	**15.6** The uterus is the hollow organ (the womb) where the woman carries the fetus before childbirth. The Latin combining form used to name the uterus is _____. A hysterectomy is the surgical removal of the uterus; this term is made from the Greek combining form _____ plus the suffix *-ectomy*, which means _____.
metr/o uterus	**15.7** The Greek word for the uterus, metra, is the origin of a third combining form for uterus: _____. The term metrorrhagia, for example, refers to irregular bleeding from the _____ not occurring during menstruation.
production milk lactogenic	**15.8** The suffix *-genic* (a combination of *gen/o* and *-ic*) pertains to origin or _____. It is used to modify the combining form *lact/o*, meaning _____, to form the adjective pertaining to the production of milk: _____.
pain -gram	**15.9** There are two combining forms meaning breast, again from Greek and Latin roots. Because the suffix *-dynia* means _____, mastodynia means breast pain. The common suffix for a record resulting from an examination technique is _____. Thus, a

ANSWERS	REVIEW
mast/o, mamm/o	mammogram is an x-ray of the breast. The two combining forms for breast are _____ and _____.
menstruation men/o menopause	**15.10** From the Greek word men, meaning month, comes the combining form that means _____, which generally occurs about once a month in the adult female. The combining form is _____. The time later in life when menstruation permanently stops (pauses) is _____.
ovari/o oophor/o -itis ovary	**15.11** Once again, the two combining forms for the ovary come from Latin and Greek roots. The adjective ovarian is built from the combining form _____, which is from the Latin word for ovary. The Greek word oophoros means egg-bearing, giving rise to the combining form _____. Recall that the common suffix for inflammation is _____. Oophoritis is an inflammation of the _____.
egg ov/i ov/o ovum or egg	**15.12** An ovum is the woman's _____, which is produced in the ovary. The two combining forms for egg are very similar: _____ and _____. Ovigenesis is the process of the formation and development of the _____.
salping/o inflammation	**15.13** The Greek word salpinx means trumpet or tube. It gives rise to the combining form _____, which refers to the uterine or fallopian tube, which carries the ovum from the ovary to the uterus. Salpingitis is an _____ of the uterine or fallopian tube.
basin pertaining to pelvic	**15.14** *Pelv/i*, a Latin combining form referring to the shape of a _____, was used to name the pelvis, a basin-like ring of skeletal bones at the base of the spine that is bordered on each side by the hip bones. The reproductive organs are contained in the space formed by these bones. Using the combining form meaning pelvis combined with the suffix -*ic*, meaning _____ ____, the term for this space is the _____ cavity.
toc/o difficult	**15.15** The combining form for birth is _____. Tocophobia, for example, is a morbid fear of childbirth. Recall that the prefix *dys*- means faulty, painful, or _____, and the suffix -*ia* refers

ANSWERS	REVIEW
condition of dystocia	to a _____ ____. Therefore, the term for a difficult childbirth is _____.
-arche menarche	**15.16** The suffix meaning beginning is _____. Using the combining form for menstruation, the term for the beginning of menstruation is _____.

 ## Self-Instruction: Anatomic Terms (Fig. 15-1)

Study the following:

TERM	MEANING
uterus *yū'tĕr-ŭs*	womb; a pear-shaped organ in the pelvic cavity in which the embryo and fetus develops
fundus *fŭn'dŭs*	upper portion of the uterus above the entry to the uterine tubes
endometrium *en-dō-mē'trē-ŭm*	lining of the uterus, which is shed approximately every 28 to 30 days in a nonpregnant female during menstruation
myometrium *mī-ō-mē'trē-ŭm*	muscular wall of the uterus
uterine tubes *yū'tĕr-in tūbz* **fallopian tubes** *fă-lō'pē-ăn tūbz*	tubes extending from each side of the uterus toward the ovary that provide a passage for ova to the uterus
adnexa *ad-nek'să*	uterine tubes and ovaries (uterine appendages)
right uterine appendage *rīt yū'tĕr-in ă-pen'dij*	right tube and ovary
left uterine appendage *left yū'tĕr-in ă-pen'dij*	left tube and ovary
ovary *ō'vă-rē*	one of two glands located on each side of the pelvic cavity that produce ova and female sex hormones
cervix *sĕr'viks*	neck of the uterus
cervical os *sĕr'vi-kăl os*	opening of the cervix to the uterus
vagina *vă-jī'nă*	tubular passageway from the cervix to the outside of the body

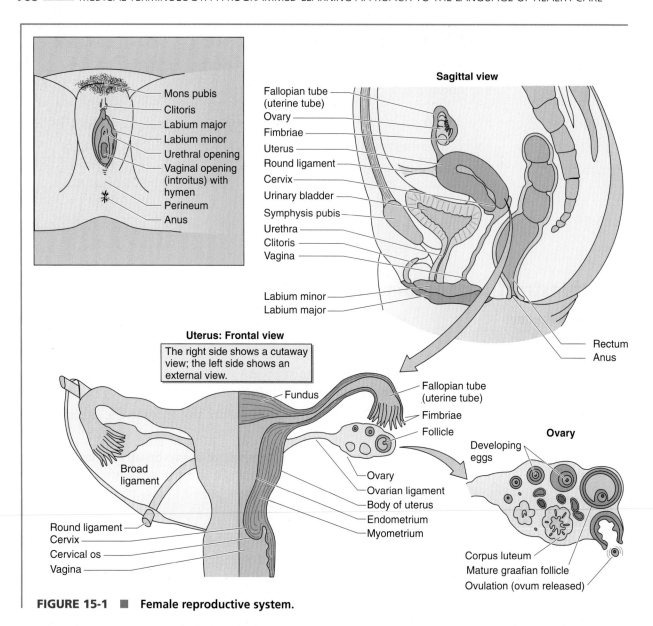

FIGURE 15-1 ■ **Female reproductive system.**

TERM	MEANING
vulva *vŭl'vă*	external genitalia of the female
labia *lā'bē-ă*	folds of tissue on either side of the vaginal opening; known as the labia majora and labia minora
clitoris *klit'ō-ris*	female erectile tissue in the anterior portion of the vulva
hymen *hī'men*	fold of mucous membrane that encircles the entrance to the vagina
introitus *in-trō'i-tŭs*	entrance to the vagina
Bartholin glands *bahr'thō-lin glanz*	two glands located on either side of the vaginal opening that secrete a lubricant during intercourse

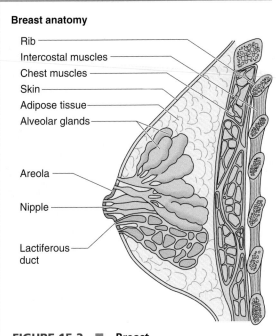

Breast anatomy

Rib
Intercostal muscles
Chest muscles
Skin
Adipose tissue
Alveolar glands

Areola

Nipple

Lactiferous
duct

FIGURE 15-2 ■ **Breast.**

TERM	MEANING
perineum *per-i-nē'ŭm*	region between the vulva and anus
mammary glands (Fig. 15-2) *mam'ă-rē glanz*	two glands in the female breasts that are capable of producing milk
mammary papilla *mam'ă-rē pă-pil'ă*	nipple
areola *ă-rē'ō-lă*	dark-pigmented area around the nipple
embryo (Fig. 15-3) *em'brē-ō*	the developing organism from fertilization to the end of the eighth week

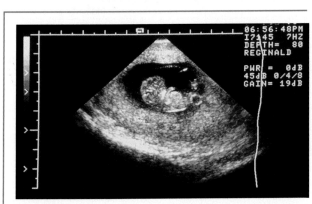

FIGURE 15-3 ■ **Two-dimensional sonogram of an 8-week embryo.**

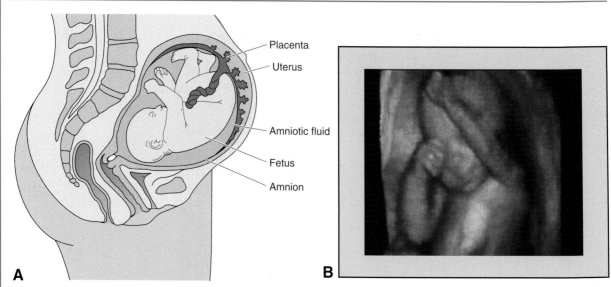

A

B

FIGURE 15-4 ■ A. Fetus in utero. B. Three-dimensional sonogram of fetus "waking up."

TERM	MEANING
fetus (Fig. 15-4) *fē'tŭs*	the developing organism from the ninth week to birth
placenta *plă-sen'tă*	vascular organ that develops in the uterine wall during pregnancy to provide nourishment for the fetus (*placenta* = cake)
amnion *am'nē-on* **amniotic sac** *am-nē-ot'ik sak*	innermost of the membranes surrounding the embryo in the uterus, filled with amniotic fluid
amniotic fluid *am-nē-ot'ik flū'id*	fluid within the amniotic sac that surrounds and protects the fetus
meconium *mē-kō'nē-ŭm*	intestinal discharges of the fetus that form the first stools in the newborn

🔷 Programmed Review: Anatomic Terms

ANSWERS	REVIEW
vulva perineum	**15.17** The external genitalia of the female are collectively called the _____. The region between the vulva in the female (the scrotum in the male) and the anus is called the _____.
labia clitoris	**15.18** The vulva consist of the folds of tissue on either side of the vaginal opening, called the _____ majora and minor, and the female erectile tissue, called the _____. The labia majora are the larger tissue folds, and within them are the labia minora, the smaller tissue folds.

ANSWERS	REVIEW
hymen	**15.19** Inward from the labia, the fold of mucous membrane encircling the entrance to the vagina is called the _____.
introitus Bartholin	**15.20** The term for the entrance to the vagina is used in medical language for the entrance to other hollow organs as well. It comes from the Latin intro-eo, meaning to go into. This term is _____. Two glands located on either side of the vaginal opening, called _____ glands, secrete a lubricant during intercourse.
cervix neck cervical os	**15.21** The vagina is a tubular passageway between the _____ and the outside of the body, where the penis is inserted during intercourse. The cervix is the _____ of the uterus. The term for the opening of the cervix to the uterus, using the Latin word os (meaning mouth) is _____ _____. The term os is used in other anatomic areas to indicate an opening to a hollow organ or canal.
uterus fundus fundi	**15.22** The cervix is the neck of the _____ (the womb), where, after conception, the embryo and fetus develop. The upper part of the uterus, above the uterine tubes, is called the _____, from the Latin word fundus, referring to the largest part of a sac farthest from the opening. The plural of fundus is _____.
uterus myometrium within endometrium	**15.23** The combining form *metr/o* refers to the _____. The suffix *-ium* refers to a structure or tissue. The combining form *my/o* means muscle. Therefore, the term for the muscular wall of the uterus is the _____. Recall that the prefix *endo-* means _____. Within the uterus is a tissue that forms its lining, which is shed during menstruation and is called the _____.
ova ovaries ovum	**15.24** Human eggs, called _____, are produced in each of the two _____. The ovaries also secrete female sex hormones. The singular of ova is _____.
fallopian appendage	**15.25** The tubes through which the ova move from the ovaries to the uterus are called the _____ or uterine tubes. The right tube and ovary collectively are called the right uterine _____. The left tube and ovary are called the left

ANSWERS	REVIEW
uterine adnexa	_____ appendage. The collective term for both uterine appendages is the _____.
uterus ovum	**15.26** Sperm deposited in the vagina during intercourse swim through the cervix into the _____. Sperm may meet an egg, or _____, in the uterus or fallopian tubes, and fertilization may occur.
embryo endometrium	**15.27** If fertilization occurs, the resultant developing organism, called an _____ for the first 8 weeks, is implanted in the lining of the uterus, called the _____.
placenta	**15.28** The vascular (blood-rich) organ that develops in the uterine wall to nourish the embryo and fetus is called the _____.
amniotic sac fluid	**15.29** The membrane sac surrounding the embryo is the _____ _____. It is filled with a protective fluid called amniotic _____.
fetus	**15.30** After 8 weeks, the developing organism is no longer called an embryo; instead, it is called a _____.
meconium	**15.31** The first stools of a newborn develop from intestinal discharges of the fetus, called _____.
mamm/o mammary	**15.32** Recall that the two combining forms for breast are *mast/o* and _____. Using the adjective form of the latter, the term for the glands in the female breast that make milk is _____ glands.
nipple	**15.33** The mammary papilla is the _____ of the breast, through which milk flows to the infant.

◆ Self-Instruction: Gynecologic Symptomatic Terms

Study the following:

TERM	MEANING
amenorrhea ă-men-ō-rē′ă	absence of menstruation
dysmenorrhea dis-men-ō-rē′ă	painful menstruation

TERM	MEANING
oligomenorrhea *ol'i-gō-men-ō-rē'ă*	scanty menstrual period
anovulation *an-ov-yū-lā'shŭn*	absence of ovulation
dyspareunia *dis-pa-rū'nē-ă*	painful intercourse (coitus) (*dys* = painful; *para* = alongside of; *eunia* = bed)
leukorrhea *lū-kō-rē'ă*	abnormal white or yellow vaginal discharge
menorrhagia *men-ō-rā'jē-ă*	excessive bleeding at the time of menstruation (menses)
metrorrhagia *mē'trō-rā'jē-ă*	bleeding from the uterus at any time other than normal menstruation
oligo-ovulation *ol'i-gō-ov'yū-lā'shŭn*	irregular ovulation

Programmed Review: Gynecologic Symptomatic Terms

ANSWERS	REVIEW
men/o discharge, without amenorrhea	**15.34** The combining form for menstruation is _____. A number of symptomatic terms for different menstrual conditions are made with this combining form. Recall that the suffix *-rrhea* means _____. The prefix *a-* means _____. Therefore, the term for being without menstrual discharge (the absence of menstruation) is _____.
painful dysmenorrhea	**15.35** The prefix *dys-* means faulty, difficult, or _____. The term for painful menstruation (menstrual discharge) is _____.
deficient oligomenorrhea	**15.36** The prefix *oligo-* means few or _____. The term for scanty (deficient) menstrual discharge is _____.
oligo-ovulation	**15.37** The same prefix (*-oligo*) is used in the term for irregular (deficient) ovulation: _____-_____.
without anovulation	**15.38** The prefix *an-* means _____. The absence of ovulation, therefore, is termed _____.
blood or bleeding menorrhagia	**15.39** The suffix *-rrhagia* means to burst forth, usually referring to _____. Excessive bleeding during menstruation is therefore called _____.

ANSWERS	REVIEW
uterus metrorrhagia	**15.40** The combining form *metr/o* means _____. Using this combining form, excessive bleeding from the uterus, other than in normal menstruation, is called _____.
leukorrhea	**15.41** The combining form *leuk/o* means white. An abnormal white or yellow discharge (from the vagina) is termed _____.
painful, difficult, or faulty dyspareunia	**15.42** Using the prefix *dys-* (meaning _____), painful intercourse is called _____.

◈ Self-Instruction: Gynecologic Diagnostic Terms: General

Study the following:

TERM	MEANING
cervicitis *ser-vi-sī'tis*	inflammation of the cervix
congenital anomalies *kon-jen'ĭ-tăl ah-nom'ah-lēz* **congenital irregularities** *kon-jen'ĭ-tăl ir-reg'yū-lār'ĭ-tēz*	birth defects that cause abnormal development of an organ or a structure (e.g., double uterus or absent vagina)
dermoid cyst *dĕr'moyd sist*	congenital tumor composed of displaced embryonic tissue (teeth, bone, cartilage, and hair); typically found in an ovary and usually benign
displacement of uterus (Fig. 15-5) *dis-plās'ment of yū'tĕr-ŭs*	displacement of the uterus from its normal position
anteflexion *an-tē-flek'shŭn*	abnormal forward bending of the uterus (*ante* = before; *flexus* = bend)
retroflexion *re-trō-flek'shŭn*	abnormal backward bending of the uterus
retroversion *re-trō-vĕr'zhŭn*	backward turn of the whole uterus; also called tipped uterus
endometriosis *en'dō-mē-trē-ō'sis*	condition characterized by migration of portions of endometrial tissue outside the uterine cavity
endometritis *en'dō-mē-trī'tis*	inflammation of the endometrium
fibroid (Fig. 15-6) *fī'broyd* **fibromyoma** *fī'brō-mī-ō'mă* **leiomyoma** *lī'ō-mī-ō'mă*	benign tumor in the uterus composed of smooth muscle and fibrous connective tissue

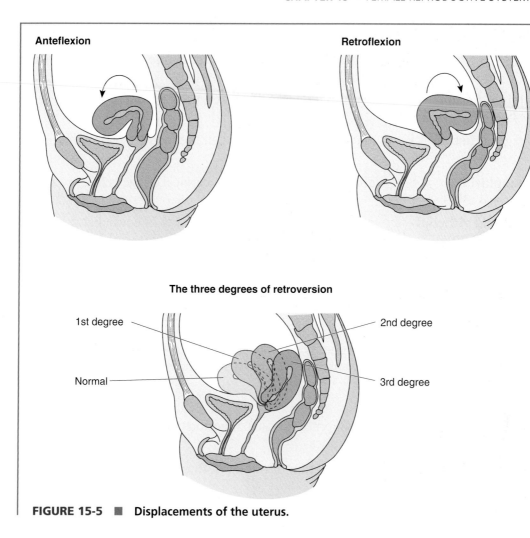

Anteflexion

Retroflexion

The three degrees of retroversion

1st degree

Normal

2nd degree

3rd degree

FIGURE 15-5 ■ **Displacements of the uterus.**

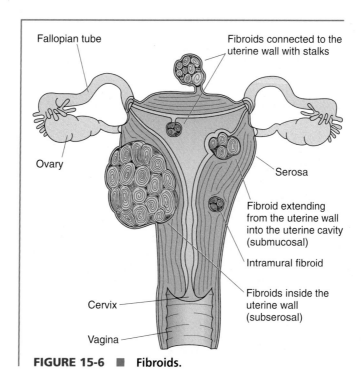

Fallopian tube

Fibroids connected to the uterine wall with stalks

Ovary

Serosa

Fibroid extending from the uterine wall into the uterine cavity (submucosal)

Intramural fibroid

Cervix

Fibroids inside the uterine wall (subserosal)

Vagina

FIGURE 15-6 ■ **Fibroids.**

TERM	MEANING
fistula *fis'tyū-lă*	abnormal passage, such as from one hollow organ to another (*fistula* = pipe)
rectovaginal fistula *rek-tō-vaj'i-năl fis'tyū-lăk*	abnormal opening between the vagina and rectum
vesicovaginal fistula *ves-i-kō-vaj'i-năl fis'tyū-lă*	abnormal opening between the bladder and vagina
cervical neoplasia *sĕr'vi-kăl nē-ō-plā'zē-ă*	abnormal development of cervical tissue cells

cervical intraepithelial neoplasia (CIN)
 sĕr'vi-kăl in'tră-ep-i-thē'lē-ăl nē-ō-plā'zē-ă
 cervical dysplasia
 (*see* Fig. 15-11B)
 sĕr'vi-kăl dis-plā'zē-ă
	potentially cancerous abnormality of epithelial tissue of the cervix, graded according to the extent of abnormal cell formation:
	    CIN-1: mild dysplasia
	    CIN-2: moderate dysplasia
	    CIN-3: severe dysplasia

carcinoma in situ (CIS) of the cervix *kar-si-nō'mă in sī'tū of the sĕr'viks*	malignant cell changes of the cervix that are localized, without any spread to adjacent structures
menopause *men'ō-pawz*	cessation of menstrual periods caused by lack of ovarian hormones
oophoritis *ō'of-ōr-ī'tis*	inflammation of one or both ovaries
parovarian cyst *par-ō-var'ē-ăn sist*	cyst of the uterine tube (fallopian tube)
pelvic adhesions *pel'vik ad-hē'zhŭnz*	scarring of tissue within the pelvic cavity resulting from endometriosis, infection, or injury
pelvic inflammatory disease (PID) *pel'vik in-flam'ă-tōr-ē di-zēz'*	inflammation of organs in the pelvic cavity; usually includes the fallopian tubes, ovaries, and endometrium; most often caused by bacteria
pelvic floor relaxation (Fig. 15-7) *pel'vik flōr rē-lak-sā'shŭn*	relaxation of supportive ligaments of the pelvic organs
cystocele *sis'tō-sēl*	pouching of the bladder into the vagina
rectocele *rek'tō-sēl*	pouching of the rectum into the vagina
enterocele *en'tĕr-ō-sēl*	pouching sac of peritoneum between the vagina and the rectum
urethrocele *yū-rē'thrō-sēl*	pouching of the urethra into the vagina
prolapse *prō-laps'*	descent of the uterus down the vaginal canal

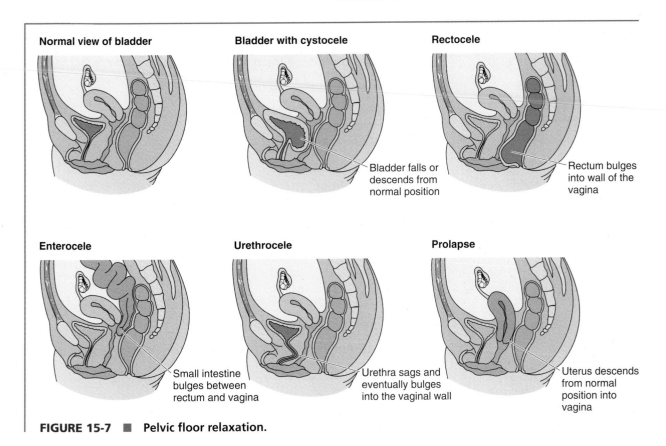

FIGURE 15-7 ■ Pelvic floor relaxation.

TERM	MEANING
salpingitis *sal-pin-jī'tis*	inflammation of a fallopian tube
vaginitis *vaj-i-nī'tis*	inflammation of the vagina with redness, swelling, and irritation; often caused by a specific organism, such as *Candida* (yeast) or *Trichomonas* (a sexually transmitted parasite)
atrophic vaginitis *ă-trof'ik vaj-i-nī'tis*	thinning of the vagina and loss of moisture because of depletion of estrogen, which causes inflammation of tissue
vaginosis *vaj-i-nō'sis*	infection of the vagina, with little or no inflammation, characterized by a milk-like discharge and an unpleasant odor; also known as nonspecific vaginitis

◆ Programmed Review: Gynecologic Diagnostic Terms: General

ANSWERS	REVIEW
-itis cervicitis	**15.43** The suffix for inflammation is _____. Inflammation of the cervix is called _____.
oophor/o oophoritis	**15.44** The two combining forms for the ovaries are *ovari/o* and _____. Using the latter, inflammation of the ovaries is termed _____.

ANSWERS	REVIEW
salping/o salpingitis	**15.45** The combining form for fallopian tube (or eustachian tube) is _____. Therefore, the term for inflammation of the fallopian tube is _____.
endometritis	**15.46** Inflammation of the endometrium is _____.
condition endometriosis	**15.47** The suffix *-osis* means increase or _____. Another condition of the endometrium, which involves endometrial tissue migrating outside the uterus, is called _____.
anomalies or irregularities dermoid	**15.48** Birth defects involving abnormal development of a structure are called congenital _____. A congenital tumor composed of displaced embryonic tissue is called a _____ cyst.
displacement anteflexion backward version	**15.49** In some women, the uterus is in a position in the abdomen that is somewhat different from normal. This atypical position is called a _____. If the uterus is bent (flexed) forward, the position is called _____. Retroflexion, however, is an abnormal _____ bending of the uterus. If the whole uterus is tipped or turned backward, it is called retro_____.
-oma leiomyoma fiber or fibrous fibromyoma fibroid	**15.50** Muscle and connective tissue in the uterus can give rise to tumors. The common suffix for a tumor is _____. Combined with *lei/o*, meaning smooth, and *my/o*, meaning muscle, the term _____ refers to a benign smooth muscle tumor, especially of the uterus. A synonymous term uses the combining forms for muscle and tumor, preceded by the combining form *fibr/o* to indicate the _____ consistency of the tissue: _____. An additional synonym simply refers to a uterine tumor that resembles fibers: _____.
fistula rectovaginal	**15.51** An abnormal passage from one organ to another is called a _____, from the Latin word fistula (pipe). An abnormal opening between the rectum and vagina is a _____ fistula. An abnormal opening between

ANSWERS	REVIEW
vesicovaginal	the bladder (*vesic/o*) and the vagina is called a _____ fistula.
men/o menopause	**15.52** Again, the combining form for menstruation is _____. A cessation (pause) of menstruation, usually occurring in older women, is called _____.
uterine or fallopian	**15.53** A parovarian cyst is a cyst in the _____ tube.
pelvic adhesions	**15.54** Scarring of tissue in the pelvic cavity resulting from endometriosis, infection, or injury can cause pelvic tissues to adhere together; this is called _____ _____.
pelvic inflammatory	**15.55** Inflammation of the pelvic cavity, including the fallopian tubes, ovaries, and endometrium, is called _____ _____ disease (PID).
cervical neoplasia dysplasia cervical intra mild moderate severe dysplasia in situ	**15.56** Neoplasia is a general term describing a new formation of abnormal tissue, which may be benign or malignant. Any new formation of abnormal cervical tissue is called _____ _____. The term describing a condition of faulty formation of tissue with cancerous potential is _____. Cervical dysplasia is also known as _____ _____epithelial neoplasia (CIN) and is classified according to the extent of abnormal cell formation. CIN-1 refers to _____ dysplasia, CIN-2 refers to _____ dysplasia, and CIN-3 refers to _____ _____. Malignant neoplasia of the cervix that is localized without any spread to adjacent structures is called carcinoma ____ _____ (CIS) of the cervix.
pelvic floor prolapse	**15.57** Pelvic organs are supported with ligaments and other connective tissue. Relaxation of these supportive tissues, called _____ _____ relaxation, may allow anatomic changes or displacements. A descent of the uterus down the vaginal canal is called a _____.
pouching rectocele	**15.58** Recall that the suffix -*cele* means hernia or _____. A pouching of the rectum (*rect/o*) into the vagina is called a _____.

ANSWERS	REVIEW
urethrocele	**15.59** A pouching of the urethra (*urethr/o*), which is the tube that carries urine to outside of the body, into the vagina is called a _____.
cystocele	**15.60** *Cyst/o* is a combining form for bladder. A pouching of the bladder into the vagina is called a _____.
pouch	**15.61** An enterocele is a _____ing sac of peritoneum between the vagina and the rectum.
-itis vaginitis atrophic	**15.62** Recall that the suffix meaning inflammation is _____. Inflammation of the vagina is called _____ and is often caused by a specific organism such as *Candida* (yeast) or *Trichomonas* (a sexually transmitted parasite). The specific kind of vaginitis involving thinning of the vagina and loss of moisture because of depletion of estrogen is called _____ vaginitis.
condition of vaginosis	**15.63** The suffix *-osis* means increase or, simply, a _____ ____. A vaginal condition involving infection but little or no inflammation is called _____.

 # Self-Instruction: Gynecologic Diagnostic Terms: Sexually Transmitted Diseases

Study the following:

TERM	MEANING
MAJOR BACTERIAL SEXUALLY TRANSMITTED DISEASES (STDs)	
chlamydia *kla-mid'ē-ă*	most common sexually transmitted bacterial infection in North America; often occurs with no symptoms and is treated only after it has spread, such as after causing pelvic inflammatory disease (PID)
gonorrhea *gon-ō-rē'ă*	contagious inflammation of the genital mucous membranes caused by invasion of the gonococcus *Neisseria gonorrhea;* the term refers to the urethral discharge characteristic of the infection, which was first thought to be a leakage of semen (*gono* = seed; *rrhea* = discharge); the genus is named for the Polish dermatologist Albert Neisser

TERM	MEANING
syphilis *sif'i-lis*	infectious disease caused by a spirochete transmitted via direct, intimate contact and that may involve any organ or tissue over time; usually manifests first on the skin, with the appearance of small, painless, red papules that erode and form bloodless ulcers called chancres

MAJOR VIRAL STDs

TERM	MEANING
hepatitis B virus (HBV) *hep-ă-tī'tis B vī'rŭs*	virus that causes an inflammation of the liver; transmitted through any body fluid, including vaginal secretions, semen, and blood
herpes simplex virus type 2 (HSV-2) (Fig. 15-8) *hĕr'pēz sim'pleks vī'rŭs tīp 2*	virus that causes ulcer-like lesions of the genital and anorectal skin and mucosa; after the initial infection, the virus lies dormant in the nerve cell root and may recur at times of stress
human immunodeficiency virus (HIV) *hyū'măn im'yū-nō-dē-fish'en-sē vī'rŭs*	virus that causes acquired immunodeficiency syndrome (AIDS), permitting various opportunistic infections, malignancies, and neurologic diseases; contracted through exposure to contaminated blood or body fluid (e.g., semen or vaginal secretions)
human papilloma virus (HPV) (Fig. 15-9) *hyū'măn pap-i-lō'mă vī'rŭs*	virus transmitted by direct sexual contact; infection can manifest on the skin or mucous membranes of the genitals
condyloma acuminatum (pl. condylomata acuminata) *kon-di-lō'mă ă-kyū'mi-nā'tŭm (kon-di-lō-mah'tă ă-kyū'mi-nā'tă)*	lesion that appears as a result of human papilloma virus; on the skin, the lesions appear as cauliflower-like warts, and on mucous membranes, they have a flat appearance; also known as venereal or genital warts

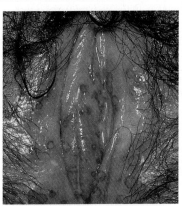

FIGURE 15-8 ■ Herpes simplex virus type 2.

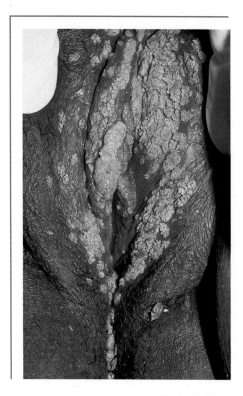

FIGURE 15-9 ■ Condylomata acuminata (genital warts) caused by human papilloma virus (HPV).

Programmed Review: Gynecologic Diagnostic Terms: Sexually Transmitted Diseases

ANSWERS	REVIEW
chlamydia	**15.64** Most sexually transmitted diseases (STDs) are caused by bacteria or viruses. The most common bacterial STD in North America is _____. Like many bacterial diseases, chlamydia gets its name from the Latin genus name for the bacteria: *Chlamydia*. It may have no symptoms until it spreads, and it can cause pelvic inflammatory disease (PID).
gonorrhea	**15.65** Another bacterial STD, the genus of which was named for the Polish dermatologist Albert Neisser, is called _____. It causes an inflammation of genital mucous membranes.
syphilis	**15.66** The bacterial STD caused by a spirochete that over time can involve any body tissue or organ is called _____.
hepatitis B	**15.67** Several viruses also cause STDs. The virus that causes inflammation of the liver, which can be spread through any body fluid, is _____ ____ virus (HBV).

ANSWERS	REVIEW
herpes simplex virus	**15.68** HSV-2 is the abbreviation for the STD virus which typically lies dormant after the initial infection but recurs at times of stress: _____ _____ _____ type 2. It causes ulcer-like lesions on genital and anorectal skin.
human immunodeficiency virus	**15.69** The virus that causes acquired immunodeficiency syndrome (AIDS) is _____ _____ _____ (HIV).
papilloma condylomata, acuminata	**15.70** HPV is the abbreviation for human _____ virus, which is characterized by lesions on the skin or mucous membranes. A condyloma is a warty growth; the plural of this term is _____. Condylomata _____ are warty growths in the genital area caused by HPV.

 ## Self-Instruction: Gynecologic Diagnostic Terms: Breasts

Study the following:

TERM	MEANING
adenocarcinoma of the breast *ad'ĕ-nō-kar-si-nō'mă of the brest*	malignant tumor of glandular breast tissue
amastia *ă-mas'tē-ă*	absence of a breast
fibrocystic breasts *fī-brō-sis'tik brests*	benign condition of the breast consisting of fibrous and cystic changes that render the tissue more dense; patient feels painful lumps that fluctuate with menstrual periods
gynecomastia *gī'nĕ-kō-mas'tē-ă*	development of mammary glands in the male caused by altered hormone levels
hypermastia *hī-pĕr-mas'tē-ă* **macromastia** *mak-rō-mas'tē-ă*	abnormally large breasts
hypomastia *hī'po-mas'tē-ă* **micromastia** *mī'kro-mas'tē-ă*	unusually small breasts
mastitis *mas-tī'tis*	inflammation of the breast; most commonly occurs in women who are breastfeeding

TERM	MEANING
polymastia *pol-ē-mas'tē-ă*	presence of more than two breasts
polythelia *pol-ē-thē'lē-ă* **supernumerary nipples** *sū-pĕr-nū'mĕr-ār-ē nip'ĕlz*	presence of more than one nipple on a breast

🔷 Programmed Review: Gynecologic Diagnostic Terms: Breasts

ANSWERS	REVIEW
mast/o condition of, without amastia	**15.71** There are two combining forms for breast: *mamm/o* and _____. The latter is used more frequently in gynecologic diagnostic terms. Recall that the suffix *-ia* means _____ _____. The prefix *a-* means _____. Thus, the condition of an absence of a breast is _____.
excessive hypermastia large macromastia	**15.72** The prefix *hyper-* means above or _____. The condition of abnormally large breasts is called _____. Recall that the prefix *macro-* means long or _____. It is used to form a synonym for hypermastia: _____.
hypo- micro- hypomastia, micromastia	**15.73** The prefix with a meaning opposite to that of *hyper-* is _____. The prefix with a meaning opposite to that of *macro-* is _____. Therefore, two terms for unusually small breasts are _____ and _____.
many polymastia condition of	**15.74** The prefix *poly-* means _____. The condition of having more than two (many) breasts is termed _____. The suffix *-ia* means _____ _____.
woman gynecomastia	**15.75** The combining form *gynec/o* means _____. The condition of a man developing mammary glands (i.e., developing like a woman) is called _____.
-itis mastitis	**15.76** Again, the suffix denoting inflammation is _____. An inflammation of the breast is called _____.
fibrocystic	**15.77** A benign condition of the breasts in which fibrous and cystic changes occur is referred to as _____ breasts.
malignant	**15.78** An adenocarcinoma of the breast is a _____ tumor of glandular breast tissue.

ANSWERS	REVIEW
	15.79 The Greek word for nipple is thele. The prefix *poly-* means
many	_____. The condition of having more than one nipple on a
polythelia	breast is called _____. These are also called
numerary	super_____ nipples.

Self-Instruction: Gynecologic Diagnostic Tests and Procedures

Study the following:

TEST OR PROCEDURE	EXPLANATION
biopsy (Bx) (Fig. 15-10) *bī'op-sē*	removal of tissue for microscopic pathologic examination
aspiration biopsy *as-pi-rā'shŭn bī'op-sē* **needle biopsy** *nēd'ĕl bī'op-sē*	needle draw of tissue or fluid from a cavity for cytologic examination

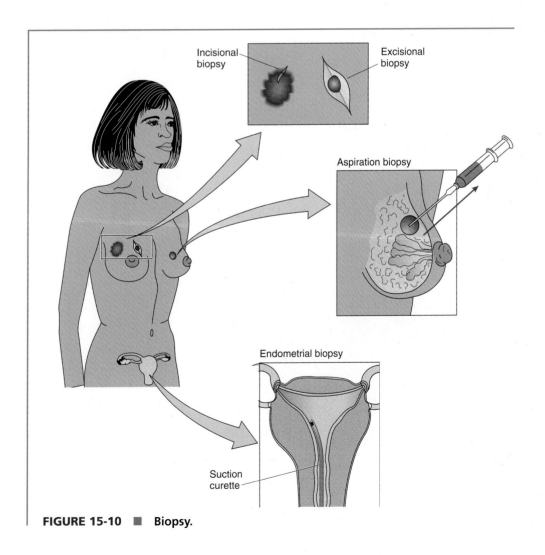

FIGURE 15-10 ▬ **Biopsy.**

TEST OR PROCEDURE	EXPLANATION
endoscopic biopsy *en′dō-skop′ik bī′op-sē*	removal of a specimen for biopsy during an endoscopic procedure (e.g., colposcopy)
excisional biopsy *ek-sizh′ŭn-ăl bī′op-sē*	removal of an entire lesion for microscopic examination
incisional biopsy *in-si′zhŭn-năl bī′op-sē*	removal of a piece of suspicious tissue for microscopic examination (e.g., cervical or endometrial biopsy)
stereotactic breast biopsy *ster′ē-ō-tak′tik brest bī′op-sē*	use of x-ray imaging, a specialized stereotactic frame, and a computer to calculate, precisely locate, and direct a needle into a breast lesion to remove a core specimen for biopsy
sentinel node breast biopsy *sen′tĭ-nel nōd bī′op-sē*	biopsy of the sentinel node (the first lymph node to receive lymphatic drainage from a tumor) in a breast with early cancer to determine metastases and, if no malignancy is found, to avoid the extensive removal of axillary nodes, which causes lymphedema (swelling under the arms); includes radionuclide imaging to locate the sentinel node (sentinel refers to guarding a point of entry)

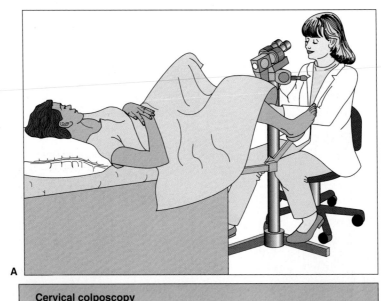

A

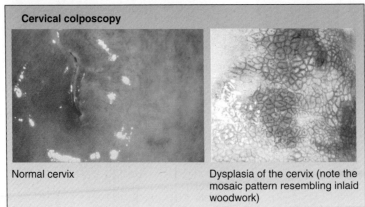

Cervical colposcopy

Normal cervix

Dysplasia of the cervix (note the mosaic pattern resembling inlaid woodwork)

B

FIGURE 15-11 ■ **A. Colposcopy. B. Photographs taken during cervical colposcopy.**

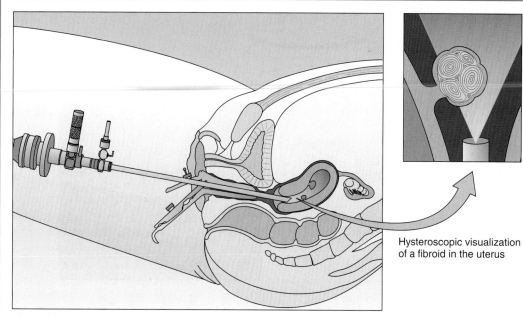

Hysteroscopic visualization of a fibroid in the uterus

FIGURE 15-12 ■ Hysteroscopy.

TEST OR PROCEDURE	EXPLANATION
colposcopy (Fig. 15-11) *kol-pos'kŏ-pē*	examination of the vagina and cervix using a colposcope, a specialized microscope which often has a camera attachment for photographs; used to document findings and for follow-up treatments
hysteroscopy (Fig. 15-12) *his-tĕr-os'kŏ-pē*	use of a hysteroscope to examine the intrauterine cavity for assessment of abnormalities (e.g., polyps, fibroids, or anomalies)
magnetic resonance imaging (MRI) *mag-net'ik rez'ō-nănts im'ă-jing*	use of nonionizing images to detect gynecologic conditions (e.g., anomalies of the pelvis or soft tissues of the breast) or to stage tumors arising from the endometrium or cervix
Papanicolaou (Pap) smear *pa-pă-ni'kō-lū (pap) smēr*	study of cells collected from the cervix to screen for cancer and other abnormalities
radiography *rā'dē-og'ră-fē*	x-ray imaging
hysterosalpingogram *his'tĕr-ō-sal-ping'gō-gram*	x-ray of the fallopian tubes after injection of a contrast medium through the cervix; used to determine tubal patency (openness)
mammogram *mam'ō-gram*	low-dose x-ray imaging of breast tissue to detect neoplasms
pelvic sonography (Fig. 15-13) *pel'vik sŏ-nog'ră-fē*	ultrasound imaging of the female pelvis

endovaginal sonogram
    en'dō-vaj'i-năl son'ō-gram
    transvaginal sonogram
    tranz-vaj'ĭ-năl son'ō-gram
	ultrasound image of the uterus, tubes, and ovaries made with the ultrasonic transducer within the vagina to detect conditions such as ectopic pregnancy or missed abortion

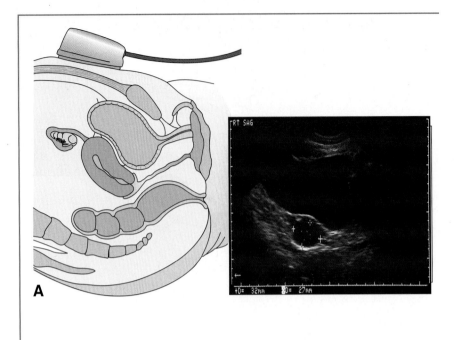

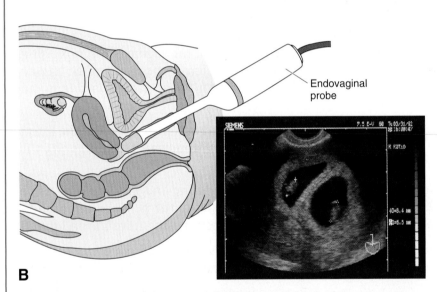

FIGURE 15-13 ▨ **Pelvic sonography. A. Transabdominal imaging procedure.** *Inset*, simple ovarian cyst. **B. Endovaginal (transvaginal) imaging procedure.** *Inset*, twin pregnancies.

TEST OR PROCEDURE	EXPLANATION
sonohysterogram *son'ō-his-tĕr-ō-gram* **hysterosonogram** *his-tĕr-ō-son'ō-gram* **saline infusion sonogram** *sā'lēn in-fyū'zhŭn son'ō-gram*	transvaginal sonographic image made as sterile saline is injected into the uterus; used to assess uterine pathology or to determine tubal patency
transabdominal sonogram *trans-ab-dom'i-năl son'ō-gram*	ultrasound image of the lower abdomen, including the bladder, uterus, tubes, and ovaries, to detect conditions such as cysts and tumors

Programmed Review: Gynecologic Diagnostic Tests and Procedures

ANSWERS	REVIEW
biopsy	**15.80** The removal of tissue from any part of the body for microscopic pathologic examination is called _____ (Bx). Several forms of biopsies can be performed in the female reproductive system.
needle	Use of a special, hollow needle to draw tissue or fluid from a cavity is called an aspiration biopsy or a _____ biopsy. If the entire lesion is removed (excised) for examination,
excisional	this is called an _____ biopsy. Removal of the biopsy specimen during an endoscopic examination is called an
endoscopic	_____ biopsy. Cutting out (incising) a small tissue
incisional	sample for examination is called an _____ biopsy.
stereotactic breast	**15.81** Use of a computer, x-ray imaging, and a specialized stereotactic frame to direct a needle into a breast lesion to remove a core specimen for biopsy is called a _____ _____ biopsy.
sentinel node biopsy	**15.82** Sentinel refers to guarding a point of entry. The first lymph node to receive lymphatic drainage from a tumor therefore is referred to as the _____ node. Removal and microscopic pathologic examination of this node in a breast with early cancer is called a sentinel _____ _____.
process colp/o colposcopy	**15.83** Recall that the suffix *-scopy* means _____ of examination with an instrument. The two combining forms for vagina are *vagin/o* and _____. Using the latter form, the term for examination of the vagina using a specialized microscope is called _____.
hyster/o hysteroscopy	**15.84** Recall that the combining forms for uterus are *metr/o*, *uter/o*, and _____. Utilize the last form in the term for use of a special microscope to examine inside the uterus: _____.

ANSWERS	REVIEW
magnetic resonance	**15.85** Gynecologic conditions are also diagnosed with nonionizing images made using _____ _____ imaging (MRI).
Pap	**15.86** The study of cells collected form the cervix to screen for abnormalities is called (in short) a _____ smear, named for Dr. Papanicolaou.
radiography record mamm/o mammogram	**15.87** The medical term for x-ray imaging is _____. Recall that the suffix *-gram* means _____. The two combining forms for breast are *mast/o* and _____. Formed from the latter, the x-ray record of breast tissue made to detect neoplasms is called a _____.
salping/o uterus hysterosalpingogram	**15.88** The combining form for fallopian tube is _____. The medical term for an x-ray of the fallopian tubes after injection of a contrast medium uses this combining form as well as *hyster/o*, which means _____. This kind of x-ray image is called a _____.
pelvic within endovaginal through transvaginal transabdominal	**15.89** Sonography is the imaging modality using ultrasound. Ultrasound imaging of the female's pelvic area is called _____ sonography. Recall that the prefix *endo-* means _____. A sonogram made with the ultrasound transducer within the vagina is called an _____ sonogram. The prefix *trans-* means across or _____. An endovaginal sonogram is also called a _____ sonogram, because the sound waves pass through the vagina. An ultrasound image of the whole lower abdomen is called a _____ sonogram.
hyster/o sonohysterogram or hysterosonogram	**15.90** Recall that the combining forms for uterus are *metr/o*, *uter/o*, and _____. Formed from the last of these combining forms, the term for a sonogram of the uterus made as sterile saline is injected into the uterus, is called a _____.

Self-Instruction: Gynecologic Operative Terms: General

Study the following:

TERM	MEANING
adhesiolysis *ad-hēz-ē-ōl'ĭ-sis* **adhesiotomy** *ad-hē-zē-ot'ŏ-mē*	breaking down or severing of pelvic adhesions
cervical conization *sĕr'vi-kăl kō-nī-zā'shŭn*	removal of a cone-shaped portion of the cervix
colporrhaphy *kol-pōr'ă-fē*	suture to repair the vagina
colporrhaphy anterior repair *kol-pōr'ă-fē an-tēr'ē-ōr rē-pār'*	repair of a cystocele
colporrhaphy posterior repair *kol-pōr'ă-fē pos-tēr'ē-ŏr rē-pār'*	repair of a rectocele
colporrhaphy A&P repair *kol-pōr'ă-fē ā and pē rē-pār'*	anterior and posterior repair of cystocele and rectocele
cryosurgery (Fig. 15-14) *krī-ō-sŭr'jĕr-ē*	method of destroying tissue by freezing; used for treating dysplasia and early cancers
dilation and curettage (D&C) (Fig. 15-15) *dī-lā'shŭn and kū-rĕ-tahzh'*	dilation of the cervix and scraping of the endometrium to control bleeding, to obtain tissue for biopsy, or to remove polyps or products of conception

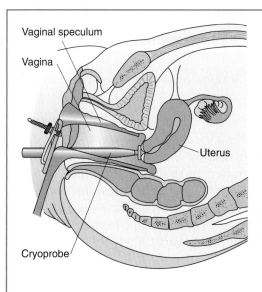

Vaginal speculum

Vagina

Uterus

Cryoprobe

A

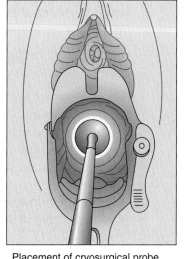

Placement of cryosurgical probe at treatment site

B

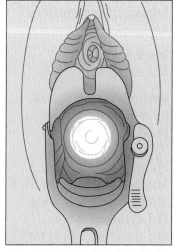

Ice crystals seen immediately after freezing treatment

C

FIGURE 15-14 ▬ **Cryosurgical procedure.**

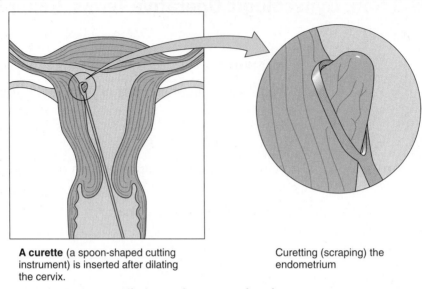

A **curette** (a spoon-shaped cutting instrument) is inserted after dilating the cervix.

Curetting (scraping) the endometrium

FIGURE 15-15 ▮ **Dilation and curettage (D&C).**

TERM	MEANING
hysterectomy *his-tĕr-ek'tŏ-mē*	removal of the uterus
abdominal hysterectomy *ab-dom'i-năl his-tĕr-ek'tŏ-mē*	removal of the uterus through an incision in the abdomen
vaginal hysterectomy *vaj'i-năl his-tĕr-ek'tŏ-mē*	removal of the uterus through the vagina
total hysterectomy *tō'tăl his-ter-ek'tŏ-mē*	removal of the uterus and the cervix
laparoscopy *lap-ă-ros'kŏ-pē*	inspection of the abdominal or pelvic cavity with a laparoscope, which is an endoscope used to examine the abdominal and pelvic regions
laparoscopic surgery *lap-ă-ro-skop'ik sŭr'jĕr-ē*	surgical procedures within the abdominal or pelvic region using a laparoscope
laser surgery *lā'zer sŭr'jĕr-ē*	use of a laser to destroy lesions or to dissect or cut tissue; used frequently in gynecology
loop electrosurgical excision procedure (LEEP) (Fig. 15-16) *lūp ē-lek-trŏ-sŭr'jik-ăl ek-sizh'ŭn prŏ-sē'jŭr* **large-loop excision of the transformation zone (LLETZ)** *larj-lūp ek-sizh'ŭn of the trans-fŏr-mā'shŭn zōn*	use of electrosurgical or radio waves transformed through a loop-configured electrosurgical device to treat precancerous cervical lesions by simultaneous excisional biopsy and treatment of affected tissue (e.g., cervical dysplasia or human papilloma virus [HPV] lesions); note that the transformation zone is the area of the cervix (between the endocervix and ectocervix), where neoplasia (new abnormal cell formation) is most likely to arise
myomectomy *mī-ō-mek'tŏ-mē*	excision of fibroid tumors

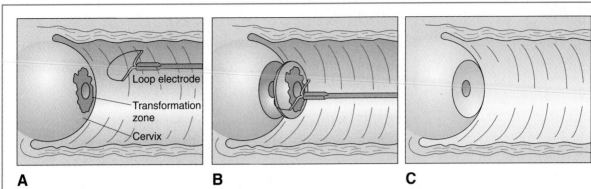

A   **B**   **C**

FIGURE 15-16 ■ **Loop electrosurgical excision procedure (LEEP) or large-loop excision of the transformation zone (LLETZ). A. Electrode approach. B. Removal of transformation zone. C. Excision site (region between endocervix and ectocervix).**

TERM	MEANING
oophorectomy *ō'of-ōr-ek'tŏ-mē*	excision of an ovary
ovarian cystectomy *ō-var'ē-ăn sis-tek'tō-mē*	excision of an ovarian cyst
salpingectomy *sal-pin-jek'tŏ-mē*	excision of a uterine tube
bilateral salpingo-oophorectomy *bi-lat'ĕr-ăl sal-ping'gō-ō-of-ō-rek'tŏ-mē*	excision of both uterine tubes and ovaries
salpingotomy *sal-pin-jek'tō-mē*	incision into a fallopian tube; often performed to remove an ectopic pregnancy
salpingostomy *sal-ping-gos'tō-mē*	creation of an opening in the fallopian tube to open a blockage
tubal ligation *tū'băl lī-gā'shŭn*	sterilization of a woman by cutting and tying (ligating) the uterine tubes

◈ Programmed Review: Gynecologic Operative Terms: General

ANSWERS	REVIEW
excision hysterectomy abdominal vaginal total hysterectomy	**15.91** Recall that the suffix *-ectomy* means _____ (or removal). Removal of the uterus is called _____. When performed through an incision in the abdomen, it is called an _____ hysterectomy. When removed through the vagina, it is called a _____ hysterectomy. The total removal of the uterus and cervix is called a _____ _____.

ANSWERS	REVIEW
myomectomy	**15.92** A tumor of muscle tissue is called a myoma. Surgical removal of fibroid tumors from the muscle tissue of the uterus is called _____.
ovary oophorectomy	**15.93** The combining form *oophor/o* means _____. Excision of an ovary is _____.
ovarian cystectomy	**15.94** Removal of an ovarian cyst is called an _____ _____.
salping/o salpingectomy	**15.95** The combining form for uterine (fallopian) tube is _____. Excision of a fallopian tube is called _____.
both both bilateral salpingo-oophorectomy	**15.96** The prefix *bi-* means two or _____. Thus, the term bilateral generally means on _____ sides. The term for excision of both uterine (fallopian) tubes and ovaries is _____ _____-_____.
incision salpingotomy	**15.97** The operative suffix *-tomy* means _____. An incision into a fallopian tube is called a _____.
opening salpingostomy	**15.98** The surgical suffix *-stomy* means the creation of an _____. The creation of an opening in the fallopian tube to open a blockage is called a _____.
tubal ligation	**15.99** Ligation means tying off. The procedure for cutting and tying the uterine tubes to cause sterilization is _____ _____.
-tomy adhesiotomy breaking down	**15.100** The surgical suffix for incision is _____. The breaking down or cutting of pelvic adhesions is called adhesiolysis or _____. The suffix *-lysis* means _____ _____ or dissolution.
cervical conization	**15.101** The surgical removal of a cone-shaped portion of the cervix is called _____ _____.
suture colp/o colporrhaphy	**15.102** The surgical suffix *-rrhaphy* means _____. The two combining forms for vagina are *vagin/o* and _____. Formed from the latter form, a suture to repair the vagina is termed _____. A repair of a cystocele

ANSWERS	REVIEW
anterior	(in the front of the vagina) is an _____ repair. The repair of a rectocele (the back of the vagina) is called a
posterior repair pouching or hernia A&P	_____ _____. Recall that -*cele* means a _____. When both the bladder and the rectum pouch into the vagina, creating both a cystocele and a rectocele, the repair of both is called an _____ repair (anterior and posterior repair).
cryosurgery	**15.103** The combining form *cry/o* means cold. Surgery that destroys tissue by freezing it is called _____. This is used for treating dysplasia and early cancers.
cervix dilation, curettage	**15.104** The D&C procedure is performed to control bleeding, to obtain tissue for biopsy, or to remove polyps or the products of conception. The _____ is dilated, and the endometrium is scraped (curettage). The abbreviation D&C stands for _____ and _____.
examination laparoscopy laparoscopic	**15.105** Recall that the suffix -*scopy* means process of _____ with a visualizing instrument. The combining form *lapar/o* refers to the abdomen generally. Thus, the examination of the abdominal and pelvic cavity with a special scope is called a _____. Surgery performed through the laparoscope is called _____ surgery.
laser	**15.106** A laser is often used in gynecologic procedures to destroy lesions or cut tissue. This is called _____ surgery.
loop electrosurgical excision transformation zone	**15.107** LEEP refers to a procedure using a loop-shaped device to make an electrosurgical excision of the transformation zone of the cervix; it is used to treat precancerous lesions, such as cervical dysplasia. LEEP is the abbreviation for _____ _____ _____ procedure. This procedure is also called LLETZ, or large-loop excision of the _____ _____.

Self-Instruction: Gynecologic Operative Terms: Breasts

Study the following:

TERM	MEANING
lumpectomy *lŭmp-ek'tŏ-mē*	excision of a breast tumor without removing any other tissue or lymph nodes; usually followed by radiation or chemotherapy if the tumor is cancerous
mastectomy (Fig. 15-17) *mas-tek'tŏ-mē*	removal of a breast
simple mastectomy *sĭm'pel mas-tek'tŏ-mē*	removal of an entire breast but with the underlying muscle and axillary lymph nodes left intact

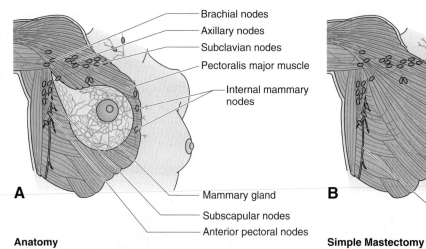

A

Anatomy
The breast, the underlying muscles, and the lymph nodes are the structures involved in breast cancer surgery. The lymph nodes, which act as barriers against bacteria or tumor cells, are useful in staging breast cancer.

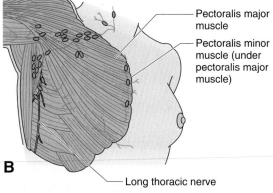

B

Simple Mastectomy
Only the breast is removed. The underlying muscle and associated lymph nodes are not removed.

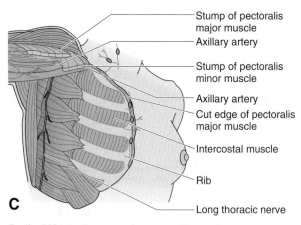

C

Radical Mastectomy
The breast, pectoralis muscles, and contents of the axilla (including lymph nodes and adipose tissue) are removed.

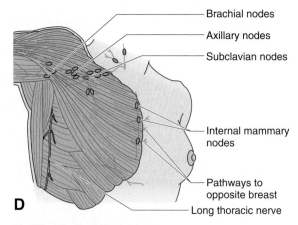

D

Modified Radical Mastectomy
The breast and lymph nodes of the axilla are removed. Occasionally, the pectoralis minor muscle is transected or removed to approach the lymph nodes.

FIGURE 15-17 ■ A. Anatomy of breast. B–D. Mastectomy alternatives.

TERM	MEANING
radical mastectomy *rad'i-kăl mas-tek'tŏ-mē*	removal of an entire breast along with the underlying chest muscles and axillary lymph nodes
modified radical mastectomy *mod'i-fīd rad'i-kăl mas-tek'tŏ-mē*	removal of an entire breast and lymph nodes of the axilla
mammoplasty *mam'ō-plas-tē*	surgical reconstruction of a breast
augmentation mammoplasty (Fig. 15-18) *awg-men-tā'shŭn mam'ō-plas-tē*	reconstruction to enlarge the breast, often by insertion of an implant
reduction mammoplasty *rē-dŭk'shŭn mam'ō-plas-tē*	reconstruction to remove excessive breast tissue
mastopexy *mas'tō-pek-sē*	elevation of pendulous breast tissue

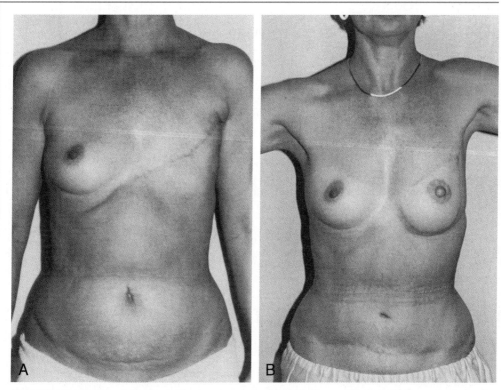

FIGURE 15-18 ■ **Augmentation mammoplasty. A. Left modified radical mastectomy in a 53-year-old woman (3 months postoperation). B. Same patient 10 months after augmentation mammoplasty.**

Programmed Review: Gynecologic Operative Terms: Breasts

ANSWERS	REVIEW
-ectomy lumpectomy	**15.108** The surgical suffix for excision (removal) is _____. The surgical removal of a breast tumor (lump) without removing other tissue or lymph nodes is called a _____.
mast/o mastectomy simple, radical mastectomy	**15.109** There are two combining forms meaning breast: *mamm/o* and _____. Formed from the latter, the term for surgical removal of a breast is _____. There are several different types of mastectomies, depending on how much tissue is removed to ensure the cancer is excised. Removal of just the breast, leaving the underlying muscle and axillary lymph nodes intact, is called a _____ mastectomy. A _____ mastectomy involves the removal of the breast as well as the underlying chest muscles and the axillary lymph nodes. A modified radical _____ removes the breast and lymph nodes only.
-plasty mamm/o mammoplasty	**15.110** Recall that the suffix for surgical reconstruction is _____. The two combining forms meaning breast are _____ and *mast/o*. Using the first of these, the term for surgical reconstruction of the breast is _____.
augmentation reduction mammoplasty	**15.111** A mammoplasty performed to enlarge the breast, usually by inserting an implant, is called _____ mammoplasty. A reconstruction performed to remove excessive breast tissue and, thereby, reduce the size of the breasts is called a _____ _____.
mast/o fixation mastopexy	**15.112** In addition to *mamm/o*, the other combining form for breast is _____. The surgical suffix *-pexy* means suspension or _____. The procedure to elevate pendulous breast tissue by fixing tissues higher is called a _____.

Self-Instruction: Gynecologic Therapeutic Terms

Study the following:

TERM	MEANING
chemotherapy *kem-ō-thār'ă-pē*	treatment of malignancies, infections, and other diseases with chemical agents that destroy selected cells or impair their ability to reproduce

TERM	MEANING
radiation therapy *rā-dē-ā'shŭn thār'ă-pē*	treatment of neoplastic disease using radiation to deter the proliferation of malignant cells
hormone replacement therapy (HRT) *hōr'mōn rē-plās'ment thār'ă-pē*	use of a hormone (e.g., estrogen or progesterone) to replace a deficiency or to regulate production
hormonal contraceptives *hōr-mōn'ăl kon-tră-sep'tivz*	hormones used to prevent conception by suppressing ovulation
oral contraceptive pill (OCP) *ōr'ăl kon-tră-sep'tiv pil*	birth control pill
contraceptive injection *kon-tră-sep'tiv in-jek'shŭn*	injection of a contraceptive hormone (e.g., Depo-Provera) into the body
contraceptive implant *kon-tră-sep'tiv im'plant*	insertion of a contraceptive capsule under the skin to provide a continual infusion over an extended period
barrier contraceptives *ba'rē-ĕr kon-tră-sep'tivz*	products that provide a physical barrier to prevent conception (e.g., condoms or diaphragms)
intrauterine device (IUD) *in'tră-yū'tĕr-in dē-vīs*	contraceptive device inserted into the uterus that prevents implantation of a fertilized egg
spermicidals *spĕr-mi-sī'dălz*	creams, jellies, lotions, or foams containing agents that kill sperm (*cid/o* = to kill)

🔷 Programmed Review: Gynecologic Therapeutic Terms

ANSWERS	REVIEW
chemotherapy	**15.113** The combining form referring to chemical agents is *chem/o*. The treatment of malignancies, infections, and other diseases with chemical agents that destroy targeted cells is called _____.
radiation therapy	**15.114** Some kinds of cancer are treated with radiation, which deters the proliferation of malignant cells. This is called _____ _____.
hormone replacement	**15.115** If a woman is deficient in the production of a hormone, such as estrogen, treatment may involve administering a replacement hormone to the person. This is called _____ _____ therapy (HRT).
contraceptives against	**15.116** Hormones administered to prevent conception and pregnancy are called hormonal _____. The prefix *contra-* means _____ or opposed to.

ANSWERS	REVIEW
contraceptive contraceptive implant	Oral _____ pills are generally called birth control pills. A hormonal contraceptive that is injected is called a _____ injection. Hormonal contraceptives also can be administered in a capsule that is placed under the skin to give a continual infusion; this is called a contraceptive _____.
barrier	**15.117** Contraceptive methods that create a physical block to prevent sperm from reaching the ovum are called _____ contraceptives (e.g., a condom or a diaphragm).
intrauterine within	**15.118** IUD is the abbreviation for _____ device, which is inserted into the uterus to prevent implantation of a fertilized egg. The prefix *intra-* means _____.
spermicidals	**15.119** Contraceptive creams, jellies, lotions, and foams that contain an agent that kills (*cid/o* means to kill) sperm are called _____.

Self-Instruction: Obstetric Symptomatic Terms

Study the following:

TERM	MEANING
gravida (Fig. 15-19) *grav'i-dă*	a pregnant woman; gravida followed by a number indicates the number of pregnancies
nulligravida *nŭl-i-grav'i-dă*	having never been pregnant
primigravida *prī-mi-grav'i-dă*	first pregnancy
para (*see* Fig. 15-19) *par'ă*	to bear; a woman who has produced one or more viable (live outside the uterus) offspring; para followed by a number indicates the number of times a pregnancy has resulted in a single or multiple birth
nullipara *nŭ-lip'ă-ră*	a woman who has not borne a child (*nulli* = none; *para* = to bear)
primipara *prī-mip'ă-ră*	first delivery (*primi* = first; *para* = to bear)
multipara *mŭl-tip'ă-ră*	a woman who has given birth to two or more children (*multi* = many; *para* = to bear)
cervical effacement *sĕr'vi-kăl ē-fās'ment*	progressive obliteration of the endocervical canal during delivery

ANSWERS	REVIEW
spontaneous habitual	expulsion occurs naturally, is called a _____ abortion (SAB). Spontaneous abortions occurring in three or more consecutive pregnancies are called _____ abortion.
incomplete missed threatened	**15.129** If the products of conception are not completely expelled, this is called an _____ abortion. If the embryo or fetus dies within the uterus but is not then naturally expelled, this is called a _____ abortion. Bleeding with the threat of miscarriage is called a _____ abortion.
ectopic pregnancy	**15.130** The term ectopic comes from a Greek word meaning out of place. A pregnancy in which the fertilized egg is implanted outside the uterus, such as in the fallopian tube, is called an _____ _____.
excessive hyperemesis gravidarum	**15.131** Many women normally experience "morning sickness" early in pregnancy, but severe nausea and vomiting can cause dehydration. The word emesis means vomit. Recall that the prefix *hyper-* means above or _____. The term for the condition of severe nausea and vomiting in pregnancy is _____ _____.
high before preeclampsia pregnancy-induced excessive	**15.132** A serious condition that can occur in pregnancy, eclampsia is characterized by _____ blood pressure and other symptoms, leading to convulsions or coma. Recall that the prefix *pre-* means _____. A condition of high blood pressure similar to eclampsia, but occurring without convulsions or coma, may precede eclampsia. It is called _____, or _____-_____ hypertension (PIH). The prefix *hyper-* means _____ or above.
Rh positive Rh	**15.133** Certain antigens may or may not be present on the surface of red blood cells; this is called the _____ factor. The presence of antigens is designated as Rh _____, and the absence of these antigens is designated as _____ negative.
	15.134 If the blood of the mother is Rh negative and the blood of the fetus is Rh positive, a reaction will occur that causes fetal red blood cell destruction. Red blood cells are also called

ANSWERS	REVIEW
condition erythroblastosis fetalis	erythroblasts. Recall that the suffix *-osis* means increase or _____. The condition that results in the fetus from this incompatibility of Rh factors is called _____ _____. A blood transfusion is usually necessary to save the fetus.
before placenta previa	**15.135** The term previa comes from a Latin word formed by the combination of *pre-*, meaning _____, and *-via*, meaning the way. If the placenta is attached in an abnormal position low in the uterus, it may obstruct the movement of the fetus out of the uterus at childbirth. This condition of a displaced placenta is called _____ _____.
abruptio placentae	**15.136** An abruption is a tearing away or detachment. The premature detachment of a normally situated placenta is called _____ _____.
amniotic meconium aspiration	**15.137** Recall that meconium staining refers to the presence of meconium in the _____ fluid. If this occurs, the fetus may suck this into its lungs, a condition called _____ _____.
head cephalopelvic	**15.138** Normally, the infant's head passes easily through the birth canal in the mother's pelvis. Recall that the combining form *cephal/o* means _____. If the infant's head is too large or the mother's pelvis is too small, a condition of _____ disproportion exists, complicating childbirth.

◈ Self-Instruction: Obstetric Diagnostic Tests and Procedures

Study the following:

TEST OR PROCEDURE	EXPLANATION
chorionic villus sampling (CVS) (Fig. 15-21) *kō-rē-on'ik vil'ŭs sam'pling*	sampling of placental tissue for microscopic and chemical examination to detect fetal abnormalities
amniocentesis (*see* Fig. 15-21) *am'nē-ō-sen-tē'sis*	aspiration of a small amount of amniotic fluid for analysis of possible fetal abnormalities

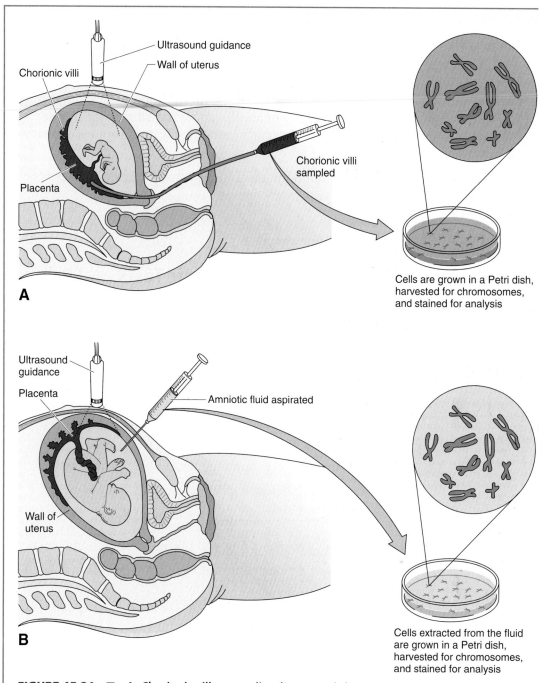

FIGURE 15-21 ■ **A. Chorionic villus sampling (9–11 weeks). B. Amniocentesis (15–18 weeks).**

TEST OR PROCEDURE	EXPLANATION
fetal monitoring *fē'tăl mon'i-tŏr-ing*	use of an electronic device for simultaneous recording of fetal heart rate and uterine contractions
pelvimetry *pel-vim'ĕ-trē*	obstetric measurement of the pelvis to evaluate proper conditions for vaginal delivery
pregnancy test *preg'nan-sē test*	test performed on urine or blood to detect the presence of human chorionic gonadotropin hormone (secreted by the placenta), which indicates pregnancy

TEST OR PROCEDURE	EXPLANATION
pelvic sonography (*see* Fig. 15-13) *pel'vik sŏ-nog'ră-fē*	ultrasound imaging of the female pelvis
endovaginal sonogram *en'dō-vaj'i-năl son'ō-gram* **transvaginal sonogram** *trans-vaj'i-năl son'ō-gram*	ultrasound image of the uterus, tubes, and ovaries made after introduction of an ultrasonic transducer within the vagina; useful for detecting pathology (e.g., ectopic pregnancy or missed abortion)
obstetric sonogram (*see* Figs. 15-3 and 15-4) *ob-stet'rik son'ō-gram*	ultrasound image of the pregnant uterus to determine fetal development

◈ Programmed Review: Obstetric Diagnostic Tests and Procedures

ANSWERS	REVIEW
aspiration amniocentesis	**15.139** Various diagnostic tests are often performed during pregnancy. Recall that the suffix -*centesis* refers to puncture for _____. Puncturing the amniotic sac and aspirating a small amount of amniotic fluid for analysis is called _____.
chorionic villus	**15.140** Another fetal sampling procedure is performed with placental tissue to detect fetal abnormalities. This is called _____ _____ sampling (CVS).
fetal monitoring	**15.141** The fetal heart rate and uterine contractions can be monitored with an electronic recording device; this process is called _____ _____.
-metry pelvimetry	**15.142** Recall that the suffix meaning process of measuring is _____. Obstetric measuring of the pelvis for conditions related to vaginal delivery is called _____.
pregnancy test	**15.143** A woman who suspects that she may be pregnant can have a _____ _____ performed with a blood or urine sample to detect whether she is pregnant.
obstetric within endovaginal transvaginal	**15.144** An ultrasound image of the pregnant uterus is called an _____ sonogram. Recall that the prefix *endo-* means _____. A sonogram made with the ultrasound transducer within the vagina is called an _____ sonogram, or a _____ sonogram (*trans* = through).

chorionic villus sampling (CVS)/746
kō-rē-on'ik vil'ŭs sam'pling

clitoris/708
klit'ō-ris

colporrhaphy/731
kol-pōr'ă-fē

colporrhaphy anterior repair/731
kol-pōr'ă-fē an-tēr'ē-ōr rē-pār'

colporrhaphy A&P repair/731
kol-pōr'ă-fē ā and pē rē-pār'

colporrhaphy posterior repair/731
kol-pōr'ă-fē pos-tēr'ē-ōr rē-pār'

colposcopy/727
kol-pos'kŏ-pē

condyloma acuminatum/721
kon-di-lō'mă ă-kyū'mi-nā'tŭm

condylomata acuminata/721
kon-di-lō-mah'tă ă-kyū'mi-nā'tă

congenital anomalies/714
kon-jen'ĭ-tăl ah-nom'ah-lēz

congenital irregularities/714
kon-jen'ĭ-tăl ir-reg'yū-lār'ĭ-tēz

contraceptive implant/739
kon-tră-sep'tiv im'plant

contraceptive injection/739
kon-tră-sep'tiv in-jek'shŭn

cryosurgery/731
krī-ō-sŭr'jĕr-ē

cystocele/716
sis'tō-sēl

dermoid cyst/714
dĕr'moyd sist

dilation and curettage (D&C)/731
dī-lā'shŭn and kū-rĕ-tahzh'

dilation and evacuation (D&E)/749
dī-lā'shŭn and ē-vak-yū-ā'shŭn

displacements of uterus/714
dis-plās'ments of yū'tĕr-ŭs

dysmenorrhea/712
dis-men-ō-rē'ă

dyspareunia/713
dis-pa-rū'nē-ă

eclampsia/743
ek-lamp'sē-ă

ectopic pregnancy/743
ek-top'ik preg'năn-sē

embryo/709
em'brē-ō

endometriosis/714
en'dō-mē-trē-ō'sis

endometritis/714
en'dō-mē-trī'tis

endometrium/707
en'dō-mē'trē-ŭm

endoscopic biopsy/726
en'dō-skop'ik bī'op-sē

endovaginal sonogram/727, 748
en'dō-vaj'i-năl son'ō-gram

enterocele/716
en'tĕr-o-sēl

episiotomy/749
e-piz-ē-oť'ŏ-mē

erythroblastosis fetalis/744
ĕ-rith'rō-blas-tō'sis fē-tā'lis

estimated date of confinement (EDC)/741
ĕs-tĭ-mā'tĕd dāt of kon-fīn'ment

estimated date of delivery (EDD)/741
ĕs-tĭ-mā'tĕd dāt of dē-liv'ĕr-ē

excisional biopsy/726
ek-sizh'ŭn-ăl bī'op-sē

external version/749
eks-tĕr'năl ver'zhŭn

fallopian tubes/707
fă-lō'pē-ăn tūbz

fetal monitoring/747
fē'tăl mon'i-tŏr'ing

fetus/710
fē'tŭs

fibrocystic breasts/723
fī-brō-sis'tik brests

fibroid/714
fī'broyd

fibromyoma/714
fī'brŏ-mī-ō'mă

fistula/716
fis'tyū-lă

fundus/707
fŭn'dŭs

gonorrhea720
gon-ō-rē'ă

gravida/740
grav'i-dă

gynecomastia/723
gī'nĕ-kō-mas'tē-ă

habitual abortion/743
hă-bi'chū-ăl ă-bōr'shŭn

hepatitis B virus (HBV)/721
hep-ă-tī'tis B vī'rŭs

herpes simplex virus type 2 (HSV-2)/721
her'pēz sim'pleks vī'rŭs tīp 2

hormonal contraceptives/739
hōr-mōn'ăl kon-tră-sep'tivz

hormone replacement therapy (HRT)/739
hōr'mōn rē-plās'ment thār'ă-pē

human immunodeficiency virus (HIV)/721
hyū'măn im'yū-nō-dē-fish'en-sē vī'rŭs

human papilloma virus (HPV)/721
hyū'măn pap-i-lō'mă vī'rŭs

hymen/708
hī'men

hyperemesis gravidarum/744
hī'pĕr-ē-mē'sis grah-vē-dar'ŭm

hypermastia/723
hī-pĕr-mas'tē-ă

hypomastia/723
hī'pō-mas'tē-ă

hysterectomy/732
his-tĕr-ek'tŏ-mē

hysterosalpingogram/727
his'tĕr-ō-sal-ping'ō-gram

hysteroscopy/727
his-tĕr-os'kŏ-pē

hysterosonogram/728
his-tĕr-ō-son'ō-gram

incisional biopsy/726
in-sizh'ŭn-năl bī'op-sē

incomplete abortion/743
in-kom-plēt' ă-bōr'shŭn

internal version/749
in-tĕr'năl ver'zhŭn

intrauterine device (IUD)/739
in'tră-yū'tĕr-in dĕ-vīs'

introitus/708
in-trō'i-tŭs

labia/708
lā'bē-ă

laparoscopic surgery/732
lap'ă-rō-skōp'ik sŭr'jĕr-ē

laparoscopy/732
lap-ă-ros'kŏ-pē

large-loop excision of the transformation zone (LLETZ)/732
larj-lūp ek-sizh'ŭn of the trans-fōr-mā'shŭn zōn

laser surgery/732
lā'zĕr sŭr'jĕr-ē

left uterine appendage/707
left yū'tĕr-in ă-pen'dij

leiomyoma/714
lī'ō-mī-ō'mă

leukorrhea/713
lū-kō-rē'ă

loop electrosurgical excision procedure (LEEP)/732
lūp ē-lek-trō-sŭr'ji-kăl ek-sizh'ŭn prō-sē'jŭr

lumpectomy/736
lŭmp-ek'tŏ-mē

macromastia/723
mak-rō-mas'tē-ă

macrosomia/742
mak-rō-sō'mē-ă

magnetic resonance imaging (MRI)/727
mag-net'ik rez'ō-nănts im'ă-jing

mammary glands/709
mam'ă-rē glanz

mammary papilla/709
mam'ă-rē pă-pil'ă

mammogram/727
mam'ō-gram

mastectomy/736
mas-tek'tŏ-mē

mastitis/723
mas-tī'tis

mastopexy/737
mas'tō-pek-sē

meconium/710
mē-kō'nē-ŭm

meconium aspiration/744
mē-kō'nē-ŭm as-pi-rā'shŭn

meconium staining/741
mē-kō'nē-ŭm stān'ing

menopause/716
men'ō-pawz

menorrhagia/713
men-ō-rā'jē-ă

metrorrhagia/713
mē-trō-rā'jē-ă

micromastia/723
mī'kro-mas'tē-ă

missed abortion/743
mist ă-bōr'shŭn

modified radical mastectomy/737
mod'i-fīd rad'i-kăl mas-tek'tō-mē

multipara/740
mŭl-tip'ă-ră

myomectomy/732
mī-ō-mek'tō-mē

myometrium/707
mī-o-mē'trē-ŭm

needle biopsy/725
nē'dĕl bī'op-sē

nulligravida/740
nŭl-i-grav'i-dă

nullipara/740
nŭ-lip'ă-ră

obstetric sonogram/748
ob-stet'rik son'ō-gram

oligomenorrhea/713
ol'i-gō-men-ō-rē'ă

oligo-ovulation/713
ol'i-gō-ov'yū-lā'shŭn

oophorectomy/733
ō'of-ōr-ek'tŏ-mē

oophoritis/716
ō'of-ōr-ī'tis

oral contraceptive pill (OCP)/739
ōr'ăl kon-tră-sep'tiv pil

ovarian cystectomy/733
ō-var'ē-an sis-tek'tō-mē

ovary/707
ō'vă-rē

oxytocin/749
ok'sē-tō'sin

Papanicolaou (Pap) smear/727
pa-pă-ni'kō-lū smēr

para/740
par'ă

parovarian cyst/716
par-ō-var'ē-an sist

pelvic adhesions/716
pel'vik ad-hē'zhŭnz

pelvic floor relaxation/716
pel'vik flōr rē-lak-sā'shŭn

pelvic inflammatory disease (PID)/716
pel'vik in-flam'ă-tōr-ē di-zēz'

pelvic sonography/727, 748
pel'vik sŏ-nog'ră-fē

pelvimetry/747
pel-vim'ĕ-trē

perineum/709
per-i-nē'ŭm

placenta/710
plă-sen'tă

placenta previa/744
plă-sen'tă prē'vē-ă

polyhydramnios/742
pol'ē-hī-dram'nē-os

polymastia/724
pol-ē-mas'tē-ă

polythelia/724
pol-ē-thē'lē-ă

preeclampsia/743
prē-ē-klamp'sē-ă

pregnancy test/747
preg'nan-sē test

pregnancy-induced hypertension (PIH)/743
preg'nan-sē-in-dūst' hī'pĕr-ten'shŭn

primigravida/740
prī-mi-grav'i-dă

primipara/740
prī-mip'ă-ră

prolapse/716
prō-laps'

radiation therapy/739
rā-dē-ā'shŭn thār-ă-pē

radical mastectomy/737
rad'i-kăl mas-tek'tŏ-mē

radiography/727
rā'dē-og'ră-fē

rectocele/716
rek'tō-sēl

rectovaginal fistula/716
rek-tō-vaj'i-năl fis'tyū-lă

retroflexion/714
re-trō-flek'shŭn

retroversion/714
re-trō-vĕr'zhŭn

Rh factor/744
r-āch fac'tŏr

Rh immune globulin/749
r-āch i-myūn' glob'yū-lin

Rh negative/744
r-āch neg'ă-tiv

Rh positive/744
r-āch pos'i-tiv

right uterine appendage/707
rīt yū'tĕr-in ă-pen'dij

ruptured membranes/742
rŭp'chūrd mem'brānz

saline infusion sonogram/728
sā'lēn in-fyū'zhŭn son'ō-gram

salpingectomy/733
sal-pin-jek'tŏ-mē

salpingitis/717
sal-pin-jī'tis

salpingostomy/733
sal-ping-gos'tŏ-mē

salpingotomy/733
sal-pin-got'ō-mē

sentinel node breast biopsy/726
sen'tĭ-nel nōd brest bī'op-sē

simple mastectomy/736
sĭm'pel mas-tek'tŏ-mē

sonohysterogram/728
son'o-his-tĕr-ō-gram

spermicidals/739
spĕr-mi-sī'dălz

spontaneous abortion (SAB)/743
spon-tā'nē-yŭs ă-bōr'shŭn

stereotactic breast biopsy/726
ster'ē-ō-tak'tik brest bī'op-sē

supernumerary nipples/724
sū-pĕr-nū'mĕr-ār-ē nip'ĕlz

syphilis/721
sif'i-lis

therapeutic abortion (TAB)/749
thār-ă-pyū'tik ă-bōr'shŭn

threatened abortion/743
thrĕ'tend ă-bōr'shŭn

tocolytic agent/749
tō-kō-lit'ik ā'jent

total hysterectomy/732
tō'tăl his-tĕr-ek'tŏ-mē

transabdominal sonogram/728
trans-ab-dom'i-năl son'ō-gram

transvaginal sonogram/727, 748
trans-vaj'i-năl son'ō-gram

tubal ligation/733
tū'băl lī-gā'shŭn

urethrocele/716
yū-rē'thrō-sēl

uterine tubes/707
yū'tĕr-in tūbz

uterus/707
yū'tĕr-ŭs

Write out the expanded term for each abbreviation:

26. IUD _____

27. HPV _____

28. CVS _____

29. D&C _____

30. HBV _____

31. EDC _____

32. HSV _____

33. STD _____

34. TAB _____

35. HRT _____

Write the letter of the matching term in the space provided:

36. removal of a uterine tube and an ovary _____ a. PID

37. white vaginal discharge _____ b. chlamydia

38. condition when baby's head is too big for birth canal _____ c. colporrhaphy

39. presence of more than one nipple on a breast _____ d. LEEP

40. implantation of a fertilized egg outside the uterus _____ e. CPD

41. most common bacterial STD in North America _____ f. leukorrhea

42. excisional biopsy _____ g. polythelia

43. painful intercourse _____ h. ectopic

44. surgical repair of cystocele _____ i. salpingo-oophorectomy

45. inflammation of entire female pelvic cavity _____ j. dyspareunia

Write the correct medical term for each of the following definitions:

46. _____ condition of benign lumps in the breast that fluctuate with menstrual cycle

47. _____ abnormal opening between the bladder and vagina

48. _____ cutting and tying the uterine tubes

49. _____ having more than two breasts

50. _____ bacterial STD caused by a spirochete

51. _____ x-ray imaging of the uterine tubes to determine patency

52. _____ study of cervical cells to screen for cancer

53. _____ condition of migration of endometrial tissue

54. _____ abnormal opening between the rectum and vagina

55. _____ surgical remedy for rectocele

Complete each medical term by writing the missing word or word part:

56. _____ pause = cessation of menstruation

57. _____rrhea = painful menstruation

58. _____rrhea = absence of menstruation

59. _____rrhea = scanty menstruation

60. _____rrhagia = excessive bleeding at the time of menstruation

61. _____rrhagia = bleeding from the uterus at any time other than during the normal menstrual period

62. _____mastia = development of mammary glands in a male

63. _____mastia = absence of a breast

64. _____mastia = unusually small breasts; a common surgical remedy is _____ mammoplasty

65. _____mastia = unusually large breasts; a common surgical remedy is _____ mammoplasty

66. masto_____ = surgical fixation of a pendulous breast

67. _____ectomy = removal of a breast

68. _____ectomy = removal of a breast lump

Identify the following terms related to abortion:

69. _____ a naturally occurring miscarriage

70. _____ a miscarriage occurring in three or more consecutive pregnancies

71. _____ fetal expulsion with parts of the placenta remaining, with bleeding

72. _____ fetal death within the uterus

73. _____ an abortion induced by mechanical means or by drugs

74. _____ bleeding with threat of miscarriage

Write the letter of the matching term in the space provided:

75. retroflexion _____   a. forward bending of the uterus

76. condylomata _____   b. toxemia of pregnancy

77. para 2 _____   c. backward bending of the uterus

78. prolapse _____   d. a pregnant woman

79. cystocele _____   e. cancer

80. gravida _____   f. genital warts

81. rectocele _____   g. woman who has given birth twice

82. eclampsia _____   h. first delivery

83. CIN-2 _____   i. protrusion of the rectum into the vagina

84. primipara _____   j. descent of uterus from normal position

85. anteflexion _____   k. dysplasia

86. CIS _____   l. pouching of the bladder into the vagina

Circle the combining form that corresponds to the meaning given:

87.	**birth or labor**	tox/o	toc/o	troph/o
88.	**vagina**	uter/o	metr/o	colp/o
89.	**uterine tube**	vagin/o	oophor/o	salping/o
90.	**menstruation**	men/o	mamm/o	mast/o
91.	**cervix**	colp/o	cervic/o	salping/o
92.	**egg**	oophor/o	ov/i	ovari/o
93.	**vulva**	episi/o	vagin/o	metr/o
94.	**uterus**	vagin/o	metr/o	oophor/o
95.	**milk**	lact/o	leuk/o	lip/o
96.	**ovary**	ov/o	oophor/o	salping/o
97.	**breast**	men/o	metr/o	mast/o
98.	**woman**	gen/o	gynec/o	hyster/o

Identify the parts of the female reproductive anatomy by writing the missing words in the spaces provided:

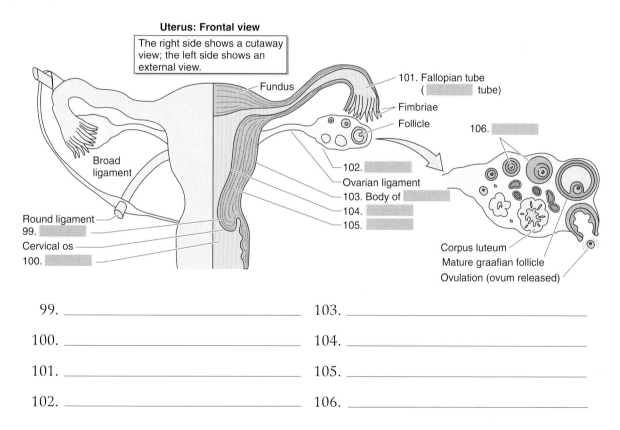

Uterus: Frontal view

The right side shows a cutaway view; the left side shows an external view.

Fundus

101. Fallopian tube
(⬚ tube)

Fimbriae

Follicle

106. ⬚

Broad ligament

102. ⬚

Ovarian ligament

103. Body of ⬚

104. ⬚

105. ⬚

Round ligament

99. ⬚

Cervical os

100. ⬚

Corpus luteum

Mature graafian follicle

Ovulation (ovum released)

99. _____	103. _____
100. _____	104. _____
101. _____	105. _____
102. _____	106. _____

Circle the correct spelling in each set of words:

107. gonorrhea	gonorhea	ghonarhea
108. dispareunia	dyspareunia	dysparunia
109. tokolytic	toecolytic	tocolytic
110. polythelia	polythellia	polytelia
111. meterorrhagia	metrorrhagia	metrorhagia
112. dialation	dyelayshun	dilation
113. salpingotomy	salpengotomy	salpigotomy
114. nulligravida	nuligravida	nulligraveda
115. meconeium	meconium	meconeum
116. macrosomia	macrosomnia	macrasomia
117. cureitage	curetage	curettage
118. eclampshea	eklampsia	eclampsia
119. menorrhea	amennorhea	amenorhea
120. abortifacient	abortafacient	abortofacent

Give the noun used to form each adjective:

121. chlamydial _____

122. areolar _____

123. syphilitic _____

124. cervical _____

125. dysplastic _____

126. endometrial _____

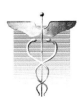

MEDICAL RECORD ANALYSIS

Medical Record 15-1

GYN CHART NOTE

S: This 44 y.o. female, gravida 2, para 2, c/o extremely heavy periods for the past several years that have been getting worse for the past 2 months and have been accompanied by moderately severe cramps. Pap smears have been normal. She has no bladder or bowel complaints.

O: On pelvic exam, the uterus is found to be retroverted and irregularly enlarged with several large fibroids palpable. There are no adnexal masses.

A: Leiomyomata uteri with secondary menorrhagia

P: Schedule vaginal hysterectomy; donate one pint of blood for autologous transfusion, if necessary

QUESTIONS ABOUT MEDICAL RECORD 15-1

1. What is the patient's OB history?
   a. has never been pregnant
   b. has been pregnant only once
   c. has had two miscarriages
   d. has been pregnant four times
   e. has had two live births

2. Identify the patient's most significant symptom:
   a. amenorrhea
   b. dyspareunia
   c. leukorrhea
   d. menorrhagia
   e. metrorrhagia

3. Which of the following was one of the objective findings?
   a. tipped uterus
   b. forward bending uterus
   c. backward bending uterus
   d. presence of several ovarian tumors
   e. migration of portions of endometrial tissue

4. What was the condition of the patient's uterine tubes?
   a. not stated
   b. normal
   c. inflamed
   d. enlarged
   e. had been removed previously

5. What was the diagnosis?
   a. congenital tumor composed of displaced embryonic tissue
   b. cyst of the uterine tube
   c. inflammation of the organs of the pelvic cavity
   d. smooth muscle tumors in the uterus
   e. ovarian tumors

6. What surgical procedure is planned?
   a. incision into the uterine tube to remove the cyst
   b. excision of the uterus
   c. excision of the ovaries
   d. dilation of the cervix and scraping of the endometrium
   e. excision of the uterine tubes and both ovaries

Medical Record 15-2

FOR ADDITIONAL STUDY

Jane Foley has seen her gynecologist, Dr. Phyllis Widetick, yearly for a routine examination and Pap smear. Every year, the results have been normal. Jane is generally a healthy, active woman. This year, however, Dr. Widetick's examination and Pap smear found a problem. When the test results were in, Jane returned for additional testing. Medical Record 14-2 is the history and physical report dictated by Dr. Widetick after her examination.

Read Medical Record 15-2 (pages 768–769) for Ms. Foley, then write your answers to the following questions in the spaces provided.

QUESTIONS ABOUT MEDICAL RECORD 15-2

1. In your own words, not using medical terminology, briefly describe the patient's chief complaint:

   _____

   _____

   _____

2. In your own words, not using medical terminology, briefly describe what a Pap smear is:

   _____

   _____

   _____

3. Explain the result of Ms. Foley's Pap smear:

   _____

   _____

   _____

4. Because of this result, Dr. Widetick used colposcopy for further testing. Translate into non-medical language what she discovered with this diagnostic procedure:

   _____

   _____

   _____

5. What was the positive finding from the biopsy? Describe this in your own words:

   _____

   _____

   _____

6. Ms. Foley underwent the following procedures. Put these in the correct sequence by numbering them from 1 to 6 in the order they were performed:

   _____ follow-up examination

   _____ visualization with colposcope

   _____ ultrasound

_____ Pap smear

_____ routine physical examination

_____ Bx

7. The sonogram _definitely_ showed what finding?

_____

What were the _possible_ findings?

_____

_____

8. In nonmedical language, define the two previous surgeries that Ms. Foley has had:

_____

_____

_____

9. How many children has Ms. Foley had? _____

10. Mark any of the following abnormal findings from the present physical examination:

   a. enlarged uterus

   b. gross reflexes

   c. eroded cervix

   d. hypertension

   e. enlarged thyroid

   f. mobile right ovarian cyst

11. Define Dr. Widetick's final diagnosis and explain what she will do next to treat Ms. Foley:

_____

_____

_____

Medical Record 15-2: For Additional Study

CENTRAL MEDICAL CENTER

211 Medical Center Drive • Central City, US 90000-1234 • PHONE: (012) 125-6784 • FAX: (012) 125-9999

TO BE ADMITTED: 9/3/20xx

HISTORY

CHIEF COMPLAINT:
Right ovarian cyst.

HISTORY OF PRESENT ILLNESS:
This is a 32-year-old Caucasian female who had a routine examination on June 21, 20xx, at which time the examination revealed the right ovary to be approximately two to three times normal size. Otherwise, all was normal. The Papanicolaou smear revealed atypical cells of undetermined significance. The patient returned for a colposcopy, and this revealed what appeared to be squamous epithelial lesions CIN 1-2. Biopsies were performed which revealed chronic cervicitis and no evidence of CIN. The patient was placed on Lo-Ovral for two cycles and then was rechecked. The right ovary continued to enlarge and got to the point where it was approximately 4 x 5 cm, floating anteriorly in the pelvis, and was fairly firm to palpation. A pelvic sonogram corroborated the clinical findings in that superior to the right adnexa was a 4 x 5 cm mass, possibly with hemorrhage into either a paraovarian cyst or possibly a dermoid cyst. The patient is to be admitted now for an exploratory laparotomy.

PAST HISTORY:
There is no history of severe medical illnesses. The patient had the usual childhood diseases and has had good health as an adult.

PREVIOUS SURGERY: The patient had a hymenotomy and dilation and curettage in 20xx

MENSTRUAL HISTORY: Menstrual cycle is 30 days, averaging a four to seven day flow.

OBSTETRICAL HISTORY: The patient is a Gravida 0.

FAMILY HISTORY:
Diabetes in the family. Mother and father are living and well

REVIEW OF SYSTEMS:
Noncontributory.

(continued)

P. Widetick, M.D.
P. Widetick, M.D.

PW:bst
D: 9/1/20xx T: 9/2/20xx

HISTORY AND PHYSICAL Page 1	PT. NAME: FOLEY, JANE J. ID NO: IP-751014 ROOM NO: 331 ATT. PHYS: P. WIDETICK, M.D.

Medical Record 15-2: For Additional Study (Continued)

CENTRAL MEDICAL CENTER

211 Medical Center Drive • Central City, US 90000-1234 • PHONE: (012) 125-6784 • FAX: (012) 125-9999

PHYSICAL EXAMINATION

GENERAL:
The patient is a well-developed, well-nourished Caucasian female who is anxious but in no acute distress.

VITAL SIGNS:
HEIGHT: 5 feet 5 inches. WEIGHT: 154 pounds. BLOOD PRESSURE: 110/82.

HEENT:
Normal.

NECK:
Supple; the trachea is in the midline. The thyroid is not enlarged.

CHEST:
LUNGS: Clear to percussion and auscultation. HEART: Regular sinus rhythm with no murmur. BREASTS: Normal to palpation.

ABDOMEN:
Soft and flat. No scars or masses.

PELVIC:
The outlet and vagina are normal. The cervix is moderately eroded. The uterus is normal size and anterior. The left adnexa is negative. The right adnexa has a firm, irregular cystic ovary that is anterior and approximately 5 x 5 cm. This is mobile and nontender.

EXTREMITIES:
Normal. Reflexes are grossly intact.

DIAGNOSIS:
Right ovarian cyst.

PLAN:
The patient is to be admitted for laparoscopy and probable ovarian cystectomy.

P. Widetick, M.D.
P. Widetick, M.D.

PW:bst
D: 9/1/20xx T: 9/2/20xx

HISTORY AND PHYSICAL PAGE 2	PT. NAME: FOLEY, JANE J. ID NO: IP-751014 ROOM NO: 331 ATT. PHYS: P. WIDETICK, M.D.

ANSWERS TO PRACTICE EXERCISES

1. vulv/itis
   R   S
   vulva (covering)/
   inflammation
2. poly/mast/ia
   P   R   S
   many/breast/condition
   of
3. ov/oid
   R S
   egg/resembling
4. toco/lysis
   CF   S
   birth or labor/breaking
   down or dissolution
5. salpingo/tomy
   CF   S
   uterine (fallopian)
   tube/incision
6. mammo/plasty
   CF   S
   breast/surgical repair or
   reconstruction
7. trans/vagin/al
   P   R   S
   across or
   through/vagina/
   pertaining to
8. hystero/rrhexis
   CF   S
   uterus/rupture
9. colpo/scopy
   CF   S
   vagina/process of examination
10. mammo/graphy
    CF   S
    breast/process of
    recording
11. metro/rrhagia
    CF   S
    uterus/to burst forth
12. ovario/centesis
    CF   S
    ovary/puncture for
    aspiration

13. men/arche
    R   S
    menstruation/beginning
14. oophor/ectomy
    R   S
    ovary/excision (removal)
15. oligo/meno/rrhea
    P   CF   S
    few or deficient/
    menstruation/discharge
16. dys/toc/ia
    P   R   S
    painful, difficult, or
    faulty/labor or
    birth/condition of
17. gyneco/logist
    CF   S
    woman/one who spe-
    cializes in the study or
    treatment of
18. hystero/salpingo/gram
    CF   CF   S
    uterus/uterine (fallop-
    ian) tube/record
19. episio/tomy
    CF   S
    vulva (covering)/incision
20. colpo/rrhaphy
    CF   S
    vagina/suture
21. hystero/spasm
    CF   S
    uterus/involuntary
    contraction
22. lacto/rrhea
    CF   S
    milk/discharge
23. ovi/genesis
    CF   S
    egg/origin or production
24. endo/cervic/al
    P   R   S
    within/cervix/
    pertaining to

25. utero/tomy
    CF   S
    uterus/incision
26. intrauterine device
27. human papilloma virus
28. chorionic villus sam-
    pling
29. dilation and curettage
30. hepatitis B virus
31. estimated date of con-
    finement
32. herpes simplex virus
33. sexually transmitted dis-
    ease
34. therapeutic abortion
35. hormone replacement
    therapy
36. i
37. f
38. e
39. g
40. h
41. b
42. d
43. j
44. c
45. a
46. fibrocystic breasts
47. vesicovaginal fistula
48. tubal ligation
49. polymastia
50. syphilis
51. hysterosalpingogram
52. Papanicolaou (Pap)
    smear
53. endometriosis
54. rectovaginal fistula
55. colporrhaphy posterior
    repair
56. menopause
57. dysmenorrhea
58. amenorrhea
59. oligomenorrhea
60. menorrhagia
61. metrorrhagia
62. gynecomastia

63. amastia
64. hypomastia or micro-mastia; augmentation mammoplasty
65. hypermastia or macro-mastia; reduction mammoplasty
66. mastopexy
67. mastectomy
68. lumpectomy
69. spontaneous abortion
70. habitual abortion
71. incomplete abortion
72. missed abortion
73. therapeutic abortion
74. threatened abortion
75. c
76. f
77. g
78. j
79. l
80. d
81. i

82. b
83. k
84. h
85. a
86. e
87. toc/o
88. colp/o
89. salping/o
90. men/o
91. cervic/o
92. ov/i
93. episi/o
94. metr/o
95. lact/o
96. oophor/o
97. mast/o
98. gynec/o
99. cervix
100. vagina
101. uterine
102. ovary
103. uterus
104. endometrium

105. myometrium
106. eggs or ova
107. gonorrhea
108. dyspareunia
109. tocolytic
110. polythelia
111. metrorrhagia
112. dilation
113. salpingotomy
114. nulligravida
115. meconium
116. macrosomia
117. curettage
118. eclampsia
119. amenorrhea
120. abortifacient
121. chlamydia
122. areola
123. syphilis
124. cervix
125. dysplasia
126. endometrium

ANSWERS TO MEDICAL RECORD ANALYSIS

Medical Record 15-1: GYN Chart Note

1. e   2. d   3. a   4. b   5. d   6. b

Medical Record 15-2: For Additional Study

See CD-ROM for answers.

APPENDIX A

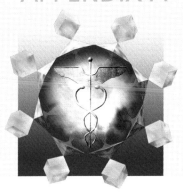

Glossary of Prefixes, Suffixes, and Combining Forms

TERM COMPONENT	MEANING	TERM COMPONENT	MEANING
a-	without	atri/o	atrium
ab-	away from	audi/o	hearing
abdomin/o	abdomen	aur/i	ear
-ac	pertaining to	bacteri/o	bacteria
acous/o	hearing	balan/o	glans penis
acr/o	extremity or topmost	bi-	two or both
-acusis	hearing condition	bil/i	bile
ad-	to, toward, or near	-blast	germ or bud
aden/o	gland	blast/o	germ or bud
adip/o	fat	blephar/o	eyelid
adren/o	adrenal gland	brachi/o	arm
adrenal/o	adrenal gland	brady-	slow
aer/o	air or gas	bronch/o	bronchus (airway)
-al	pertaining to	bronchi/o	bronchus (airway)
albumin/o	protein	bronchiol/o	bronchiole (little airway)
-algia	pain	bucc/o	cheek
alveol/o	alveolus (air sac)	capn/o	carbon dioxide
ambi-	both	carb/o	carbon dioxide
an-	without	carcin/o	cancer
an/o	anus	cardi/o	heart
andr/o	male	cata-	down
angi/o	vessel	-cele	pouching or hernia
ankyl/o	crooked or stiff	celi/o	abdomen
ante-	before	-centesis	puncture for aspiration
anti-	against or opposed to	cephal/o	head
aort/o	aorta	cerebell/o	cerebellum (little brain)
appendic/o	appendix	cerebr/o	cerebrum (largest part of brain)
aque/o	water	cerumin/o	wax
-ar	pertaining to	cervic/o	neck or cervix
-arche	beginning	cheil/o	lip
arteri/o	artery	chol/e	bile
arthr/o	joint	chondr/o	cartilage (gristle)
articul/o	joint	chrom/o	color
-ary	pertaining to	chromat/o	color
-ase	an enzyme	chyl/o	juice
-asthenia	weakness	circum-	around
ather/o	fatty paste	col/o	colon
-ation	process	colon/o	colon

TERM COMPONENT	MEANING	TERM COMPONENT	MEANING
colp/o	vagina (sheath)	femor/o	femur
con-	together or with	fibr/o	fiber
conjunctiv/o	conjunctiva (to join together)	gangli/o	ganglion (knot)
contra-	against or opposed to	gastr/o	stomach
corne/o	cornea	-gen	origin or production
coron/o	circle or crown	gen/o	origin or production
cost/o	rib	-genesis	origin or production
crani/o	skull	gingiv/o	gum
crin/o	to secrete	gli/o	glue
cutane/o	skin	glomerul/o	glomerulus (small ball)
cyan/o	blue	gloss/o	tongue
cyst/o	bladder or sac	glott/o	opening
cyt/o	cell	gluc/o	sugar
dacry/o	tear	glyc/o	sugar
dactyl/o	digit (finger or toe)	gnos/o	knowing
de-	from, down, or not	-gram	record
dent/i	teeth	-graph	instrument for recording
derm/o	skin	-graphy	process of recording
dermat/o	skin	gynec/o	woman
-desis	binding	hem/o	blood
dextr/o	right or on the right side	hemat/o	blood
dia-	across or through	hemi-	half
diaphor/o	profuse sweating	hepat/o	liver
dips/o	thirst	hepatic/o	liver
dis-	separate from or apart	herni/o	hernia
doch/o	duct	hidr/o	sweat
duoden/o	duodenum	hist/o	tissue
-dynia	pain	histi/o	tissue
dys-	painful, difficult, or faulty	hormon/o	hormone (an urging on)
-e	noun marker	hydr/o	water
e-	out or away	hyper-	above or excessive
-eal	pertaining to	hypo-	below or deficient
ec-	out or away	hypn/o	sleep
-ectasis	expansion or dilation	hyster/o	uterus
ecto-	outside	-ia	condition of
-ectomy	excision (removal)	-iasis	formation of or presence of
-emesis	vomiting	-iatrics	treatment
-emia	blood condition	-iatry	treatment
en-	within	-ic	pertaining to
encephal/o	entire brain	-icle	small
endo-	within	ile/o	ileum
enter/o	small intestine	immun/o	safe
epi-	upon	infra-	below or under
epididym/o	epididymis	inguin/o	groin
episi/o	vulva (covering)	inter-	between
erythr/o	red	intra-	within
esophag/o	esophagus	ir/o	iris (colored circle)
esthesi/o	sensation	irid/o	iris (colored circle)
eu-	good or normal	-ism	condition of
ex-	out or away	iso-	equal or like
exo-	outside	-ist	one who specializes in
extra-	outside	-itis	inflammation
fasci/o	fascia (a band)	-ium	structure or tissue

TERM COMPONENT	MEANING	TERM COMPONENT	MEANING
jejun/o	jejunum (empty)	narc/o	stupor or sleep
kerat/o	hard or cornea	nas/o	nose
ket/o	ketone bodies	nat/i	birth
keton/o	ketone bodies	necr/o	death
kinesi/o	movement	neo-	new
kyph/o	humped-back	nephr/o	kidney
lacrim/o	tear	neur/o	nerve
lact/o	milk	ocul/o	eye
lapar/o	abdomen	-oid	resembling
laryng/o	larynx (voice box)	-ole	small
lei/o	smooth	olig/o	few or deficient
-lepsy	seizure	-oma	tumor
leuc/o	white	onc/o	tumor or mass
leuk/o	white	onych/o	nail
lex/o	word or phrase	oophor/o	ovary
lingu/o	tongue	ophthalm/o	eye
lip/o	fat	-opia	condition of vision
lith/o	stone	opt/o	eye
lob/o	lobe (a portion)	orch/o	testis (testicle)
-logist	one who specializes in the study or treatment of	orchi/o	testis (testicle)
		orchid/o	testis (testicle)
-logy	study of	or/o	mouth
lord/o	bent	orth/o	straight, normal, or correct
lumb/o	loin (lower back)	-osis	condition or increase
lymph/o	clear fluid	oste/o	bone
-lysis	breaking down or dissolution	ot/o	ear
macro-	large or long	-ous	pertaining to
-malacia	softening	ovari/o	ovary
mamm/o	breast	ov/i	egg
-mania	abnormal impulse (attraction) toward	ov/o	egg
		ox/o	oxygen
mast/o	breast	pachy-	thick
meat/o	opening	palat/o	palate
-megaly	enlargement	pan-	all
melan/o	black	pancreat/o	pancreas
men/o	menstruation	para-	alongside of or abnormal
mening/o	meninges (membrane)	-paresis	slight paralysis
meningi/o	meninges (membrane)	patell/o	knee cap
meso-	middle	path/o	disease
meta-	beyond, after, or change	pector/o	chest
-meter	instrument for measuring	ped/o	child or foot
metr/o	uterus	pelv/i	hip bone
-metry	process of measuring	-penia	abnormal reduction
micro-	small	per-	through or by
mono-	one	peri-	around
morph/o	form	perine/o	perineum
multi-	many	peritone/o	peritoneum
muscul/o	muscle	-pexy	suspension or fixation
my/o	muscle	phac/o	lens (lentil)
myc/o	fungus	phag/o	eat or swallow
myel/o	bone marrow or spinal cord	phak/o	lens (lentil)
myos/o	muscle	pharyng/o	pharynx (throat)
myring/o	eardrum	phas/o	speech

TERM COMPONENT	MEANING
-phil	attraction for
-philia	attraction for
phleb/o	vein
phob/o	exaggerated fear or sensitivity
phon/o	voice or sound
phor/o	to carry or bear
phot/o	light
phren/o	diaphragm or mind
plas/o	formation
-plasia	formation
-plasty	surgical repair or reconstruction
-plegia	paralysis
pleur/o	pleura
-pnea	breathing
pneum/o	air or lung
pneumon/o	air or lung
pod/o	foot
-poiesis	formation
poly-	many
post-	after or behind
pre-	before
presby/o	old age
pro-	before
proct/o	anus and rectum
prostat/o	prostate
psych/o	mind
-ptosis	falling or downward displacement
pulmon/o	lung
purpur/o	purple
py/o	pus
pyel/o	basin
pylor/o	pylorus (gatekeeper)
quadri-	four
radi/o	radius or radiation (especially x-ray)
re-	again or back
rect/o	rectum
ren/o	kidney
reticul/o	a net
retin/o	retina
retro-	backward or behind
rhabd/o	rod shaped or striated (skeletal)
rhin/o	nose
-rrhage	to burst forth
-rrhagia	to burst forth
-rrhaphy	suture
-rrhea	discharge
-rrhexis	rupture
salping/o	uterine (fallopian) tube or eustachian tube
sarc/o	flesh
schiz/o	split or division
scler/o	hard or sclera

TERM COMPONENT	MEANING
scoli/o	twisted
-scope	instrument for examination
-scopy	process of examination
seb/o	sebum (oil)
semi-	half
sial/o	saliva
sigmoid/o	sigmoid colon
sinistr/o	left or on the left side
sinus/o	hollow (cavity)
somat/o	body
somn/o	sleep
somn/i	sleep
son/o	sound
-spasm	involuntary contraction
sperm/o	sperm (seed)
spermat/o	sperm (seed)
sphygm/o	pulse
spin/o	spine (thorn)
spir/o	breathing
splen/o	spleen
spondyl/o	vertebra
squam/o	scale
-stasis	stop or stand
steat/o	fat
sten/o	narrow
stere/o	three-dimensional or solid
stern/o	sternum (breastbone)
steth/o	chest
stomat/o	mouth
-stomy	creation of an opening
sub-	below or under
super-	above or excessive
supra-	above or excessive
sym-	together or with
syn-	together or with
tachy-	fast
tax/o	order or coordination
ten/o	tendon (to stretch)
tend/o	tendon (to stretch)
tendin/o	tendon (to stretch)
test/o	testis (testicle)
thalam/o	thalamus (a room)
thorac/o	chest
thromb/o	clot
thym/o	thymus gland or mind
thyr/o	thyroid gland (shield)
thyroid/o	thyroid gland (shield)
-tic	pertaining to
toc/o	labor
tom/o	to cut
-tomy	incision
ton/o	tone or tension
tonsill/o	tonsil
top/o	place

TERM COMPONENT	MEANING
tox/o	poison
toxic/o	poison
trache/o	trachea (windpipe)
trans-	across or through
tri-	three
trich/o	hair
-tripsy	crushing
troph/o	nourishment or development
tympan/o	eardrum
-ula	small
-ule	small
uln/o	ulna
ultra-	beyond or excessive
uni-	one
ur/o	urine
ureter/o	ureter
urethr/o	urethra

TERM COMPONENT	MEANING
urin/o	urine
uter/o	uterus
uvul/o	uvula
vagin/o	vagina (sheath)
varic/o	swollen or twisted vein
vas/o	vessel
vascul/o	vessel
ven/o	vein
ventricul/o	ventricle (belly or pouch)
vertebr/o	vertebra
vesic/o	bladder or sac
vesicul/o	bladder or sac
vitre/o	glassy
vulv/o	vulva (covering)
xanth/o	yellow
xer/o	dry
-y	condition or process of

ENGLISH TO TERM COMPONENT

MEANING	TERM COMPONENT
abdomen	abdomin/o, celi/o, lapar/o
abnormal	para-
abnormal reduction	-penia
above	hyper-, super-, supra-
across	dia-, trans-
adrenal gland	adrenal/o
after	post-, meta-
again	re-
against	anti-, contra-
air	aer/o, pneum/o, pneumon/o
air sac	alveol/o
airway	bronch/o, bronchi/o
all	pan-
alongside of	para-
alveolus	alveol/o
anus	an/o
anus and rectum	proct/o
aorta	aort/o
apart	dis-
appendix	appendic/o
arm	brachi/o
around	circum-, peri-
artery	arteri/o
atrium	atri/o
attraction for	-phil, -philia
away	e-, ec-, ex-
away from	ab-
back	re-
backward	retro-

MEANING	TERM COMPONENT
bacteria	bacteri/o
basin	pyel/o
before	ante-, pre-, pro-
beginning	-arche
behind	post-, retro-
below	hypo-, infra-, sub-
bent	lord/o
between	inter-
beyond	meta-, ultra-
bile	bil/i, chol/e
bile duct	choledoch/o
binding	-desis
birth	nat/i, toc/o
black	melan/o
bladder	cyst/o, vesic/o, vesicul/o
blood	hem/o, hemat/o
blood condition	-emia
blue	cyan/o
body	somat/o
bone	oste/o
bone marrow	myel/o
both	ambi-, bi-
brain	cerebr/o (largest part of brain), encephal/o (entire brain)
breaking down	-lysis
breast	mamm/o, mast/o
breathing	-pnea, spir/o
bronchus	bronch/o, bronchi/o
bud	-blast, blast/o
burst forth	-rrhage, -rrhagia

MEANING	TERM COMPONENT
calculus	lith/o
cancer	carcin/o
carbon dioxide	capn/o, carb/o
carry	phor/o
cartilage	chondr/o
cavity (sinus)	atri/o, sin/o
cell	cyt/o
cerebellum	cerebell/o
cervix	cervic/o
change	meta-
cheek	bucc/o
chest	pector/o, steth/o, thorac/o
child	ped/o
circle	coron/o
clear fluid	lymph/o
clot	thromb/o
colon	col/o, colon/o
colon, sigmoid	sigmoid/o
color	chrom/o, chromat/o
colored circle	irid/o, ir/o
condition	-osis
condition of	-ia, -ism, -ium, -y
contraction, involuntary	-spasm
coordination	tax/o
cornea	corne/o, kerat/o
correct	ortho-
creation of an opening	-stomy
crooked	ankyl/o
crown	coron/o
crushing	-tripsy
cut (to cut)	tom/o
death	necr/o
deficient	hypo-, olig/o
development	troph/o
diaphragm	phren/o
different	hetero-
difficult	dys-
digit (finger or toe)	dactyl/o
dilation or expansion	-ectasis
discharge	-rrhea
disease	path/o
dissolution	-lysis
division	schiz/o
down	de-
downward placement	-ptosis
dry	xer/o
duct	doch/o
duodenum	duoden/o

MEANING	TERM COMPONENT
ear	aur/i, ot/o
eardrum	myring/o, tympan/o
eat or swallow	phag/o
egg	ov/i, ov/o
enlargement	-megaly
enzyme	-ase
epididymis	epididym/o
equal	iso-
esophagus	esophag/o
eustachian tube	salping/o
examination	-scopy
excessive	hyper-, super-, supra-, ultra-
excision (removal)	-ectomy
expansion or dilation	-ectasis
extremity	acr/o
eye	ocul/o, ophthalm/o, opt/o
eyelid	blephar/o
falling	-ptosis
fallopian tube	salping/o
fascia	fasci/o
fast	tachy-
fat	adip/o, ather/o, lip/o, steat/o
faulty	dys-
fear, exaggerated	phob/o
femur	femor/o
few	olig/o
fiber	fibr/o
fixation	-pexy
flesh	sarc/o
foot	pod/o, ped/o
form	morph/o
formation	-plasia, plas/o, -poiesis
formation of	-lasis
four	quadri-
from	de-
fungus	myc/o
ganglion	gangli/o
gas	aer/o
germ or bud	-blast, blast/o
gland	aden/o
glans penis	balan/o
glassy	vitre/o
glomerulus	glomerul/o
glue	gli/o
good	eu-
groin	inguin/o
gums	gingiv/o
hair	trich/o
half	hemi-, semi-
hard	kerat/o, scler/o
head	cephal/o

MEANING	TERM COMPONENT	MEANING	TERM COMPONENT
hearing	acous/o, audi/o	narrow	sten/o
hearing condition	-acusis	near	ad-
heart	cardi/o	neck	cervic/o
heat	therm/o	nerve	neur/o
hernia	-cele, herni/o	net	reticul/o
hip bone	pelv/i	new	neo-
hormone	hormon/o	normal	eu-, ortho-
humped-back	kyph/o	nose	nas/o, rhin/o
ileum	ile/o	not	de-
incision	-tomy	nourishment	troph/o
increase	-osis	oil	seb/o
inflammation	-itis	old age	presby-
instrument for examination	-scope	one	mono-
instrument for measuring	-meter	one who specializes in	-ist
instrument for recording	-graph	one who specializes in the study or treatment of	-logist
jejunum (empty)	jejun/o	opening	glott/o, meat/o
joint	arthr/o, articul/o	opening, creation of	-stomy
juice	chyl/o	opposed to	anti-, contra-
ketone bodies	ket/o, keton/o	order	tax/o
kidney	nephr/o, ren/o	origin	gen/o, -gen, -genesis
kneecap	patell/o	out	e-, ec-, ex-
knowing	gnos/o	outside	ecto-, exo-, extra-
labor	toc/o	ovary	oophor/o, ovari/o
large	macro-	oxygen	ox/o
larynx	laryng/o	pain	-algia, -dynia
left or on the left side	sinistr/o	painful	dys-
lens	phac/o, phak/o	palate	palat/o
light	phot/o	pancreas	pancreat/o
like	iso-	paralysis	-plegia
lip	cheil/o	paralysis, slight	-paresis
liver	hepat/o, hepatic/o	perineum	perine/o
lobe	lob/o	peritoneum	peritone/o
loin (lower back)	lumb/o	pertaining to	-ac, -al, -ar, -ary, -eal, -ic, -ous, -tic
long	macro-	pharynx	pharyng/o
lung	pneum/o, pneumon/o, pulmon/o	place	top/o
male	andr/o	pleura	pleur/o
many	multi-, poly-	poison	tox/o, toxic/o
measuring, instrument for	-meter	portion	lob/o
measuring, process of	-metry	pouching	-cele
meninges	mening/o, meningi/o	presence of	-iasis
menstruation	men/o	process	-ation
milk	lact/o	process of	-y
mind	psych/o, phren/o, thym/o	production	gen/o, -gen, -genesis
mouth	or/o, stomat/o	prostate	prostat/o
movement	kinesi/o	protein	albumin/o
muscle	muscul/o, my/o, myos/o	pulse	sphygm/o
nail	onych/o	puncture for aspiration	-centesis

MEANING	TERM COMPONENT	MEANING	TERM COMPONENT
purple	purpur/o	stiff	ankyl/o
pus	py/o	stomach	gastr/o
pylorus	pylor/o	stone	lith/o
radius	radi/o	stop or stand	-stasis
record	-gram	straight	orth/o
recording, process of	-graphy	striated	rhabd/o
		structure	-ium
rectum	proct/o, rect/o	study of	-logy
red	erythr/o	study of, one who specializes in the	-logist
resembling	-oid		
reticulum	reticul/o		
retina	retin/o	stupor	narc/o
rib	cost/o	sugar	gluc/o, glyc/o, glycos/o
right or on the right side	dextr/o	surgical repair or reconstruction	-plasty
rod shaped	rhabd/o	suspension	-pexy
rupture	-rrhexis	suture	-rrhaphy
sac	cyst/o, vesic/o, vesicul/o	swallow	phag/o
safe	immun/o	sweat	hidr/o
saliva	sial/o	sweat, profuse	diaphor/o
same	homo-	tear	dacry/o, lacrim/o
scale	squam/o	teeth	dent/i
sclera	scler/o	tendon	ten/o, tend/o, tendin/o
sebum	seb/o	tension	ton/o
secrete	crin/o	testis (testicle)	orch/o, orchi/o, orchid/o, test/o
seizure	-lepsy	thalamus	thalam/o
self	auto-	thick	pachy-
sensation	esthesi/o	thirst	dips/o
sensitivity, exaggerated	phob/o	three	tri-
		three-dimensional or solid	stere/o
separate from	dis-		
sigmoid colon	sigmoid/o		
sinus	sinus/o	throat	pharyng/o
skeletal	rhabd/o	through	dia-, per-, trans-
skin	cutane/o, derm/o, dermat/o	thymus gland	thym/o
skull	crani/o	thyroid gland	thyr/o, thyroid/o
sleep	hypn/o, somn/i, somn/o	tissue	hist/o, -ium
slow	brady-	to or toward	ad-
small	-icle, micro-, -ole, -ula, -ule	together	con-, sym-, syn-
small intestine	enter/o	tone	ton/o
smooth	lei/o	tongue	gloss/o, lingu/o
softening	-malacia	tonsil	tonsill/o
sound	phon/o, son/o	topmost	acr/o
sheath	vagin/o	trachea	trache/o
specializes, one who	-ist	treatment	-iactrics, -iatry, -iatr/o
		treatment of, one who specializes in the	-logist
speech	phas/o		
sperm	sperm/o, spermat/o		
spinal cord	myel/o		
spine	spin/o	tumor	-oma, onc/o
spleen	splen/o	twisted	scoli/o
split	schiz/o	two	bi-
sternum	stern/o	ulna	uln/o

MEANING	TERM COMPONENT	MEANING	TERM COMPONENT
under	infra-, sub-	voice	phon/o
upon	epi-	voice box	laryng/o
ureter	ureter/o	vomiting	-emesis
urethra	urethr/o	vulva	vulv/o, episi/o
urine	ur/o, urin/o	water	aque/o, hydr/o
uterine tube	salping/o	wax	cerumin/o
uterus	hyster/o, metr/o, uter/o	weakness	-asthenia
vagina	colp/o, vagin/o	white	leuc/o, leuk/o
vein	phleb/o, ven/o	windpipe	trache/o
vein, swollen or twisted	varic/o	with	con-, sym-, syn-
		within	en-, endo-, intra-
ventricle	ventricul/o	without	a-, an-
vertebra	vertebr/o, spondyl/o	woman	gynec/o
vessel	angi/o, vas/o, vascul/o	word, phrase	lex/o
vision, condition of	-opia	yellow	xanth/o

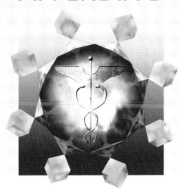

Abbreviations and Symbols

Abbreviations and symbols that appear in **red font** are considered "Dangerous Abbreviations" and should not be used.

ABBREVIATION OR SYMBOL	MEANING
ā	before
A	anterior; assessment
A&P	auscultation and percussion
A&W	alive and well
AB	abortion
ABG	arterial blood gas
a.c.	before meals
ACE	angiotensin-converting enzyme
ACS	acute coronary syndrome
ACTH	adrenocorticotropic hormone
AD	right ear
ad lib.	as desired
ADH	antidiuretic hormone
ADHD	attention-deficit/hyperactivity disorder
AIDS	acquired immunodeficiency syndrome
AKA	above-knee amputation
alb	albumin
ALS	amyotrophic lateral sclerosis
ALT	alanine aminotransferase (enzyme)
a.m.	morning
amt	amount
ANS	autonomic nervous system
AP	anterior-posterior
APKD	adult polycystic kidney disease
aq	water
AS	left ear
ASD	atrial septal defect
AST	aspartate aminotransferase (enzyme)
AU	both ears
AV	atrioventricular
Ⓑ	bilateral

ABBREVIATION OR SYMBOL	MEANING
BAEP	brainstem auditory evoked potential
BAER	brainstem auditory evoked response
BCC	basal cell carcinoma
BD	bipolar disorder
b.i.d.	twice a day
BKA	below-knee amputation
BM	bowel movement
BMP	basic metabolic panel
BP	blood pressure
BPH	benign prostatic hypertrophy; benign prostatic hyperplasia
BRP	bathroom privileges
BS	blood sugar
BUN	blood urea nitrogen
Bx	biopsy
c̄	with
C	Celsius; centigrade
C&S	culture and sensitivity
CABG	coronary artery bypass graft
CAD	coronary artery disease
cap	capsule
CAT	computed axial tomography
CBC	complete blood count
cc	cubic centimeter
CC	chief complaint
CCU	coronary (cardiac) care unit
CF	cystic fibrosis
CHF	congestive heart failure
CIN	cervical intraepithelial neoplasia
CIS	carcinoma in situ
cm	centimeter
CMP	comprehensive metabolic panel

ABBREVIATION OR SYMBOL	MEANING
CNS	central nervous system
c/o	complains of
CO	cardiac output
CO_2	carbon dioxide
COPD	chronic obstructive pulmonary disease
CP	cerebral palsy; chest pain
CPAP	continuous positive airway pressure
CPD	cephalopelvic disproportion
CPR	cardiopulmonary resuscitation
CSF	cerebrospinal fluid
CSII	continuous subcutaneous insulin infusion
CT	computed tomography
CTA	computed tomographic angiography
cu mm or mm³	cubic millimeter
CVA	cerebrovascular accident
CVS	chorionic villus sampling
CXR	chest x-ray
d	day
D&C	dilation and curettage
D&E	dilation and evacuation
DC	discharge; discontinue; doctor of chiropractic
DDS	doctor of dental surgery
DJD	degenerative joint disease
DKA	diabetic ketoacidosis
DO	doctor of osteopathy
DPM	doctor of podiatric medicine
dr	dram
DRE	digital rectal exam
DTR	deep tendon reflex
DVT	deep vein thrombosis
Dx	diagnosis
ECG	electrocardiogram
echo	echocardiogram
ECT	electroconvulsive therapy
ECU	emergency care unit
ED	erectile dysfunction
EDC	estimated date of confinement
EDD	estimated date of delivery
EEG	electroencephalogram
EGD	esophagogastroduodenoscopy
EKG	electrocardiogram
EMG	electromyogram
ENT	ear, nose, and throat
EPS	electrophysiological study
ER	emergency room
ERCP	endoscopic retrograde cholangiopancreatography
ESR	erythrocyte sedimentation rate

ABBREVIATION OR SYMBOL	MEANING
ESWL	extracorporeal shock wave lithotripsy
ETOH	ethyl alcohol
EUS	endoscopic ultrasonography
F	Fahrenheit
FBS	fasting blood sugar
Fe	iron
FH	family history
fl oz	fluid ounce
FS	frozen section
FSH	follicle-stimulating hormone
Fx	fracture
g	gram
GAD	generalized anxiety disorder
GERD	gastroesophageal reflux disease
GH	growth hormone
GI	gastrointestinal
gm	gram
gr	grain
gt	drop
gtt	drops
GTT	glucose tolerance test
GYN	gynecology
h	hour
H&H	hemoglobin and hematocrit
H&P	history and physical
HAV	hepatitis A virus
HBV	hepatitis B virus
HCT or Hct	hematocrit
HCV	hepatitis C virus
HD	Huntington disease
HEENT	head, eyes, ears, nose, and throat
HGB or Hgb	hemoglobin
HIV	human immunodeficiency virus
hpf	high-power field
HPI	history of present illness
HPV	human papilloma virus
HRT	hormone replacement therapy
h.s.	hour of sleep
HSV-1	herpes simplex virus type 1
HSV-2	herpes simplex virus type 2
Ht	height
HTN	hypertension
Hx	history
I&D	incision and drainage
ICD	implantable cardioverter defibrillator
ICU	intensive care unit
ID	intradermal
IM	intramuscular

ABBREVIATION OR SYMBOL	MEANING
IMP	impression
IOL	intraocular lens
IP	inpatient
IUD	intrauterine device
IV	intravenous
IVP	intravenous pyelogram
IVU	intravenous urogram
JCAHO	Joint Commission on Accreditation of Healthcare Organizations
kg	kilogram
KUB	kidneys, ureters, bladder
L	liter
Ⓛ	left
L&W	living and well
LASIK	laser-assisted in situ keratomileusis
lb	pound
LEEP	loop electrosurgical excision procedure
LH	luteinizing hormone
LLETZ	large-loop excision of transformation zone
LLQ	left lower quadrant
LP	lumbar puncture
lpf	low-power field
LTB	laryngotracheobronchitis
LUQ	left upper quadrant
m	meter
ⓜ	murmur
MCH	mean corpuscular (cell) hemoglobin
MCHC	mean corpuscular (cell) hemoglobin concentration
MCV	mean corpuscular (cell) volume
MD	medical doctor; muscular dystrophy
mg	milligram
MI	myocardial infarction
ml or mL	milliliter
mm	millimeter
mm³ or cu mm	cubic millimeter
MPI	myocardial perfusion image
MRA	magnetic resonance angiography
MRI	magnetic resonance imaging
MS	multiple sclerosis; musculoskeletal
MSH	melanocyte-stimulating hormone
MUGA	multiple-gated acquisition (scan)

ABBREVIATION OR SYMBOL	MEANING
MVP	mitral valve prolapse
NAD	no acute distress
NCV	nerve conduction velocity
NG	nasogastric
NK	natural killer (cell)
NKA	no known allergy
NKDA	no known drug allergy
noc.	night
NPO	nothing by mouth
NSAID	nonsteroidal antiinflammatory drug
NSR	normal sinus rhythm
O	objective
O₂	oxygen
OA	osteoarthritis
OB	obstetrics
OCD	obsessive-compulsive disorder
OCP	oral contraceptive pill
OD	right eye; doctor of optometry
OH	occupational history
OP	outpatient
OR	operating room
ORIF	open reduction, internal fixation
OS	left eye
OU	both eyes
oz	ounce
p̄	after
P	plan; posterior; pulse
PA	posterior-anterior
PACU	postanesthetic care unit
PaCO₂	partial pressure of carbon dioxide
PaO₂	partial pressure of oxygen
Pap	Papanicolaou (smear)
PAR	postanesthetic recovery
p.c.	after meals
PCI	percutaneous coronary intervention
PD	panic disorder
PDA	patent ductus arteriosus
PE	physical examination; pulmonary embolism; polyethylene
PEFR	peak expiratory flow rate
per	by or through
PERRLA	pupils equal, round, and reactive to light and accommodation
PET	positron-emission tomography
PF	peak flow
PFT	pulmonary function testing
pH	potential of hydrogen

ABBREVIATION OR SYMBOL	MEANING
PH	past history
PI	present illness
PID	pelvic inflammatory disease
PIH	pregnancy-induced hypertension
p.m.	after noon
PLT	platelet
PMH	past medical history
PMN	polymorphonuclear (leukocyte)
PNS	peripheral nervous system
p.o.	by mouth
post-op or postop	postoperative
PPBS	postprandial blood sugar
PR	per rectum
pre-op or preop	preoperative
p.r.n.	as needed
PSA	prostate-specific antigen
PSG	polysomnography
pt	patient
PT	physical therapy; prothrombin time
PTCA	percutaneous transluminal coronary angioplasty
PTH	parathyroid hormone
PTSD	posttraumatic stress disorder
PTT	partial thromboplastin time
PUD	peptic ulcer disease
PV	per vagina
PVC	premature ventricular contraction
Px	physical examination
q	every
q.d.	every day, daily
qh	every hour
q2h	every 2 hours
q.i.d.	four times a day
q.o.d.	every other day
qt	quart
R	respiration
®	right
RA	rheumatoid arthritis
RBC	red blood cell; red blood count
RLQ	right lower quadrant
R/O	rule out
ROM	range of motion
ROS	review of symptoms
RP	retrograde pyelogram
RRR	regular rate and rhythm
RTC	return to clinic
RTO	return to office
RUQ	right upper quadrant
Rx	recipe; prescription

ABBREVIATION OR SYMBOL	MEANING
$\bar{s}$	without
S	subjective
SA	sinoatrial
SAB	spontaneous abortion
SAD	seasonal affective disorder
SC	subcutaneous
SCA	sudden cardiac arrest
SCC	squamous cell carcinoma
SH	social history
Sig:	instruction to patient
SLE	systemic lupus erythematosus
SOB	shortness of breath
SPECT	single-photon emission computed tomography
SpGr	specific gravity
SQ	subcutaneous
SR	systems review
$\bar{\bar{s}}\bar{s}$	one-half
STAT	immediately
STD	sexually transmitted disease
SUI	stress urinary incontinence
suppos	suppository
SV	stroke volume
Sx	symptom
T	temperature
T_3	triiodothyronine
T_4	thyroxine
T&A	tonsillectomy and adenoidectomy
tab	tablet
TAB	therapeutic abortion
TB	tuberculosis
TEDS	thromboembolic disease stockings
TEE	transesophageal echocardiogram
TIA	transient ischemic attack
t.i.d.	three times a day
TM	tympanic membrane
TMR	transmyocardial revascularization
tPA or TPA	tissue plasminogen activator
Tr	treatment
TSH	thyroid-stimulating hormone
TURP	transurethral resection of the prostate
TV	tidal volume
Tx	treatment; traction
UA	urinalysis
UCHD	usual childhood diseases
URI	upper respiratory infection
US or U/S	ultrasound
UTI	urinary tract infection

ABBREVIATION OR SYMBOL	MEANING
VC	vital capacity
VCU or VCUG	voiding cystourethrogram
V/Q	ventilation/perfusion
VS	vital signs
VSD	ventricular septal defect
V_T	tidal volume
w.a.	while awake
WBC	white blood cell; white blood count
WDWN	well developed, well nourished
wk	week
WNL	within normal limits
Wt	weight
x	times; for
x-ray	radiography
y.o. or y/o	year old
yr	year
♀	female
♂	male

ABBREVIATION OR SYMBOL	MEANING
#	number; pound
°	degree; hour
↑	increase; above
↓	decrease; below
✓	check
θ	none; negative
♀	standing
♀	sitting
o⃨	lying
×	times; for
>	greater than
<	less than
i	one
ii	two
iii	three
iv	four
I, II, III, IV, V, VI, VII, VIII, IX, and X	uppercase Roman numerals 1–10

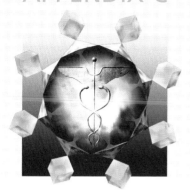

Commonly Prescribed Drugs

The following alphabetical list of commonly prescribed drugs (trade and generic) is based on listings of prescriptions dispensed in the United States during 2005. The classification and major therapeutic uses for each are also provided. Trade drug names begin with a capital letter; the generic names accompany them in parentheses. All generic names are set in lowercase.

NAME	CLASSIFICATION	MAJOR THERAPEUTIC USES
acetaminophen and codeine	nonsteroidal antiinflammatory drug (NSAID) (analgesic/antipyretic) and opiate (narcotic) combination	moderate to severe pain, fever
AcipHex (rabeprazole)	proton-pump inhibitor (PPI) (gastric acid secretion inhibitor)	peptic ulcer disease (PUD), gastroesophageal reflux disease (GERD)
Actonel (risedronate)	bisphosphonate (bone resorption inhibitor)	osteoporosis, Paget disease
Actos (pioglitazone)	oral antidiabetic	type 2 diabetes mellitus
acyclovir	antiviral	viral infections
Adderall XR (amphetamine mixed salts)	central nervous system (CNS) stimulant	attention-deficit/hyperactivity disorder (ADHD)
Advair Diskus (salmeterol and fluticasone)	β_2-adrenergic agonist (bronchodilator) and glucocorticoid (antiinflammatory) combination	asthma
Abilify (aripiprazole)	antipsychotic	schizophrenia, bipolar disorder
albuterol aerosol	β_2-adrenergic agonist (bronchodilator)	asthma, bronchitis
Allegra (fexofenadine)	antihistamine	allergy
Allegra D (fexofenadine and pseudoephedrine)	antihistamine and decongestant combination	allergy with nasal congestion
allopurinol	xanthine oxidase inhibitor	gout
Alphagan P (brimonidine) ophthalmic solution	α_2-adrenergic agonist (antihypertensive)	glaucoma
alprazolam	benzodiazepine (anxiolytic, sedative, hypnotic)	anxiety
Altace (ramipril)	angiotensin-converting enzyme (ACE) inhibitor	hypertension, congestive heart failure (CHF)
Amaryl (glimepiride)	oral antidiabetic	type 2 diabetes mellitus
Ambien (zolpidem)	sedative; hypnotic	insomnia
amitriptyline	antidepressant	depression
amoxicillin	penicillin (antibiotic)	bacterial infections

NAME	CLASSIFICATION	MAJOR THERAPEUTIC USES
Aricept (donepezil)	acetylcholinesterase inhibitor	Alzheimer disease
atenolol	cardioselective β-blocker (antihypertensive, antiarrhythmic, antianginal)	hypertension, angina pectoris, cardiac arrhythmias
atenolol and chlorthalidone	cardioselective β-blocker (antihypertensive, antiarrhythmic, antianginal) and diuretic combination	hypertension
Augmentin (amoxicillin and clavulanate)	penicillin (antibiotic) and β-lactamase inhibitor combination	bacterial infections
Avalide (irbesartan and hydrochlorothiazide)	angiotensin-receptor blocker (antihypertensive) and diuretic combination	hypertension
Avandia (rosiglitazone)	oral antidiabetic	type 2 diabetes mellitus
Avapro (irbesartan)	angiotensin-receptor blocker (antihypertensive)	hypertension
Avelox (moxifloxacin)	fluoroquinolone (antibiotic)	bacterial infections
Aviane (levonorgestrel and ethinyl estradiol)	oral contraceptive	birth control
azithromycin	macrolide (antibiotic)	bacterial infections
baclofen	skeletal muscle relaxant	muscle spasms and spasticity
Bactroban (mupirocin)	topical antibiotic	bacterial skin infections
benazepril	angiotensin-converting enzyme (ACE) inhibitor	hypertension
Benicar (olmesartan medoxomil)	angiotensin-receptor blocker (antihypertensive)	hypertension
benzonatate	nonnarcotic antitussive	cough
Biaxin (clarithromycin)	macrolide (antibiotic)	bacterial infections
bupropion SR	atypical antidepressant	depression
buspirone	anxiolytic	anxiety
butalbital, acetaminophen, and caffeine	sedative barbiturate; analgesic/antipyretic; central nervous system (CNS) stimulant combination	muscle tension headache
carisoprodol	skeletal muscle relaxant	skeletal muscle spasms and spasticity
Cartia XT (diltiazem)	calcium-channel blocker	hypertension, angina pectoris, cardiac arrhythmias
Celebrex (celecoxib)	COX-2 inhibitor (nonsteroidal anti-inflammatory drug [NSAID])	pain, inflammation, fever, arthritis
cephalexin	cephalosporin (antibiotic)	bacterial infections
Cialis (tadalafil)	phosphodiesterase (type 5) enzyme inhibitor	erectile dysfunction (ED)
ciprofloxacin	fluoroquinolone (antibiotic)	bacterial infections
citalopram	selective serotonin reuptake inhibitor (SSRI) (antidepressant)	depression
Clarinex (desloratadine)	antihistamine	allergy
clindamycin	antibiotic	bacterial infections
clonazepam	benzodiazepine (sedative/hypnotic, anticonvulsant, anxiolytic)	epilepsy, seizures, anxiety (panic disorder)

NAME	CLASSIFICATION	MAJOR THERAPEUTIC USES
clonidine	α_2-adrenergic agonist (antihypertensive)	hypertension
clotrimazole and betamethasone	topical antifungal and glucocorticoid (steroid) combination	fungal infections, some parasites
Combivent (ipratropium and albuterol) inhalation aerosol	anticholinergic and β_2-adrenergic agonist combination (bronchodilators)	asthma, chronic bronchitis, emphysema
Concerta (methylphenidate) extended release	central nervous system (CNS) stimulant	attention-deficit/hyperactivity disorder (ADHD)
Coreg (carvedilol)	cardioselective β-blocker (antihypertensive, antiarrhythmic, antianginal)	hypertension, congestive heart failure (CHF)
Cosopt (dorzolamide hydrochloride and timolol maleate) ophthalmic solution	carbonic anhydrase inhibitor and β-blocker combination	intraocular pressure
Coumadin (warfarin sodium)	anticoagulant	thromboembolic disorders
Cozaar (losartan)	angiotensin-receptor blocker (antihypertensive)	hypertension
Crestor (rosuvastatin)	HMG-CoA reductase inhibitor (statin)	hyperlipidemia, hypercholesterolemia
cyclobenzaprine	skeletal muscle relaxant	skeletal muscle spasms and spasticity
Cymbalta (duloxetine hydrochloride)	selective serotonin and norepinephrine reuptake inhibitor (SSNRI)	major depression, diabetic peripheral neuropathic pain
Depakote (divalproex)	anticonvulsant	epilepsy, migraine prophylaxis, bipolar mania
Detrol LA (tolterodine)	anticholinergic	overactive bladder
diazepam	benzodiazepine (sedative/hypnotic, anticonvulsant, anxiolytic)	anxiety, skeletal muscle spasm, epilepsy, seizures
diclofenac	nonsteroidal antiinflammatory (NSAID)	pain, inflammation, fever
Digitek (digoxin)	cardiac glycoside	congestive heart failure (CHF), cardiac tachyarrhythmias
digoxin	cardiac glycoside	congestive heart failure (CHF), cardiac tachyarrhythmias
Dilantin (phenytoin)	hydantoin (anticonvulsant)	epilepsy, seizures
diltiazem	calcium-channel blocker	hypertension, angina pectoris, cardiac arrhythmias
Diovan (valsartan)	angiotensin-receptor blocker (antihypertensive)	hypertension
Diovan HCT (valsartan and hydrochlorothiazide)	angiotensin-receptor blocker and diuretic combination (antihypertensive)	hypertension
Ditropan XL (oxybutynin)	anticholinergic (urinary antispasmodic)	overactive bladder
doxazosin	α_1-adrenergic antagonist (antihypertensive, vasodilator)	benign prostatic hyperplasia (BPH), hypertension
doxycycline	tetracycline (antibiotic)	bacterial, rickettsial, chlamydial infections

NAME	CLASSIFICATION	MAJOR THERAPEUTIC USES
Effexor XR (venlafaxine)	antidepressant	depression
Elidel (pimecrolimus) topical cream	immunosuppressant agent	atopic dermatitis
enalapril	angiotensin-converting enzyme (ACE) inhibitor	hypertension, congestive heart failure (CHF)
Endocet (oxycodone and acetaminophen)	opiate (narcotic) and nonsteroidal antiinflammatory (NSAID) (analgesic/antipyretic) combination	moderate to severe pain
estradiol	estrogen	contraception, menstrual irregularity, hormone replacement, vaginal atrophy
etodolac	nonsteroidal antiinflammatory drug (NSAID) (analgesic/antipyretic)	pain, inflammation, fever, arthritis
Evista (raloxifene)	selective estrogen-receptor modulator (SERM)	prevention and treatment of osteoporosis
famotidine	H_2 receptor antagonist	peptic ulcer disease (PUD), gastroesophageal reflux disease (GERD)
fexofenadine	antihistamine	allergy
Flexeril (cyclobenzaprine)	skeletal muscle relaxant	skeletal muscle spasms and spasticity
Flomax (tamsulosin)	α_1-adrenergic antagonist (antihypertensive, vasodilator)	benign prostatic hypertrophy (BPH)
Flonase (fluticasone) nasal spray	glucocorticoid (antiinflammatory, immunosuppressant)	allergic rhinitis
Flovent (fluticasone) oral inhalation	glucocorticoid (antiinflammatory, immunosuppressant)	asthma control
fluconazole	antifungal	fungal infections
fluoxetine	selective serotonin reuptake inhibitor (SSRI) (antidepressant)	depression
folic acid	vitamin	nutritional supplement
Fosamax (alendronate)	bisphosphonate (bone resorption inhibitor)	osteoporosis, Paget disease
fosinopril	angiotensin-converting enzyme (ACE) inhibitor	hypertension
furosemide	diuretic	hypertension, edema associated with congestive heart failure (CHF) or renal disease
gabapentin	anticonvulsant	postherpetic neuralgia, epilepsy (partial seizures)
gemfibrozil	antihyperlipidemic	hypertriglyceridemia, hyperlipidemia
glipizide	oral antidiabetic	type 2 diabetes mellitus
glyburide	oral antidiabetic	type 2 diabetes mellitus
glyburide and metformin	oral antidiabetic (combination product)	type 2 diabetes mellitus
GlycoLax (polyethylene glycol)	laxative	constipation

NAME	CLASSIFICATION	MAJOR THERAPEUTIC USES
Humalog (insulin lispro)	insulin; antidiabetic	types 1 and 2 diabetes mellitus
Humulin (insulin preparation)	insulin; antidiabetic	types 1 and 2 diabetes mellitus
hydrochlorothiazide	diuretic	hypertension, edema associated with congestive heart failure (CHF) or renal disease
hydrochlorothiazide and bisoprolol	diuretic and cardioselective β-blocker combination (antihypertensive)	hypertension
hydrochlorothiazide and triamterene	potassium-sparing diuretic combination	hypertension, edema in congestive heart failure (CHF)
hydrocodone and acetaminophen	opiate (narcotic) and nonsteroidal antiinflammatory (NSAID) (analgesic/antipyretic) combination	moderate to severe pain
hydroxyzine	antihistamine	allergy, insomnia
Hyzaar (losartan and hydrochlorothiazide)	angiotensin-receptor blocker and diuretic combination (antihypertensive)	hypertension
ibuprofen	analgesic; nonsteroidal antiinflammatory (NSAID)	pain, inflammation, fever
Imitrex (sumatriptan succinate)	triptan (antimigraine agent)	migraine headache
isosorbide mononitrate	coronary vasodilator (antianginal)	angina pectoris
Klor-Con (potassium chloride)	potassium salt; electrolyte supplement	potassium deficiency
Lamictal (lamotrigine)	anticonvulsant	epilepsy, seizures
Lanoxin (digoxin)	cardiac glycoside	congestive heart failure (CHF), cardiac tachyarrhythmias
Lantus (insulin glargine)	insulin; antidiabetic	types 1 and 2 diabetes mellitus
Lescol XL (fluvastatin)	HMG-CoA reductase inhibitor (statin)	hyperlipidemia, hypercholesterolemia
Levaquin (levofloxacin)	fluoroquinolone (antibiotic)	bacterial infections
Levitra (vardenafil)	phosphodiesterase (type 5) enzyme inhibitor	erectile dysfunction (ED)
levothyroxine	thyroid hormone	hypothyroidism
Levoxyl (levothyroxine sodium)	thyroid hormone	hypothyroidism
Lexapro (escitalopram)	selective serotonin reuptake inhibitor (SSRI) (antidepressant)	depression
Lidoderm (lidocaine) patch	local anesthetic	postherpetic neuralgia
Lipitor (atorvastatin)	HMG-CoA reductase inhibitor (statin)	hyperlipidemia, hypercholesterolemia
lisinopril	angiotensin-converting enzyme (ACE) inhibitor	hypertension
lisinopril and hydrochlorothiazide	angiotensin-converting enzyme (ACE) inhibitor and diuretic combination	hypertension
lithium	antimanic	manic episodes of bipolar disorder

NAME	CLASSIFICATION	MAJOR THERAPEUTIC USES
lorazepam	benzodiazepine (sedative/hypnotic, anticonvulsant, anxiolytic)	anxiety, preoperative sedation, epilepsy, seizures
Lotrel (amlodipine and benazepril)	calcium-channel blocker and angiotensin-converting enzyme (ACE) inhibitor combination	hypertension
lovastatin	HMG-CoA reductase inhibitor (statin)	hyperlipidemia, hypercholes-terolemia
Lunesta (eszopiclone)	hypnotic	insomnia
Macrobid (nitrofurantoin)	antibiotic	bacterial infections of urinary tract
meclizine	anticholinergic	motion sickness, vertigo
metformin	oral antidiabetic	type 2 diabetes mellitus
methotrexate	antineoplastic	neoplastic and immunological disorders
methylprednisolone	glucocorticoid (antiinflammatory, immunosuppressant)	inflammation, immunological disorders, allergies
metoclopramide	prokinetic; antiemetic	gastroesophageal reflux disease (GERD), gastroparesis, nausea, vomiting
metoprolol	cardioselective β-blocker (antihyper-tensive, antiarrhythmic, antianginal)	hypertension, angina pectoris
metronidazole	antibacterial, antiprotozoal	bacterial infections, protozoal infections
Miacalcin (calcitonin)	hormone	osteoporosis, Paget disease
minocycline	antibiotic	bacterial infections
mirtazapine	atypical antidepressant	depression
Mobic (meloxicam)	nonsteroidal antiinflammatory drug (NSAID)	osteoarthritis
morphine	opiate agonist	pain
mupirocin	topical antibiotic	bacterial skin infections
nabumetone	nonsteroidal antiinflammatory drug (NSAID)	pain, inflammation, fever
naproxen	nonsteroidal antiinflammatory drug (NSAID)	pain, inflammation, fever
Nasacort (triamcinolone) AQ topical nasal spray	glucocorticoid (antiinflammatory, immunosuppressant)	allergic rhinitis
Nasonex (mometasone) topical nasal spray	glucocorticoid (antiinflammatory, immunosuppressant)	allergic rhinitis
Nexium (esomeprazole)	proton-pump inhibitor (PPI) (gastric acid secretion inhibitor)	peptic ulcer disease (PUD), gastroesophageal reflux disease (GERD)
Niaspan (niacin)	vitamin	dyslipidemia
nifedipine	calcium-channel blocker	hypertension, angina pectoris
nitrofurantoin	antibiotic	bacterial infections of urinary tract
NitroQuick (nitroglycerin)	antianginal	coronary vasodilator
nortriptyline	tricyclic antidepressant	depression

NAME	CLASSIFICATION	MAJOR THERAPEUTIC USES
Norvasc (amlodipine)	calcium-channel blocker	hypertension, angina pectoris
nystatin	antifungal	fungus
omeprazole	proton-pump inhibitor (PPI) (gastric acid secretion inhibitor)	peptic ulcer disease (PUD), gastroesophageal reflux disease (GERD)
Omnicef (cefdinir)	cephalosporin (antibiotic)	bacterial infections
Ortho Evra (norelgestromin and ethinyl estradiol)	contraceptive patch	birth control
Ortho Tri-Cyclen Lo (norgestimate and ethyl estradiol)	oral contraceptive	birth control
oxycodone and aceta-minophen	opiate (narcotic) and nonsteroidal antiinflammatory drug (NSAID) (analgesic/antipyretic) combination	moderate to severe pain
OxyContin (oxycodone)	opiate (narcotic) analgesic	moderate to severe pain
Patanol (olopatadine)	ophthalmic antihistamine	allergic conjunctivitis
Paxil (paroxetine)	selective serotonin reuptake inhibitor (SSRI) (antidepressant)	depression
Penicillin VK (penicillin V potassium)	penicillin (antibiotic)	bacterial infections
phenazopyridine	urinary analgesic	urinary tract pain
phenobarbital	barbiturate (sedative/hypnotic, anticonvulsant, anxiolytic)	insomnia, epilepsy, seizures, anxiety
phentermine	anorexiant; decongestant; central nervous system (CNS) stimulant	nasal congestion, obesity, attention-deficit/hyperactivity disorder (ADHD)
phenytoin	hydantoin (anticonvulsant)	epilepsy, seizures
Plavix (clopidogrel)	antiplatelet agent	reduction in stroke or myocardial infarction risk by excessive clot prevention
potassium chloride	potassium salt; electrolyte supplement	potassium deficiency
Pravachol (pravastatin)	HMG-CoA reductase inhibitor (statin)	hyperlipidemia, hypercholesterolemia
prednisone	glucocorticoid (antiinflammatory, immunosuppressant)	inflammation, immunological disorders, allergy
Premarin (conjugated estrogens)	estrogen derivative	hormone replacement
Prempro (estrogen and medroxyprogesterone)	estrogen/progestin	hormone replacement
Prevacid (lansoprazole)	proton-pump inhibitor (PPI) (gastric acid secretion inhibitor)	peptic ulcer disease (PUD), gastroesophageal reflux disease (GERD)
Prilosec (omeprazole)	proton-pump inhibitor (PPI) (gastric acid secretion inhibitor)	peptic ulcer disease (PUD), gastroesophageal reflux disease (GERD)
promethazine	antihistamine; sedative; antiemetic	allergy, motion sickness, nausea
promethazine and codeine	antihistamine and opiate (narcotic) antitussive combination	cold and cough

NAME	CLASSIFICATION	MAJOR THERAPEUTIC USES
propoxyphene and acetaminophen	opiate (narcotic) analgesic and non-steroidal antiinflammatory drug (NSAID) (analgesic/antipyretic) combination	mild to moderate pain
propranolol	β-blocker	hypertension, angina pectoris, cardiac arrhythmias, migraine headache prophylaxis
Proscar (finasteride)	5α-reductase inhibitor	benign prostatic hyperplasia (BPH)
Protonix (pantoprazole)	proton-pump inhibitor (PPI) (gastric acid secretion inhibitor)	peptic ulcer disease (PUD), gastroesophageal reflux disease (GERD)
Pulmicort (budesonide) inhalant	glucocorticoid (antiinflammatory, immunosuppressant)	asthma
quinapril hydrochloride	angiotensin-converting enzyme (ACE) inhibitor	hypertension, congestive heart failure (CHF)
quinine	antimalarial	malaria, nocturnal leg cramps
ranitidine	H_2 receptor antagonist	peptic ulcer disease (PUD), gastroesophageal reflux disease (GERD)
Rhinocort Aqua (budesonide) nasal spray	glucocorticoid (antiinflammatory, immunosuppressant)	allergic rhinitis
Risperdal (risperidone)	atypical antipsychotic (neuroleptic)	psychoses (e.g., schizophrenia)
Seroquel (quetiapine)	atypical antipsychotic (neuroleptic)	psychoses (e.g. schizophrenia)
Singulair (montelukast)	leukotriene-receptor antagonist	asthma
Skelaxin (metaxalone)	skeletal muscle relaxant	skeletal muscle spasms and spasticity
Spiriva (tiotropium bromide) inhaler	anticholinergic	bronchospasm, as seen in bronchitis, emphysema, or chronic obstructive pulmonary disease (COPD)
spironolactone	potassium-sparing diuretic	hypertension, edema
Strattera (atomoxetine)	selective norepinephrine reuptake inhibitor (SNRI)	attention-deficit/hyperactivity disorder (ADHD)
Synthroid (levothyroxine)	thyroid product	hypothyroidism
Tamiflu (oseltamivir)	antiviral	viral infections
temazepam	benzodiazepine (hypnotic)	insomnia
terazosin	α_1-adrenergic antagonist (antihypertensive, vasodilator)	benign prostatic hypertrophy (BPH)
tetracycline	antibiotic	bacterial infections
tizanidine	central sympatholytic (α_2-adrenergic agonist)	muscle spasticity
Topamax (topiramate)	anticonvulsant	epilepsy (partial seizures)
Toprol-XL (metoprolol)	cardioselective β-blocker (antihypertensive, antiarrhythmic, antianginal)	hypertension, angina pectoris, congestive heart failure (CHF)
tramadol	opioid analgesic	chronic pain

NAME	CLASSIFICATION	MAJOR THERAPEUTIC USES
tramadol and aceta-minophen	opioid analgesic and nonsteroidal antiinflammatory drug (NSAID) (analgesic/antipyretic) combination	acute pain
trazodone	atypical antidepressant	depression
triamcinolone	glucocorticoid (antiinflammatory, immunosuppressant)	inflammation, immunological disorders, allergy
TriCor (fenofibrate)	fibric acid derivative	hyperlipidemia, hypertriglyc-eridemia, hypercholesterolemia
Trileptal (oxcarbazepine)	anticonvulsant	epilepsy (partial seizures)
trimethoprim and sulfa-methoxazole (TMP-SMX or co-trimoxazole)	antibacterial and sulfonamide (antibiotic) combination	bacterial infections
Trimox (amoxicillin)	penicillin (antibiotic)	bacterial infections
Tussionex (hydrocodone and chlorpheniramine)	narcotic antitussive and antihistamine combination	cough and cold
Ultracet (tramadol and acetaminophen)	opioid analgesic and nonsteroidal antiinflammatory drug (NSAID) (analgesic/antipyretic) combination	acute pain
Valtrex (valacyclovir)	antiviral	herpes viruses
verapamil	calcium-channel blocker	hypertension, cardiac arrhyth-mias, angina pectoris
Viagra (sildenafil)	phosphodiesterase (type 5) enzyme inhibitor	erectile dysfunction (ED)
Vigamox (moxifloxacin hydrochloride)	ophthalmic solution	antibacterial
Vytorin (ezetimibe and simvastatin)	cholesterol absorption inhibitor and HMG-CoA reductase inhibitor (statin) combination	hyperlipidemia, hypercholes-terolemia
warfarin	anticoagulant	thromboembolic disorders
Wellbutrin SR (bupropion)	atypical antidepressant	depression
Xalatan (latanoprost) oph-thalmic solution	prostaglandin	glaucoma
Yasmin 28 (drospirenone and ethinyl estradiol)	oral contraceptive	birth control
Zetia (ezetimibe)	cholesterol absorption inhibitor	hypercholesterolemia
Zithromax (azithromycin dihydrate)	macrolide (antibiotic)	bacterial infections
Zocor (simvastatin)	HMG-CoA reductase inhibitor (statin)	hyperlipidemia, hypercholes-terolemia
Zoloft (sertraline)	selective serotonin reuptake inhibitor (SSRI) (antidepressant)	depression
Zyprexa (olanzapine)	atypical antipsychotic (neuroleptic)	psychoses (e.g., schizophrenia)
Zyrtec (cetirizine)	antihistamine	allergy

RxList Top 300 Drugs of 2005, www.rxlist.com/top200.htm

Stedman's Medical Dictionary for the Health Professions and Nursing, 5th edition, appendix listing of *Commonly Prescribed Drugs and Their Applications*. Baltimore: Lippincott Williams & Wilkins, 2005.

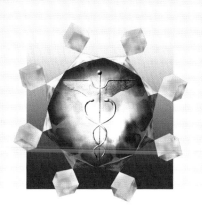

Figure Credits

FIGURE 4-21 ■ Photo courtesy of 3M™ Scotchcast Products, St. Paul, MN.

FIGURE 4-22 ■ From Bucholz RW, Heckman JD. *Rockwood & Green's Fractures in Adults*. 5th ed. Philadelphia: Lippincott Williams & Wilkins, 2001.

FIGURE 4-23 ■ Photo courtesy of Trulife, Jackson, MI.

FIGURE 4-24 ■ Courtesy of Smith & Nephew Systems, Inc., Memphis, TN.

FIGURE 4-25 ■ Photo courtesy of Trulife, Jackson, MI.

FIGURE 4-26 ■ Courtesy of RGP Prosthetic Research Center, San Diego, CA.

FIGURE 5-1 ■ Photo courtesy of Orange Coast College Cardiovascular Technology Program, Costa Mesa, CA.

FIGURE 5-2 ■ PTCA courtesy of Medtronic Interventional Vascular, San Diego, CA.

FIGURE 5-5 ■ Doppler color flow courtesy of Siemens Medical Solutions, Inc., Ultrasound Division, Mountain View, CA.

FIGURE 5-6 ■ Courtesy of Welch Allyn, Skaneateles Falls, NY.

FIGURE 5-10 ■ From *Roche Lexikon Medizin*. 3rd ed. Munich, Germany: Urban & Schwarzenburg, 1993:877.

FIGURE 5-14 ■ **C.** Photo from Sheldon GF. *Boyd's Introduction to the Study of Disease*. 11th ed. Philadelphia: Lea & Febiger, 1992:90.

FIGURE 5-15 ■ From Pillitteri A. *Maternal and Child Nursing*. 4th ed. Philadelphia: Lippincott Williams & Wilkins, 2003.

FIGURE 5-16 ■ **B.** Quinton Cardiology equipment courtesy of Cardiac Science, Inc, Bothell, WA.

FIGURE 5-17 ■ Quinton Cardiology equipment courtesy of Cardiac Science, Inc, Bothell, WA.

FIGURE 5-18 ■ **B.** Courtesy of Cook, Incorporated, Bloomington, IN. **C.** Courtesy of Philips Medical Systems.

FIGURE 5-19 ■ Courtesy of Toshiba America Medical Systems, Inc.

FIGURE 5-20 ■ Courtesy of Siemens Medical Solutions, Inc., Ultrasound Division, Mountain View, CA.

FIGURE 5-23 ■ Courtesy of Philips Medical Systems, Shelton, CT.

FIGURE 5-24 ■ **A.** Redrawn from About Your Pacemaker. Sylmar, CA: Siemens Pacesetter, p. 18. **B.** Courtesy of Philips Medical Systems, Shelton, CT.

FIGURE 6-2 ■ White and red blood cells from Lee GR, et al. *Wintrobe's Clinical Hematology*. 9th ed. Philadelphia: Lea & Febiger, 1993.

FIGURE 6-4 ■ From Lee GR, Foerster J, Lukens JN. *Wintrobe's Clinical Hematology*. 10th ed. Philadelphia: Lippincott Williams & Wilkins, 1999.

FIGURE 6-5 ■ From Lee GR, et al. *Wintrobe's Clinical Hematology*. 9th ed. Philadelphia: Lea & Febiger, 1993;1:758.

FIGURE 6-8 ■ From LifeART. Image copyright © 2006 Lippincott Williams & Wilkins. All rights reserved.

FIGURE 7-7 ■ From Sheldon GF. *Boyd's Introduction to the Study of Disease*. 11th ed. Philadelphia: Lea & Febiger, 1992:340.

FIGURE 7-10 ■ Courtesy of Felix Wang, MD, University of California at Irvine, Irvine, CA.

FIGURE 7-11 ■ Courtesy of VIASYS Respiratory Care.

FIGURE 7-12 ■ Reprinted by permission of Nellcor Puritan Bennett Inc., Pleasanton, CA.

FIGURE 7-13 ■ Courtesy of Felix Wang, MD, University of California at Irvine, Irvine, CA.

FIGURE 7-16 ■ Photo courtesy of Respironics, Inc., Murrysville, PA.

FIGURE 7-17 ■ Coach 2 incentive spirometer courtesy of Smiths Medical, Carlsbad, CA. Patent nos. 5,984,873 and D403,769.

FIGURE 7-18 ■ Courtesy of MAQUET, Inc., Bridgewater, NJ.

FIGURE 8-3 ■ Inset from Haines DL. *Neuroanatomy: An Atlas of Structures, Sections, and Systems*. 4th ed. Baltimore: Williams & Wilkins, 1995:29.

FIGURE 8-4 ■ From Haines DL. *Neuroanatomy: An Atlas of Structures, Sections, and Systems*. 4th ed. Baltimore: Williams & Wilkins, 1995:131,237.

FIGURE 8-5 ■ From Pillitteri A. *Maternal and Child Nursing*. 4th ed. Philadelphia: Lippincott Williams & Wilkins, 2003.

FIGURE 8-9 ■ Courtesy of Saied M. Tohamy, MD.

FIGURE 8-10 ■ Courtesy of Mission Regional Imaging, Mission Viejo, CA.

FIGURE 8-11 ■ From Pillitteri A. *Child Health Nursing: Care of the Child and Family. Philadelphia.* Lippincott Williams & Wilkins, 1999.

FIGURE 8-12 ▦ From Haines DL. *Neuroanatomy: An Atlas of Structures, Sections, and Systems*. 4th ed. Baltimore: Williams & Wilkins, 1995:29.

FIGURE 8-13 ▦ Used by permission of Cadwell Laboratories, Inc., Kennewick, WA.

FIGURE 8-14 ▦ Courtesy of VIASYS Respiratory Care.

FIGURE 8-15 ▦ Images courtesy of Philips Medical Systems, Shelton, CT.

FIGURE 8-16 ▦ Courtesy of Newport Diagnostic Center, Newport Beach, CA.

FIGURE 8-18 ▦ Photo courtesy of VIASYS Neurocare, Madison, WI.

FIGURE 8-20 ▦ Courtesy of Carl Zeiss Surgery, Inc.

FIGURE 8-22 ▦ Photo courtesy of Varian Medical Systems, Palo Alto, CA.

FIGURE 8-23 ▦ Copyright © 2006 Integra LifeSciences Corporation. Reprinted with permission.

FIGURE 9-3 ▦ From Weber J, Kelly J. *Lippincott's Learning System: Health Assessment in Nursing*. Philadelphia: Lippincott Williams & Wilkins, 1997:188.

FIGURE 9-4 ▦ From Weber J, Kelly J. *Lippincott's Learning System: Health Assessment in Nursing*. Philadelphia: Lippincott Williams & Wilkins, 1997:188.

FIGURE 9-5 ▦ From Sheldon GF. *Boyd's Introduction to the Study of Disease*. 11th ed. Philadelphia: Lea & Febiger, 1992:640.

FIGURE 9-6 ▦ From Weber J, Kelly J. *Lippincott's Learning System: Health Assessment in Nursing*. Philadelphia: Lippincott Williams & Wilkins, 1997:188.

FIGURE 9-7 ▦ Courtesy of Felix Wang, MD, University of California at Irvine, Irvine, CA.

FIGURE 9-8 ▦ Photo courtesy of Medtronic Diabetes.

FIGURE 10-4 ▦ From Tasman W, Jaeger E. *The Wills Eye Hospital Atlas of Clinical Ophthalmology*. 2nd ed. Philadelphia: Lippincott Williams & Wilkins, 1997:254.

FIGURE 10-5 ▦ Used by permission of ApaGrafix, Inc., Marietta, GA.

FIGURE 10-7 ▦ From Tasman W, Jaeger E. *The Wills Eye Hospital Atlas of Clinical Ophthalmology*. 2nd ed. Philadelphia: Lippincott Williams & Wilkins, 1997:254.

FIGURE 10-8 ▦ Courtesy of Ellman International, Hewlett, NY (Robert Baran, MD, photographer).

FIGURE 10-9 ▦ From *Roche Lexikon Medizin*. 3rd ed. Munich, Germany: Urban & Schwarzenburg, 1993.

FIGURE 10-13 ▦ **B**, **C**, and **D**. Courtesy of Welch Allyn, Skaneateles Falls, NY.

FIGURE 10-14 ▦ Courtesy of Nikon, Inc., Melville, NY.

FIGURE 10-15 ▦ Courtesy of Keeler Instruments, Inc., Broomall, PA.

FIGURE 10-16 ▦ Courtesy of Lumenis, Inc.

FIGURE 10-17 ▦ Used by permission of ApaGrafix, Inc., Marietta, GA.

FIGURE 11-2 ▦ Courtesy of Welch Allyn, Skaneateles Falls, NY.

FIGURE 11-3 ▦ Courtesy of Welch Allyn, Skaneateles Falls, NY.

FIGURE 11-4 ▦ Courtesy of Welch Allyn, Skaneateles Falls, NY.

FIGURE 11-6 ▦ Photo courtesy of Bio-logic Systems.

FIGURE 11-7 ▦ Courtesy of Welch Allyn, Skaneateles Falls, NY.

FIGURE 11-8 ▦ Photo provided by Cochlear Ltd, Englewood, CO.

FIGURE 12-5 ▦ From Lindsay KL, Reynolds TB, Hoefs JC, Sanmarco ME. Ascites. *West J Med*. 1981;134:415. Used by permission of BMJ Publishing Group.

FIGURE 12-6 ▦ From Bickley, LS, Szilagyi P. *Bates' Guide to Physical Examination and History Taking*. 8th ed. Philadelphia: Lippincott Williams & Wilkins, 2003.

FIGURE 12-14 ▦ From Smeltzer SC, Bare BG. *Textbook of Medical-Surgical Nursing*. 9th ed. Philadelphia: Lippincott Williams & Wilkins, 2000.

FIGURE 12-15 ▦ Endoscope and fiberoptics courtesy of Olympus America, Inc., Lake Success, NY. Photographs courtesy of Mission Hospital Regional Medical Center, Mission Viejo, CA.

FIGURE 12-17 ▦ From Ratcliff KM. Esophageal foreign bodies. *Am Fam Physician*. 1991;44:827.

FIGURE 12-18 ▦ Courtesy of William Brandt, M.D.

FIGURE 12-20 ▦ **A**. Courtesy of Siemens Medical Solutions, Inc., Ultrasound Division. **B**. Courtesy of Mission Regional Medical Center, Mission Viejo, CA.

FIGURE 13-3 ▦ From McClatchey KD, Alkan S, Hackel E, et al. *Clinical Laboratory Medicine*. 2nd ed. Baltimore: Lippincott Williams & Wilkins, 2001:538.

FIGURE 13-4 ■ From McClatchey KD, Alkan S, Hackel E, et al. *Clinical Laboratory Medicine*. 2nd ed. Baltimore: Lippincott Williams & Wilkins, 2001:539.

FIGURE 13-5 ■ From Sheldon GF. *Boyd's Introduction to the Study of Disease*. 11th ed. Philadelphia: Lea & Febiger, 1992:436.

FIGURE 13-7 ■ Courtesy of Mission Regional Imaging, Mission Viejo, CA.

FIGURE 13-10 ■ Courtesy of ACMI Corporation, Southborough, MA.

FIGURE 13-11 ■ Courtesy of ACMI Corporation, Southborough, MA.

FIGURE 14-3 ■ From Rubin E, Farber JL. *Pathology*. 3rd ed. Philadelphia: Lippincott Williams & Wilkins, 1999.

FIGURE 14-6 ■ From Weber J, Kelley J. *Health Assessment in Nursing*. 2nd ed. Philadelphia: Lippincott Williams & Wilkins, 2003.

FIGURE 14-8 ■ Courtesy of Laurence J. and Richard D. Underwood, San Clemente, CA.

FIGURE 15-3 ■ Courtesy of Siemens Medical Solutions, Inc., Ultrasound Division, Mountain View, CA.

FIGURE 15-4 ■ **B.** Courtesy of Dr. Saied M. Tohamy.

FIGURE 15-11 ■ From Rubin E, Gorstein F, Schwarting R, Strayer DS. *Rubin's Pathology: Clinicopathologic Foundations of Medicine*. 4th ed. Philadelphia: Lippincott Williams & Wilkins, 2004.

FIGURE 15-13 ■ Sonograms courtesy of Siemens Medical Solutions, Inc., Ultrasound Division, Mountain View, CA.

FIGURE 15-18 ■ From Georgiade GS, et al. *Textbook of Plastic, Maxillofacial and Reconstructive Surgery*. 2nd ed. Baltimore: Williams & Wilkins, 1992:853, 863.

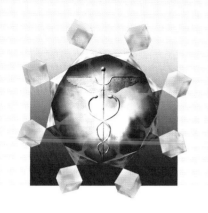

Index

Page numbers followed by an *f* denote figures.

A

a-, 13
AB. *See* Abortion
ab-, 13
Abbreviations
  blood, 299–300
  cardiovascular, 250–251, 260
  ear, 543
  endocrine, 466
  error-prone, 67, 78–79, 90–91
  expanded terms for, 89, 138
  eye, 508
  gastrointestinal, 600
  H&P, 44–45
  highlighted terms for, 87–88
  integumentary, 128
  lymphatic, 299–300
  male reproductive system, 687–688
  matching of, 89–90
  medical record, 67–69, 81–85
  musculoskeletal system, 185–186
  nervous system, 419–420
  obstetric history, 741*f*
  obstetrical, 751
  patient care, 69
    documentation of, 45–47, 69
  pharmaceutical, 69–73
  prescription, 74–77
  psychiatry, 419–420
  respiratory system, 350
  urinary system, 649, 656
Abdomen
  anatomic divisions of, 569–571, 569*f*–570*f*, 609–610
  clinical divisions of, 569–571, 569*f*–570*f*, 610
  CT of, 589
  distention of, 572*f*
  pain in, 570*f*
  sonography of, 589, 591*f*, 637
Abdominal aorta, images of, 622*f*
Abdominal hysterectomy, 732
Abdominal paracentesis, 595
abdomin/o, 25, 560
ABG. *See* Arterial blood gas

Abortifacient, 749
Abortion (AB), 743
  TAB, 749
Above-the-knee prosthesis, 184*f*
Abruptio placentae, 744
Abscess, 115
Absence seizure, 390
Absorption, gastrointestinal, 559
-ac, 8, 20
a.c. *See* Before meals
Accessory organs
  endoscopy of, 588, 588*f*
  gastrointestinal-system related, 579–581, 581*f*, 587*f*
Accommodation, 491
ACE. *See* Angiotensin-converting enzyme
Acne, 114, 115*f*
acous/o, 526
Acoustic neuroma, 533
Acquired immunodeficiency syndrome (AIDS), 286
acr/o, 25
Acromegaly, 454, 455*f*
Acronyms
  blood, 299–300
  cardiovascular, 250–251
  ear related, 543
  endocrine, 466
  eye related, 508
  gastrointestinal, 600
  integumentary, 128
  lymphatic, 299–300
  male reproductive, 687–688
  musculoskeletal, 185–186
  for nervous system, 419–420
  obstetrical, 751
  psychiatry related, 423419–420
  for respiratory system, 350
  for urinary system, 649, 656
ACS. *See* Acute coronary syndrome
ACTH. *See* Adrenocorticotropic hormone
-action, 19
Active immunity, 282
-acusis, 526

Acute, 64
Acute coronary syndrome (ACS), 227
AD. *See* Right ear
ad-, 13
ad lib. *See* As desired
aden/o, 25
Adenocarcinoma, of breast, 723
Adenohypophysis, 447
Adenoid, 322
Adenoidectomy, 344
ADH. *See* Antidiuretic hormone
ADHD. *See* Attention-deficit/hyperactivity disorder
Adhesiolysis, 731
Adhesiotomy, 731
adip/o, 101
Adnexa, 707
Adrenal glands, 442*f*–443*f*, 446
  diagnostic terms, 453–454, 453*f*
Adrenal virilism, 454
Adrenalectomy, 463
Adrenalin, 446
Adrenocorticotropic hormone (ACTH), 447
Adult polycystic kidney disease (APKD), 632
aer/o, 24, 526
Aerotitis media, 532
Affect, 409
After meals (p.c.), 75
After noon (pm), 75
Agnosia, 388
Agranulocyte, 278
ai-, 14
AIDS. *See* Acquired immunodeficiency syndrome
Airways, 318*f*
-al, 8, 20
Alb. *See* Albumin
Albinism, 114
Albumin (Alb), 637
albumin/o, 622
Albuminuria, 628
-algia, 18
Alopecia, 112